LAVIN'S

Radiography for Veterinary Technicians

Radiography for Veterinary Technicians

Sixth Edition

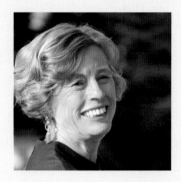

Marg Brown, RVT, BEd Ad Ed

Formerly of Seneca College of Applied Arts
and Technology
King City, Ontario;
Formerly of Penn Foster College
Scranton, Pennsylvania;
Active Member
Ontario Association of Veterinary Technicians, Association
of Veterinary Technician Educators, National Association
of Veterinary Technicians in America

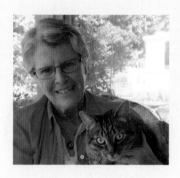

**Lois C. Brown, RTR (Can/USA), ACR,
MSc., P.Phys**

President
Xray Imaging Consultants Ltd.
Orangeville, Ontario

ELSEVIER

ELSEVIER

3251 Riverport Lane
St. Louis, Missouri 63043

LAVIN'S RADIOGRAPHY FOR VETERINARY TECHNICIANS,
SIXTH EDITION

ISBN 978-0-323-41367-1

Previous editions copyrighted 2014, 2007, 2003, 1999, 1994.

International Standard Book Number: 978-0-323-41367-1

Content Strategist: Brandi Graham
Senior Content Development Manager: Ellen Wurm-Cutter
Senior Content Development Specialist: Maria Broeker
Publishing Services Manager: Jeff Patterson
Senior Project Manager: Jodi M. Willard
Design Direction: Brian Salisbury

Printed in Canada

Last digit is the print number: 9 8 7 6 5 4 3 2 1

Contributors

Darryl Bonder, DVM
Nuclear Medicine, Toronto Equine Hospital
Mississauga, Ontario

Stephanie Holowka, MRT(R), MRT(MR), MRSO(MRSC™)
Lead Technologist, MEG and 3-Dimensional Imaging
Diagnostic Imaging
The Hospital for Sick Children
Toronto, Ontario

Robert F. Hylands, DVM
Westbridge Veterinary Hospital
Mississauga, Ontario

Evelyn Kelly, RTR, ACR, RN, BSc, MSc
Radiological Technologist, Nurse, Instructor;
President
Ev Kelly Services
Toronto, Ontario

Susan MacNeal, RVT, CVDT, BSC
Professor, Veterinary Technician
Georgian College
Orillia, Ontario

Amanda Barr, BA, RVT
Registered Veterinary Technician;
Adjunct Instructor, Veterinary Technician Program
Platt College
Riverside, California

Laura L Black, LVT, BAAS
Associate Professor of Veterinary Technology
Veterinary Technology Distance Learning Program
San Juan College
Farmington, New Mexico

Carla Mayers Bletsch, DVM
Associate Professor and Attending Veterinarian
Veterinary Technology Program in the Veterinary, Imaging
    and Surgical Technologies Department
Columbus State Community College
Columbus, Ohio

Crystal Brown, CVT, BS
Clinical Coordinator, Instructor, SCNAVTA Advisor
Veterinary Technology
Brown Mackie College—Boise
Boise, Idaho

Stephanie Brown, LVT
Instructor, Coordinator of Instructional Activities
Veterinary Technology
Tri-County Technical College
Pendleton, South Carolina

Ryan Cheek, MS, RVTg, VTS (ECC)
Instructor, Veterinary Technology
Gwinnett Technical College
Lawrenceville, Georgia

Amy D'Andrea, MEd, RVT
National Director of Veterinary Education
Heritage College
Denver, Colorado

Donna Fortin Davidson, DVM
Assistant Professor
Veterinary Technology
New England Institute of Technology
East Greenwich, Rhode Island

Susan Dibbley LVT, LAT, BTIS, MA
Program Director, Veterinary Technology
Wayne County Community College District/Wayne State
    University
Detroit, Michigan

Cathy Hall-Patch, AHT, RVT
Senior Lecturer
Thompson Rivers University
Kamloops, British Columbia

Sharlene Halozan, RVT
Registered Veterinary Technician
Northern College, Veterinary Technician Program
Haileybury, Ontario, Canada;
VEC-South (Veterinary Emergency Clinic South)
CTVEC (Central Toronto Veterinary Emergency and
    Referral Clinic)
Toronto, Ontario

James E. Hurrell, DVM
Director, Penn Foster Veterinary Academy
Penn Foster College
Scottsdale, Arizona

Myra Jones, DVM
Associate Veterinarian
Gettysburg Animal Hospital Inc.
Gettysburg, Pennsylvania

James E Krickhan, RVT, AAS
Chair, Veterinary Technology Program
Stautzenberger College
Brecksville, Ohio

R. Michele Lopez, RVT, BS
Program Director
Veterinary Technology Department
San Joaquin Valley College, Fresno
Fresno, California

Jennifer Louise Martin, DVM
Director, On-Campus and Distance Learning Veterinary
    Technology Programs
Veterinary Technology
Colby Community College
Colby, Kansas

Rachel McGinty, RVT
Veterinary Technician Instructor, Veterinary Technology
Vet Tech Institute at Bradford School
Columbus, Ohio

Deborah Peters-Piotrowski, LVT, MaEd
Lab Assistant Adjunct Instructor
Division of Veterinary and Natural Sciences
Medaille College
Buffalo, New York

Heather Riggs, CVT, BA
Certified Veterinary Technician, Colorado;
Program Chair
Veterinary Technology
Broadview University Orem
Orem, Utah

Tracy Ross, RVT
College Senior Lecturer
Veterinary Technology
University of Guelph, Ridgetown Campus
Ridgetown, Ontario

Amy Johnson Staton, EdD, LVT
Instructor of Veterinary Technology
Agriculture Sciences
Morehead State University
Morehead, Kentucky

Allene N. Taylor, CVT
Certified Veterinary Technician
Instructor of Veterinary Technology
Johnson College
Scranton, Pennsylvania

Amanda L. Teter, VMD
Assistant Director
Veterinary Academy
Penn Foster College
Scottsdale, Arizona

Stacey Thompson, B.Sc., RVT
Registered Veterinary Technician
McKee-Pownall Equine Services
Campbellville, Ontario

Jennifer Wakeling, DVM
Faculty Instructor, Veterinary Technology
Douglas College
Coquitlam, British Columbia

We are excited to present the sixth edition of *Lavin's Radiography for Veterinary Technicians*. As with the previous text, it continues to focus on teaching the science of imaging used in veterinary medicine and veterinary technology programs. The purpose of the book is to instill a working knowledge of radiologic science as it applies to producing a diagnostic quality image, to prepare radiography students in veterinary technology programs for the certification exam, to assist in the training of veterinary students, and to provide a base from which practicing radiographers can make informed decisions about technical factors and diagnostic image quality in the workplace. This text is a mainstay for teaching radiographic anatomy and positioning of all species. It will be a valuable reference for technicians when they have finished their training as well as for veterinarians. This 6th edition provides a thorough yet practical level of imaging and positioning coverage to equip individuals with the knowledge they need to produce high-quality images on the first attempt.

New Features

The textbook has been totally revised with new photographs, radiographs, and a consistent style of color line drawings along with tables and boxes. Application Information boxes have been added and provide practical information to help prepare the veterinary technician for on-the-job challenges. Review questions are now included in the textbook at the end of each chapter. A comprehensive glossary in which key words and other terms are defined is included on the accompanying Evolve website in the Student Resources along with completely revised Review Questions.

A major goal of this edition has been to ensure that each chapter is unique yet succinct so that important information is easy to understand and is found in the text without the need to reference other sources. Part One puts theory into practice, and each of the chapters in Part Two have been expanded to include not only essential positioning information but also anatomic references to support the technician in understanding normal anatomic features so that the veterinarian receives accurate images for diagnosis.

Organization

This text is divided into two major parts: diagnostic imaging, and radiographic positioning and related anatomy.

Part One: Diagnostic Imaging

It is particularly pleasant to present to you the results of many research excursions into the ever evolving world of veterinary imaging. This edition presents the field of imaging in an ever-evolving and current text.

With the advent of digital imaging and the Internet, the veterinary profession has embraced technology with enthusiasm. Advances in technology were taking place even as this text was being written, and new technologies were incorporated into this sixth edition as they evolved.

Employment opportunities for veterinary technicians and technologists are also expanding into the fields of imaging—opportunities that were unavailable in previous years. Knowledge of the many disciplines of x-ray imaging is vital to today's veterinary technician.

There are 17 separate yet interrelated disciplines in the field of medical imaging, and these new disciplines are currently being installed in veterinary hospitals and clinics. The discipline of imaging is driven by the larger field of medical imaging and, from that, new protocols are developed for inclusion into veterinary practices.

New Features of Part One

Part One of this text has been completely revised for this sixth edition. It presents the technical side of imaging as clearly and succinctly as possible, with little emphasis on theory and greater emphasis on the practical application of the rules and laws that guide our daily lives. We have rearranged the chapters to be more readily available as the student progresses through the course of study.

Chapters 1 and 2 explain the mechanics and the science of x-rays and present the inner workings of the radiography unit, from the source of electricity to the production of x-rays and how we use them. Images of rotating anodes and the principles of transformers, resistance, conductance, and rectification are presented with actual case studies of possible problems and potential solutions.

Chapter 3 introduces radiation biology and protection. In this edition, this topic is presented earlier in the text to more closely align with a course of study. The various harmful effects of radiation are introduced along with methods by which to eliminate the possibility of overexposure of both the patient and the operator.

Chapters 4 to 7 present a new look at the other side of imaging—the receptor. Film and intensifying screens are explained in a completely new way, with the many variables and explanations of this part of imaging explained in detail. Films and screens are still used in many facilities and the veterinary technician must be prepared to deal with any problems and artifacts that develop as these technologies age.

Chapter 8, which introduces and explains the world of digital imaging, has been completely updated for this edition to include the latest technology in use today. This new technology is exciting and fascinating, but 'caveat emptor' remains the watchword.

Chapter 9 presents quality control and quality assurance. This chapter discusses the many tests available to the technician/veterinarian to ensure that the x-ray unit is performing correctly and what tests can be done to explain any problems to the service person.

Chapters 10 to 14 explore specialized imaging. As veterinary clinics and hospitals become more sophisticated, these modalities are being incorporated into many practices. The veterinary technician should be aware of these modalities and the advances to diagnostic information that they represent.

Ultrasound, magnetic resonance imaging, and nuclear medicine are nonradiation imaging modalities; protocols and diagnostic units are being specifically designed for veterinary use. These modalities are ideal to confirm difficult pathologies, trauma, or rate of healing. These chapters have been completely revised for this edition and include image galleries that present a variety of images described in the chapter.

Part Two: Radiographic Positioning and Related Anatomy

As with the previous edition, this part is divided into the varied positioning of small animals, namely small animal abdomen, thorax, forelimb, pelvis and hind limbs, spine, and skull. In addition, comprehensive chapters on small animal dental radiography, special procedures, large animal radiography, and avian and exotic radiography are included, making this a one-source reference for radiography in these areas.

The major goal of this section is to clearly include the information required for accurate positioning so that other texts do not need to be referenced. Both routine and ancillary views are included. Each chapter includes an outline, learning objectives, key terms, where to measure, the location of the central ray, the borders to include, a step-by-step approach to positioning, further comments and tips to ensure that the perfect image is obtained, and a further description of the anatomy related to that part. Technician notes scattered throughout the chapters help to emphasize important points.

In practice, radiation safety is often compromised, with veterinary medicine being practically the only health science field in which the radiographer feels the need to restrain the patient while obtaining the image. The major emphasis in our chapters is on nonmanual restraint techniques that improve safety and radiation protection for the radiographer. May our patients also benefit greatly.

The positioning views are accompanied by high-quality color photographs and graphic color drawings that visibly indicate the anatomic features and radiographs. Anatomy is an important feature that will help students learn through the integrative application of radiography and anatomy and ensure that optimized images are presented to the veterinarian. To avoid confusion with actual positioning, related descriptive anatomy that students are expected to know is included in the appendixes on the Evolve website.

Additional Learning Resources

The Evolve Student Resources include review questions, crossword puzzles, and fill-in-the-blank exercises, as well as five appendixes and a comprehensive glossary. A full complement of support materials for teaching and learning are also available and include a complete collection of all images in the text.

Radiography is an exciting field in which the radiographer plays an important part in ensuring an accurate diagnosis. With the tools and information presented here, each image should be perfect.

Welcome to the sixth edition. We hope that you enjoy learning from it as much as we enjoyed writing it.

Marg Brown
Lois C. Brown

Acknowledgments

Thanks to everyone who has contributed to the production of this edition. I appreciate all of your contributions and input, and hope I have not forgotten anyone.

I wish to continue recognizing my former colleagues of the Veterinary Technology program at Seneca College in King City, Ontario, who are a support system always willing to help. I would like to make a special tribute to Ace, who unfortunately has passed away. He was a fantastic model willing to be subjected to various positions. Spud and Sam were also ideal and continue to be our models. Unless otherwise indicated, the positioning photographs included in the previous edition were taken at Seneca College and provided courtesy of Katerina White. Many thanks to Emma Brown, RVT, Jocelyn Affleck, RVT, and Chris Brown, DVM, the models' owners; to Peggy Casey, RVT, Lucy de Los Reyes, RVT, and Sue Gourley, RVT, co-radiography instructors; and to the other technicians. Many radiographic images included in the previous edition were also taken at Seneca College.

I would like to thank my students. Thanks to you and your enthusiasm, questions, and willingness to learn, I have never worked a day in my life. You were a constant source of motivation and joy. I learned and continue to learn from all of you.

Special thanks to Sue MacNeal, RVT, CVDT, BSc, for the dentistry chapter. Thanks also to those of you who gave me great input on what should be changed and helped review the chapters. Your guidance and the images you provided have been essential to helping us improve the content and layout. A big thank you to Cathy Hall Patch, RAHT; Stacey Thompson, BSc; RVT; Jo Ann Kennedy, BSc.Ag. RVT, VTS Equine; Cally Merritt, RVT; Lynda Forgie, RVT; Dr Meg Thompson, DVM; Carolyn Bennett, AHT; Evelyn Kelly, RN, MRT(R), ACR, BSc; Ashley Jenner, RVT; and Julia Bitan, RVT. To the contributors to the previous edition—Shannon Brownrigg, RVT; Sue Carstairs, DVM; G.K. Smith, DVM; and Mandy Wallace, DVM—thank you. I also wish to continue to express my appreciation to those who contributed to our previous photo gallery. Jeanne Robertson, your graphic images continue to be awesome.

Of course huge credit is extended to the editing team at Elsevier, especially Brandi Graham, Maria Broeker, and Jodi Willard. Your inspiration, suggestions, and patience have helped make this book an essential resource. Lois, your perspective and enthusiasm continue to amaze me.

Marg Brown

In this sixth edition, the input from many experts in their field who put their lives aside and contributed to the "renovation" of the sixth edition deserve our gratitude.

Stephanie Holowka, M.R.T.(R), M.R.T. (MR), MRSO (MRSC™), was especially involved with the computed tomography, magnetic resonance imaging and the new positron emission tomography section. Stephanie's encyclopedic and enthusiastic knowledge of these imaging disciplines answered many questions. Her thorough enjoyment of discovery of the veterinary aspect of imaging was always refreshing as we visited veterinary MRI suites, CT suites, and the PET. unit at Thames Valley Imaging in London, Ontario. Jane Sykes, R.T.(R), willingly shared the images that we have presented in this edition.

Robert Hylands, DVM, was so very helpful in rewriting the ultrasound chapter and including comparative images.

Darryl Bonder, DVM, RSO, has contributed images and expertise to both the fifth edition and now the reworking of the sixth edition in the field of veterinary nuclear medicine.

Thanks also go to the equipment engineers and the many veterinary hospitals and clinics we visited to research the various aspects of imaging, from wet processing to the evolution of digital imaging. Once again the assistance of the staff at Raymax Medical Corporation was invaluable in reviewing the manuscripts of the first two chapters.

The many contributors of images and experiences would fill several pages, and to those people, veterinarians, technicians, technical educators and other staff members I, once again, offer my special thanks. Thanks also to Evelyn Kelly, who willingly took on the job of filling out the definitions in the glossary.

Finally, the careful constructive criticism of our fifth edition reviewers and the suggestions they made helped immensely to guide the content of the sixth edition. The expertise of our editors and their staff certainly kept us on track and led to this new and totally revised sixth edition.

Lois C. Brown

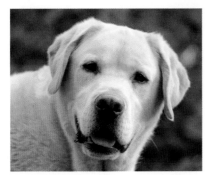

Ace—the face (June 2008–December 2015). A real hooligan who loved people, attention, and food—not necessarily in that order.

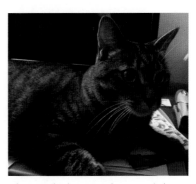

I Curious Tiberius—the literary—always providing assistance.

Contents

PART ONE

Diagnostic Imaging

In Part One you will be introduced to the technical side of imaging. The main emphasis is on the practical applications of rules and laws guiding the principles of radiography. You will learn about the inner workings of the radiographic unit. Film, digital, and specialized imaging are also addressed. Identifying radiographic artifacts and quality control testing techniques are also included.

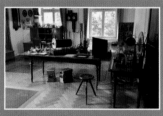

Wilhelm Roentgen's laboratory. (Photo courtesy of Röntgen-Kuratorium Würzburg e. V., Röntgenring 8, 97070 Würzburg.)

CHAPTER 1
The Basics of Atoms and Electricity

Lois C. Brown, RTR (Can/USA), ACR, MSc, P.Phys

All bodies are transparent to this agent. For brevity's sake I shall use the expression 'rays' and to distinguish them from others of this name I shall call them 'x-rays.'

—Wilhelm Roentgen, Physicist, University of Wurzberg, 1845–1923

OUTLINE

LEARNING OBJECTIVES

When you have finished this chapter, you will be able to:

1. Describe the events related to the discovery of x-rays.
2. List the properties of x-rays.
3. Understand the relationship between atoms and elements.
4. Describe the basics of atomic theory.
5. Understand the relationship between matter and energy.
6. Describe the basics of the table of the elements.
7. Define x-ray photons as waves and particles.

APPLICATIONS

This chapter provides basic information that will be expanded on in subsequent chapters.

KEY TERMS

Key terms are defined in the Glossary on the Evolve website.

Atomic theory
Atoms
Diagnostic imaging
Electricity
Electromagnetic spectrum

Elements
Energy
Fluorescence
Frequency
Heterogeneous

Matter
Nuclear energy
Nucleus
Particles
Polyenergetic

Thermal energy
Thermionic emission
Wavelength
X-rays

The Discovery of X-Rays

X-rays were discovered by German scientist Wilhelm Conrad Roentgen in 1895. He was working in his laboratory and setting up experiments for the next morning when he discovered a platinocyanide plate glowing a few feet from where he was working.

The fortuitous decision by Roentgen to understand what caused the plate to glow, how to prevent it from glowing (by removing the radiation source), and how to categorize the rays that caused the glow was the beginning of the profession that we know as diagnostic imaging.

Roentgen named the rays "x-rays" because of their unknown nature ("x" in science denotes an unknown quantity). He was also the first person to patent the phenomenon at a registry office.

As Roentgen developed his experiments and identified the characteristics of the new rays that he was investigating, he listed 12 unique properties (Table 1.1). He thought that these were just the beginning of a list of properties, but such was the thoroughness of his experiments and his scientific investigation that to this day no one has added to the original list. It is important that we learn the contents of the list, as we will encounter these characteristics throughout the balance of the text.

Elements and Atomic Theory

An element is the smallest particle of a substance. Elements are arranged on a table of the elements (Fig. 1.1). This table was put together to understand the nature of the atoms, which make up the elements contained within the table. Scientists realized early on that some elements were much more stable than others and some were very unstable. Throughout the text various elements will be described in relation to their position on this table.

An atom consists mainly of empty space, but the units within the atom, and the atom itself, are very small. The smallest particle of an element is an atom (Fig. 1.2). An atom consists of a nucleus containing protons and neutrons. Protons have a positive electrical charge, and neutrons have no charge. Circling around the nucleus are negatively charged electrons. The electrons are held "in orbit" by the positive electrical charge of the protons and their own negative charge. They are arranged in very definite "rings," with specific numbers of electrons in each ring matched with specific numbers of protons within the nucleus. As the numbers of protons within an atom's nucleus increases, the number of corresponding electrons also increases. With this increase the number of rings of electrons increases and, because of the distance from the nucleus, the electrical charge holding the electrons within the rings lessens to the point that individual electrons may leave their orbits, or they can be "boiled off" if heat is applied to the element. Boiling electrons off the filament of the cathode is the first step in creating x-rays.

> ### ◆ APPLICATION INFORMATION
>
> When the x-ray generator is turned on and heat is applied to the cathode of the x-ray tube, electrons are boiled off in an effect called *thermionic emission*. When the exposure switch is closed, it is the energy of the electrons—drawn across from the cathode to the anode and interacting with the anode—that produces x-rays.

TABLE 1.1	Roentgen's List of Unique Properties of X-Rays
PROPERTIES OF X-RAYS	**NOTES**
Are invisible	One cannot hear, smell, or see x-rays.
Are electrically neutral	X-rays carry neither a positive or negative charge.
Have no mass	X-rays have no resistance or force when put into motion.
Travel at the speed of light in a vacuum	X-rays move at 186,000 miles/second in a vacuum (3×10^8 meters/second).
Cannot be focused by a lens	The beam will pass through the lens unchanged.
Form a polyenergetic (heterogeneous beam)	Multiple photon energies are contained within one exposure. Peak kilovoltage (kVp) is the maximum energy in one exposure. One exposure equals the energy used to produce one image.
Can be produced in a range of energies (kV)	The useful range for diagnostic imaging is 25–125 kV; 25–40 is used in specialized imaging.
Travel in straight lines	Individual photons travel in a divergent (straight line) beam from the x-ray tube.
Cause fluorescence in certain substances	Fluorescence is useful to intensify the effect of radiation on a film with the use of intensifying screens.
Can cause chemical changes to occur in radiographic and photographic film	Depending on the energy of the photons, x-rays either penetrate matter or are absorbed by it, and therefore an image can occur on film.
Can be absorbed or scattered by tissues in the body; can produce scattered and secondary radiation	Based on the energy of the x-rays and on the composition and thickness of the tissues being exposed, characteristic radiation may be produced when the photon interacts with matter.
Can cause chemical and biological damage to living tissue	Through excitation and ionization (removal of electrons) of atoms comprising cells, damage to cells may occur.

Periodic Table of Elements

Period	I A																	VIII A
													III A	IV A	V A	VI A	VII A	
1	1 H	II A																2 He
2	3 Li	4 Be											5 B	6 C	7 N	8 O	9 F	10 Ne
3	11 Na	12 Mg	III B	IV B	V B	VI B	VII B ———		VIII	———	I B	II B	13 Al	14 Si	15 P	16 S	17 Cl	18 Ar
4	19 K	20 Ca	21 Sc	22 Ti	23 V	24 Cr	25 Mn	26 Fe	27 Co	28 Ni	29 Cu	30 Zn	31 Ga	32 Ge	33 As	34 Se	35 Br	36 Kr
5	37 Rb	38 Sr	39 Y	40 Zr	41 Nb	42 Mo	43 Tc	44 Ru	45 Rh	46 Pd	47 Ag	48 Cd	49 In	50 Sn	51 Sb	52 Te	53 I	54 Xe
6	55 Cs	56 Ba	* 71 Lu	72 Hf	73 Ta	74 W	75 Re	76 Os	77 Ir	78 Pt	79 Au	80 Hg	81 Tl	82 Pb	83 Bi	84 Po	85 At	86 Rn
7	87 Fr	88 Ra	** 103 Lr	104 Rf	105 Db	106 Sg	107 Bh	108 Hs	109 Mt	110 Ds	111 Rg	112 Uub	113 Uut	114 Uuq	115 Uup	116 Uuh	117 Uus	118 Uuo

*Lanthanoids	*	57 La	58 Ce	59 Pr	60 Nd	61 Pm	62 Sm	63 Eu	64 Gd	65 Tb	66 Dy	67 Ho	68 Er	69 Tm	70 Yb
**Actinoids	**	89 Ac	90 Th	91 Pa	92 U	93 Np	94 Pu	95 Am	96 Cm	97 Bk	98 Cf	99 Es	100 Fm	101 Md	102 No

FIG. 1.1 A periodic table of the elements. (From Ziessman HA, O'Malley JP, Thrall JH. *Nuclear Medicine: The Requisites in Radiobiology*, 4th ed. London: Elsevier; 2014.)

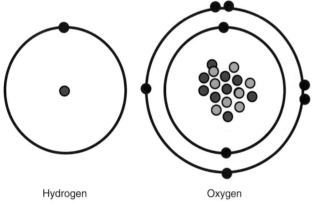

Hydrogen   Oxygen

FIG. 1.2 Two examples of elements. The hydrogen element has 1 proton inside the nucleus and 1 electron orbiting the nucleus. The oxygen atom has 8 protons, 8 neutrons within the nucleus, and 8 electrons orbiting the nucleus.

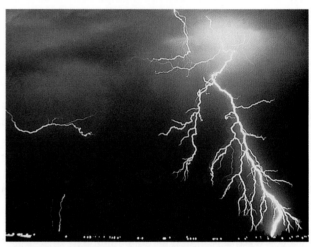

FIG. 1.3 Lightning is an excellent example of electrical energy. The negatively charged electrons build up in the clouds until they are attracted by the powerful force of the positive earth.

Matter and Energy

Every element on earth has substance, either matter (mass) or energy. It is the conversion of matter into energy that we use to create x-rays. The principle characteristic of matter is mass or weight. Weight involves gravity. The principle characteristic of energy is movement or motion (Fig. 1.3).

The combination of matter and energy in the universe is a constant. Matter can become energy. Energy can become matter. Neither can be created or destroyed. Each can only be changed in form from one to the other.

◆ APPLICATION INFORMATION

The production of x-rays depends on the tungsten wire in the negatively charged cathode. As energy is infused into the wire, creating heat, electrons are emitted from the wire. These electrons are drawn across to the positively charged anode as packets of energy when the switch is closed and the circuit is complete.

? POINTS TO PONDER

- Dr. Einstein said it best when he developed his famous formula $E = MC^2$.
- E = energy; M = mass (or matter), c^2 = the speed of light, which is a constant.
- This means that everything that has mass can be changed into energy, and energy can be converted to mass. Neither can be created or destroyed.
- This matters to the production of x-rays because the electrons that are boiled off the cathode in the x-ray tube will be absorbed into whatever they encounter.

The Electromagnetic Spectrum

There are several types of energy: mechanical, chemical, thermal, nuclear, electromagnetic, and electrical. Electrical energy and electromagnetism are the two major types of energy used in x-ray technology. This is evident when we turn on the power to the x-ray generator at the electrical box, and

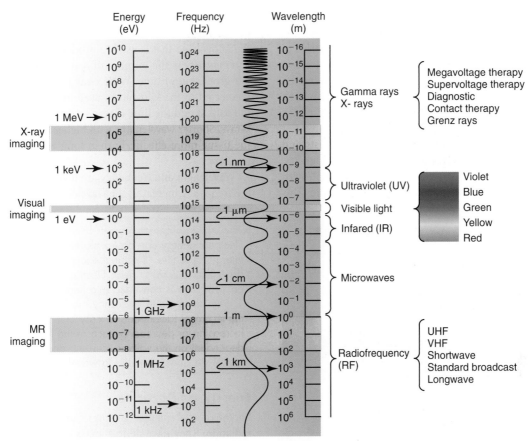

FIG. 1.4 The entire electromagnetic spectrum is much larger than just the visible light portion. This chart shows the values of energy, frequency, and wavelength for all portions and identifies the three imaging windows. (From Bushong SC. *Radiologic Science for Technologists*, 11th ed. St Louis: Elsevier; 2017.)

the energy (both electrical and electromagnetic) is directed to the production of x-rays.

The electrical spectrum covers a vast number of energies. We are concerned with the portions that involve radiation and visible light. In Fig. 1.4 the portion of the spectrum that involves radiation is near the top of the scale, whereas the visible light area is below that and divides into all the colors of the rainbow (Fig. 1.5).

The Dual Nature of X-Rays

X-rays can be described as waves because they move in waves and have wavelength and frequency. A wave has height (amplitude) and moves at the speed of light.

At other times during the discussion of x-radiation, the concept is changed to x-rays as particles. These particles are photons of pure energy. A photon is the smallest quantity of any type of electromagnetic radiation. An x-ray photon is a unit of pure energy. X-ray photons travel in waves at the speed of light.

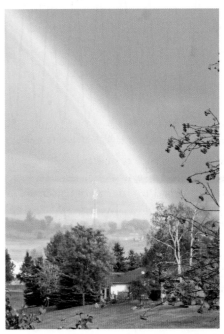

FIG. 1.5 A rainbow shows all the colors in the *visible* light portion of the electromagnetic spectrum.

◆ APPLICATION INFORMATION

Waves and particles of energy are important in the production of radiation. Setting the voltage and current on the x-ray generator controls the nature of the quantity and energy of the x-rays produced.

Energy as Wavelengths and Frequencies

Watching waves on the seashore is an excellent example of energy transformed into waves (Fig. 1.6). There are crests and troughs, and there is a measurable distance between the crests or the troughs. There is a time factor between each crest and trough. That time factor is the frequency of the waves (Fig. 1.7).

A *sinusoidal (sine) wave* is the tracing of the crests and troughs that the waves describe as they travel through the ocean. Sine waves have a high point and a low point, with time being the constant that runs through the middle. This is very important when we set x-ray technical factors and choose the time over which the x-rays will be produced and the kilovoltage that is used to produce them.

Frequency is the number of waves passing a given point per given unit of time. With x-ray production, frequency is connected to the kilovoltage used to penetrate the tissue of the patient and the time that is set for the production of the x-rays. Shorter wavelengths with higher frequencies penetrate the tissue more effectively than long wavelengths with low frequency.

Wavelength and frequency are inversely related so that as the frequency increases, the wavelength decreases (Fig. 1.8).

Energy as Particles

Photons are the smallest quantity of any type of electromagnetic radiation. They have neither mass nor electrical charge but

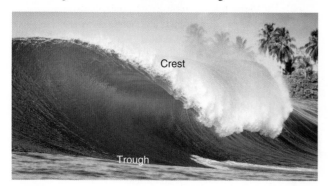

FIG. 1.6 Energy represented by waves on the ocean. The power of the wind creates waves with frequency and wavelength. This image represents one wave with a crest and a trough. (Copyright 2015 petesphotography/ Getty Images.)

Time line (1 second)

Short wavelength — high-frequency wave

Time line (1 second)

Crest

Trough

Long wavelength — low-frequency wave

FIG. 1.7 If waves have a short wavelength, they will pass a fixed point frequently (short wavelength/high frequency). If the waves have a long wavelength, they will pass that given point less often (long wavelength/ low frequency).

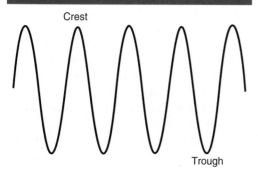

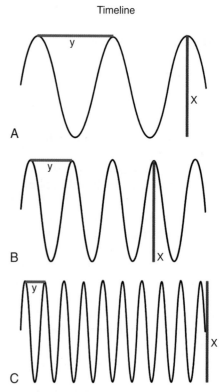

Timeline

A

B

C

FIG. 1.8 These three sine waves have different wavelengths (y). The shorter the wavelength, the higher the frequency as measured over a constant time. The height of the wave from crest to trough is the amplitude (x). **A,** Long wavelength. **B,** Medium wavelength. **C,** Shorter wavelength.

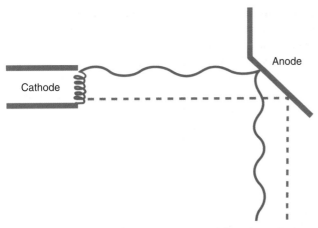

Cathode

Anode

FIG. 1.9 In an x-ray tube, energy is emitted from the cathode as particles. The photons of energy are magnetically drawn to the anode when the circuit is activated.

interact with matter as though they are a particle (Fig. 1.9). It is this energy that has been produced within the cathode to create the potential x-ray beam. A photon may be pictured as a small bundle of energy, just as an atom is the smallest quantity of an element. This is particularly true when using high-frequency energies such as x-rays or gamma rays. The photon particle carries a specific energy that is dependent on frequency. The energy and the frequency are directly proportional. If the energy is doubled, then the frequency is doubled. When described as particles, it is possible to mathematically quantify the relationship between frequency and photons and the amount of energy required to perform work.

Summary

Roentgen discovered x-rays in the late 1800s and described the nature of the phenomenon completely. The electromagnetic spectrum describes all forms of energy and categorizes it on a table depending on wavelength, with x-rays near the top of the scale and light near the middle of the scale.

The table of the elements categorizes all of the elements known at this time. Throughout the text we will describe some of these elements and show how their place on the table is important.

Scientists realized that x-rays can act as continuous waves or as particles (photons of energy) depending on their activity. Sinusoidal (sine) waves are examples of how x-rays behave as waves. Each wave has a crest and a trough, and there is an important relationship between the crests and the troughs.

REVIEW QUESTIONS

1. X-rays are described as:
   a. Invisible, but they travel in straight lines at the speed of light
   b. Electrically neutral unless they are emitted from a charged source
   c. Visible through a lens during x-ray exposure
   d. Causing electrical changes in photographic film

2. An element is the smallest part of a substance. Which of the following statements is true?
   a. The element is combined with a proton.
   b. The smallest part of an element is an atom.
   c. The element is composed of neutrons and particles.
   d. Electrons circle the element in random order.

3. The electrons are held in place by:
   a. The neutral charge of the neutrons
   b. Their own attachment to the nucleus
   c. The ionization of the atom
   d. The positive charge of the protons

4. On the table of the elements:
   a. The elements are arranged alphabetically.
   b. The order of the elements depends on when they were discovered.
   c. The elements are arranged in specific groups.
   d. All the known substances are listed with the radioactive ones at the beginning.

5. Matter and energy are basic to every substance on earth. Which of the following statements is true?
   a. The principle characteristic of matter is mass or weight.
   b. The principle characteristics of energy are time and space.
   c. Matter represents motion and frequency.
   d. Energy cannot be created out of atoms and molecules.

6. The electromagnetic spectrum represents:
   a. The color wheel and the electrical properties of light
   b. The vast spectrum from x-rays to radiowaves
   c. The intensity of light and the darkness of radiation
   d. Electricity, wavelength, and frequency

7. Energy can be represented by both:
   a. Waves and particles
   b. Waves and frequencies
   c. Mass and matter
   d. Matter and waves

8. A sinusoidal wave represents x-ray energy as waves. Which of the following statements is true?
   a. It contains the energy of the x-ray beam.
   b. It is an uneven wave so cannot be measured.
   c. It has frequency and amplitude in its definition.
   d. It represents the motion of the x-ray timer.

9. Energy as particles is represented as:
   a. Units of motion or as packets
   b. Individual movements of atoms within a substance
   c. Particles within the nucleus of the atom
   d. Waves with frequencies and structure

10. Photons are described as:
    a. Electromagnetic radiation that has a positive electrical charge
    b. Negatively charged electrons in the nucleus or the atom
    c. Negatively charged protons within the nucleus of the atom
    d. Electromagnetic radiation that has no electrical charge

Answers to Review Questions can be found on the Evolve website.

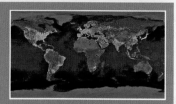

The representation of the distribution of electricity of the world. (Courtesy U.S. National Aeronautics and Space Administration [NASA].)

CHAPTER **2**

Diagnostic X-Ray Production

Lois C. Brown, RTR (Can/USA), ACR, MSc., P.Phys

I did not think; I investigated.
—Wilhelm Roentgen, Physicist, University of Wurzberg, 1845–1923

OUTLINE

LEARNING OBJECTIVES

When you have finished this chapter, you will be able to:

1. Describe the functions of each part of the x-ray tube.
2. List the four criteria necessary to produce x-rays.
3. Understand the construction of the x-ray tube.
4. Describe the anode heel effect and what causes it.
5. Discuss the line focus principle and anode heat bloom.
6. Distinguish between single-phase, three-phase, and high-frequency generators.
7. Understand potential difference.
8. Be familiar with direct and alternating current.
9. Know the difference between transformers and rectifiers.
10. Understand heat dissipation and know how to interpret the cooling charts.
11. Describe the activation of the single-stage and two-stage exposure switches.

APPLICATIONS

The application of the information in this chapter is relevant to the following areas:

1. Production of radiation using electricity
2. The use of electricity in radiography and all the other imaging modalities
3. The application of switches, circuit breakers, transformers, and rectifiers in the production of radiation
4. The use of transformers to increase and decrease the voltage of the incoming power to the x-ray unit
5. The application of electricity in all aspects of work in every area of the profession

KEY TERMS

Key terms are defined in the Glossary on the Evolve website.

Alternating current
Amperage
Anode
Anode heel effect
Bremsstrahlung radiation
Cathode
Characteristic radiation
Circuit
Circuit breaker
Current
Direct current

Exposure switch
Filament
Focal spot
Focal spot bloom
Generator
Ground
Heat bloom
Heat dissipation
Hertz
High frequency
Line focus principle

Line voltage compensator
Off-focus radiation
Photons
Potential difference
Power
Pulses (timer)
Rectifier
Resistance
Rotating anode
Rotor
Space charge effect

Stationary anode
Target
Thermionic emission
Transformer
Unsharpness
Voltage
Watt
Waveform
X-ray tube

The x-ray unit consists of a closed circuit with four main criteria:

1. It must have enough power to eventually produce x-rays.
2. It must have selections where the power can be increased or decreased as necessary.
3. The power must travel in the same direction through the x-ray tube.
4. There must be a way to produce free electrons and with enough energy to produce x-rays.

The main component in this x-ray circuit is the x-ray tube itself, and this is the structure that actually produces the x-rays. The x-ray tube contains two major components: a cathode and an anode. The cathode is a thin tungsten wire that is coiled and placed in a focusing cup. When it is heated, it produces a cloud of electrons. This is called *thermionic emission* (emission due to heating). The anode is a tungsten plate that is beveled on the outer rim so that the electrons are directed downward toward the patient.

When the exposure switch is closed the electrons are drawn across to the anode by electromagnetic force, where they are stopped very suddenly by the density of the metal of the anode. They react immediately by (1) losing speed, and (2) converting the forward motion to energy, which results in heat and x-rays (99% heat and 1% x-rays).

In order for these reactions to take place and produce radiation, the x-ray tube requires a vast amount of power. The standard power in the veterinary facility will not be enough to activate most x-ray units. Transformers must be installed in the veterinary facility and within the x-ray unit itself to boost the power from the incoming power lines. Step-up transformers increase the power to the cathode side of the x-ray tube.

The power supplied by the electric companies in North America and around the world is an alternating current. This means that the power fluctuates from positive to negative 120 times every second. In North America this is called *60 hertz*; one positive and one negative pulse is one cycle—120 positive and negative fluctuations gives us 60 cycles.

The power going through the x-ray tube must not fluctuate. Rectifiers change the alternating current to direct current. A rectifier circuit is placed in the x-ray circuit to correct the fluctuation and cause all of the current to remain positive. This way the current always flow through the circuit from the cathode to the anode in one direction.

Once the transformers and the rectifiers are in place, the unit is ready to produce x-rays. The filament circuit heats the cathode to reach temperatures in excess of 2200° C (3900° F). The x-ray tube receiving this power is constructed not only to produce photons, which are pure energy, but also to convert those photons into x-rays.

This chapter will explore the x-ray circuit starting with the x-ray tube and then continuing to the rest of the circuit and how each component works to produce the final result.

The X-Ray Tube

The x-ray tube consists of a glass enclosure that houses a cathode and an anode (Fig. 2.1). The glass enclosure is a special heat-resistant glass. Pyrex is one brand of glass manufactured for x-ray tubes. The standard x-ray tube is approximately 30 cm long and approximately 20 cm in diameter. The external housing enlarges the tube to about 50 cm long and 30 cm in diameter.

Every x-ray tube is shielded with a metal covering, which restricts any radiation from exiting the tube other than at the tube port.

The Cathode

The cathode of the x-ray tube typically has two filaments (Fig. 2.2). The large filament (typically 1.4 mm wide and 1 cm in length) is used when large body parts are examined; the small filament (typically 0.7 mm in width and 0.75 mm in length) is used for detailed work such as extremities and small pocket pets. These filaments are labeled on the x-ray unit as large and small focus. Which filament is used is determined by

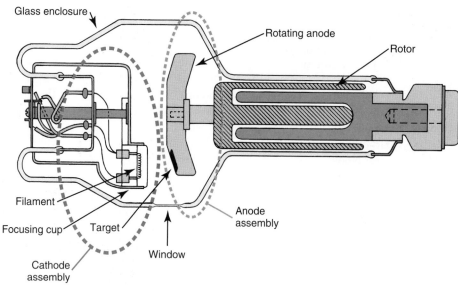

FIG. 2.1 Cutaway of a typical x-ray tube to visualize the anode and the cathode. Note that the cathode is offset from the anode so the electron beam is directed toward the outer ring of the rotating anode. The angle of the anode will deflect the beam at 90 degrees toward the patient. (From Bushong SC. *Radiologic Science for Technologists*, 11th ed. St Louis: Elsevier; 2017.)

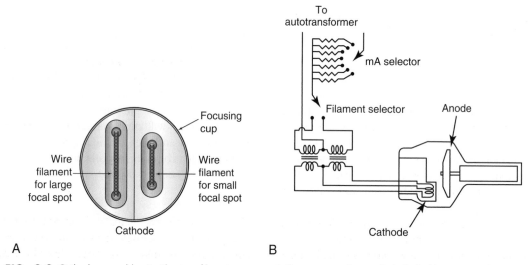

FIG. 2.2 Cathode assembly. **A**, The two filaments are much like an incandescent light bulb filament. **B**, The wiring diagram for the filament selector and the cathode assembly. Note that the cathode is offset so the photon beam is directed toward the beveled edge of the anode. (**A** from Fauber TL. *Radiographic Imaging and Exposure*, 5th ed. St. Louis: Mosby; 2017; **B** from Fauber TL. *Radiographic Imaging and Exposure*, 4th ed. St. Louis: Mosby; 2013.)

the milliamperage setting on the x-ray generator by the operator.

The filaments are made of thoriated tungsten, which can withstand very high temperatures without melting. The melting point of tungsten is 3410° C (6170° F). Therefore it can withstand many x-ray exposures without melting.

The filaments are very carefully positioned opposite the outer rim of the anode in a small cup-shaped device called the *focusing cup* in such a way that they are aimed directly at the anode. The focusing cups are slightly negatively charged to focus the electrons that are boiled off the cathode filaments

(Fig. 2.3). The beveled edges of the focusing cups are designed to focus on very small areas on the anode. It is here, on the focal spot of the anode, that x-rays are produced, and it is from here that the exceptional amount of heat must be dissipated.

When the circuit is activated, the exposure switch is closed and the filament transformer sends electricity to the cathode. The cathode temperature quickly rises, and electrons are "boiled off" the cathode filament in a reaction called *thermionic emission*. The cloud of electrons that is produced is called a *space charge*, and the whole process is called *space charge effect*.

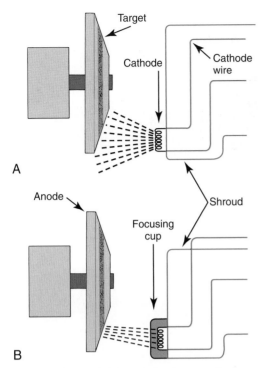

FIG. 2.3 A, Without a slightly negative charge on the focusing cup, the electron beam spreads beyond the anode. (Similar charges repel one another in a mutually electrostatic repulsion.) **B,** With a negatively charged focusing cup, the entire electron beam is directed toward the target. (From Bushong SC. *Radiologic Science for Technologists,* 11th ed. St Louis: Elsevier; 2017.)

The Anode

The anode is the partner to the cathode in the x-ray tube. It consists of a tungsten "target" upon which the electrons (now photons of energy) are focused. This very small area is called the *focal spot,* and it is this area where the x-rays are produced and sent in a downward projection to the patient.

There are two varieties of anode: rotating and stationary. Small-animal installed x-ray units use rotating anodes, and large-animal portable units use stationary anodes. The anode material is tungsten or a tungsten molybdenum alloy. Tungsten has a high atomic number (74) and is well positioned on the table of the elements to absorb electrons and heat (Fig. 2.4).

The Rotating Anode

The rotating anode is mounted on a stem that in turn is mounted on ball bearings. The entire structure rotates very rapidly once the circuit is closed, and the anode is prepared to receive electrons. On the beveled front edge of the rotating anode is the target of the x-ray tube.

The anode stem mechanically supports the electron target. It serves as a thermal dissipater by directing the heat emitted in the production of x-rays along the stem, as well as rotating so that the electrons (which are now traveling at tremendous speed across the gap toward the anode and are now called *photons*) are not always focused on the exact same spot.

The outer edge of the disk is beveled at a very specific angle in order to direct the x-rays down toward the patient being radiographed. This angle is important because it creates

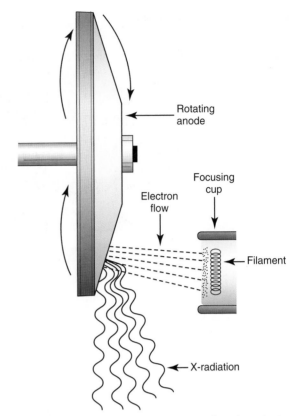

FIG. 2.4 A rotating anode receiving electrons from the cathode and converting them to x-radiation, which is directed toward the patient. The composition of the anode is a tungsten molybdenum alloy to assist in dissipating heat. (From Fauber TL. *Radiographic Imaging and Exposure,* 5th ed. St Louis: Mosby; 2017.)

the deflection by which the x-rays travel toward the patient. The angle is fixed when the x-ray tube is manufactured, and it is not adjustable. The angle is usually between 11 and 15 degrees depending on the supplier.

The Rotor Circuit

The rotor circuit is activated at the same time as the filament transformer starts to heat the cathode (Fig. 2.5). The rotor circuit causes the rotation of the anode and will reach speeds of 3200 to 3600 revolutions per minute. The inside of the rotor shaft contains very-high-grade stainless steel bearings that are manufactured to withstand extremely high temperatures as heat is dissipated from the rotating anode. As the x-ray tube ages, these bearings can distort and develop flat edges as they become very hot during the exposure and then rest in one position after the exposure. Because the bearings move rapidly when the rotor is turning, the noise made by the flattened sides of the bearings can become extreme. If the bearings seize and the rotor does not rotate, the heat is directed to one tiny spot on the anode, the focal spot. The accumulated heat will crack the overheated anode. Usually at this point safety interlocks prevent further exposures.

The veterinary technician should always listen for the noise of the rotating anode before the exposure. If no noise is heard, the exposure should not be attempted and service should be called.

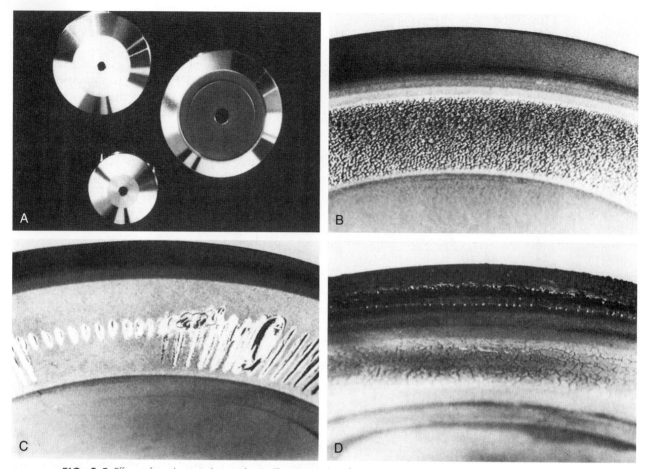

FIG. 2.5 Effects of overheating the anode. **A,** Three examples of new anodes. **B,** Effect of etching due to slow rotation of the anode due to bearing damage. **C,** Effect of repeated overload or overheating of the anode. **D,** Effect of exceeding maximum heat storage capacity. (Courtesy Philips Medical Systems.)

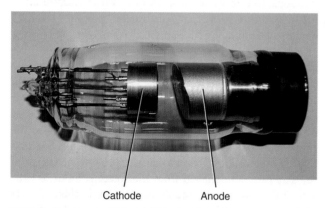

Cathode   Anode

FIG. 2.6 A large-animal portable x-ray tube with a stationary anode, with a tungsten target embedded in a copper shield for faster dissipation of heat. The cathode filaments are offset within the surrounding shield so they are aimed directly at the center of the anode.

The Stationary Anode

Equine portable x-ray units, dental x-ray units, and fluoroscopy C-arms have stationary anodes (Fig. 2.6). Because a lot of heat is produced during the exposure, the stationary anode must have an efficient method of dissipating heat. The stationary anode is composed primarily of copper with a wide stem

and a tungsten insert to handle the high amount of heat produced during the exposure. The targeted end of the stationary anode is angled to direct the beam to the patient. Because the anode is not rotating to dissipate the heat, the operator must be careful to follow the warning and ready lights on the unit so the heat may dissipate between exposures.

The Anode Heel Effect

Because so few x-rays are produced per exposure, it is important that the x-ray beam is used efficiently. The bevel of the angled anode limits the amount of x-rays being produced beyond the edge of the anode. The intensity of the radiation is greater on the cathode side than on the anode side (Fig. 2.7). This effect, called the *anode heel effect,* becomes important when a patient is thicker on one end of its anatomy than on the other.

The thicker end of the animal should be placed on the cathode side to take advantage of the greater amount of radiation at that end. In Fig. 2.7, the end of the table with the higher amount of radiation would be to the right. With any new or unfamiliar installation, it is important to note the anode and cathode positions of the x-ray tube and to ascertain the correct orientation. If unsure, a call to the vendor or the installer will answer the question.

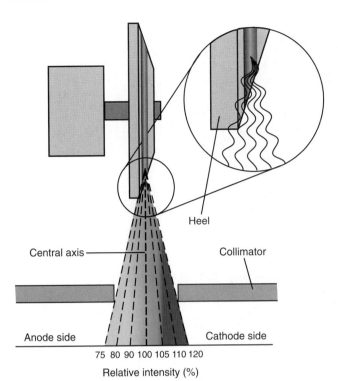

FIG. 2.7 The anode heel effect. The radiation on the cathode side of the central ray is more powerful than the radiation from the anode side of the central ray. (From Bushong SC. *Radiologic Science for Technologists*, 11th ed. St Louis: Elsevier; 2017.)

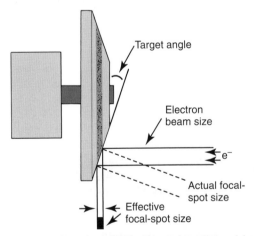

FIG. 2.8 The line focus principle. The electrons travel toward the anode and are converted into x-rays as they encounter the target. The x-rays are directed downward toward the patient. Because of the angle of the anode, the effective central ray is narrower than the primary beam, making the focal spot effectively smaller. (From Bushong SC. *Radiologic Science for Technologists*, 11th ed. St Louis: Elsevier; 2017.)

The Line Focus Principle

The line focus principle describes how the electrons interact with the anode and change direction so the x-rays are directed toward the patient being radiographed. The angle of the bevel on the outer edge of the anode and the resulting change of direction of the radiation is called the *line focus principle* (Fig. 2.8).

If the angle of the anode is less than 15 degrees from the vertical, the resulting x-ray beam will be very narrow and the image will have higher resolution. An angle of less than 15 degrees and multiple exposures will heat the area around the focal spot to the point where that area will also produce x-rays, effectively enlarging the focal spot. The images will lose resolution as the focal spot enlarges (*focal spot bloom*). It would be very unusual for this to happen in a veterinary hospital, but it could be a problem in a larger setting in which special procedures such as fluoroscopy or angiography are practiced.

If the angle is greater than 15 degrees, the beam will be wider, resulting in less heat focused on a very small focal spot and decreasing the "bloom" effect on the focal spot. The typical angle for x-ray tubes in North America is 11 degrees, which provides a very narrow x-ray beam and therefore allows for high resolution.

Off-Focus Radiation and Heat Bloom

When the exposure switch is closed, the interactions between the electrons and the anode are in effect and produce x-rays throughout the length of the exposure. The stream of electrons interacts not only with the actual target but also with the areas of the anode immediately adjacent to the target. Occasionally the electrons "bounce" off the target anode and are then attracted back to the anode but at a point beyond the focal spot (Fig. 2.9A).

It is very important to ensure that the area of the glass envelope of the tube is supplied with a collar of lead so that any extra focal radiation, or radiation produced outside the actual focal spot, is absorbed by the collar and does not appear on the image as an artifact (Fig. 2.9B).

Off-focus radiation effects can also occur if the kilovoltage is set higher than necessary and the collimation is inadequate. (Collimation will be discussed in Chapter 6.)

Electricity

Now that we have learned about the x-ray tube and its position in the x-ray circuit, it is time to learn about electricity and the factors that generate the power to activate the x-ray tube.

The Wall Switch

Before the on/off switch for the x-ray unit itself is the wall switch (Fig. 2.10). It is very important—and in fact, the law in most countries—that the x-ray unit is installed with a separate wall switch mounted at eye level (about 5 feet) above the floor within reach of the x-ray generator. This is in place so that if there is an equipment malfunction and the x-ray unit timer does not terminate the x-ray exposure, the power can then be shut off from the disconnect switch on the wall.

The Electric Circuit

The wall switch is the main access to the electricity that will eventually generate x-rays. The electricity that is used in the production of x-rays travels in wires that have the capacity to contain the necessary amount of voltage and current. Electricity always flows in a *circuit* (Fig. 2.11). In other words

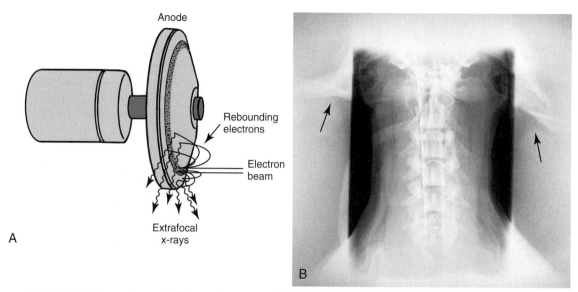

FIG. 2.9 A, The production of off-focus radiation. **B,** Off-focus radiation (extra focal radiation) has produced an image of the dog's ears beyond the limits of the collimator *(arrows).* (**A** from Bushong SC. *Radiologic Science for Technologists,* 11th ed. St Louis: Elsevier; 2017; **B** from Bushong SC. *Radiologic Science for Technologists,* 10th ed. St Louis: Elsevier; 2013.)

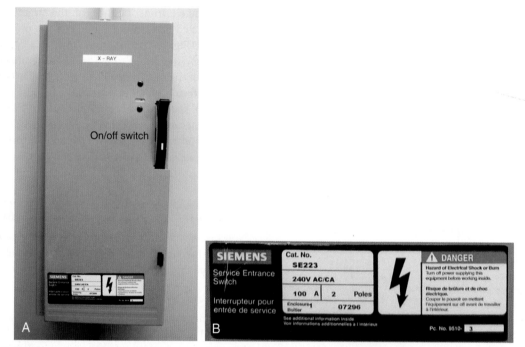

FIG. 2.10 A, The wall switch must be mounted at eye level and as close as possible to the control panel. **B,** The label on the outside notes the voltage (240V) and the current rating (100 amps) for this switch box.

it needs to be connected in a "circle." Any interruption of the circuit will cause the electricity to stop flowing.

Four important factors are involved in transmitting the electricity to the x-ray tube (Fig. 2.12):

1. *Current* (I): Milliamperage is the unit used to measure the electric current that activates the x-ray tube.
2. *Voltage* (V): Voltage is the speed with which the electrons in the electric current transfer energy along the circuit. *High voltage* (kV) produces short-wavelength/high-frequency, highly penetrating x-rays.

3. *Resistance* (R): Resistance is the factor that slows the current as it travels through a wire. A wire that is large in diameter will have low resistance. A wire that is small in diameter will have high resistance (Fig. 2.13). Very-large-diameter or long cables that are used in the x-ray unit will "leak" electric current. This is known as *line loss.*
4. *Time:* A timer controls the length of time that the x-rays are produced. This is determined by the setting on the control panel.

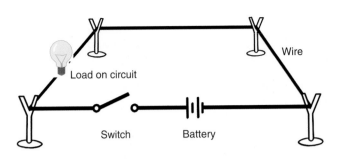

FIG. 2.11 The electric circuit. Electricity must always travel in a circle or circuit. In this drawing the power source is a battery and the light bulb is the load on the circuit. A break in the circuit (when the switch is open) will cause the electricity to stop flowing.

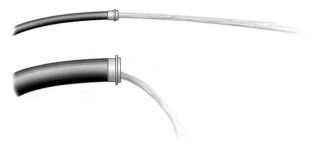

FIG. 2.13 Principle of resistance. Different-sized fire hoses provide various amounts of resistance depending on their diameters. With the same amount of water flowing through the hose, the smaller-diameter hose provides greater resistance (and therefore a more forceful exit) than the larger-diameter hose.

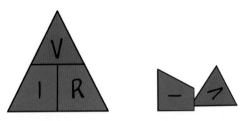

FIG. 2.12 The Ohm's law triangle. The electric circuit components are interrelated. If one component is not functioning, there is no current. Time is the shadowy fourth component as the current flows over time. (*V*, Voltage; *I*, current; *R*, resistance.)

⬥ **APPLICATION INFORMATION**

If the cables used to attach the x-ray generator are excessively long, the line loss will seriously affect the factors used to create the x-ray image. It is important to keep the cables as short as possible.

Two x-ray clinics owned by the same veterinarian had the same x-ray units installed: identical tube, x-ray unit, and generator, as well as identical processing. The technicians traveled between clinics and found that the technical factors in one clinic were nearly double those of the other clinic. The consultant identified "line loss" as the problem. The cables in one clinic were three times longer than those at the other clinic.

Potential Difference

Potential difference will cause the electrons to flow from the start of the circuit (at the generator) through the x-ray tube as part of the circuit. If we use a garden hose as an analogy, the hose is connected to a generator (the faucet). When the hose is stored, there is very little water throughout the hose itself but a great deal of potential ability to contain water from the faucet. When the faucet is turned on to allow water to flow, there is a potential difference along the length of the hose. One end has no water and the other has a lot of water, with more coming in all the time. The "potential difference"

is the measurement of the full end of the hose compared with the empty end of the hose.

In radiography the potential difference between the cathode and anode of the x-ray tube causes the electrons to flow from the cathode to the anode when the exposure switch is closed.

Line Voltage Compensator

The line voltage compensator is standard equipment on every unit. On some older units still in use today, a compensator is mounted on the control panel (Fig. 2.14). In older units and in areas of the country in which the incoming line voltage is not always as stable as it should be or the incoming power lines to a facility are limited or restricted, the compensator can stabilize the incoming power line to the x-ray unit. It is usually connected through the kilovolt (kV) meter and is a method of increasing or decreasing the incoming power line voltage. The veterinary technician should always check the line voltage meter on an older unit before positioning the patient and making an exposure. If it is low or high, it must be adjusted before setting the technical factors. Newer units compensate automatically through an internal compensator.

⬥ **APPLICATION INFORMATION**

A veterinary hospital was opened in an industrial mall on the outskirts of a large city. The images were excellent, and the techniques were consistent for the first 5 years. Unexpectedly, the veterinary technician noticed that intermittent images were so underexposed as to be unreadable. He called in a consultant, who discovered an intermittent severe voltage drop on the line. After tracing the problem to the transformer on the roof of the building, it was discovered that an auto body shop specializing in trim work and welding had illegally tapped into the veterinary clinic's transformer on the roof of the building. Every time the shop used the welding equipment and the veterinarian used the radiography unit at the same time, the voltage dropped and the resulting images were underexposed.

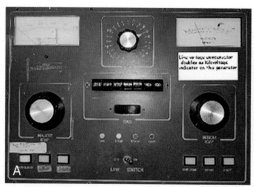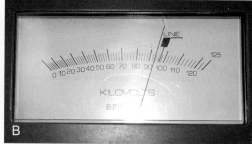

FIG. 2.14 A, The line voltage compensator on an older-model Bennett x-ray generator circa 1985-1990. **B,** Close-up of the compensator readout on the Bennett generator. The knob on the side of the unit must be turned until the needle is centered on the black bar.

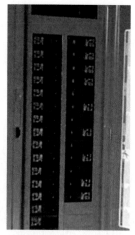

FIG. 2.15 An example of a circuit breaker panel. Each switch represents a circuit within the building so that power can be interrupted in one area and maintained everywhere else. A #2 wire from the electrical panel to the x-ray unit will disconnect the x-ray unit from the panel if an overload occurs.

Circuit Breakers: Amperage and Ground

When the power first arrives at the x-ray unit, it immediately encounters the circuit breaker (Fig. 2.15). This is a power supply to the x-ray unit. A series of switches are connected to the power lines going out to each room in the facility. A circuit breaker will accept current (amperage) up to a certain point (its rating). If the maximum quantity of power exceeds the rating, the circuit breaker disconnects, and power to the electronic device is interrupted until it is manually reset.

Because the nominal voltage coming into most buildings is 110 volts, it must be doubled to 220 volts in order to provide enough power to supply the x-ray circuit. This is done by connecting two 110-volt power lines coming into the building to the x-ray unit.

Current (Amperage)

The current in a radiography generator is labeled as milliamperage (mA). If the current demanded by the x-ray generator is in excess of what is available, an overload light is displayed and no exposure is possible until the factors are reduced. An exposure is still possible on a very old unit, but the unit will produce only its maximum mA and not necessarily the mA requested by the operator. It is very important that the operator is aware of the correct settings and the maximum rating of the x-ray unit.

Circuit breakers are a very important part of the x-ray unit and must never be bypassed because of inadequate service from the installer/manufacturer or the power company.

Ground

A grounding wire provides an alternative route for the electricity to flow if the circuit is broken inappropriately. The original electrical circuit is directed to a ground wire attached to an object that will absorb excess electrons and therefore redirect the current flow. The flow of electrons will stop with the broken circuit, but the excess electrons that are still flowing will be redirected to the ground wire. In most cases the ground wire is a green wire within the switch box (Fig. 2.16).

Direct Current and Alternating Current

Direct Current

A flashlight is an example of direct current (Fig. 2.17). The batteries installed in a flashlight need to be in a certain orientation so that when the switch connects the circuit, the unit produces light through the light bulb.

Direct current requires a source situated very close to the end user. If power is to be transmitted over vast distances, then a source that transmits a very low current paired with a very high voltage is less expensive and much more efficient.

Alternating Current

Alternating current produces one positive pulse and then one matching negative pulse (Fig. 2.18). In North America the pulses are paired at 120 cycles (one positive [+ve] cycle and one negative [−ve] cycle) per second. This transmission of power from the power station to any end point (e.g., a veterinary hospital) requires the use of transformers (see

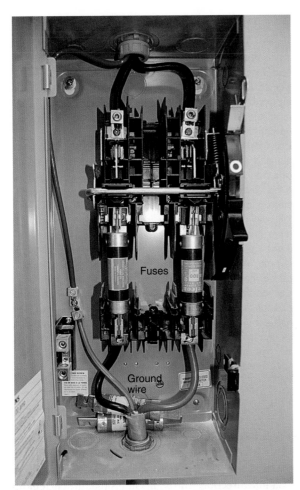

FIG. 2.16 On the inside of the box two fuses are connected to the two 110-volt lines to provide 220 volts to the radiography unit. The ground wire is green and is located to the left side of the box in this installation.

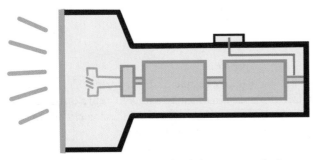

FIG. 2.17 A flashlight is an example of direct current. The batteries carry the voltage. When the switch is closed, the current flows through the batteries and the contact plate to the light bulb, which emits radiant energy in the form of light.

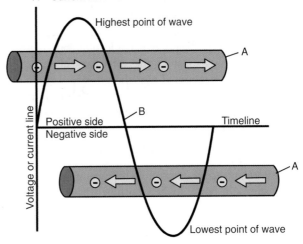

The sinusoidal waveform of alternating current
A = Current flow   B = The flow of current over time

FIG. 2.18 An example of alternating current. The electrons flow through the coil (**A**) creating one positive portion and (**B**) one negative portion of one cycle.

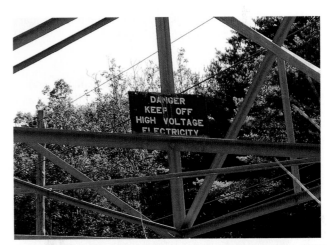

FIG. 2.19 An example of hydroelectric transmission lines alongside a New York highway. The sign warns potential climbers of the high voltage being transmitted through the lines.

1,000,000 amperes at 1 volt (Fig. 2.19). Using transformers at each end of the journey alters the voltage as required. The shortest time on a single-phase, fully rectified generator is based on 60 full cycles per second. The 60 positive pulses and 60 rectified negative pulses provide a fastest time of 1/120 of a second.

Transformers

Transformers are placed in the x-ray circuit to either increase or decrease the power necessary to produce x-rays. The autotransformer is used to provide the voltage requested by the veterinarian when she sets the kV on the control panel. The high-voltage transformer increases the current to the amount requested by the operator when setting the mA on the control panel. The filament transformer reduces the current to the right amount to heat the cathode filament and produce

Fig. 2.20). Transformers step up (increase) the power at one end of the journey and then step down (decrease) the power at the destination.

For example, to send 1 million watts of power across a grid to provide electricity to a neighborhood, it is much easier and more efficient to send 1 ampere at 1,000,000 volts than the electron cloud (thermionic emission) so the electrons can be drawn across to the anode and produce x-rays and heat.

The power that is generated to activate x-ray units and other electronic devices originates at a power plant. The power is transmitted over vast distances, with transformer stations along the way to boost the power that is lost through transmission. What matters most to the veterinary clinic is the transformer that is mounted near the veterinary clinic and supplies power to the entire clinic (Fig. 2.20). Quite often the local transformer station is within a few miles of the veterinary hospital, and an auxiliary transformer is mounted on a hydroelectric pole or within a transformer on the ground just outside the clinic.

Transformers receive power from the incoming power lines and transform the power to the x-ray tube. They use the turns of a wire around a central core or around two magnetic cores in close proximity to each other to either increase or decrease the voltage in a circuit. There is a direct relationship between the windings on one side of the transformer and the windings on the other side of the transformer. In a step-up transformer, 100 turns on the primary coil and 200 turns on the secondary coil produce twice the voltage. In a step-down transformer, 100 turns on the primary coil and 50 turns on the secondary coil produce half the voltage (Fig. 2.21).

Rectifiers

The rectifying circuit ensures that the current that travels through the x-ray tube does so in the same direction as a direct current. Four diodes are paired in the circuit. In each

pair one diode allows the current to flow and one diode prevents it from flowing. The second pair repeats this when the current alternates, thereby maintaining the current flow in the same direction. The end result is that the current flows in one direction through the x-ray tube and is fully rectified.

If one of the rectifiers stops working, the current on that portion of the alternating current is prevented from reaching the x-ray tube, and the images will be too light by exactly one-half the density.

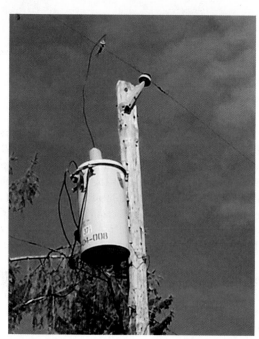

FIG. 2.20 The transformer mounted on a hydroelectric pole outside a veterinary hospital in New York State.

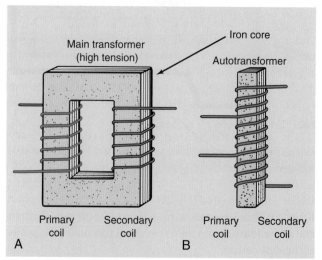

FIG. 2.21 Example of two simple types of transformer. **A**, Closed core transformer. **B**, Autotransformer. (Modified from Bushong SC. *Radiologic Science for Technologists*, 11th ed. St Louis: Elsevier; 2017.)

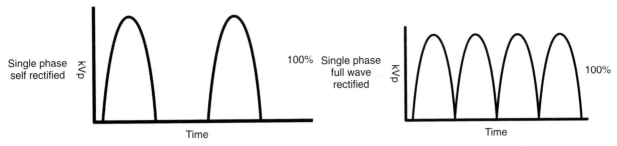

FIG. 2.22 A, A single-phase generator produces a waveform that rises and falls throughout the exposure. The negative portion of the waveform does not go through the x-ray tube, and therefore one half of the exposure is lost. **B,** A fully rectified single-phase generator changes the negative phase to positive; the full waveform is used during the exposure.

◆ APPLICATION INFORMATION

A veterinary hospital with a simple x-ray unit called a consultant to investigate why the images started to turn out with exactly half the density that was expected. Everything seemed to be working well except that the milliampere-seconds (mAs) had to be doubled to produce a properly exposed image.

Upon investigation the consultant discovered that one half of the rectifying circuit had malfunctioned, so the film was only receiving one half of the expected radiation.

Single-Phase Circuits

The original single-phase x-ray units were equipped with basic auototransformers, timers, and simple rectifying circuits. These units had a fastest time of 1/120 of a second, but there was a voltage drop during each pulse.

Some units had no rectifiers and were described as *self-rectified units*. The timers used the pulses of 120 cycles/second but, since there was no rectification, the radiation was produced only during the positive pulses. Therefore the fastest time was 1/60 of a second. The problem that arose was the long exposure time due to the low power of these units and the loss of power as the voltage dropped during the exposure with the completion of each pulse (Fig. 2.22).

Three-Phase Circuits

One solution to the dips of power in the waveform of the single-phase x-ray units was to add two more pulses of power offset from the first pulse and also from each other to make the drop in power much less significant (Fig. 2.23). This change considerably reduced the ripple effect in the power and made the output of the x-ray unit much more efficient.

The problem that now occurred was that the x-ray unit became much more sophisticated and required a great deal more power when it was installed. These units are not normally used in veterinary medicine except in large veterinary hospitals, where very high milliamperes (mA) combined with short times (seconds) are necessary to image large-animal chests and abdomens.

High-Frequency Pulses

Another less expensive and better alternative to the power drop problem is to use high-frequency pulses. In this case

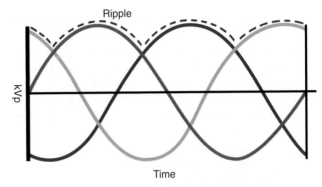

FIG. 2.23 An example of a three-phase circuit. The circuit now has three overlapping cycles and therefore very little loss of power when each cycle reaches zero. The small fluctuation at the top of the waveform is called a *ripple*.

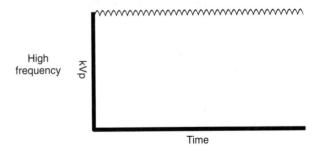

FIG. 2.24 A waveform from a high-frequency generator. There is a 3% ripple with virtually continuous output.

many phases are overlapped continuously, and the ripple stays very low (around 2% to 3%) with continuous output. High-frequency units cost a little more than the original single-phase units, but the benefit of more x-rays for each exposure allows the operator to reduce the overall exposure time, saving wear and tear on the x-ray unit and reducing the overall dose. Today virtually all new x-ray units installed in North American Veterinary Hospitals are high-frequency units (Fig. 2.24).

The X-Ray Unit

Components of the X-Ray Unit

The x-ray unit consists of three component parts:
1. The x-ray table and x-ray tube
2. The x-ray generator (control panel)
3. The high-voltage transformer

The high-voltage transformer (sometimes called the high-tension transformer) is located beneath the x-ray table (Fig. 2.25). It is connected to the hospital power lines and uses the power supplied to the hospital by the outside power lines. The x-ray generator receives its power from the high-voltage transformer and sends it through the circuit to the rectifiers and then to the x-ray tube (Fig. 2.26). The x-ray tube is the most important part of the x-ray machine because it is here that the x-rays are produced.

The x-ray generator and the high-voltage transformer are matched as a pair. If one of these components malfunctions, they must both be replaced. The x-ray generator is separate from the x-ray table and the x-ray tube (Fig. 2.27). The x-ray tube can be replaced on its own but must be recalibrated to match the generator.

A word of caution: The milliamperage (mA) knob on the generator panel is connected directly to the high-voltage transformer. It is very dangerous to try to service this knob if it becomes loose or is broken. A qualified service electrician must be contacted to service the generator or serious injury or death may result.

The x-ray unit requires a dedicated power line. It cannot share a power line or source with another piece of equipment that draws a lot of power. If another unit (such as a sterilizer or clothes dryer) is installed on the same line, the draw will reduce the power to the x-ray unit, and the transformers will not be able to compensate for the loss of power. The resulting image will be underexposed.

On some units the generator is mounted above the table (Figs. 2.28 and 2.29). This is fine if the staff are reasonably tall, but it can be awkward if the technician is short because the readouts can be difficult to see.

Large-Animal Portable X-Ray Units

Equine veterinarians must have the facility to travel to their patients and radiograph them on site. To do this, a small version of a full-sized x-ray unit has been developed. These units are not as powerful as the small-animal units, and they do not have the milliamperage of the larger units. However, because equine legs and feet are usually the areas of concern, the units are quite adequate.

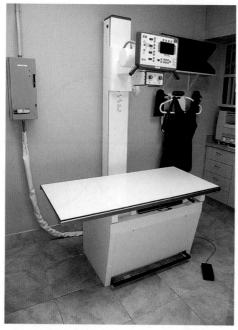

FIG. 2.25 The Sedecal veterinary x-ray unit. The transformer is beneath the table; note that the operator controls are mounted in front of the x-ray tube. This configuration may pose a challenge with staff members who are short. In this case the generator panel may be relocated to a stand at one end of the table.

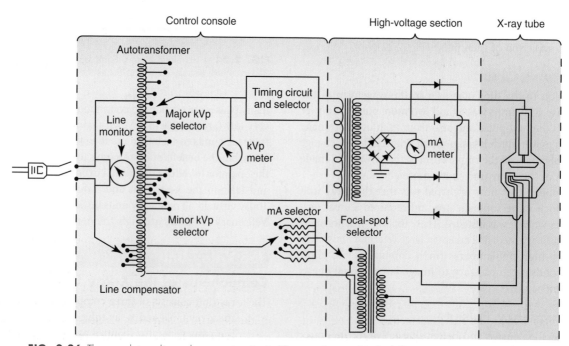

FIG. 2.26 The complete radiography generator circuit. (Courtesy Raymax Medical Corporation, Brampton, Ontario.)

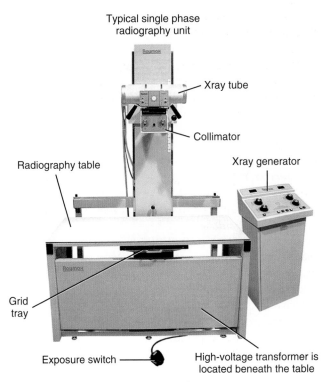

Typical single phase
radiography unit

Xray tube

Collimator

Xray generator

Radiography table

Grid
tray

Exposure switch

High-voltage transformer is
located beneath the table

FIG. 2.27 Typical x-ray unit with a separate generator.

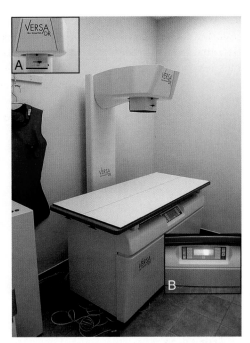

FIG. 2.29 A, The Innovet line of high-frequency generators. Note that the cables are contained within the tube stand. B, *(Inset)* Technique selection is located on the front of the table. The x-ray generator and transformer are located beside the table.

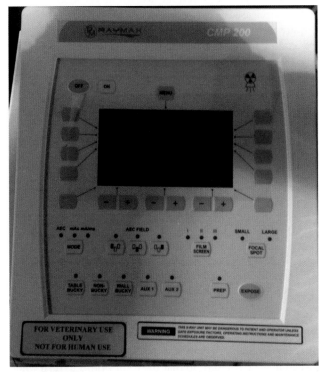

FIG. 2.28 The operator console of a high-frequency generator with anatomical programming. This unit is the size of a computer keyboard and may be mounted at the front of the x-ray tube or on a stand at the end of the table.

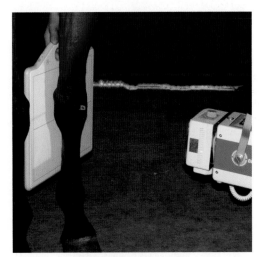

FIG. 2.30 Wireless digital equine imaging. The laser *(red dot)* ensures the correct distance, and the lack of electrical cords simplifies the imaging process. The assistant holding the digital plate wears a lead apron and lead gloves. If a film cassette is used, a cassette holder would be in place with the assistant standing well out of the beam. The veterinarian holding the shielded x-ray unit is also wearing a lead apron and lead gloves.

These units can also be used in a small-animal veterinary hospital. Because the milliamperage is limited on these smaller units, longer time factors must be used to achieve the correct milliampere-seconds. Using the inverse square law, the ideal distance is 30 inches (76 cm)

to compensate for the lower output of the x-ray unit (Fig. 2.30).

In a large-animal unit, the generator, transformers, and x-ray tube are all miniaturized and compressed into a very small space (Fig. 2.31A). The newest unit on the market features a completely wireless system that combines digital radiography and portable large-animal radiography (Fig. 2.31B).

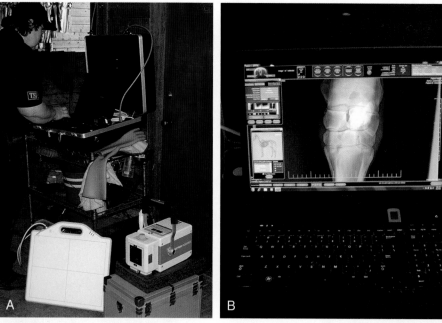

FIG. 2.31 A, The United Radiology Systems battery-operated x-ray unit paired with a Thales digital wireless plate. B, The image is delivered wirelessly to the computer from the digital plate.

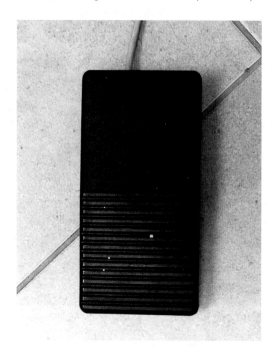

FIG. 2.32 Two-stage exposure switch. The switch plate is depressed halfway to initiate the rotor circuit and then all the way to initiate the x-ray exposure.

X-Ray Production

The Exposure Switch

The exposure switch sets the sequence of events in motion to produce the x-ray exposure. Most small-animal x-ray units have one two-stage exposure switch (Fig. 2.32). The *first* stage activates the rotating anode and boosts the filament circuit. The *second* stage activates the exposure, and x-rays are produced.

The exposure switch should be tested on a regular basis (semiannually) to ensure that it disconnects when the foot pedal is released. This "dead man" safety factor is a legal requirement to ensure that the x-ray beam is terminated at the end of an exposure. Tube heat overload is an indication that the x-ray tube is overheated and will require time to cool before another exposure is attempted. This occurrence is very common on large-animal mobile units. Waiting for the "ready" signal is a very important part of the radiography protocol and prolongs the life of the x-ray tube by not overheating it continually.

♦ **APPLICATION INFORMATION**

If the first-stage switch is activated and the sound of boiling liquid (actually oil) is heard, the exposure switch must be released immediately. It is likely that the x-ray tube has "shorted out" and the filament circuit is overheating the cooling oil in the x-ray tube housing. This situation is very unsafe because the tube could explode if the full force of the tube voltage (kV) were applied.

Exposure Switch Variations

There are several variations of exposure switches. A single-stage switch may be wired in so that the rotor begins to turn when the generator is turned on. This is not ideal because the rotor should be activated only when the exposure is about to be made. If this is the case, the unit should be turned off between exposures and activated only when the exposure is about to be made. A single-stage foot switch may also be wired in so the rotor is initiated when the foot switch is depressed. There will be a safety delay until the rotating anode achieves the necessary speed. This installation is not efficient and should be revised as soon as possible because animals being radiographed

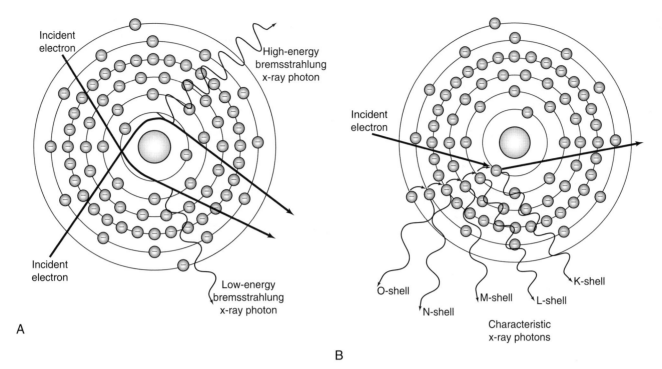

FIG. 2.33 A, Bremsstrahlung radiation. Radiation resulting from an interaction of an electron and a tungsten atom. The electron misses the nucleus but loses some energy as it swings around the nucleus and travels in a different direction. The energy lost is emitted as bremsstrahlung radiation. **B,** Characteristic radiation. The electron interacts directly with an inner orbital electron of the tungsten atom. The energy lost is emitted as a photoelectric effect characteristic of the tungsten atom. (From Fauber TL: *Radiographic Imaging and Exposure,* 5th ed. St. Louis: Mosby; 2017.)

are not necessarily cooperative and initiating the exposure depends on timing for minimal patient movement or, for certain views, full inspiration or full expiration.

Another variation is the hand switch. Most human units are activated with a hand switch, and the technologist stands behind a screen and instructs the patient. The hand switch may be replaced with a foot switch when such a unit is sold to a veterinary facility. Occasionally the hand switch is still active on a unit with an added foot switch. This can be useful if there is a problem with the foot switch; the hand switch can be used while the service engineer is on the way.

Producing X-Rays

Electrons are "boiled off" the cathode filament as it is heated up, ready for the x-ray exposure. At the same time the rotating anode reaches speeds of 3000 to 10,000 revolutions per minute (rpm). When the exposure switch is closed, the electrons are attracted to the anode at very high speeds, and their energy is transferred to the tungsten atoms in the anode to produce x-rays. Many electrons travel from the cathode to the anode, and various interactions take place during the time of the exposure. This produces an x-ray beam of a number of different energies, and this heterogeneous beam is important for diagnostic images.

Two common interactions take place. In *bremsstrahlung interactions* the incoming electron avoids hitting a tungsten electron but travels very close to its nucleus. In doing this it is redirected into a different path and loses some energy, which is emitted as an x-ray photon. The name comes from the term for "braking," as in losing speed rapidly (Fig. 2.33A).

Characteristic interactions occur when an incoming electron interacts with an electron from the inner shell of the tungsten atom (the K-shell). If the incoming electron ejects the inner shell electron, it leaves a space that is rapidly filled by electrons from the next ring in a roller-coaster effect. As each electron drops into place, it emits a small amount of radiation. The K-shell electron now travels on as an x-ray photon with properties *characteristic* of tungsten. This radiation has the strongest effect on the exposure because a strong incoming electron is required to oust the K-shell electron from its orbit. Once the K-shell electron leaves its orbit, all other electrons move in to fill the vacant spaces. An L-shell electron drops into the K-shell ring, an M-shell electron drops into the L-shell ring, etc. Each time an electron drops into the next ring, it loses energy, which is also emitted as x-rays (Fig. 2.33B).

Heat Dissipation

When the x-ray beam is generated, the exposure to the image detector is only 1% x-rays and 99% heat. This heat must be dissipated quickly before the next exposure. When the target is exposed to radiation over a number of exposures in a short time, the anode can become exceptionally hot, usually 1000° to 2000° C (1832° to 3632° F). With repeated exposures the focal spot will dissipate heat into the area immediately surrounding it—this will enlarge the effective focal spot. The descriptive term for this is *heat bloom.*

Each x-ray tube is supplied with an anode cooling chart when it is installed. This chart graphically illustrates the cooling period necessary between exposures to prevent overheating

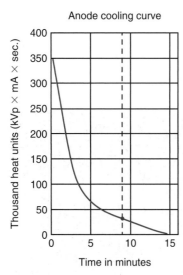

FIG. 2.34 An anode cooling chart. This chart shows that at maximum heating this tube requires 15 minutes to cool between exposures. If 32,000 heat units are applied to the tube, it will take approximately 6 minutes to complete cooling (15 − 9 = 6).

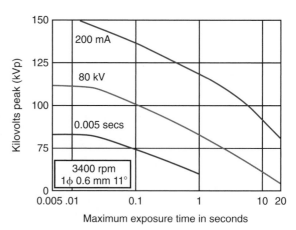

FIG. 2.35 A tube rating chart for the small focus on a single-phase 150 kV, 200 mA unit. (From Bushong SC. *Radiologic Science for Technologists*, 11th ed. St Louis: Elsevier; 2017.)

of the x-ray tube. Large-animal portable units typically have a safety shutoff that prevents overheating. In Fig. 2.34 the anode cooling chart indicates that an interval of 15 minutes should be allowed to dissipate 350,000 heat units. The maximum heat units for this x-ray tube are 350,000 units. Using this chart, if 100,000 heat units are produced, read to where the line crosses the blue curve (approx. 4 minutes) and subtract that number (4) from the maximum allowable 15 minutes (15 − 4 = 11). Therefore at 100,000 heat units, it will take 11 minutes for the tube to cool sufficiently for another exposure to be made safely.

To calculate heat units, multiply as follows: Using the chart in Fig. 2.34:

$$kV \times mA \times Seconds \times Number\ of\ exposures = Heat\ units$$

For example:

At $80\,kV \times 200\,mA \times 0.20\ seconds \times 10\ exposures$
$= 32,000\ heat\ units$

Heat dissipation requires $15 - 9 = 6$ minutes

When multiple exposures are necessary, the technician should be aware of how quickly the heat is dissipated and what the limits of exposure are for the particular unit in the facility. Each unit sold is supplied with both charts. Overheating is not likely to occur in a veterinary clinic because many concurrent exposures rarely happen rapidly during the course of the day. However, the technician should be aware that this can occur if multiple exposures are made with an older x-ray tube. It can also occur with large-animal portable units if many exposures are being taken rapidly, such as during prepurchase examinations.

The Tube Rating Chart

An additional chart that is useful to determine the maximum exposure on an x-ray unit is the tube rating chart. This chart indicates the x-ray tube limits based on the equation mA × kV × time for the x-ray unit. In Fig. 2.35 the maximum exposure at 200 mA is 80 kV and 0.005 seconds. This would not be a suitable unit for a clinic whose patients included very large dogs, but it may work very well for a cat clinic.

Each x-ray tube that is sold comes with a tube rating chart specific to it. It is important that the tube rating chart is referred to if a very large animal is to be radiographed using an old x-ray tube with a low tube rating. High technical factors may easily exceed the limits of the x-ray tube.

Focal Spot Bloom

Focal spot bloom affects the sharpness of the image. When the anode is bombarded with radiation, it becomes very hot. The heat dissipates through the surrounding metal, but if the exposures continue throughout the day and the tube is not allowed to cool, the outer edges of the focal spot become hot enough to expand the size of the focal spot, even though the heating effect of each individual exposure does not exceed the rating chart. A focal spot that started the day at 0.3 mm × 1 cm after several exposures can bloom to 0.45 or 0.5 mm. This will cause the image to lose sharpness, reducing resolution. The cause of the unsharpness is the increased area of the focal spot, as illustrated in Fig. 2.36A. The effect is demonstrated in Fig. 2.36B.

Focal spot bloom may also occur on a very old x-ray tube. The edges of the focal spot become enlarged and the images start to lose sharpness.

Minimum Power Supply Requirements

A power rating chart allows the electrician to communicate with the vendor of the x-ray unit to make sure that the power supplied by the veterinary hospital is sufficient to run the installed x-ray unit (Table 2.1).

When an x-ray unit is purchased, the veterinary hospital will receive a minimum power rating chart. This chart outlines

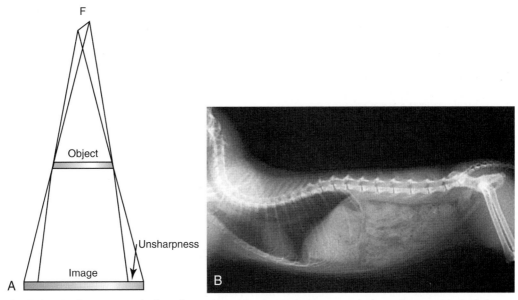

FIG. 2.36 A, The geometrical effect of an enlarged focal spot. **B,** The image loses resolution and lack of sharpness predominates. (**A** from Fauber TL. *Radiographic Imaging and Exposure*, 5th ed. St. Louis: Mosby; 2017.)

TABLE 2.1	Minimum Power Requirement Chart				
X-ray unit rating	Max kilovoltage (kV)	100	125	125	125
	Milliamperage (mA)	200	200	300	400
Power supply from wall	Power supply	60	60	100	100
	Disconnect fuse	40	50	80	80

the minimum power required to run this unit correctly using all of the stations supplied. This rating chart is usually attached to the unit itself. The salesperson must instruct the purchaser about the safest and most efficient use of the x-ray unit. If the power supply coming into the building is provided at only 80 amperes and fused at 60 amperes, then the power will not run a unit that is rated at 100 amperes and fused at 80 amperes. It is very important to make sure that the electric circuit is equipped to handle the requirements of new x-ray equipment.

◆ APPLICATION INFORMATION

A consultant was called in to diagnose a problem on a brand-new x-ray machine in which the images for large dogs were always light. If the technician increased the settings, the circuit breaker tripped and turned the machine off. The consultant discovered that the electrical panel was rated at 80 amperes and fused at 60 amperes. The x-ray machine required 100 amperes and fused at 80 amperes. The electrical circuit was not equipped to handle the technical factors necessary to x-ray large dogs.

Summary

In this chapter we have reviewed the parts of the electrical circuit that are required for an x-ray unit to function. The most important parts of the unit are the x-ray tube, the generator, the rectifiers, the transformers, and the exposure switch, all of which enable the technician to select the correct technical factors to produce an image and ensure that the current travels through the x-ray tube in the correct direction.

The filament transformer, which is activated before the exposure, ensures that the cathode of the x-ray tube is heated correctly in order to produce the free electrons necessary to close the circuit and produce x-rays. The anode attracts the electrons, which are drawn across to the target area, producing 99% heat and 1% x-rays.

The main interactions that produce the photons of x-rays are bremsstrahlung and characteristic radiation. The line focus principle ensures that the x-rays are directed toward the object being radiographed. The anode heel effect uses the more powerful part of the x-ray beam at the cathode end of the x-ray tube.

REVIEW QUESTIONS

1. A transformer is used to step up or step down electricity; it receives:
   a. High voltage and low amperage
   b. High amperage and low voltage
   c. High wattage and low resistance
   d. Low wattage and high resistance
2. In x-ray technology, potential difference refers to the difference between:
   a. The charge between the cathode and the anode of the x-ray tube
   b. The technical factors used with large dogs compared with cats
   c. The voltage and the amperage in an electric circuit
   d. The power ratings of two different x-ray units

3. The purpose of a transformer is to:
   a. Transform the voltage to enable the unit to power up
   b. Maintain the voltage and decrease the current
   c. Increase the voltage in a step-up transformer
   d. Decrease the voltage in a step-up transformer
4. Rectifiers are used in the x-ray circuit to ensure that:
   a. A direct current flows in the x-ray circuit
   b. An alternating current flows through the x-ray tube
   c. The current flows through the x-ray tube in a continuous direction
   d. The voltage is maintained in the x-ray circuit
5. The high-frequency x-ray unit is _____ efficient than a/an _____ unit.
   a. less, equine mobile
   b. less, single-phase
   c. less, three-phase
   d. more, single-phase
6. The cathode in the x-ray tube is a coiled _____. It is made of _____.
   a. tube, aluminum
   b. tube, tungsten
   c. wire, copper
   d. wire, tungsten
7. The filament circuit is used to:
   a. Boost the current to the x-ray transformer
   b. Send voltage to the cathode to heat it
   c. Increase the current to the collimator light
   d. Increase the intensity of the electron beam
8. The anode rotates in order to:
   a. Dissipate the heating effect of the electrons as they hit the target
   b. Dissipate the heat emitted in the production of x-rays
   c. Decrease the size of the focal spot to form a clearer image
   d. Increase the size of the focal spot and increase contrast
9. X-rays are produced when _____ electrons are attracted to _____ by an electromagnetic force.
   a. negative, a negative cathode
   b. negative, a positive anode
   c. positive, a negative anode
   d. positive, a positive anode

10. Heat builds up on the anode and must be dissipated by:
    a. A long tungsten stem and a rhodium filter
    b. A rotating anode or a thick copper stem
    c. A rotating anode or an aluminum coil
    d. A rotating anode and a tungsten alloy target
11. The rotor circuit is responsible to activate:
    a. The rotating anode
    b. The x-ray filament
    c. The internal rectifiers
    d. The production of x-rays
12. The exposure switch must _____ and _____.
    a. activate a two-stage exposure, will not reexpose until the door is closed
    b. be depressed to activate the exposure, will continue to expose until it is released
    c. expose only when the correct factors are set, must not reexpose until the switch is released and reactivated
    d. terminate when the exposure is complete, must not reexpose until the switch is released and reactivated
13. The line voltage compensator is situated_____ and controls the _____.
    a. on the incoming line; incoming voltage
    b. on the autotransformer; incoming voltage
    c. at the on/off switch; incoming current
    d. at the filament transformer; current to the cathode
14. A ground wire is installed in every generator. Which of the following statements is correct?
    a. It prevents electric shock if there is a fault in the line.
    b. It uses the excess electrons after the exposure.
    c. It always feeds the on/off switch to the generator.
    d. It provides an alternative route for the electricity.
15. Direct current is necessary to produce x-rays; the current must flow through the x-ray tube:
    a. From the cathode to the anode without interruption
    b. From the anode to the cathode without interruption
    c. From the transformer circuit directly to the x-ray tube
    d. From the filament circuit to the anode in one direction only

Answers to Review Questions can be found on the Evolve website.

CHAPTER 3

Radiobiology and Radiation Protection for the Patient and the Worker

Lois C. Brown, RTR (Can/USA), ACR, MSc., P.Phys

Research is to see what everybody else has seen, and to think what nobody else has thought.

—Albert Szent-Gyorgyi, Hungarian scientist, 1893–1986

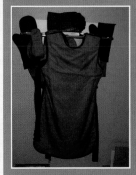

Correct storage of leaded accessories is important.

OUTLINE

LEARNING OBJECTIVES

When you have finished this chapter, you will be able to:

1. Understand radiation risks.
2. List the effects of excess radiation doses.
3. Define stochastic and deterministic effects.
4. Describe radiation and DNA.
5. Discuss radiation exposure and radioactivity.
6. Describe radiation-protective apparel.
7. Know the laws and regulations regarding radiation protection.

APPLICATIONS

The application of the information in this chapter is relevant to the following areas:

1. Protecting the hospital or clinic staff from primary, secondary, and scattered radiation
2. Protecting the patients and their owners from radiation dose

KEY TERMS

Key terms are defined in the Glossary on the Evolve website.

'ALARA' principle
Distance
DNA molecules
Dosimeters
Fluoroscopy
Gonadal shields
Half-life
International Commission
   on Radiological
   Protection (ICRP)

Linear energy transfer
Meiosis
Mitosis
Must/should
National Council on
   Radiation Protection and
   Measurements (NCRP)
Nonradiation worker
Nonstochastic effects
Organogenesis

RAD
Radiation dosimeter
Radiation Emitting Devices
   Act
Radiation worker
Radioactive decay
Radioactive disintegration
Radiography
Radionuclides
REM

Roentgen
Secondary radiation
Shielding
Stochastic effects
Thermoluminescent
   dosimeters
Time

This chapter discusses the various methods of radiation protection and the means by which veterinary health care workers can ensure they are protected from excess amounts of radiation. Each staff member should be encouraged to use the guidelines within this chapter and to check the specific guidelines that relate to his or her geographical area. Included throughout the chapter are quotations from both the National Council on Radiation Protection and Measurements (NCRP) in the United States and Safety Code 28 in Canada. International radiation protection is administered by the International Commission of Radiological Protection (ICRP).

Employees within a veterinary facility must be educated regarding radiation protection. All of the regulations are very similar, and a copy of the appropriate regulations should be available in the veterinary hospital for employees to review when necessary. In most countries, it is the law that, during the initial interview for any prospective employee, the employer must discuss the fact that the clinic uses radiation in the diagnosis of patients. This includes all personnel and not just the employees who will work directly with radiation.

Radiation doses to workers and patients within the veterinary facility must be reduced to a level *as low as reasonably achievable* (ALARA). This is a universal principle. It is very easy to become lax in the strict standards set out in the law because radiation in the radiography room is invisible. Protecting the staff and the patients from excess amounts of radiation over the course of a career is vital.

All of the handbooks on radiation protection are available online by typing in the handbook number, or hard copies may be ordered from the various organizations. (Contact information for the various organizations is listed at the end of this chapter.)

Radiobiology

Cell Biology in Brief

There are millions of cells in the bodies of the veterinary patient. Each animal stays alive by these cells dividing and subdividing in a process known as *mitosis*. This process occurs throughout the life of every living being. The exception to this are the genetic cells, which are involved in procreation and divide in a process called *meiosis*.

The energy contained in radiation will disturb the natural sequencing of these processes and can have various effects depending on what stage of cell division is occurring and which cells are affected. There are also various gradations within these effects, and it should be noted that these effects are demonstrated over many cells, not just an isolated cell.

It is also important to be aware that radiation dose is cumulative. Even though the effect of a single exposure or even multiple exposures is not felt immediately, the radiation does affect the cells, and a late-effect consequence may be the result of carelessness throughout one's career if excessive exposures are not avoided. The mammalian body is roughly 80% to 95% water. It is the interaction between the fluid in the body and x-radiation that primarily affects the cells.

When a radiation disaster strikes at a nuclear plant anywhere in the world today, the many precautions that have been established since the radiation disasters at Hiroshima, Nagasaki, Chernobyl, and Fukushima are very effective in containing the fallout and preventing radiation illness and death. Although the amounts of radiation in diagnostic imaging are considerably lower than in national disasters, it is important to be aware of the potentially devastating effects of excess exposure, even in small amounts, over the course of a career.

Radiation Effects

There are two main types of radiation effects: stochastic (somatic) effects and deterministic (nonstochastic) effects.

Stochastic effects occur by chance and may occur without a threshold level of dose. The probability of this type of effect is proportional to the dose, and its severity is independent of the dose. These late-term effects usually do not appear right away but often appear many years after the initial exposure or appear as a genetic effect that causes mutations in offspring from the initial victim of the dose. The effects of such amounts of radiation are stochastic in nature because the radiation is delivered intermittently over long careers. It must be understood that exposure reactions are cumulative. Even if a person is not immediately affected by a very low dose, the cumulative result of a repeated dose over a long career in radiation can be devastating. The most common stochastic effect is cancer. Other stochastic effects are cataracts, hyperthyroidism and hypothyroidism, and sterility.

Deterministic effects (nonstochastic effects) are noticeable in the short term. Several documented effects are noticeable immediately and are very rare in a diagnostic imaging setting. Erythema is the most common effect and will cause reddening of the skin, radiation burns, and tissue necrosis. A common nonstochastic effect is sunburn.

Radiation effects are mainly demonstrated in the DNA of the cell. This is the most vulnerable area, and the cell is particularly vulnerable during cell division. Radiation is nonselective. It affects the area of the cell upon which it arrives. DNA molecules, and particularly the nucleus of the cell, may be affected by the disintegration of the side rails of the DNA double helix. Four effects may occur when DNA is affected by radiation:

1. The radiation may pass through the cell and not affect a critical point. Mitosis may be suspended, but the cell is not damaged.
2. The cell may display no immediate effects, but damage may have occurred internally that will affect the individual later, when mitosis (cell division) occurs. In this case cell division may not occur successfully and the cell dies.
3. Cell damage may be obvious, with portions of the DNA compromised.
4. Cell death may occur from the "hit," severely damaging the molecule.

Diagnostic radiation workers are not as concerned about the massive cell damage that occurs with radiation therapy doses and nuclear disasters. The main concern in diagnostic imaging are the latent effects (stochastic). To produce these latent effects, the radiation dose over time must be substantial. There are currently no recorded cases of death after diagnostic x-ray exposure. The principal effects experienced by radiation personnel who do not take the necessary precautions consist of radiation-induced malignancy and genetic effects.

Early radiation workers did develop malignancies from radiation exposure before implementation of the safety precautions that are in effect today. Marie Curie, one of the original researchers in radiation in the early 1900s, died of radiation-induced cancer. Her household items, even her cookbooks, are still contaminated with radiation today. This is because she lived and worked with radiation—even in her home while she was cooking.

The doses that cause severe radiation sickness are far above any that would be delivered in a veterinary hospital. These types of effects result from radiation accidents, usually at a nuclear facility. Severe radiation sickness is usually threefold, and often the person cannot recover. Death from these effects is inevitable. The effects are listed here to show how cells are devastated by severe amounts of radiation:

- Hemopoietic effect (disturbance of blood cell formation)
- Gastrointestinal effect (the effect on the gastrointestinal system)
- Central nervous system effect (the effect on the nervous system and brain)

Radioactivity

This section is particularly applicable to nuclear medicine, but the radiographer also should be aware of radioactivity in the earth and atmosphere. Certain atoms exist in an abnormally excited state characterized by an unstable nucleus. The nucleus becomes unstable as a result of an imbalance of neutrons and protons with reference to the number of electrons encircling the atom. To reach stability, the nucleus of the atom spontaneously emits particles and energy (decays) and transforms itself into another atom with a stable and proper ratio. This process is called *radioactive disintegration* or *radioactive decay*. The atoms that emit particles and energy in order to become stable are called *radionuclides*. The radionuclides may be in the form of solids, liquids, or gases. These unstable atoms are used in the field of imaging called *nuclear medicine.*

Nuclear medicine technicians use radioisotopes, which are administered to patients by injection, inhalation, or oral consumption (see Chapter 14). Isotopes are variants of atoms of a particular chemical element that have differing numbers of neutrons. If the isotope is radioactive, it is called a radioisotope. Radioisotopes may be produced artificially in machines such as particle accelerators and nuclear reactors. For example, seven radioisotopes of the element barium have been artificially produced within nuclear reactors. Radioisotopes were also produced naturally during the formation of the earth, and because they are very slow to decay, they are still emitting radiation today. An example is uranium, which ultimately decays to radium, which in turn decays to radon. Other isotopes, such as carbon (C^{14}), are produced continuously in the upper atmosphere by the action of cosmic radiation.

Each radioisotope has its own pattern of decay. The energies of particles or waves emitted have unique characteristics that can be associated with that specific radionuclide. The decay rate of a radionuclide is called its *half-life*. A half-life is the amount of time it takes for half of the radioactive atoms to disintegrate or decay into a stable form.

Intensity of Radiation

All types of radiation have the ability to penetrate tissue and transfer energy. This ability is called *linear energy transfer (LET)* and describes the amount of energy imparted to the target. In radiography, LET is a measure of the rate at which energy is transferred from ionizing radiation into the tissue of the patient. The higher the value of the LET, the greater the amount of energy being transferred to tissue per interaction. If large amounts of energy are transferred rapidly, the ability of the particle to penetrate is reduced because the energy decreases rapidly. However, this also means that the risk of potential damage to the target material is increased because the energy is absorbed into the tissue.

Alpha and beta particles (weaker radiation) have high LET with low penetrability. These are commonly the secondary and scattered radiations from which the health care worker requires protection. X-rays and gamma rays have low LET with higher penetrability. This means that their ability to travel

TABLE 3.1	Tissue Compositions and Radiosensitivities		
TISSUE	**ABUNDANCE IN THE BODY**	**RADIOSENSITIVITY**	**EFFECTS OF OVERDOSE**
Lymphoid tissue	Minimal	High	Atrophy
Bone marrow	4%	High	Hypoplasia
Gonads	Minimal	High	Atrophy
Skin	3%	Intermediate	Erythema
Gastrointestinal tract	3%	Intermediate	Ulcers
Eyes (cornea)	Minimal	Intermediate	Cataract
Growing bone	4%	Intermediate	Growth arrest
Organs	12%	Intermediate	Nephrosclerosis/ascites
Muscle	43%	Low	Fibrosis
Fat	14%	Low	Atrophy
Brain	Minimal	Low	Necrosis
Skeleton	10%	Low	Transection

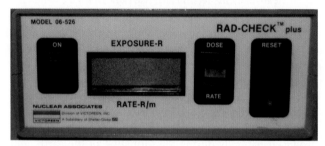

FIG. 3.1 A simple radiation dosimeter. This unit is shielded to measure cumulative x-rays, beta rays, and gamma rays. It will measure both a single exposure and a fluoroscopic exposure of continuous radiation.

through matter is high, producing less immediate effects on the tissue through which they pass. X-rays and gamma rays are produced in the radiography department. The patient's body absorbs the photons of radiation according to the density of the tissue exposed to the x-ray beam (Table 3.1).

Bone is much denser than soft tissue or fat. Bone efficiently absorbs the radiation reaching it and therefore prevents the image receptor from being exposed. This explains why bony areas are white on the image. Fat and air, which are radiolucent, allow the radiation to penetrate through to the image receptor and show up as black or dark areas on the image receptor.

Learning how to optimize images by varying the settings on the machine is discussed in Chapter 6. It is important to note that the higher the kilovoltage (kV), the higher the energy of the x-ray beam and thus the greater the amount of scattered and secondary radiation and the potential risk to the x-ray worker. When a technique chart is developed, the kilovoltage should be optimized to penetrate the body part, and then the milliamperes/seconds (mAs) value should be set to provide the correct density on the film.

Radiation-Monitoring Equipment

Measurement of Radiation Doses

Radiation doses are measured by means of a dosimeter (Fig. 3.1). Radiation is emitted from objects over which we have

no control, such as the sun and even the concrete in the pavement we walk on or the walls in our houses. The fluorescent lights in our clinics and hospitals are activated by ballasts, which ionize the gas within the light tubes and produce light.

If radiation is measured with an incorrect meter, these levels can be alarming because the meters are set to a random sensitivity level and are exceptionally sensitive. When beta, gamma, and x-ray levels are measured, it is important to use a shielded dosimeter specifically set to measure these types of radiation.

Types of Dosimeters

Handlers who are regularly required to work within the radiography room or who may be exposed to radiation during the course of their work are required to wear a personal radiation dosimeter (Fig. 3.2A). Personal radiation dosimeters capture the radiation dose from x-ray, beta, and gamma radiation and maintain it until it is read by a dosimetry service. Several companies supply personal dosimeters, with the most common types as follows:

- **Thermoluminescent dosimeters (TLDs).** A TLD demonstrates radiation exposure by measuring the intensity of light emitted from a crystal within the detector when the crystal is heated. The intensity of light emitted is dependent on the radiation exposure (thermo = heat; luminescence = light) (see Fig. 3.2D).
- **Optically stimulated luminescence (OSL).** An OSL contains sensitive elements that absorb radiation and store some of the energy in the form of excited electrons. The dosimeter is read by stimulating the sensitive elements using light-emitting diodes, which release some of the stored energy as light. The amount of released light is measured and used to determine the radiation exposure received by the dosimeter's user during the wearing period (see Fig. 3.2C) (obtained from the National Dosimetry Services website: www.hc-sc .gc.ca).

The radiation protection officer or his or her designate replaces the dosimeters at specific time intervals so they may be read

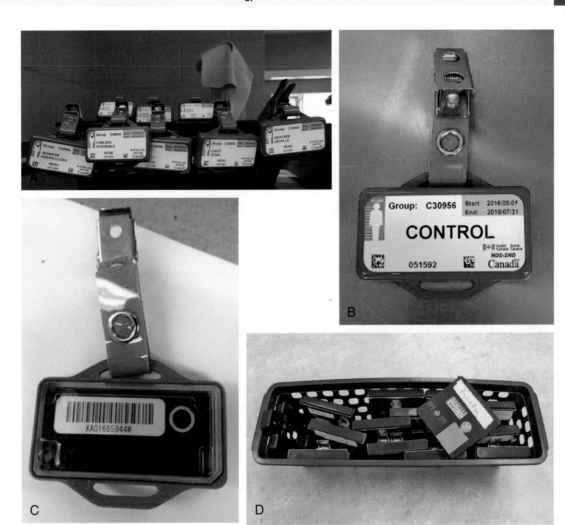

FIG. 3.2 A, Radiation dosimeters at a veterinary clinic. These units are stored outside of the x-ray room away from any possible extraneous radiation exposure. **B,** The control dosimeter is kept in the original packaging well away from any possible exposure within the facility. If the dosimeter indicates a radiation exposure, this would mean that all of the dosimeters were exposed during shipping. **C,** The reverse side of the dosimeter indicating the facility and wearer's identification. This is read by the dosimetry service and prevents misidentification. **D,** Thermoluminescent dosimeters stored outside the radiography room.

by an outside independent company. They can be read monthly, quarterly, or biannually.

Spare dosimeters may be maintained for visiting personnel or for dose studies in certain areas. These dosimeters should be labeled and noted on the remittance form when they are sent in to be read.

Control dosimeters are kept in the container received in the mail and removed from any possible radiation exposure (see Fig. 3.2B). The dosimeters are sent back to the laboratory along with the control. If the control dosimeter registers a radiation dose, then it is likely that all of the other dosimeters in the package received the same dose during shipping.

Use of Dosimeters

The rules of use apply to all dosimeters (Box 3.1). When a health care worker is issued a dosimeter, his or her personal information is required by the facility to which the service is registered. This process enables the dosimetry service to combine reports from other employers in order to calculate total exposure for an annual reading. If the worker is employed at more than one site, he or she must wear a different dosimeter at each site. In this way incidents can be tracked to a specific site.

Radiation Exposure

Recommended Dose Limits for Radiation Workers and Nonradiation Workers

Specified dose limits apply to both radiation workers and nonradiation workers. There is no dose discrimination between men and women of reproductive capacity. Once pregnancy has been confirmed, the woman's fetus should be protected from all types of x-ray exposure. X-ray radiation worker dose limits specifically apply only to irradiation resulting directly from their occupation and do not include radiation from medical diagnosis and background radiation. Dose limits for nonradiation workers are considerably higher than those for

BOX 3.1	Dosimeter Guidelines

- A dosimeter must not be taken home.
- A dosimeter must be stored in a location where it is not likely to be exposed to radiation.
- A dosimeter must not be stored where it will be exposed to heat and/or sunlight.
- A dosimeter must be worn only at the site to which it is registered.
- A dosimeter should be worn attached to the thyroid collar outside the leaded apron by any worker who is potentially exposed to radiation.
- A dosimeter must never be shared with another worker.
- A dosimeter must not be worn on a jacket or laboratory coat that might then be removed and hung in a radiation area.
- If the dosimeter is to be worn during fluoroscopic examinations, a second dosimeter should be worn attached to the thyroid collar outside the apron. These dosimeters must be clearly marked and must never be exchanged.
- Visitors and new staff must be provided with personal dosimeters, and service personnel working on x-ray equipment must also wear personal dosimeters.
- Each facility is responsible for posting the results of the dosimetry readings as they are received. Reports should be kept as a medical record according to the protocol of the facility.

BOX 3.2	Employer Prerequisites Necessary to Maintain Radiation Safety

- A health and safety representative has the power to review any and all testing procedures that in any way affect the occupational, biological, chemical, or physical health and safety of any worker.
- The employer must provide information regarding any potential or existing hazards to any worker.
- A health and safety committee has the power to identify hazardous situations in the workplace and make recommendations to establish monitoring programs that will improve the present status of safety to the workers.
- The committee will designate a member representing workers who shall monitor the testing procedures to ensure the safety of the workers.
- An employer shall ensure that equipment, materials, and protective devices are provided in good condition to the workers and are used as proscribed.
- An employer must appoint a competent safety officer who will supervise the handling, storage, use, and disposal of any article, device, equipment, or biological, chemical, or physical agent. The safety officer will prepare and post a written health and safety report in a conspicuous location and review and maintain it annually.

TABLE 3.2	Maximum Permissible Dose Recommendations

	AMOUNT
Occupational Exposure Limits	
Annual	50 mSv
Cumulative	10 mSv × Age
Public Exposure	
Effective dose limit, continuous or frequent	1 mSv
Effective dose limit, infrequent exposure	5 mSv
Embryo or Fetus Exposures Monthly	
Equivalent dose limit for the embryo or fetus	0.5 mSv
Negligible Individual Dose (Annual)[d]	
Effective dose	0.01 mSv

Note: All dose limits exclude medical exposures and exposures to natural sources.
For further information on this table, refer to NCRP Report #148, Table 2.1. http://ncrponline.org/publications/reports/ncrp-reports-148/.

radiation workers because radiation workers wear protective garments over the most sensitive areas of their anatomy.

The Radiation Emitting Devices (RED) Act in Canada, the National Council on Radiation Protection and Measurements (NCRP), and International Commission of Radiological Protection (ICRP) clearly state the dose limits for radiation and nonradiation workers (Table 3.2 and Boxes 3.2 and 3.3).

The ICRP specifies the allowable doses and should be consulted for further information (www.icrp.org).

The Occupational Health and Safety Acts (Canada, United States, and International)

The Occupational Health and Safety Acts specify that it is the employer's responsibility to ensure that the health care worker is protected against any excessive radiation exposure. Several sections refer specifically to radiation protection of the health care worker. All of the legislation is similar across international borders. The terms *must* and *should* in the Canadian Safety Code are *shall and should* in the American report (NCRP Report No. 148). **Shall and *must* are mandatory in both countries; *should* is optional.**

These sections of legislation apply to radiography and to all other modalities addressed in this text, including nuclear medicine and positron emission tomography:

1. A supervisor shall ensure that a worker is instructed in the use of the protective devices and that he or she uses or wears these devices appropriately.
2. The supervisor must advise the worker of any potential of actual danger of which he or she may be aware and take every precaution to protect the workers under his or her advisement, including providing written instructions regarding any unusual circumstance concerning dangers in the workplace.
3. The worker shall observe all the provisions of the Health and Safety Act of the country in which he or she is employed. Report to the supervisor any defect in any

of the measures provided to ensure the safety of the workers.

4. No worker shall remove any protective device required by the regulations or by his or her employer without providing adequate temporary protection. No worker shall engage in any act that would render the protective devices installed to be ineffective or nonexistent.

5. Every person who supplies any equipment shall ensure that the equipment is in good condition and complies with the safety measures outlined in this act.

6. Where a biological, chemical, or physical agent is used in a workplace, the local legal authority must be notified and shall decree whether the use is prohibited, limited, or subject to the safety conditions outlined in his or her directive.

7. A distributor must provide clear written instructions as to the use of any hazardous physical agent that he or she manufactures or designs to be used in the workplace.

8. Where an employer has an item described in subsection (1) in the workplace, the employer must ensure that the workers are aware of any potential hazard and are thoroughly instructed as to the proper use and maintenance of that item.

9. The employer must post prominent notices identifying and warning of the hazardous physical properties of the item in the place in which the item is to be used or operated.

10. Notices must be written in English and whatever appropriate languages are prescribed.

BOX 3.3   Further Legislation Regarding the Employer and the X-Ray Worker

1. If a worker exceeds the allowable dose, the employer shall investigate the cause and shall communicate the process of the investigation and the outcome and corrective measures taken to ensure compliance with the legal authority in that jurisdiction.

2. In each facility the owner of the radiation-emitting equipment or source must either assume the duties of the designated competent person or assign those duties in writing to an officer designate. That individual will ensure that the directives of the appropriate government body are carried out. Further duties include the training of the staff of the facility regarding radiation protection. He or she will also ensure that appropriate measures are in place to protect the patients and members of the general public who visit the clinic.

3. It is recommended that the equipment in a veterinarian's office be tested every 2 years. This testing will include, but is not limited to, accuracy of kilovoltage, half-value layer, milliampere linearity, reproducibility, timer accuracy, and collimator accuracy (see Chapter 9).

4. In addition to the responsible user of the diagnostic facility, a radiation protection (safety) officer must be delegated to act as advisor regarding all matters directly connected to the radiation protection aspects of the facility during the initial stages of construction, during installation of equipment, and during subsequent operations.

5. The specific duties of the radiation protection officer are outlined in the relevant act. They include the provision of a determination of responsibility and monitoring of radiation doses emitted by the equipment and received by both personnel and patients.

Legislation Regarding Radiation Doses to the Health Care Worker

It is the responsibility of the radiation worker to read the entire act in terms of its context before making a claim against any employer or section of this text. Each country provides legal direction specific to radiation workers within their borders, and it is the responsibility of the individual worker to be familiar with these legal directions. A radiation worker is defined as an individual who "could be exposed to radiation from manmade sources *during their work*." The nonradiation worker includes the rest of the population. The doses allowed for the radiation worker assume that the individual has been supplied with and is wearing protective devices on the parts of his or her body that would be susceptible to radiation damage (e.g., leaded aprons, thyroid collar).

Radiation Units

Radiation units were named as they were discovered. Recently the names have been changed to follow an international naming code, and the quantities have also been altered. The names and quantities in Table 3.3 are the most common in a veterinary practice.

TABLE 3.3   The Most Common Units of Dose in a Veterinary Practice

Radiation units were named as they were discovered. Recently the names were changed to follow an international naming code. When this occurred, the quantities were also altered. The names and quantities that are mentioned here are the most common in a veterinary practice.

NAME	QUANTITY	SYMBOL	SI UNITS	EQUIVALENTS
Roentgen	Exposure (dose)	R	Coulomb/kg (C/kg)	$1\ R = 258 \times 10^{-4}\ C/kg$
RAD	Absorbed dose	rad	Gray (Gy)	$1\ rad = 0.01\ Gy$
REM	Effective dose	rem	Sievert (Sv)	$1\ rem = 0.01\ Sv$
Curie	Radioactivity	Ci	Becquerel (Bq)	$1\ Ci = 3.73 \times 10^{10}\ Bq$

The following radiation units are of most concern to veterinary personnel:

1. **Absorbed dose.** The RAD (Radiation Absorbed Dose) changed to the gray (Gy), which measures the amount of radiation absorbed per unit mass of matter. This usually concerns biologic effects and are not mentioned in diagnostic imaging because the effects are minimal.
2. **Dose equivalent.** The REM (Radiation Equivalent Man/Mammal) changed to the sievert (Sv). This is the unit measured by the radiation-monitoring dosimeters that are worn by personnel who regularly are exposed to minimal amounts of radiation during the course of their work.
3. **Measured radiation.** The Roentgen, the dose output of the x-ray unit, changed to the air kerma (Gy_a). This is the dose measured by service personnel calibrating the x-ray unit. Most meters still measure in roentgens and milliroentgens.

Dosimeters are usually read in REM (Sv) and usually display both units on their reports. Both the NCRP in the United States and the RED Act in Canada use the dose limits developed by the ICRP. Table 3.2 is a summary of the maximum permissible dose recommendations for ionizing radiation. **Persons under 18 years of age are not allowed to work in radiographic areas.**

Principles of Radiation Protection

Once Roentgen had discovered the potential of the "x-ray," its value to medicine was immediately recognized. Shortly thereafter, the detrimental effects of radiation were also identified.

The science of health physics develops protocols to protect health care workers, x-ray radiation workers, patients, and the general public. The three cardinal rules for radiation protection are *time, distance,* and *shielding.* Reducing the time of exposure, increasing the distance between the source of the radiation and the subject, and placing a shield or barrier between the operator and the source are the three primary methods for reducing exposure.

Protection from radiation is important for any individual. Particular attention should be paid to males or females who have the ability to reproduce. This group includes all males of any age and all females before menopause. In all geographical areas it is illegal to employ a radiation worker under the age of 18 years.

One consideration that must be emphasized is protection of the pregnant veterinary worker. Research indicates that the severity of the response of the fetus to radiation is related to both dose and time. The second to the tenth week of pregnancy is the period of major organogenesis and therefore is the most critical time. Because it is quite possible that a female may not yet be aware that she is pregnant, protection of any female of childbearing age is essential.

Time

Exposure refers to two different occurrences: exposure rate and exposure time.

RULE: Exposure = Exposure rate × Exposure time

The exposure rate to an operator during radiographic examinations is obtained either by holding a patient during radiography or by standing too close to the x-ray table when the exposure is produced. This is measured by a personal radiation dosimeter worn by the operator. In veterinary medicine, the dosimeter must be worn on the thyroid collar when the operator is handling the patient. This will track the dose from secondary and scattered radiation. The radiation dosimeter is not meant to track primary radiation.

Every precaution must be taken to limit exposure time, or the time that the operator is exposed to radiation. Exposure time is measured by the radiation dosimeter, which measures an immediate dose—either a per-exposure dose or a fluoroscopic (real-time) dose. There is no delay in this reading. A radiation dose measured over time results in a given amount of exposure. The dosimeter will measure a dose over time, and a monitoring company will read the dosimeter and email a report to the facility.

During fluoroscopy (real-time imaging), the veterinarian is trained to pulse the exposure rather than leaving it on continuously. Pulsing the exposure limits the time of the exposure and thus the dose to the patient and to any staff member who must restrain the patient. A 5-minute reset timer on the fluoroscopy unit notifies the veterinarian exactly how much exposure time has elapsed during each procedure. Many facilities note the time elapsed for each procedure on the patient's chart so the dose calculation may be completed easily if a question arises regarding the examination.

Distance (The Inverse Square Law)

To calculate the intensity of radiation at a particular point (distance) away from the source, one must know the following three things:

- The intensity of the radiation (I_1) at a fixed distance from the source (focal point) (e.g.,. 123 mR)
- The fixed distance (D_1) (e.g., 100 cm)
- The calculated distance (D_2) (or the distance at which the intensity is to be calculated) (e.g., 140 cm)

Calculate using the formula:

$$\frac{I_1}{I_2} = \left[\frac{D_2}{D_1}\right]^2$$

For example, if I sit 1 foot away from a lamp, the intensity of the light reaching me is 1×. If I move to 2 feet from the source (2×), the intensity of the light reaching me is now decreased to one fourth of its original value. This is the application of the *inverse square law,* and it must be observed whenever a patient is being radiographed.

The rule of distance is also important when a new facility is planned or renovations are contemplated (Fig. 3.3). Enlarging an x-ray room means that the technicians can stand farther away from the patient and still be able to react if the patient moves or requires repositioning.

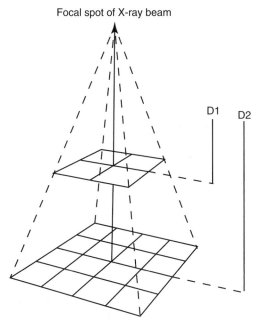

Focal spot of X-ray beam

D1   D2

FIG. 3.3 The intensity of radiation is inversely proportional to the square of the distance (D₁ and D₂) of the object from the source.

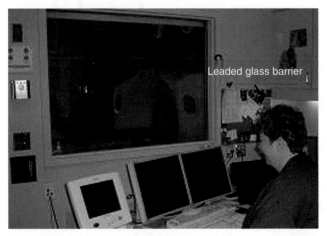

Leaded glass barrier

FIG. 3.4 An example of a leaded glass window between the operator of a CT unit and the CT unit.

Shielding

RULE: Positioning a shield or barrier between the health care worker and the radiation source greatly reduces the level of radiation exposure (Fig. 3.4).

Ideally the operator exposes the patient while standing behind a shield or barrier. In some cases doing so is not possible because the veterinary patient must be restrained and cannot be anesthetized. Shielding material is usually defined with reference to the thickness of lead. Other construction materials may be used, but they are commonly calculated according to their comparison with lead. For example, at 100 kV, 2.20 centimeters of concrete is equal to 0.79 mm of lead. Large sheets of lead may be purchased for construction. The minimum thickness is usually 0.79 mm (¹⁄₃₂ inch). Calculations for the shielding of x-ray rooms are beyond the scope of this text. Legally, in every country, the barriers (walls, ceiling, floor, and doorways) must be designated radiation barriers.

The maximum amount of radiation that may affect these barriers over the course of time must be calculated to ensure that the appropriate protection is installed before the first exposure of the imaging equipment. The necessary calculations may be carried out only by radiation-trained personnel or a medical radiation physicist. The calculations for each barrier must be submitted to and approved by the appropriate legal authority (Fig. 3.5).

If the equipment in the room is changed by either upgrading or downgrading, a new set of plans must be submitted. If the adjoining areas of the facility are changed, a new set of calculations must be submitted. Any room containing an x-ray generator must be designated with the appropriate legal signage (Fig. 3.6).

Radiation-Protective Devices

Leaded Protection Materials

Shielding material used to protect the patient is usually in the form of leaded drapes and/or gonadal shields (Figs. 3.7 and 3.8). Leaded aprons are typically measured for their effectiveness at 125 kV.

In film screen radiography the cassette may be divided, and the area to be radiated is then restricted so leaded dividers can be used to limit scattered radiation from fogging the unexposed part of the cassette (Fig. 3.9).

Leaded gloves, leaded aprons, and thyroid protectors must be worn by the health care workers present in the room during the radiographic examination (Fig. 3.10). Leaded glass goggles are also available to protect the lenses of the eyes from scattered and/or secondary radiation (Fig. 3.11).

Movable leaded barriers are available as added protection in imaging rooms where the workers are exposed to a higher amount of radiation than their colleagues (Fig. 3.12).

Use and Care

The lead used in aprons, leaded blockers, and drape shields is usually manufactured in thin sheets that are then layered together to achieve the correct amount of radiation protection. The sheets of leaded rubber are very thin and must be handled carefully in order to last for many years. Guidelines for the use and care of protective devices are included in Box 3.4.

If a patient must be supported or restrained during an imaging procedure, the x-ray worker should stay as far away from the source of the radiation as possible. Whenever possible, a nonradiation worker should be asked to restrain the patient. Nonradiation workers should be rotated throughout the shift so that no one worker is continuously exposed to radiation.

Lead Specifications

Radiographic and fluoroscopic leaded aprons must provide attenuation equivalent to at least 0.5 mm of lead at 150 kV. The lead equivalency must be permanently marked on the apron. **NOTE:** Most leaded aprons are rated at 125 kV. To meet 150 kV standard, an extra layer of lead needs to be added to the basic apron during manufacturing.

ABC Animal Hospital
92 Barkley Lane
Meow City, Indiana 46777

Plans Prepared on April 28/16

Above: Roof 1.58 cm FR Drywall; .4 cm Steel, 4 cm Concrete, 2 cm Asphalt
Below: Grade 10 cm Concrete

Scale 1:25
X = Focal Spot   .79 mm (1/32 in) lead added

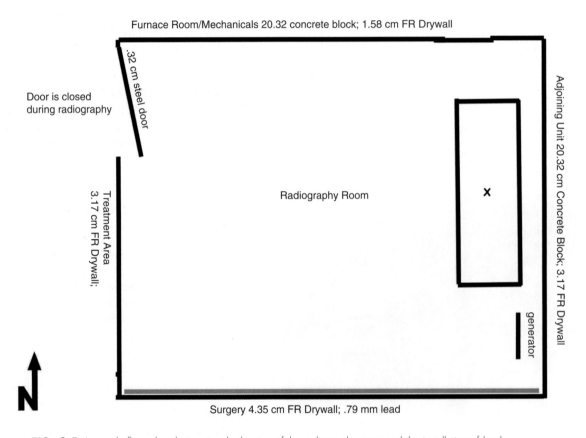

FIG. 3.5 A sample floor plan designating the barriers of the radiography room and the installation of lead.

Protective gloves must provide attenuation equivalent to at least 0.25 mm of lead at 150 kV. This protection must be provided throughout the glove, including the fingers and the wrist.

◆ APPLICATION INFORMATION

There are many different shapes and designs of protective mitts or gloves. It is important to ensure that the hands and fingers are covered during the radiation exposure if it is necessary to restrain the patient. For further information on patient restraint and safe handling practices, please review all of Part Two of this text.

Further Methods to Reduce Radiation Exposure to the Veterinary Handler

Immobilization Equipment

Equipment to restrain and/or immobilize the patient during any imaging procedure should be available in each imaging suite. Such equipment includes radiolucent foam blocks, cloth restraints, and tie-downs (Fig. 3.13). The patient should not be held in place by any person who is not fully clothed in protective apparel and shielded from the direct beam by accurate collimation. (See also Part Two regarding protection and positioning with nonmanual restraint.)

CAUTION X-RAYS

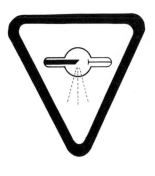

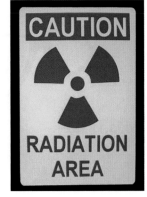

ATTENTION RAYONS X

A   B

FIG. 3.6 A, A legal door sign in Canada warning of the potential for radiation in the room behind it. The image denotes an early x-ray tube. **B,** A legal door sign in the United States. This sign also warns of nuclear isotopes in both the United States and Canada.

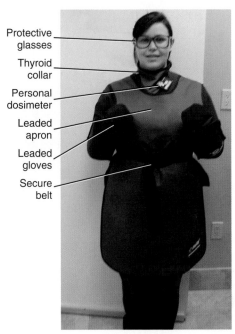

Protective glasses
Thyroid collar
Personal dosimeter
Leaded apron
Leaded gloves
Secure belt

FIG. 3.7 Radiation-protective wear. The apron is secured across the shoulders with a hook-and-loop (Velcro) band so that it will remain in place while the technician is positioning a patient.

Veterinary Facilities Inspection Checklist

Fig. 3.14 provides a checklist for a typical facility. It is available on the Evolve website for any facility to download and post.

Radiation Safety Websites

General sites for additional radiation safety training include:
- Occupational Health and Safety Act (www.osha.gov)
- X-Ray Safety Regulation (www.radiationsafety.ca)
- Radiation Emitting Devices Act (Safety Codes 20A and 35) (http://laws-lois.justice.gc.ca)
- Radiation Protection in Veterinary Medicine (Safety Code 28) (www.hc-sc.gc.ca)
- International Commission on Radiological Protection (www.icrp.org)
- National Council on Radiation Protection and Measurements (ncrponline.org/)
- U.S. Nuclear Regulatory Commission, Radiation Information Regarding Disposal of Nuclear Waste (https://www.nrc.gov/waste.html)

BOX 3.4	Use and Care of Protective Devices

- Aprons should be hung up by the shoulders when not in use.
- Aprons should not be folded or creased under any circumstances.
- Aprons should be cleaned regularly with warm water and a mild soap.
- The leaded apron should fit correctly. It should have a method to secure it on the wearer's shoulders so it does not fall off the shoulder during use. Simply adding a strap with a piece of hook-and-loop (Velcro) to the shoulder units of the apron will ensure that it stays in place when the handler bends forward. If the apron is worn during fluoroscopy, it should wrap around the technologist's back. In this way, protection is ensured while the technologist is in the room during continuous radiation.
- Thyroid collars should always be worn in conjunction with the leaded apron. They should be treated with the same care as the leaded aprons.

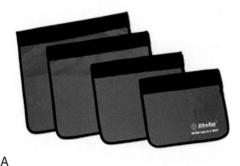

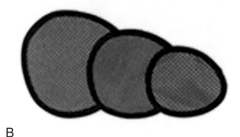

A   B

FIG. 3.8 A, Leaded shields used to protect the patient from excess or scattered radiation, to shield the detector from excess scatter, and to be placed on the patient to act as a mild restraint. **B,** Gonadal shields to be used to protect gonadal areas, particularly with breeding animals.

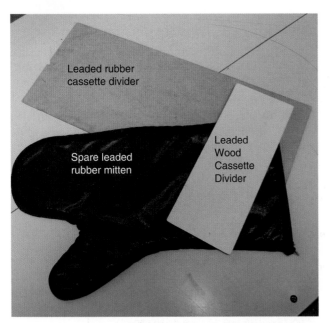

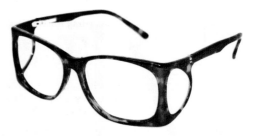

FIG. 3.11 Radiation glasses. These are made with leaded glass lenses and can also be ordered as prescription glasses. They are fairly heavy and should always be worn with a neck strap, as they are quite fragile.

FIG. 3.9 Various blockers that can be used to protect the image detector from scattered or secondary radiation. Collimation is vital in digital imaging.

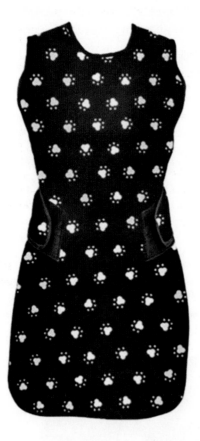

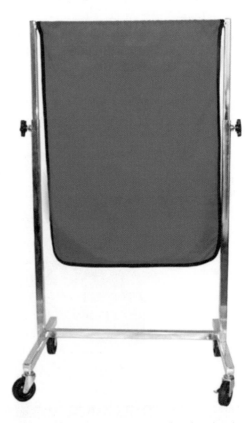

FIG. 3.12 A leaded screen. This unit can be placed in the room so that the technician can stand behind it when the exposure is made. This does not replace a leaded apron.

FIG. 3.10 An example of a leaded apron. It must be tied around the waist and secured on the shoulders so that the radiation worker is protected when they are in the room during a radiation exposure

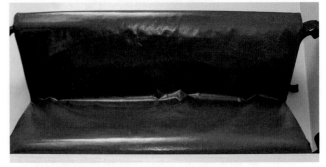

FIG. 3.13 Foam block used to assist in positioning patients.

Checklist regarding the safety of and the information provided to radiation workers.

_____ X-ray source not operated for the irradiation of a worker [section 4]

_____ Informed Workers in Writing (at time that employment begins) that worker is employed as an x-ray worker (i.e. higher dose equivalent limit), informed workers of those dose equivalent limits, and if female, limit for pregnant x-ray workers [section 9;1]

_____ Employer created and maintains a list of x-ray workers [section 9;2]

_____ Dose is ALARA and within dose equivalent annual limits [section 10;1]

_____ Employer takes every precaution reasonable to ensure mean dose equivalent received by the abdomen of a pregnant x-ray worker does not exceed 5 mSv during the pregnancy [section 10;2]

_____ X-ray warning signs or devices posted in conspicuous locations (i.e.door signs) [section 11;1]

_____ Label on X-ray control stating that the machine is a source of x-rays [section 11;2]

_____ Locks/interlocks in areas where air kerma may exceed 100 microGrays in one hour [section 11;3, i]

_____ Barriers and warning signs if the x-ray source is portable or mobile and is so used and where air kerma may exceed 100 microGrays in one hour [section 11;3, ii]

_____ Structural or other shielding shall be installed as per Ministry of Health plan approval [section 11;4, i]

_____ Diaphragms, cones and adjustable collimators used to limit size of beam [section 11;4, ii]

_____ Each x-ray worker has approved dosimeter [section 12;1]

_____ X-ray Worker using dosimeter as instructed by employer [section 12;2]

_____ Employer ensures dosimeter is read accurately [section 12;3]

_____ Employer furnishes worker the record of dosimeter results [section 12;3]

_____ Employer verifies dosimeter results as reasonable and informs MoL otherwise [section 12;4]

_____ Employer retains dosimeter results for at least 3 years [section 12;5]

_____ Copy of X-ray regulations posted and available to workers [OSHA section 22;2, i]

FIG. 3.14 Checklist for a typical facility in Canada. *ALARA*, as low as reasonably achievable; *MOL*, Ministry of Labour; *OSHA*, Occupational Safety and Health Act.

Summary

In this chapter we explored the regulations that have been put into effect to protect radiation workers, nonradiation workers, and patients undergoing radiographic examination from harmful doses. Protective apparel and its use and care have been discussed. The world of the radiation worker is much safer today than it was when the early pioneers were exploring this exciting new field.

REVIEW QUESTIONS

1. Radiation workers should always reduce radiation doses by following the:
   a. ALARA principle
   b. The least dose principle
   c. The no dose–image gently formula
   d. The principle of radiation doses

2. The radiation dose that workers are subjected to today is _____ than the _____ doses of early researchers.
   a. far higher, high
   b. far higher, low
   c. far less, high
   d. far less, low

3. When radiation strikes a cell, the most vulnerable area is the:
   a. Cell wall
   b. DNA
   c. Mitochondria
   d. Mitosis

4. If there is damage to the DNA, one of the outcomes is:
   a. Cell damage disrupting the cell walls
   b. Cell death from damage to the entire cell
   c. Cell death from other effects
   d. No change because the DNA can mend itself

5. Late-occurring effects are evident long after the damage has occurred. They are:
   a. Latent effects
   b. Nonstochastic effects
   c. Radiation effects
   d. Stochastic effects
6. Radiation exposure to veterinary workers is usually due to:
   a. Primary and secondary radiation
   b. Scattered and primary radiation
   c. Scattered and secondary radiation
   d. Secondary and stochastic radiation
7. Isotopes are variants of elements. They have differing numbers of:
   a. Electrons
   b. Neutrons
   c. Nuclei
   d. Protons
8. Linear energy transfer is defined as:
   a. The type of energy available only through radioactive disintegration
   b. The ability of radiation to affect DNA
   c. The ability of radiation to affect tissue
   d. The ability of radiation to transfer energy into tissue
9. X-rays and gamma rays have:
   a. High LET with high penetrability
   b. High LET with low penetrability
   c. Low LET with higher penetrability
   d. Low LET with low penetrability
10. Bone is much denser than fat so it absorbs more radiation than fat.
    a. True
    b. False
11. Three methods of radiation protection are:
    a. Distance, leaded aprons, and leaded gloves
    b. Time, distance, and shielding
    c. Time, inverse square law, and distance
    d. Time, LET, and shielding
12. The most susceptible tissue is tissue that is rapidly dividing; which of the following is true?
    a. Postpubertal adolescents would be highly affected.
    b. Prepubertal children would be most affected.
    c. This includes the healing of surgical wounds.
    d. This includes the tissue in a 2- to 10-week fetus.
13. Shielding of radiography rooms is essential in all installations; which of the following is true?
    a. Most radiation therapy suites are excused from this regulation.
    b. This applies to all imaging suites where ionizing radiation is used.
    c. This applies to only dental and nuclear medicine suites.
    d. This applies to only units that use over 90 kilovolts.

14. Leaded aprons are composed of thin sheets of leaded rubber; which of the following is true?
    a. The rubber is flexible and not likely to split if folded.
    b. The rubber is heavy and does not react to bending or splitting.
    c. The sheets of rubber are fragile and will split apart over time.
    d. The leaded apron should be hung up when not in use.
15. Radiation dosimeters must be issued to every radiation worker; which of the following is true?
    a. Personal dosimeters should be hung in the x-ray room when not in use.
    b. These are personal dosimeters and must not be shared with other workers.
    c. They can be shared by people who job-share.
    d. They should be taken home at the end of each shift to ensure they are safe.
16. The radiation worker is described as:
    a. A person who works in the same building where radiation is produced
    b. A worker who does not work with radiation but may be exposed to it
    c. A worker who works with radiation during his or her normal duties
    d. The employer of people who work with radiation
17. An employer is legally bound to instruct new employees that:
    a. There is equipment that produces radiation on site
    b. There is a radiation source but they will not be exposed to it
    c. They are in a facility where there is a radiation source for radiography
    d. They are not obligated to work with radiation
18. When maximum doses allowed are listed, there is no discrimination between men and women of reproductive age.
    a. True
    b. False

Answers to Review Questions can be found on the Evolve website.

CHAPTER **4**
Imaging on Film

Lois C. Brown, RTR (Can/USA), ACR, MSc., P.Phys

I love creating images, of course, because I'm an artist.
—Steve McQueen, American actor, 1930–1980

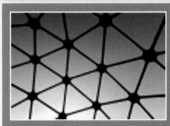

Imaging on film, any film, is similar to building a geodesic dome.

OUTLINE

LEARNING OBJECTIVES

When you have finished this chapter, you will be able to:

1. Identify cassettes, screens, and film, and understand how they work together to produce an image.
2. Understand the purpose of screen and film speed and screen colors and how they affect the image.
3. List the characteristics of various commercial cassettes and screens.
4. Understand latent image formation.

APPLICATIONS

The application of the information in this chapter is relevant to the following areas:

1. Producing x-ray images (radiographs) for evaluation and diagnosis
2. The selection of intensifying screens that will serve the requirements of the animal hospital
3. Ensuring that the film selected is compatible with the intensifying screens
4. The selection of appropriate storage space for both unused film and cassettes and film in use

KEY TERMS

Key terms are defined in the Glossary on the Evolve website.

Artifacts
Calcium tungstate
Cassette
Conversion efficiency
Crossover effect

Emulsion
Film base
Film/screen contact
Generator
Halation

Image receptor
Intensification factor
Intensifying screens
Latent image
Light spectrum

Luminescence
Manifest image
Resolution
Screen characteristics
Supercoat

Every x-ray image is produced using two completely separate systems: (1) the x-ray generator, which produces the x-rays; and (2) the receptor, which receives the x-rays and produces the actual image. Chapters 1 and 2 discussed the functions of the x-ray unit and how x-rays are produced via an electrical circuit through the x-ray tube. This chapter introduces the other side of imaging—the image receptor.

> **? POINTS TO PONDER**
>
> It is very important to remember the two separate components of the x-ray system. If one component is changed (e.g., the receptor), it is not always necessary to change the second component (e.g., the generator, transformer, table, or x-ray tube).

When we review various image receptors, we are immediately aware of how much imaging has changed over the years (Fig. 4.1). Since Roentgen's discovery of x-rays just over

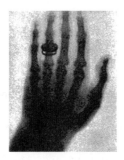

FIG. 4.1 Imaging then. The first radiograph—the hand of Mrs. Roentgen. It also contains the first artifact; can you identify it?

100 years ago, the field of imaging has evolved to encompass areas that could not have been imagined in the 1800s (Fig. 4.2).

As new concepts evolve, new units are manufactured and tested in the marketplace. Such testing always leads to upgrades as each new x-ray unit is challenged by its supporters and its competitors. Every unit that is successful in the veterinary clinic has some merit. It may be smaller or larger or faster or more efficient to use, but each design is changed as the imaging community demands even more convenience and better imaging. The age and appearance of the generator make little difference to the final image. As long as the technical factors are correct and the generator is calibrated correctly and produces consistent results, a 50-year-old generator will produce the same image as a brand-new generator.

X-ray film was the common receptor until a few years ago. Computers have now taken over the medical imaging world, and veterinary hospitals and clinics are rapidly following this trend. The concept of simplifying the selection of technical factors beyond the control of the operator and allowing the computer to manipulate the image reflects the lack of knowledge of the commercial vendor and the operator regarding technical factors and how they unify to produce an optimized image.

The term *photography* derives from the Greek words *phos* (*photós*), meaning "light," and *gráphein,* meaning "to write." From this the term *radiographer* denotes the technician or technologist who "writes with radiation." Obtaining a superior image and maintaining good imaging practices is achievable only if the technician has a basic understanding of technical factors and a solid background in image production and radiation protection.

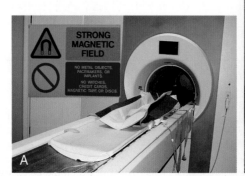
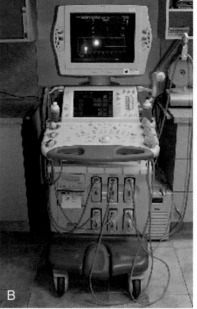

FIG. 4.2 Imaging now. Magnetic resonance imaging **(A)** evolved from radiography and ultrasound **(B)**, although neither modality uses x-rays to produce images.

Just as a camera must be set correctly to record the perfect image, so must the x-ray generator. A local camera store would be seriously remiss if they sold a digital camera with the concept that there is no need for operator training and support, or if the camera store told the proud new owner that there is no need to adjust the settings because every image can be optimized with postprocessing. In both photography and diagnostic imaging, the image data cannot be created with postprocessing if they are not recorded correctly.

There are three receptor components to every film-based imaging system: the cassette (the film holder), the intensifying screen (permanently installed within the cassette), and the film. Each item is an integral part of the imaging system. Each one is laterally important, so we will start from the outside and move inward.

X-Ray Cassettes

The x-ray cassette is a film holder designed to contain one pair of intensifying screens (attached to the front and back of the inside of the cassette) and one sheet of film of the appropriate size, which is placed between the screens (Fig. 4.3).

The cassette front is the "tube" side of the cassette and is located adjacent to the patient when it is in position. The cassette back is the side farthest from the object of interest. The cassette back usually contains the intensifying screen information and also contains the opening device. When the cassettes are opened, they are placed on the counter with the front side down.

Early cardboard and later plastic holders were used to encase the thinner and more flexible film because, unlike photography, the radiation penetrated the film holder. These holders were vulnerable to repetitive handling, and it soon became evident that a more substantial product was necessary. However, the early film holders are still in use in some facilities that radiograph very small animal extremities and small birds (Fig. 4.4).

With the introduction of intensifying screens, the entire package needed to be protected by a holder that was sturdy and unbendable because the emulsion of the intensifying screen could be damaged if it was folded or bent. The metal/Bakelite x-ray cassette was introduced in the 1930s. These film holders were substantial and addressed the problem of protection for the film. Transporting cassettes to and from the processing area required wheeled transport because multiple cassettes were very heavy. Manufacturers finally developed a cassette that met all the necessary criteria.

An x-ray film cassette must:
- Be sturdy so it doesn't crack under the heavy weight of a patient or several cassettes in a pile
- Not break apart in very cold conditions (equine radiography)
- Withstand considerable abuse during the course of many years of service
- Be inflexible and not warp if the patient's weight is unevenly distributed on the front
- Have secure latches that do not come undone inappropriately, exposing the film to light
- Have a radiolucent front that will not produce artifacts on the film
- Have a balanced weight from back to front so the cassette does not warp with age
- Contain a leaded foil or steel back to absorb scattered radiation emitted from the patient
- Contain some method of ensuring that the x-ray film is in good contact across the entire intensifying screen on both sides of the cassette (usually either foam or

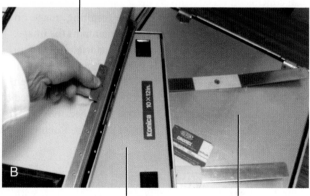

Kodak always yellow on back

Konica cassette
Double deck

Wolf cassette with
DuPont Hi Plus screens

FIG. 4.3 A, Cassette fronts. These labels indicate the screen type within the cassette and also the placement of the mask for the film identifier. **B,** Cassette backs from three different manufacturers. Sometimes the screens of one vendor are mounted within a cassette made by a different company. The labels on the back of the cassette should always be compared with the screen stencil stamped onto the screen itself. Note that the cassette front shows where the film identifier is located; the cassette back identifies the type of intensifying screen enclosed.

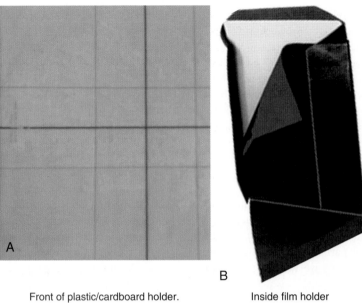

Front of plastic/cardboard holder.

Inside film holder with flap folded out and single screen installed.

FIG. 4.4 Film holders were originally made of cardboard and, later, plastic. They usually had a paper liner and can still be used for small body parts (wings and rodent's feet).

felt); film/screen contact is essential to high resolution (see Chapter 9)

- Have material on the outside that is washable and impervious to cleaning solutions, blood, and other effluents

Intensifying Screens

Very soon after discovering x-rays, Roentgen noticed that a paper covered with barium platinocyanide reacted quickly to the x-rays, converting them to light. Because he already knew that film is more sensitive to light than to x-rays, the logical conclusion was to convert the x-rays to light after they penetrate the patient and to record the resulting image on glass plates coated with an emulsion that maintains the image.

Barium platinocyanide was the first material used as an intensifying screen. Other physicists carried on his research, and in February 1897 the first commercial intensifying screen was developed. Thomas Edison, a fastidious inventor, applied for the first U.S. patent, but intensifying screens became widely used throughout the world within months of Roentgen's discovery of x-rays.

Screen Composition

The modern intensifying screen is composed of a base with an emulsion painted onto it. Often there is an adhesive layer that glues the emulsion to the base. Originally, the base was composed of cardstock (cardboard), which was easily damaged. Currently the base is a plastic/polymer, which is virtually indestructible within the hospital. The emulsion adheres to the base with an adhesive layer.

Screen Characteristics

Film has an infinite resolution. Film that is contained in the appropriate light-tight film holder and exposed and processed under perfect conditions will produce a near-perfect, high-resolution image. Problems arise because of the exposure time necessary to acquire that image. Patients are not always cooperative, hearts beat, lungs move ribs, and abdominal contents gurgle their way through the system. Original exposures in the late 1800s were measured in minutes rather than fractions of a second.

Intensifying screens provide a faster, more efficient method of image production. An added benefit of intensifying screens is the enhancement of contrast. When film alone is used on body parts greater than 10 centimeters, the amount of radiation required to expose the film causes scattered and secondary radiation to reduce the contrast dramatically. Visualization of the anatomy is compromised, making diagnosis from the film nearly impossible.

When x-ray photons penetrate the front of the cassette and arrive at the intensifying screen, they are immediately converted to light by the phosphor in the emulsion of the screens. The intensity and color of the light depend on the components of the phosphor. This is one of the most important areas of imaging with film/screens.

The speed (or rate) at which the x-rays are converted to light by the individual phosphors is called the *intrinsic conversion efficiency* of the phosphor. Each screen is rated by how quickly or how slowly the conversion occurs. This number determines the speed of the screen (screen speed), or how quickly that particular screen converts radiation to light. A calcium tungstate emulsion (the older technology) has a 30%

to 40% conversion efficiency, whereas a rare earth emulsion (the newer technology) has a 50% to 60% conversion efficiency. This means that less exposure time is required to produce an image on film that uses rare earth intensifying screens than on film that uses calcium tungstate screens.

The concept of screen speed classifications was introduced in order to compare the screens produced by each manufacturer. A standard film and rigidly controlled processing was used to test the system speeds. The speed of the system was measured by the amount of radiation required to produce a certain specific density (1.0) on a film (Fig. 4.5). A density of 1.0 is exactly in the center of the visible density range and is the density imaged in the middle of the ilium or in the center of the cranium of a lateral skull on a correctly exposed radiograph. (See Chapter 9 for more information on uniform density.)

A measurement of the exposure needed to produce a density of 1.0 *with* intensifying screens compared with the exposure needed *without* the use of intensifying screens is called *the intensification factor (IF)*. One example of a reduction in exposure time are the technical factors required for a radiograph of a bird's wing. All other factors being equal, the time required with no intensifying screens is approximately 0.03 seconds, whereas the time required using 400-speed intensifying screens is 0.003 seconds.

$$IF = \frac{\text{Exposure without screens}}{\text{Exposure with screens}}$$
$$= \frac{.03}{.003}$$
$$IF = 10$$

This type of calculation is useful if no screen/cassette is available. Usually it is used when very high resolution is necessary to visualize very small, thin body parts.

Until the 1970s calcium tungstate ($CaWO_4$) was the phosphor of choice for producing intensifying screens. In the 1970s a scientist at 3M in Minnesota experimented with phosphors while conducting research to collect light from distant stars, and she identified several phosphors as being very efficient at capturing light photons. These phosphors all belonged to a group of elements known as the *rare earths,* so-called because of the difficulties encountered when mining them from the earth. This discovery was shared throughout 3M, and it marketed the first rare earth radiographic intensifying screens in the late 1970s. Kodak and DuPont followed soon after. In the early days, 3M produced system speeds of up to 1200; due to a number of factors, however, the company settled on a 400-speed system.

Rare earth phosphors produce three to four times the amount of visible light per absorbed photon than the calcium tungstate phosphors. This means that the technical factors and thus the amount of radiation necessary to produce the same image density (optical density [OD] 1.0) may be reduced by a factor of 3 or 4. An examination requiring 0.10 seconds with calcium tungstate phosphors would now be perfectly acceptable at 0.025 seconds with rare earth phosphors. The older calcium tungstate screens are still available but are not recommended for use in any medical or veterinary facility.

The Blue/Green Question

Until 1981 all radiography film was manufactured to react to blue light from the blue light–emitting intensifying screens (Fig. 4.6). In 1981 Kodak introduced the rare earth lanthanum oxide intensifying screens, which emitted green light. This event threw the imaging world into chaos. Now the competitive film companies, who were just perfecting the blue systems, had to "play catch-up" and manufacture two completely different emulsions—an intensifying screen emulsion and a companion film emulsion. In addition, Kodak introduced the 24 cm × 30 cm x-ray cassette, which replaced the standard 10 inch × 12 inch (25 cm × 30 cm) cassette. The

FIG. 4.5 An example of density 1.0 + base + fog. This density on a film is exactly midway between completely black (density 3.00) and completely clear (density .10). For a further explanation, see Chapter 9.

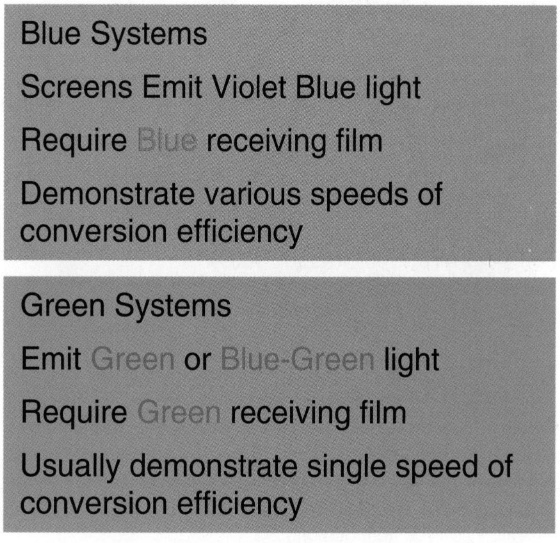

Blue Systems

Screens Emit Violet Blue light

Require Blue receiving film

Demonstrate various speeds of conversion efficiency

Green Systems

Emit Green or Blue-Green light

Require Green receiving film

Usually demonstrate single speed of conversion efficiency

FIG. 4.6 Blue systems vs. green systems.

added metric cassette was a marketing ploy that confuses people to this day. The green screen technology was definitely a superior imaging system, and the research dollars spent to improve this system have given it an advantage over the blue systems.

At the time of this writing, blue systems are being phased out and eventually will not be supported as the production of blue-receiving film slows down and eventually ceases. Research into blue systems ended in the mid to late 1980s, which means that the technology used to produce any blue-emitting screens is at least 35 years old. It is vitally important to know which color system is in place at the veterinary facility. Ordering or accepting a delivery of incorrect film and trying to optimize imaging is a very common problem in the radiography room.

More About Color

A rainbow is the result of light traveling through the atmosphere. Each of the colors of the rainbow is refracted at a slightly different angle (Fig. 4.7), resulting in a perfect spectrum of color. Every time light is refracted, whether through a prism of glass, a sudden shower, or a perfect diamond, the colors remain in the same orientation and order. This arrangement is known as the *visible light spectrum*. Infrared light is at the far "outside" of the curve, and blue and ultraviolet light are on the "inside" of the curve. Violet morphs to blue and then to green, yellow, orange, and red. This order is important when investigating x-ray film and intensifying screens and when setting up a darkroom and using a safelight (see Chapter 7). If the film reacts to only the blue-green side of the spectrum, it will not react to the deepest red part of the spectrum. If it

reacts to green, it will react to an orange-yellow color because there is a yellow component in the color green (blue + yellow = green).

The early intensifying screens were made of calcium tungstate ($CaWO_4$), which emits a very pretty blue-violet light. When the rare earth phosphors were developed, the striking difference (apart from their rapid conversion efficiency) was the bright green-yellow color of their phosphor emission. This changed the entire world of imaging. The x-ray film that had been developed to respond to blue light did not "see" the extended yellow-green portion of the spectrum. Therefore a new film had to be developed that responded both to blue light and to yellow-green light.

Green-sensitive film "sees" the blue light portion of the green screens, but blue film does not react to the green portion of the green-emitting screens. If the incorrect film is used, the technical factors will need to be increased because the imaging is not optimized. This increases patient and staff radiation dose considerably and results in a less-than-optimal film. If blue film is inserted between green screens, the images will be a dull gray, lacking contrast that does not improve even if the technical factors are raised or lowered.

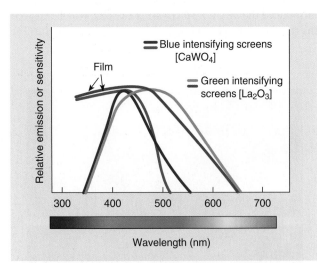

FIG. 4.7 The importance of spectral matching. The film must be able to "see" the light emitted from the intensifying screen. In this case blue light is emitted and blue film overlaps the emission and therefore reacts to the light. The film would not "see" green light as it is too far removed to the right of the spectrum to be activated. It does, however, "see" a small amount of the blue light because there is a blue component in the green light. (Modified from Bushong SC. *Radiologic Science for Technologists*, 10th ed. St Louis: Elsevier; 2013.)

ultraviolet range. These screens had limited success and were mostly successful with extremities and thinner body parts. They do show up in the veterinary market occasionally but are no longer produced, and the UV film is no longer sold.

The film to be used with these screens, if one attempts to use them, is blue-receiving film; this film is no longer marketed. They do not respond well to the light of green-emitting screens, even though there is a minor blue component in the green light. Ideally the screens should be replaced.

We will visit this topic again when we discuss radiographic film, both blue-receiving film and green-receiving film. The concept is important and frequently confused.

Screen Speed

The conversion efficiency of the phosphor reflects the components of the x-ray screen; unfortunately, not all screens are created equal (Fig. 4.8). Green-screen technology has two screen speeds: fast response to radiation and slow response to radiation (Table 4.1). (A medium-speed screen was available but not in general use and is now mainly phased out.) The phosphor thickness is a factor in the screen speed, but so is the thickness of the emulsion. Slower-speed systems have thinner emulsions. Faster systems with thicker emulsions produce more photons of light per incident ray than the slower systems. Faster systems reduce the radiation dose to the patient, but they also reduce the *spatial resolution* (the ability to see very fine detail). The slower the screen speed, the more detail is evident on the image (higher resolution).

To produce the same density on the film every time, more radiation must be used to produce an image from a slow screen than from a faster screen. The screen type does not influence contrast—only film and technical factors influence contrast. Over time, many applications were developed using a variety of screen speeds, and mixing and matching screens became quite common. This interchanging of screens was known as *asymmetrical systems,* and 3M was the company best known for this technology.

Cassette Identification vs. Screen Identification

Cassette/screen manufacturers place labels on the back of the cassettes to notify the user which screens have been installed. 3M cassettes are often labeled 2/6 or 6/12; this labeling denotes an asymmetrical system.

Screens are always labeled in very fine print on the edge, usually along the long side. The imprinting is very tiny and sometimes hard to read, but it is essential that the operator is aware of the phosphor emission color and the screen designation. Cassettes do have the screen type labeled on the back, but occasionally screens are replaced in cassettes and the labels are not changed. The positive identification is on the screen stencil (Fig. 4.9).

TABLE 4.1	The Influence of Slow Screens vs. Fast Screens on Images	
FACTOR	**SLOW SCREEN SPEED RESPONSE TO RADIATION**	**FAST SCREEN SPEED RESPONSE TO RADIATION**
Technique	Increase technical factors	Decrease technical factors
Dose	Higher dose	Lower dose
Resolution	Better resolution	Lower resolution
Contrast	No difference	No difference
Density	Lighter image if factors are not adjusted	Darker image if factors are not adjusted

400 speed
Green emitting screens presently slowed to ~300 speed

200 speed
Green emitting screens presently slowed to ~100 speed

400 speed
Green emitting screens presently remains at 400 speed

600 speed
Green emitting screens

FIG. 4.8 The backs of various cassettes and screen speeds.

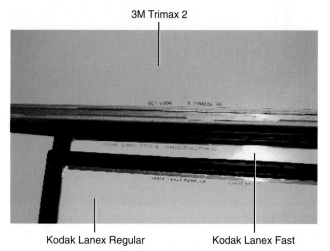

3M Trimax 2

Kodak Lanex Regular   Kodak Lanex Fast

FIG. 4.9 Screen stencils: 3M and Kodak. The numbers identify when the screen was manufactured and the batch number.

Luminescence and Phosphorescence

Intensifying screens react to the incoming radiation by a process called *luminescence*. The photons of the x-ray beam are converted to light when they reach the emulsion of the screen.

There are two types of luminescence: fluorescence and phosphorescence. Fluorescence is an instantaneous reaction that lasts exactly as long as the phosphor is stimulated. Phosphorescence occurs when the phosphor continues to emit light after the stimulation has ceased (Fig. 4.10). Phosphorescence is not desirable in medical imaging and is termed *screen lag or afterglow*.

Screen Aging Response

As intensifying screens age over time, the response of the phosphor reduces in brightness and speed. A screen that responded to the incoming radiation 100% when new will respond only 50% after 15 or 20 years. The response of the screen, both in brightness and over time, is called *screen speed*. Technical problems arise as the products age, particularly with the technique chart (Fig. 4.11). If older screens from various manufacturers are used in one clinic, the screen speed may differ widely, and the images produced can vary in density and contrast. This is often the reason why a particular cassette is discarded because "it doesn't work properly." Actually, it may be reacting to the x-ray beam correctly according to its manufacture, original screen speed, and age. It is very important to know which screens are in use at the veterinary facility and whether they are matched for screen speed and age.

If a facility has a mixture of various manufacturers' screens, there is most likely a wide variation in the speeds of the intensifying screens. In this case adherence to a standard technique chart is impossible, as is the production of consistent, optimized radiographs. Intensifying screens are often replaced in cassettes, but the change is not necessarily noted on the outside of the cassette. A cassette label on the back of the cassette may note that it contains Quanta 111 Screens installed in 1982, but the actual screens may be Fuji HR or Kodak Lanex Regular and installed very recently (see Chapter 9).

Speed Response Differences

In order to compare screen speeds, the manufacturers agreed on a numbering system that is still used today. The DuPont (E.I. DuPont de Nemours) Hi Speed Screen is used as a baseline and called 100-speed class. Table 4.2 lists the common manufacturers with the names and speeds of their systems.

It must be remembered that each manufacturer has its own concept of the speed of its particular phosphor "recipe," so the speeds are not all exactly the same; this is why we use the term *"speed class."* For example, Kodak Lanex screens are a true 400-speed, whereas DuPont Quanta 111 screens in the 400-speed class are actually closer to 350-speed. More radiation must be used with the Quanta 111 screens than with the Kodak Lanex screens to produce the same density on a film.

3M Corporation originally developed the technology to use the rare earth phosphors for intensifying screens and therefore had many more varieties and combinations than are listed in Table 4.2. Old Agfa screens, often donated by medical facilities to veterinary clinics, demonstrated phosphorescence and would fog the film in the cassette as it waited to be used. Agfa's Ortho 400s had the most frequent problems. DuPont rare earth screens were never very good, with poor resolution and very flat contrast, and the emulsions tended to absorb moisture (see Chapter 9).

As screens age, their response to radiation may slow down. Screens of various companies lose their speed over time in and at various rates. Fig. 4.11 lists the average speed loss of screens from six major manufacturers over a 30-year period.

If there is a problem with imaging, the first place to investigate is always the film/screen combination. It is common for the incorrect film to be ordered or even supplied by the film vendor. Checking the film/screen combination is the easiest place to start the investigative process.

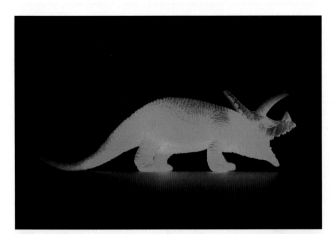

FIG. 4.10 An example of *phosphorescence*. The light from the sun causes the crystals to glow, which remains long after the excitation of the crystals. The effect that the screens must have is *fluorescence*, which means the crystals stop glowing immediately after the stimulation is removed. (Copyright myshkovsky/Getty Images.)

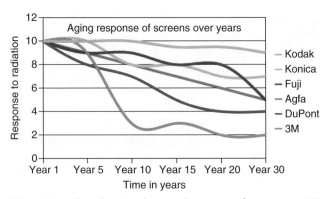

FIG. 4.11 Chart depicting the typical responses of screens over 30 years. The Lanex screens retain their original speed throughout their lifetime. Most other screens deteriorate in speed. This is not the result of a controlled experiment, but rather an observation over 50 years of imaging consultation.

TABLE 4.2	Screen Manufacturers and Their Speed Classifications			
MANUFACTURER	**SCREEN NAME**	**SPEED CLASS**	**COLOR OF PHOSPHOR**	**RARE EARTH?**
Agfa	Ortho Fine	100	Green	Yes
	Ortho Medium	200	Green	Yes
	Ortho 400*	400	Green	Yes—no longer available
	Ortho	400	Green	Yes
DuPont	Par	50	Blue	These screens were produced from 1960-1980 and are now obsolete. The speed of the screens has diminished to the point that they should no longer be used, ever.
	Hi Speed	100	Blue	
	Hi Plus +	200	Blue	
	Lightning Plus	150	Blue	
	Quanta 11	300	Blue	Yes—no longer in use. These were very "noisy" screens and were either dumped onto the vet/chiropractor/osteopath market or scrapped.
	Quanta 111	400	Blue	Yes
	Quanta V	400	Green	Yes. These were manufactured only by DuPont and are no longer available; they had very poor contrast.
	Quanta UV	400	Ultraviolet	Yes. These were available only around 1985–1989. They produced good imaging for extremities but very poor imaging for abdomens. they were removed from the medical market around 1990.
Fuji	G4	200	Green	Yes
	G8	300	Green	Yes
	G12	400	Green	Yes
	HR	400	Green	Yes
Kodak	Xomat	200	Blue	No
	Fine	100	Blue	No
	Lanex Fine	100	Green	Yes
	Lanex Med	200	Green	Yes
	Lanex Regular	400	Green	Yes
	Lanex Fast	600	Green	Yes
Konica	KMC	200	Blue	Yes, with type HB film
	KMC	400	Blue	Yes with type A film
	KF	100	Green	Yes
	KM	300	Green	Yes
	KR	400	Green	Yes
	KS	600	Green	Yes
3M Corp[†]	2 or 3	100	Green	Yes
	6	200	Green	Yes
	12	400	Green	Yes

*Old Agfa screens often donated to a veterinary clinic demonstrated phosphorescence and would fog the film in the cassette as it waited to be used. Agfa's Ortho 400s had the most frequent problems.
[†]3M corporation developed the technology to use the rare earth phosphors for intensifying screens and therefore had many more varieties and combinations than are listed here.
With assistance from Leo Reina, X-ray Cassette Repair Company, dba Reina Imaging, Crystal Lake, Illinois.

Radiography Film

Several companies manufacture film, and several more cut and sell the film. The one standard among all these companies is the film size (Table 4.3).

Film is sold in very specific sizes to match the sizes of the cassettes. It is important to know what size cassette is in use in the facility and then order the appropriate size film. Kodak's introduction of the 24 cm × 30 cm film and cassette made the industry even more complicated. Film price is based on the square inch of the product. A box of 25 cm × 30 cm film (traditionally 10 inches × 12 inches, or 120 square inches) is more expensive than the 24 cm × 30 cm (113 square inches) film introduced by Kodak and now sold universally. Film that is 25 cm × 30 cm will fit into a 24 cm × 30 cm cassette only if it is cut down to size in the darkroom; 1 cm must be removed from the long side. This is a lengthy procedure and unnecessary if the correct size is originally ordered. It is

TABLE 4.3	Film and Cassette Sizes (Metric vs. Inch)*	
FILM SIZE (inches)	**FILM SIZE (centimeters)**	**TYPICAL IMAGING USE**
6 × 8	18 × 24	Extremities, pocket pets,
8 × 10	20 × 25	Equine and extremities, pocket pets
	24 × 30	Equine and feline, also skull and extremities
10 × 12	25 × 30	Equine and feline, also skull and extremities
11 × 14	28 × 35	General radiography
	30 × 35	General radiography
14 × 17	35 × 43	General radiography

*Some of the inch sizes do not have an equal-sized metric partner, as is the case with the cm sizes.

expensive to order the incorrect film in terms of both time and money.

The Development of Film-Based Imaging

Cellulose nitrate was introduced as a film base in 1914 (Fig. 4.12A). A major problem with this material was its flammability; several tragic hospital fires occurred in which patients and staff died because of the noxious emissions from the breakdown of x-ray products. A nonflammable base, cellulose triacetate, was introduced in the 1920s. One problem with cellulose triacetate that did not show up until years later was its tendency to shrink when stored for long periods (Fig. 4.12B).

The old emulsions on the original film bases took a very long time to react to light or x-rays, with some exposures taking as long as 10 minutes. Processing the images was also a lengthy procedure. So along with the new film bases, more efficient emulsions were investigated.

The cellulose triacetate base was used into the 1960s, when E.I. DuPont de Nemours introduced the film base that is in use today. Along the way the company also invented nylon, Dacron, Kevlar, and many other related substances, but their major achievement in imaging was the invention of Mylar. Mylar has been used in medical imaging for about 50 years. Before the introduction of Mylar, the film would tear apart and be destroyed if it became caught in a processor. With the introduction of a film base that was nontearing and inflammable, x-ray film became virtually indestructible.

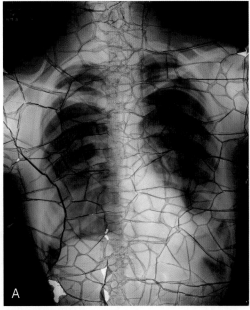 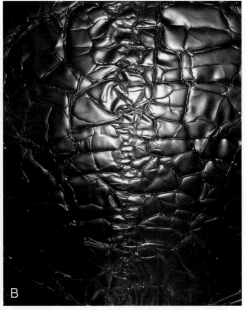

FIG. 4.12 A, Cellulose acetate base; human chest radiograph. **B,** The film base has slowly shrunk over a period of 40 years, buckling and bubbling the fragile emulsion layer. The lesson here is that older radiographs are not necessarily archival quality. The emulsion can still separate from the base or can change color as the sulfides become evident.

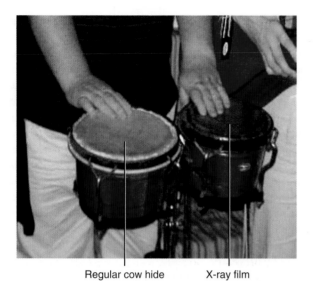

Regular cow hide   X-ray film

FIG. 4.13 One use for recycled radiography film! This is a band in Cuba. Used x-ray film has many uses, including fencing and fence posts, lawn chairs, and fashion jewelry. It is very important to find a recycler for used x-ray film; it should not go to a landfill. (Courtesy James Duhaime, St Clair Veterinary Facilities, Toronto.)

When it is time to dispose of used film, the veterinary technician should always make sure that the recycler is actually destroying the film by shredding, or the facility should remove all patient identifiers from each film before it is shipped from the veterinary hospital.

Composition of Radiography Film

The x-ray film base is translucent and flexible. Light-sensitive film emulsion coats either one side of the base (single-emulsion film) or two sides of the base (double-emulsion film) (Fig. 4.14). Between the base and the emulsion is an adhesive layer that is so thin it is basically incorporated into the emulsion layer. The supercoat is a hard protective gelatin layer on top of the emulsion that protects the image from the rigors of processing. This is only somewhat effective, so film should always be handled with respect because the emulsion on a preexposed film and the image on a postexposed film are very tenuous and easily compromised.

Halation is the effect of light reflecting off the back of the film base and affecting the image by causing a shadow effect. Double-emulsion film contains a dye layer that prevents a crossover effect, a type of halation in which the light of one intensifying screen affects the opposite emulsion (Figs. 4.15 and 4.16). Single-emulsion film requires an anticurl/

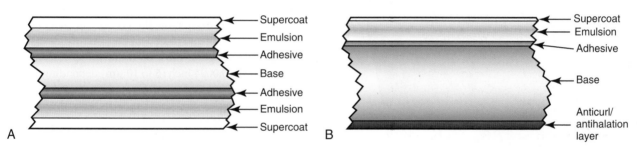

FIG. 4.14 Cross-section of double-emulsion film **(A)** and single-emulsion film **(B)**. (Modified from Fauber TL. *Radiographic Imaging and Exposure*, 5th ed. St. Louis: Mosby; 2017.)

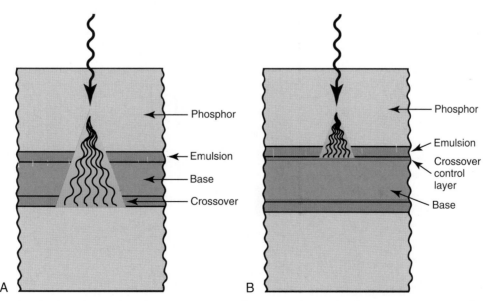

FIG. 4.15 Dye layer *(orange layer)* that prevents crossover from one emulsion to the other. **A,** Crossover occurs when the film has no dye layer to prevent light from the top screen affecting the film emulsion on the opposite side. **B,** The dye layer prevents the light from the top screen affecting the light from the bottom screen. This occurs only with double-emulsion film.

antihalation layer on the nonemulsion side. The antihalation layer is removed during film processing. Single-emulsion film is easily identified even in the darkroom under safelight conditions. The side with the emulsion is dull, and the side with the anticurl/antihalation layer is very shiny.

Double-emulsion film is used in general radiography. Single-emulsion film is used in special applications, such as high-resolution imaging (extremities and equine) and in laser imaging printing for computed tomography, magnetic resonance imaging, nuclear medicine, and positron emission tomography if the veterinarian needs a hard-copy image from these modalities.

Film Base

The base material that holds the emulsion of the film must be strong yet flexible. It must bend without stretching, and it must be stable throughout changes in temperature and

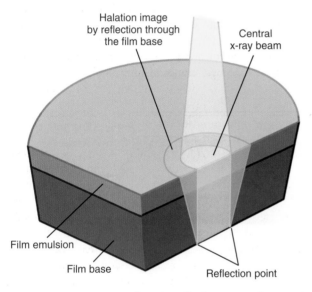

FIG. 4.16 The halation effect. If the film has two emulsions and no antihalation layer, there will be a crossover effect.

humidity. It must be rigid enough to hang on an illuminator and yet flexible enough to travel through an x-ray processor. Most of all, it must be consistently and uniformly optically translucent. It must permit the transmission of light without adding any artifacts to the final x-ray image. The film base must also be thin enough so there is no crossover effect (reflection) from one side of the image to the other when the image is produced.

In the 1960s it was discovered that the addition of a slight blue tint to the film base enabled the radiologist reading the images to work for longer periods without experiencing eyestrain and headaches from the glare of the illuminators transmitted through the lightly exposed or unexposed portions of the film (see Chapter 6).

Film Emulsion

The emulsion is the material that is coated onto the film base by means of an adhesive material that binds it to the film base. Film emulsion starts with gelatin—the same gelatin used in cooking and Jell-O. The gelatin used in this application is of very high quality and is completely translucent. The photosensitive products within the emulsion are mainly silver bromide (about 95% to 98%), silver iodide, and silver chloride. There is very little silver chloride in film emulsion today. Collectively, the term *silver halide* is used to describe the components of the emulsion (Fig. 4.17).

The gelatin base must allow the processing chemicals to infiltrate the emulsion and react with the silver halide crystals to produce the image. It must be uniform, its thickness is usually 0.0002 to 0.0004 inch (5 to 10 μm) depending on the manufacturer, and it must be flexible enough to permit bending without stretching as the film winds its way through an automatic processor.

The Supercoat

The outside of the film is protected by a tough coating of hard protective gelatin (the supercoat) that has been treated to prevent tearing, scratching, and abrasions to the film as it is loaded into the cassettes and then processed either manually

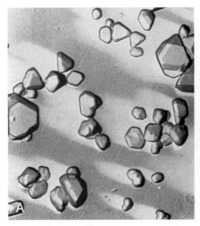
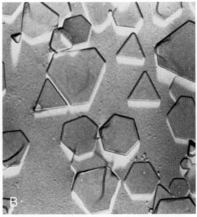

FIG. 4.17 Magnified portion of the film emulsion. **A,** Old technology silver halide crystals. **B,** New technology using tabular grain silver halide crystals. (Courtesy Carestream Health.)

or automatically. It is not very thick, and rough handling and scratching can damage the supercoat. This supercoat also protects the film from diffusing its dye into the screens. If the film does not meet quality control specifications, the supercoat is not applied and it is sold as "white box film."

It is important to note that once the film is wet, the gelatin absorbs moisture and the supercoat becomes vulnerable to scratches and abrasions.

Latent Image Formation

The film emulsion with the silver halide particles suspended in a gelatinous layer also contains sensitivity specks (centers), small physical imperfections within the network of the silver halide. It is these small areas that become magnets for the silver particles to adhere to one another and form an image.

It is important to note that if the silver halide were perfect and without any imperfections (sensitivity specks), the image would not form and the film would exit the processor with no discernible image. Therefore when film is first manufactured, it must remain in the warehouse for a time to allow the sensitivity specks to settle within the emulsion. This process is called *aging* or *seasoning*.

According to theory, the latent image is formed within the emulsion of the x-ray film when the x-rays and light activate the silver particles in the film emulsion. The silver particles are attracted to the sensitivity specks by electromagnetism. It is believed that there must be at least three silver atoms to each sensitivity speck in order for the image to form. The term *latent image* refers to the image that is formed but is invisible until processed either manually or in an automatic processor. This new arrangement of silver halide particles is called the *lattice network*. It is a tenuous arrangement and may be easily destroyed.

The pattern of a lattice network is much like a geodesic dome (Fig. 4.18). The joints of the bars are the sensitivity specks. High-detail film contains more sensitivity specks than general radiography film and therefore produces a more detailed image. The silver compounds wait until they are processed to produce a manifest image.

The lattice network forms very much like the seeding of clouds to cause rain (Fig. 4.19). The water droplets require impurities in the clouds to form rain; these impurities can be added naturally by the wind raising dust clouds or mechanically by an airplane dropping dust onto the cloud. With film, the impurities (sensitivity specks) are built into the film emulsion, and the catalyst to start the process of latent image formation is the introduction of photons of light and x-rays. The actual physical process is still somewhat a mystery, but it is known that the image forms around the sensitivity specks electromagnetically and that at least three freed silver atoms must be deposited for a clump of black metallic silver to be formed by chemical development later during processing.

The latent image is fragile, and the network is very easy to break. Dropping a cassette from a table can destroy the network and cause an artifact of streaks radiating from the point of impact. Time will also cause the latent image to start to fade, although it does take a fairly long time (in excess of 24 hours) to fade completely. The lattice network will form a denser (darker) image the more it is exposed to radiation, light, and heat. A continuous heavy pressure on unexposed film will prevent the lattice network from forming or will break down what has already formed, leaving a clear area outlining the area of the pressure. Therefore film and cassettes should always be stored in an upright position in the darkroom and never flat on the counter.

Base + Fog

When the film is originally manufactured, it will process completely clear except for the base + fog that is inherent in the film manufacturing. After the film seasons, or matures, to the point that it can be sold and put into practice, it will develop a low fog level. Brand-new film out of a new box will have a very low optical density (OD), usually 0.10 to 0.15. This optical density is the evidence that the sensitivity specks are active and will convert any light or radiation into metallic silver during processing. Whenever film density is discussed, the base color and the fog level are always included as part of the image (e.g., density 1.0 + base + fog).

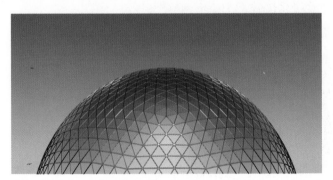

FIG. 4.18 A geodesic dome. The pattern is similar to the lattice network that forms when an image is produced on a film. The joints are the sensitivity specks drawing the silver ions together to form the network, or lattice. (Copyright photoart23D/Getty Images.)

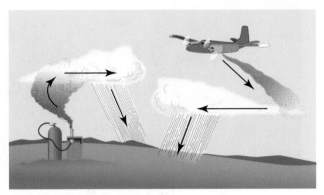

FIG. 4.19 Seeding of clouds by human intervention. The moisture gathers on the dust until it becomes so heavy that it starts to rain. This is similar to the sensitivity specks distributed throughout the film emulsion. Once the emulsion is activated by the x-rays, the sensitivity specks form "collection points" where the latent image forms

The base + fog level is usually minimal in unexposed film. However, if the film is exposed to unsuitable storage conditions (e.g., heat, air heavy with a chemical odor) and then exposed to radiation, the base + fog will be dark enough to compromise the radiograph because the clear areas will no longer be visible, having been replaced by a fog density of 0.20 to 0.29.

The Response of Film to Light

Film Color

Modern film responds to the light emitted from the intensifying screens. This light may be either blue or green, and this causes the most confusion in any veterinary facility. It is also one of the most important concepts in the practice of film/screen imaging.

Blue-emitting screens require blue-receiving film (Fig. 4.20A). Confusion arises when the blue dye used in the base "mixes" with the yellow color of the emulsion. The blue-receiving film then becomes physically green in color. Green-receiving film is physically violet. This was agreed to by the film manufacturers to differentiate between blue-receiving film and green-receiving film (Fig. 4.20B). Rather than preventing confusion, however, this step added to the confusion; to this day, green-receiving film is physically violet and blue-receiving film is physically green.

Film Speed

It is always good practice to examine every box of film delivered from the supplier to ensure that the correct film has been shipped. The type of film and the code number are clearly marked on the front and/or side of the film box.

It is common to find hospitals using a half-speed film in old blue-screened cassettes when they could decrease the dose just by changing the film they put into the cassettes (Table 4.4).

TABLE 4.4	Common Film Types and Their Speed		
COMPANY	**FILM TYPE**	**FILM SPEED**	**FILM COLOR**
Carestream	T-mat-G/RA	Full-speed	Green
Carestream	CSB	Full-speed	Blue
Fuji	HRS	Full-speed	Green
Fuji	RX	Full-speed	Blue
3M	UD+	Full-speed	Green

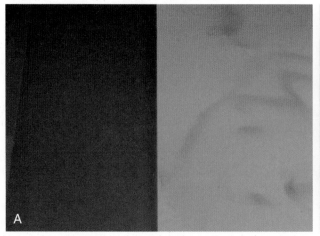

FIG. 4.20 Two film/screen systems are available on the market today. Green is the preferred color, but some facilities still use blue. Four brands of film are illustrated here, two blue and two green. **A,** Blue light–receiving film is physically green. The image is "blue" film from two different companies. **B,** Green light–receiving film is physically violet. The image is "green" film from two different companies.

Swapping out the screens to green-emitting screens can save money (green is less expensive than blue) and improve imaging using modern technology. The imaging research on blue systems ended many years ago. If a facility is going to stay with film-screen imaging, the cassettes should be replaced with ones containing green-emitting screens or, at the very least, the screens within the cassettes should be replaced.

It is important to remember that half-speed film stored away somewhere may arrive at your facility. Because half-speed film reacts 50% slower to stimulation, it will produce an image that is 50% lighter than it should be given the technical factors used for a 400-speed system.

The other film that may be available today in certain geographical locations is extremity film and/or single-emulsion film. Single-emulsion film has emulsion on one side and an antihalation layer on the other side. Single-emulsion film reacts to radiation and light from the screens only on the side with the emulsion, and it is far slower than double-emulsion film. Single-emulsion film is used for certain specific applications in which exceptional detail is required. It may be used in some equine practices when tiny spurs, spicules, or hairline fractures are suspected. It can also be used in wildlife practices to diagnose fractures in reptiles or on the wings of birds. Single-emulsion film requires considerably higher doses of radiation to produce an image and therefore is definitely not recommended for routine veterinary examinations. The most common use of single-emulsion film up until a few years ago was human breast imaging; thus it is typically available only in 8 in × 10 in, 24 cm × 30 cm, and 10 in × 12 in sizes.

Other films, such as duplicating film and laser film, are not in wide practice in veterinary medicine.

Film Speed and White Box Film

Film speed is the most difficult factor to control in the production of the film itself. Mixing emulsions is a little like following a recipe from a list of dissimilar ingredients. Depending on the manufacturer, many different components are mixed in with a lot of gelatin.

If the mix is slightly "off" either way, the film may react a little too quickly or a little too slowly to exposure by radiation. Each manufacturer has a specific benchmark for the reaction time of the film, and each batch of film is tested against this benchmark. If the speed of the film is within ±10% of the perfect speed, it is accepted and boxed with the manufacturer's label. At this point the film is in huge rolls about 2 feet (0.61 m) in diameter and about 80 to 100 feet (24.4-30.5 m) in length.

If the speed of the entire roll of film is beyond the 10% parameter up to a point of nonacceptance as defined by each manufacturer (usually ±25%), it is sold as "white box" film (Fig. 4.21). This film remains unfinished—it is not given a supercoat to prevent the dye within the emulsion from leaching out onto the screens. This means that over time the dye will stain the screen and reduce its speed by coloring the screen emulsion.

FIG. 4.21 Two examples of "white box" packaged film. The film in these packages was manufactured in Belgium (Agfa film) and finished in the United States. Other film may be manufactured in the United States (Kodak film).

White box film is cut to various sizes and boxed in white boxes with a film dealer's label. Because white box packagers deal only with originally rejected film, they may easily mix films of different speeds in one box. A box of 100 sheets may contain film that failed the quality control standards because it was too "slow" mixed in with film that failed because it was too "fast." It is important to remember this process when images never seem to be quite right, with some images too dark and other images too light for the same size animal under the exact same exposure and processing conditions. The easiest solution is to purchase film with the original manufacturer's label on the box. The few dollars saved by buying white box film is not necessarily a cost saving when a diagnosis is missed because of poor image quality or an uncertain speed.

Typically, the original manufacturer is identifiable on the white box by the location indicated on the label. Because it is law that the country in which the film is manufactured be noted on every product, the label will state "Manufactured in USA" (Kodak film, now Carestream) or "Manufactured in Belgium" (Agfa film). This information serves only for general interest and does not reflect on the product of either manufacturer.

Storage of Film, Cassettes, and Screens

Proper storage of the products used for imaging is very important. The film and chemicals must be stored on a rotating basis so that the first product in is the first product out. This is also known as *FIFO storage.*

Film

Film boxes must always be stored on edge and not flat on a counter. Film is sensitive to pressure both before and after it has been exposed to radiation. Dropping a cassette with exposed film can destroy the lattice network and ruin the

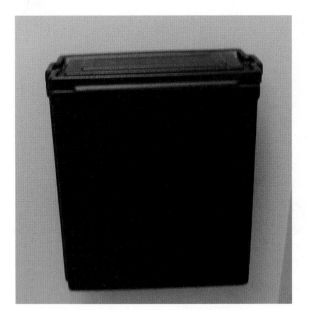

FIG. 4.22 Open boxes of film should be stored in a light-tight film bin. This box should be hung on the wall so the film boxes inside remain upright.

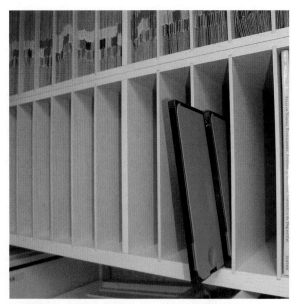

FIG. 4.23 Cassettes should be stored upright on a counter or in a cabinet protected from radiation.

image. Heavy pressure on the film can also destroy the film's capability to form a lattice network, resulting in no image in the area of the pressure.

Film must be protected from light leaks and from radiation (Fig. 4.22). It is important to note the expiration date on the boxes. If the facility has several different sizes of cassettes and film, some of the film may age beyond its expiration date.

When a film is manufactured and finally presented to the market, it has aged and is ready to be used. The emulsion on the film is an unstable entity ready to react within fractions of a second to any stimulus. Heat, chemical fumes, light leaks, and aging will darken the film without any exposure to radiation. It is important to store film at room temperature and in a dry atmosphere. Film that has aged beyond its expiration date starts to darken as the fog level rises. At first this darkening does not interfere with the image. As the fog level rises, however, the darkening increases dramatically and the resulting image loses contrast because the clear areas of the film will no longer be visible.

Cassettes and Screens

Cassettes should be stored upright in a cupboard or in the darkroom without the possibility of exposure to radiation (Fig. 4.23). They should not be stored on the floor, where they could be knocked over or subjected to spills and liquids. They should not be stored in a pile on a counter because the pressure of one cassette on top of another will affect the film. In addition, pulling a cassette out from under a pile of cassettes exerts extra wear and poses the risk of damage to the cassettes.

Cassettes should be loaded with film and ready to be used. It is important to ensure that the correct film is used

in each cassette. The cassettes should be kept closed in the darkroom in order to protect the integrity of the screens. Humidity and dust adversely affect the screen and compromise the image.

Screens should be protected when the film is being removed from the cassette. Sliding the film in the cassette will cause wear artifacts on the screen. If the film is not readily removable, the cassette should be held on edge to allow the film to separate from the screen naturally (Fig. 4.24).

Other Equipment and Accessories

We will examine the tabletop, the grid, and the illuminators in other discussions of equipment and accessories (see Chapter 5), technical factors (see Chapter 6), and processing and processing artifacts (see Chapters 7 and 9).

Summary

An optimized system is possible only if the correct products are matched, purchased, and used correctly. This chapter discussed various x-ray cassettes and screen types along with some of the problems inherent in selecting the correct combination to produce an optimized image. Screen/film combinations and the blue vs. green problems were reviewed. Latent image formation, base + fog, and general film fog were discussed, and the importance of correctly storing and handling these products was outlined.

Image Gallery

Figs. 4.25 to 4.37 illustrate what can go wrong with film, cassettes, and screens.

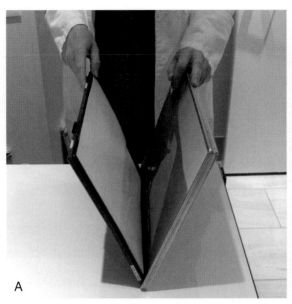
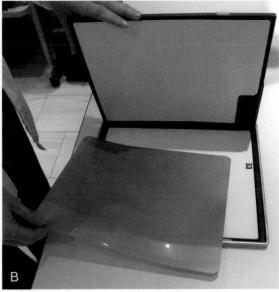

FIG. 4.24 Two ways to remove film from a cassette. **A,** Stand the cassette on edge and let the film fall away from the screen. Then lay the cassette on its front and remove the film from the cassette. **B,** The film may be removed by lifting it from the cassette as shown. DuPont cassettes have a small spring that lifts the film away from the bottom screen.

Magnetized rubber back   Metal foil fixed to back of screen

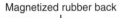
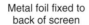
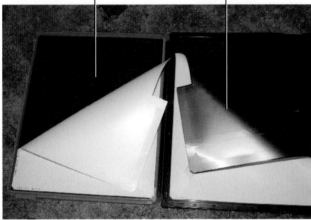

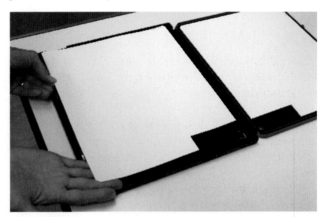

FIG. 4.26 The foil-backed screen is not firmly attached to the cassette front and can be lifted up and moved forward on two strips of radiolucent polyethylene. The manufacturer's philosophy was that the front screen would be pulled forward by the magnetic rubber and provide excellent film/screen contact across the entire cassette. This did not work well and the film/screen contact was imperfect, especially on larger cassettes. See Fig. 4.29.

FIG. 4.25 Agfa cassette with the screens peeled back to demonstrate the structure of the cassette beneath the screen. The front screen has metal foil attached to the back. The back of the cassette has a magnetic rubber sheet.

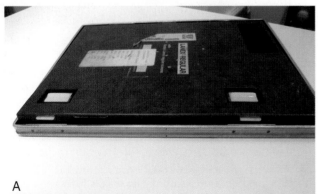
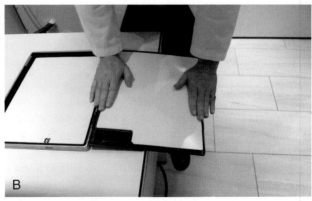

FIG. 4.27 **A,** DuPont cassettes are opened when the locks are released. The back of the cassette is slightly curved and is supposed to spring up so the cassette can be opened and the film removed. Over time the cassettes lose the "spring" opening and become more difficult to open. **B,** To correct this problem, open the cassette and lay the back over the edge of a flat surface. Very carefully and slowly press down on the side suspended from the table and the side still on the table. The pressure needs to be firm but not hard. Gently press and release four or five times. Now close the cassette and reopen. The back should now spring up correctly.

FIG. 4.28 Kodak cassettes have a rubber surround that is vulnerable to cracking and breaking. These cassettes have come completely apart at the hinge back and are not reparable. Even if taped with heavy tape (such as duct tape), they cannot be taped tightly enough to provide excellent screen contact. The screens can be removed from each half of the cassette and placed into an intact cassette. Using another Kodak cassette is not recommended because opening it completely will compromise the rubber hinge. When removing the screens, be very careful to keep the screen intact and not bent or creased, because this will render an artifact on the image. Kodak screens are excellent and have a long life with little deterioration of speed, so they are worth retrieving.

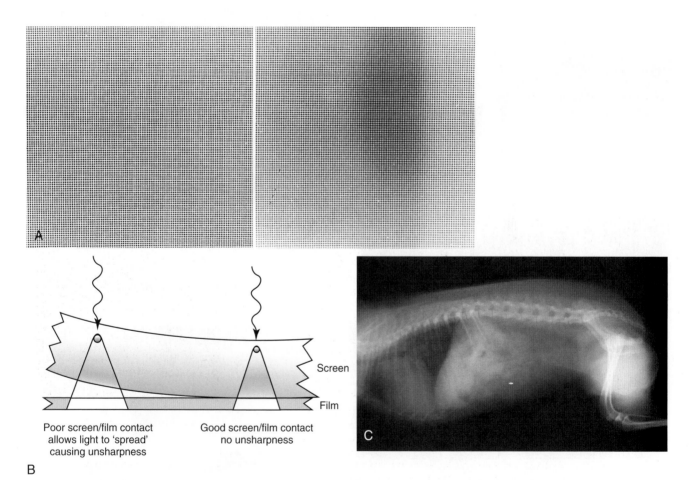

FIG. 4.29 **A,** Two images of a film screen contact mesh test tool. The image on the left shows a test image with excellent screen contact. The image on the right demonstrates poor screen contact *(larger darkened area)* on the upper right. **B,** Poor screen contact produces a darkened area of the film. If the film is lifted away from the screen for any reason during the exposure, there will be an area that lights up the screen but spreads very slightly around the specific area because of the lack of good contact. This area of penumbra will translate onto the image as a fuzziness or blurriness. **C,** An image taken using an Agfa screen/cassette with particularly poor screen contact. (From Fauber TL. *Radiographic Imaging and Exposure,* 4th ed. St. Louis: Mosby; 2013.)

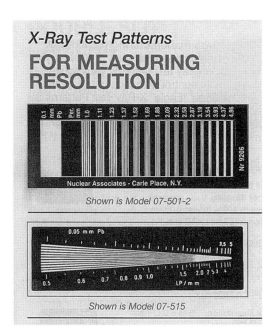

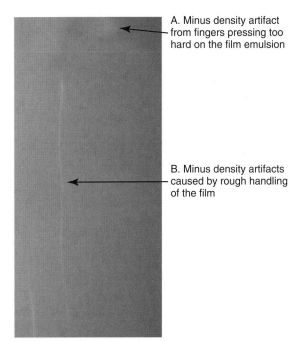

A. Minus density artifact from fingers pressing too hard on the film emulsion

B. Minus density artifacts caused by rough handling of the film

FIG. 4.30 A resolution test tool. The tool consists of two different scales, but each lists the line pairs per millimeter demonstrated on the film. A line pair consists of one white line and one black line. This tool is placed on the top of a cassette to test the resolution of the film screen system. The exposed film is processed and checked with a small magnifier. The line pairs will visually blend together when the highest resolution is reached. This tool is not used for digital systems. Typically the highest resolution for film screen imaging is nine line pairs. The highest resolution for film/screen extremity imaging is 15 to 20 line pairs.

FIG. 4.31 A, Processed film demonstrating a density 1.0 + base + fog. On the film are two major artifacts: a minus-density artifact from damp fingers handling the film as it is placed in the processor. The salts from sweat will loosen the emulsion, which will float away in the processor and leave fingerprint evidence. **B,** A long vertical minus-density artifact in which the film was roughly dragged out of the film box, destroying the ability of the emulsion to form a lattice network across this trauma line. Film must be handled with care from the time the box is opened until it is processed, dried, and ready for viewing.

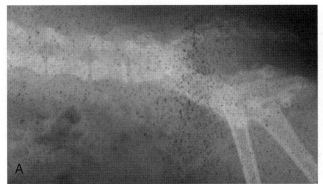

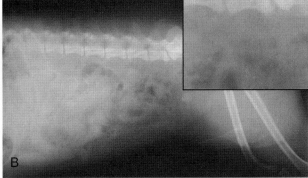

FIG. 4.32 A, Overuse of commercial screen cleaners build up residue on the screen, which eventually causes artifacts on the film as they case plus-density artifacts across the image. The artifacts are actually areas of the film that were affected by the components of the screen cleaner that caused the silver in the emulsion to coagulate. **B,** Intensifying screen emulsion becomes physically worn after many years of films being drawn across its surface and is not able to uniformly convert x-rays to light to expose the film. The lighter areas on the film replicate the wear areas of the screen. The inset demonstrates an enlarged part of the indistinct image due to screen wear.

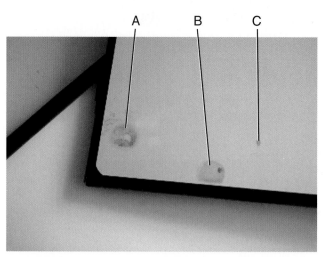

FIG. 4.33 Using the incorrect screen cleaner (e.g., for example, cleaner manufactured by a company other than the screen manufacturer) can cause severe yellowing of the screen. This causes a loss of speed because the light emitted from the screen is an altered color.

FIG. 4.34 Chemical stains on a cassette. These may be wiped off if the screen has a cellulose supercoat. Typically they penetrate the emulsion of the screen and are permanent. **A** and **B** are caused by drips from manual processing that have penetrated the emulsion. **C,** A small drip may look like pathology on an image until the veterinarian notices that every view is demonstrating the same "pathology" on the same place on the film whether or not there is overlying anatomy.

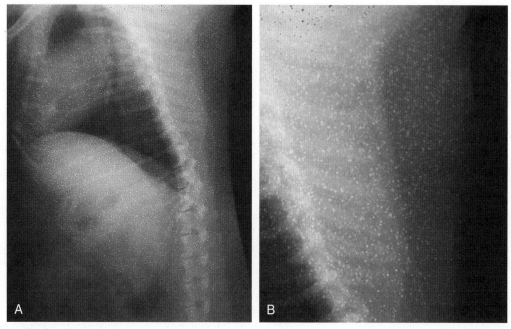

FIG. 4.35 A, The result of DuPont using water-based screen emulsion. The screens worked well in hospitals because the atmosphere in most hospitals is fairly dry. Once the screens were used in private clinics and particularly veterinary hospitals, the water-based emulsion absorbed moisture from the air and swelled to the point where the lattice network was destroyed as soon as the exposure was made and the film stayed in the cassette for any length of time waiting to be processed. This also occurred with films that were preloaded into cassettes waiting to be used. The pin points exerted such pressure that the ability of the film emulsion to form a lattice network was compromised. The screens are not repairable and must be replaced. New screens can be purchased and placed into the cassette. **B,** A close-up of the particularly compromised screen. The swellings are most visible on the UV screens. With Quanta 111 screens the swellings are not always visible but usually can be felt as tiny pin points. The presence of the swellings is always evident.

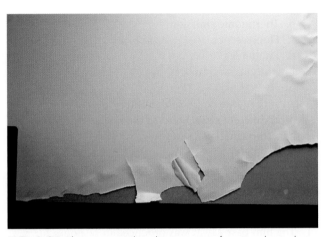

FIG. 4.36 The screen emulsion has torn away from its polyester base. This was a particular problem with DuPont UV screens.

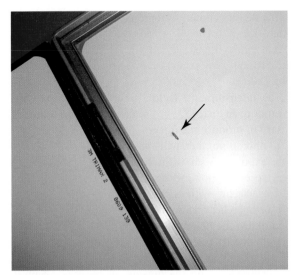

FIG. 4.37 A piece of hay in a cassette. This can be a problem with large-animal veterinarians trying to change films in a darkened room in a barn.

REVIEW QUESTIONS

1. There are two completely separate components to an imaging system; they are:
   a. X-ray generator and imaging receptor
   b. The x-ray tube and the generator
   c. The generator and the film
   d. The x-ray tube and the processing unit
2. It is very important that the x-ray generator is the latest model available.
   a. False
   b. True
3. A good technique chart and knowledge of image production is essential because:
   a. The technique chart supplied by the vendor is always correct
   b. The technique chart set up by the previous tech is always the best
   c. Setting correct technical factors is essential to good imaging
   d. Technical factors change over the years and service is not always available
4. The x-ray cassette is a sophisticated film holder. Which of the following statements is true?
   a. It can be made of any plastic as long as it is bendable.
   b. It must be sturdy and have a strong reliable closure.
   c. The film can be held loosely in place as long as it is light-tight.
   d. The intensifying screens are placed in the cassette by the technician.

5. The front of the x-ray cassette:
   a. Must absorb scattered radiation
   b. Should have a reflective coating to match the screen
   c. Should have an adhesive layer to hold the film in place
   d. Must be radiolucent and free of artifacts
6. The purpose of an intensifying screen is to:
   a. Enhance the x-ray beam to make it stronger
   b. Convert the x-ray beam to x-ray photons
   c. Convert the primary x-ray beam to light photons
   d. Change the x-ray beam to scattered radiation
7. The intensifying screen is composed of a _____ and a(n) _____.
   a. base, emulsion layer
   b. cardboard base, adhesive layer
   c. polyester base, supercoat
   d. cardboard base, emulsion layer
8. Conversion efficiency is _____ at which the x-ray photons are converted _____.
   a. the rate, to x-rays
   b. the speed, to silver
   c. the speed, to polyphotons
   d. the speed, to light
9. Screen speed is defined by the:
   a. Intrinsic nature of the photons
   b. Conversion efficiency of the phosphor
   c. Atomic mass of the phosphor
   d. Comparison of rare earth elements
10. Rare earth elements are so named because they are _____ and _____ efficient than standard phosphors.
    a. difficult to mine from the earth, more
    b. really rare and not easily found, more
    c. rare gases that have to be processed, less
    d. difficult to mine from the earth, less

11. The density chosen to represent a midline density is:
    a. −1.0
    b. 1.0
    c. 10
    d. 2.0
12. The intensification factor is the _____ necessary to produce an image _____ screens vs. the exposure necessary to produce the image _____ screens.
    a. photon number, with, without
    b. exposure, with, without
    c. speed, without, with
    d. electricity, with, without
13. Imaging relies on a sound knowledge of the colors of the rainbow; the following is true:
    a. It doesn't matter because we can't see color in the dark.
    b. Ultraviolet, on the outside of the curve, cannot be affected by infrared.
    c. Ultraviolet is in the middle of the curve; infrared is on the outside of the curve.
    d. The color of the light that film emulsion reacts to must match the screen color.
14. The introduction of green light–emitting screens:
    a. Was a natural progression in screen technology but created confusion
    b. Was really unnecessary because we already had good systems
    c. Did not change the film industry because we could still use the same film
    d. Changed the look of the image and clarified film ordering and stocking
15. The green-receiving film will "see" blue light:
    a. But will not "see" the green color, so the film will be light
    b. But needs the green light to produce an optimum image
    c. But it will not make use of it when it produces the image
    d. But requires the full spectrum to produce an optimum image
16. Knowledge of the system speed is critical to produce the correct amount of radiation:
    a. To determine which cassette will be used to radiograph the animal
    b. To optimize imaging and produce a diagnostic radiograph
    c. To set the technical factors and calculate the weight of the animal
    d. And determine the rate of conversion efficiency of the photons
17. Luminescence is the reaction of the screen to the photons; the reaction is called:
    a. Fluorescence
    b. Phosphorescence
    c. Thermionic
    d. Light speed
18. If the screen continues to emit light after the photon source is removed, the effect is called:
    a. Phosphorescence
    b. Thermionic emission
    c. Fluorescence
    d. Photon lag
19. Intensifying screens age _____ and _____ over time.
    a. at the same rate, maintain their speed
    b. at different rates, increase the rate of reaction
    c. at the same rate, slow down
    d. at different rates, slow down
20. A knowledge of screen color and speed assists in optimizing imaging and ensuring uniformity of images.
    a. True
    b. False
21. The film base Mylar was produced in response to:
    a. Increase profits for the photo products division of the DuPont company
    b. The need for a more efficient bonding agent for the emulsion to adhere to
    c. A need for a stable, nonflammable, nontearable support for the emulsion
    d. A need to find a nonflammable substitute for cellulose acetate
22. Two types of film are _____ emulsion and _____ emulsion film.
    a. double-, extremity
    b. triacetate, polyester
    c. polyester, general radiography
    d. double-, single-
23. Screen speed is determined by the _____ of the emulsion and the _____ of the silver halide crystals.
    a. color, weight
    b. thickness, color
    c. thickness, size
    d. reaction, speed
24. Film emulsion is composed of mainly:
    a. Silver iodide crystals and gelatin
    b. Silver halide crystals and sensitivity specks
    c. Carbon halides and silver atoms
    d. Silver carbide and silver halide
25. The supercoat is an added top layer that:
    a. Prevents any further radiation from affecting the film
    b. Prevents the image from overdeveloping
    c. Sets the image once it is processed
    d. Protects the emulsion during processing
26. The lattice network is so named because:
    a. The latent image forms as a network held together by sensitivity centers
    b. The lattice network forms before the film is exposed as a preexposure
    c. The latent image will replace the lattice network so it must be in place
    d. A confluence of sensitivity specks will make up the beginning of the image

27. The combination of the color of the film base and the initial aging of the film:
    a. Is not a part of the image
    b. Does not affect the overall film density
    c. Is called base + fog
    d. Only affects the image before processing

28. If a film is exposed to alternative energy, it will acquire a density before exposure. Which of these statements is true?
    a. This may be caused by heat, light, or chemical fumes.
    b. This density does not affect the overall image.
    c. Film fog is a natural part of imaging.
    d. Fogging a film is not important in image production.

29. The following factor distinguishes a fogged film as opposed to overexposed film.
    a. The two factors cannot be separated.
    b. The density decreases if the technique is changed.
    c. Fogged film feels "different" when it exits the processor.
    d. The density does not change if the technique is altered.

30. Blue-receiving film is physically _____; green-receiving film is physically _____.
    a. green, violet
    b. blue, green
    c. violet, green
    d. green, blue

31. The following method is used to determine the color of the screens in order to use the correct film:
    a. The cassette is opened and the stencil is read.
    b. The color is obvious when the cassette is opened.
    c. The cassette is placed open on the table and exposed to radiation.
    d. A blue or green label is attached to the back of the cassette.

32. White box film is so called because:
    a. It is sold off in batches; it is no different from regular film
    b. It did not meet the quality control standards of the parent company
    c. The companies that sell it are overstocked
    d. It is mainly blue film that is being phased out and so it needs to be sold

33. New unused boxes of film should be stored:
    a. Upright in an area unaffected by radiation and heat
    b. Upright wherever there is room in the clinic
    c. Lying flat on the darkroom counter
    d. Lying flat on the darkroom shelf so it is available

34. X-ray film has an expiration date, which should be:
    a. Within 5 years of the date noted on the box
    b. Checked carefully and then noted when the box is empty
    c. Ignored as it is used by the supplier and not the facility
    d. Noted and adhered to by the facility staff

35. The standard film sizes are important to the ordering process because:
    a. The film sizes all match the cassette sizes in the facility
    b. All film sizes may be either in centimeters or inches and fit the cassettes equally
    c. The film sizes are critical to the size of the cassette
    d. 10 in × 12 in film will fit into a 24 cm × 30 cm cassette

Answers to Review Questions can be found on the Evolve website.

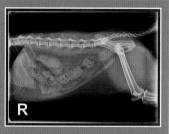

Correct measuring, correct positioning, and correct technique = Optimum imaging

CHAPTER 5
Producing the Image

Lois C. Brown, RTR (Can/USA), ACR, MSc., P.Phys

Pleasure in the job puts perfection in the work.
—Aristotle, Greek critic, Philosopher, physicist, and zoologist, 384–322 BC

OUTLINE

LEARNING OBJECTIVES

When you have finished this chapter, you will be able to:

1. Recognize exposures on film.
2. Define film fog.
3. Define density and contrast.
4. Know the difference between subject contrast and radiographic contrast.
5. Understand the importance of correct patient measurement.
6. Know how to establish a technique chart.
7. Develop a technique chart.
8. Record your exposures in a radiography log book.

APPLICATIONS

The application of the information in this chapter is relevant to the following area:

1. Producing optimized images (radiographs) for evaluation and diagnosis

KEY TERMS

Key terms are defined in the Glossary on the Evolve website.

Contrast
Density
Direct Radiation
Expiration date
Fog
Grid tray
Inverse square law

Kilovoltage
Log book
Measurement
Milliamperage
Optimized image
Positioning
Primary beam

Quality/quantity
Radiographic contrast
Remnant radiation
Scattered radiation
Secondary radiation
Source image distance (SID)
Subject contrast

Tabletop
Technique chart
Time
Tissue fluence

The main objective of all imaging systems is to demonstrate the differences in tissue density. Air, water, fat, tendons, muscle, and bone all have different tissue densities, and it is this differentiation, this contrast, that must be optimized. This chapter will deal only with producing images for film/screen combinations. Digital imaging and computed radiography are to be found in Chapter 8.

The Technique Chart

There are several ways to set up a technique chart, and the charts in animal hospitals can range from hand scribbles on the wall to sophisticated laminated and colorful charts. Every imaging department is slightly different, and all of the factors discussed in previous chapters must be taken into consideration. Just because a technique chart works in one clinic does not mean that it will produce optimized images in a neighboring facility.

Most equipment suppliers will supply a technique chart with a new radiographic unit. Some of these charts have been set up by salespeople who have no concept of all the factors that are components of the image. Therefore some charts are suitable and some are not. Typically, if the images are good for a 10-cm abdomen measured and positioned correctly, then the chart may be extrapolated and should produce optimized images for any size animal for that particular unit and the film/screen combination that accompanies it.

The production of an optimized radiograph is an art and a science. The x-ray generator is the same basic unit now as it was 60 years ago. On a correctly calibrated radiography unit, 70 kilovolts is still 70 kV, and 200 milliamperes is 200 mA; all the rest is cosmetics. If the generator has the variables necessary to produce good radiography, there is no need to replace it because a new imaging system is introduced or because it is old and not as attractive as the newer models. As long as the unit is correctly calibrated and the parts and service are available to keep it that way, there is no need to upgrade to a different unit.

A technique chart is a guide. It should be developed to work with a specific system (film and intensifying screens) in a specific radiography room. The technique charts in this chapter are suggestions only. Slight variations in power supplies, film/screen combinations, or x-ray unit setup may necessitate some adjustment but, if all the rules are followed, these charts will provide good basic imaging.

These technique charts are in use in many hospitals and clinics and have proven to produce excellent images when the radiography units are calibrated correctly and the rules for positioning and measuring are followed exactly. If the technique chart is correctly set up and the patient is measured correctly, the image should never be too light or too dark. The flow chart in Fig. 5.9 can be used to evaluate and correct any technical difficulties. A technique chart can be developed to work with any x-ray unit from a large-animal portable unit to a highly sophisticated medical model.

This chapter explores the development of these technique charts. Two charts are presented in which we have followed the rules of chart development, and these charts are arranged so the technician can choose the type of chart that matches the model of the generator in use. The third chart is a large-animal portable chart and is an example used by the owners of the Poskom veterinary unit. All large-animal units are supplied with a technique chart to be used with that specific x-ray unit. If the unit is to be used as a small-animal unit, the company usually supplies a technique chart for small-animal radiography.

The Radiography Unit

Every complete x-ray unit is composed of three individual components: an x-ray tube, a generator, and a high-tension transformer. In a small-animal facility, the other necessary component is the radiography table.

Some radiography units have add-ons for convenience, such as a cassette holder or a recessed control at the table side, but these are not necessary. The only two components that must be matched every time are the generator and the high-tension transformer.

Quite frequently a tabletop becomes scratched, broken, or marred in some way (Fig. 5.1). Most tabletops can be removed and replaced with a new medical-grade, radiolucent tabletop. The new tabletop should be attached to the frame of the table with hook-and-loop tape to facilitate removal for cleaning or if a kitten escapes and goes exploring beneath the x-ray table.

The factors to consider when selecting an x-ray table are stability, height, ability to install a grid tray and, most important, radiolucency. The x-ray photons must be transmitted through the tabletop without superimposing an image of the grain of the tabletop onto the radiograph. Test for table lucency by placing a cassette beneath the tabletop, without the grid. Use 50 kV and 4 mAs to produce a 1.0 density image.

The cassettes exposed during an examination should be removed from the radiography room and placed well out of possible exposure by direct or scattered radiation.

Technical Factors

To produce a radiographic image, the contrast that separates the tissue densities must be optimized. The four factors of exposure—kilovoltage (kV), milliamperage (mA), time

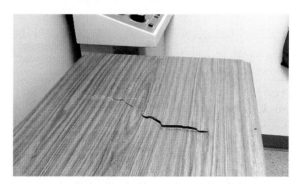

FIG. 5.1 A badly damaged tabletop. This crack will show up on any image that is exposed with the cassette in the grid tray.

(seconds), and distance (inches or centimeters)—must be manipulated in such a way that the tissue absorption of radiation is exactly correct to demonstrate anatomy and pathology and to minimize any external artifact that may obscure the desired result.

Radiographic Contrast vs. Subject Contrast

What constitutes the variables that provide contrast in an image? There are two main areas in which contrast may be manipulated (Table 5.1):

- The patient's thickness and shape (subject contrast)
- The mechanical variables available to enhance contrast (radiographic contrast)

Please note that the factors that manipulate radiographic contrast in a digital system are quite different than with imaging on film. See Chapter 8 for more on digital and computerized images.

Distance, Kilovoltage, Milliamperage, and Time

Three factors that are set on the x-ray unit are kilovoltage, milliamperage, and time. A fourth factor, distance, is set at the x-ray table. All of these factors are interdependent in terms of film/screen imaging. A change in one factor dramatically affects the other three. In common practice, mA and time are combined and called *mAs*.

Distance and the Inverse Square Law

The inverse square law is a rule that refers to distance. It states that "the intensity of the radiation at a location is inversely proportional to the square of its distance from the source of the radiation" (Fig. 5.2). The lesson learned here is that the distance between the x-ray tube and the image receptor (film or digital plate) is critical.

If the original distance is 40 inches (100 cm) and we halve it to 20 inches (50 cm), the intensity of the radiation is four times higher. This can be a very useful tool if the x-ray unit has low power and the body part that we need to examine is thick.

In most small-animal hospitals the distance between the x-ray tube and the receptor is preset and marked on the x-ray tube column. Forty inches (100 cm) is the normal preset distance. Occasionally this is altered because of the limitation

of the ceiling height or the height of the tabletop. This alteration must be considered when the technique chart is established. At this point the inverse square law is useful:

$$\frac{\text{Original mAs}}{\text{New mAs}} = \left[\frac{\text{New source image distance (SID)}}{\text{Original source image distance (SID)}}\right]^2$$

For example: If the technique chart calls for 20 mAs at 40 inches and the x-ray tube height is 36 inches:

$$\frac{20 \text{ mAs}}{X} \times \left[\frac{(36 \text{ inches})}{(40 \text{ inches})}\right]^2$$

$$\frac{20 \text{ mAs}}{X} \times \frac{1296}{1600}$$

$$20 \times .81 = 16.2 \text{ or } 16 \text{ mAs}$$

The mAs would be reduced to 16 mAs, and the density on the image would be the same as one exposed at 40 inches.

The film is exposed in one of two ways in a small-animal clinic. The cassette is placed either on the tabletop or into a grid tray beneath the tabletop. The grid tray usually sits approximately 3 inches (7.6 cm) below the tabletop, and the technique chart must be adjusted not only for the tube–tray distance (source image distance, or SID) but also because of the grid, which is addressed in Chapter 6. The operator is often encouraged to change the height of the x-ray tube, lowering it when the cassette is placed in the grid tray and raising it when the film is on the tabletop. This change of x-ray tube height is not necessary if the technique chart is adjusted slightly to compensate for the extra 3-inch (7.6-cm) distance, because it must already be adjusted to account for the grid. The grid factor formula is detailed in Table 5.2 and discussed further in Chapter 6.

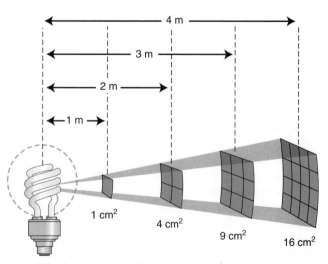

FIG. 5.2 The inverse square law. The intensity of radiation at a location is inversely proportional to the square of the distance. For example, doubling the distance from 2 meters to 4 meters increases the area covered by a factor of four. At 2 meters it is 4 squares; at 4 meters it is 16 squares. (From Johnston J, Fauber T. *Essentials of Radiographic Physics and Imaging,* 2nd ed. St Louis: Mosby; 2016.)

TABLE 5.1	Subject and Radiographic Contrast Components	
SUBJECT CONTRAST (ALL FACTORS CONCERNING A PATIENT)	**RADIOGRAPHIC CONTRAST (ALL FACTORS CONCERNING THE EQUIPMENT)**
Patient thickness	Kilovoltage
Body part being examined	Milliampere-seconds
Bone-to-muscle-to-fat-to-fluid ratio	Distance
Use of contrast media (barium, etc.)	Film/screen combinations
	Processing parameters
	Grid, filters
	Collimation
	Anode heel effect

◆ **APPLICATION INFORMATION**

Quite frequently the small amount that the tube is raised and lowered is confused in the facility, and often the tube is mistakenly lowered for the tabletop exposures and raised for the grid tray exposures. It is far preferable to compensate for the extra SID by adjusting the technique chart for both the grid and the distance, leaving the x-ray tube stationary.

Kilovoltage, Milliamperage, and Time

Kilovoltage, milliamperage, and time are often referred to as the *factors controlling the quality of the radiation* (kV) and the *quantity of the radiation* (mAs). In the case of kV, quality refers to an increase in the penetrating power. When the kV is increased, the beam is said to be "hardened." This means that fewer low-energy x-rays are produced and more high-energy x-rays are produced. This leaves the x-ray beam with more capability to penetrate denser tissue. Kilovoltage mainly affects contrast in the image. It also affects density because setting the kilovoltage too high will blacken the film and so eliminate any contrast.

When the mAs is increased, the density of the image is directly affected because a greater quantity of photons are produced, which in turn yields an increased number of x-rays. The increase in the number of x-rays is directly proportional to the amount of the increase in mAs. For example, if we increase the mAs from 20 to 40, we are producing twice the number of x-ray photons and therefore doubling the density on the radiograph. The mAs value primarily affects density; however, this value will also eliminate contrast if set far too high or far too low, and then the overall image will be black or clear.

Billiards Analogy

The best analogy for understanding the interaction of the technical factors is represented in the game of pool. A certain number of balls are racked or positioned on a felt-covered table. A cue ball is aimed at the prepositioned balls, and the cue stick is used to hit the cue ball and scatter the racked balls to put them into play (Fig. 5.3). In radiography, the x-ray photons projected from the cathode of the x-ray tube are the balls on the table. The cue ball and some of the other balls travel straight through the mass of balls to the other end of the table. (This is called the *primary radiation.*) The scattered balls move according to how much energy is transferred down the cue stick and at what angle that energy is transferred.

The milliamperage (mA) represents the number of balls on the table. If there are a lot of balls on the table, there will be a high number of interactions and a greater potential to have a high-density or dark film image. If there are very few balls on the table, a light film will result. ***The mAs value is responsible for density.*** It is directly proportional—doubling the mAs doubles the density on the film. There is no higher math to calculate when determining how to optimize an image using mAs.

The *kilovoltage (kV)* is the power behind the cue stick. It is how hard the balls are hit and how much energy is transferred to the balls. If the balls are hit very hard (high kV), more of the balls travel straight through and reach the end of the table. The high-energy scattered balls bounce off the sides and ends of the table, and as they do they transfer a little energy to the table side and move off to interact with other balls or the other side of the table until they come to rest. Each interaction, whether it be with table edges or with other balls, subtracts energy from the initial moving ball until all the balls finally come to rest.

In the world of radiation, the primary beam is the useful beam with varying energies but enough to penetrate the patient and reach the detector (either film or detector plate). The radiation that reaches the film or detector is called *remnant radiation.* Energy is transferred when the photons bounce off one another or bounce off the atoms within the patient. This deflected energy becomes *scattered radiation,* or *secondary radiation,* and is either visualized on the image as nonuseful

TABLE 5.2	Grid Factor Formula
GRID RATIO	**MULTIPLY MAS BY**
5 : 1	2
8 : 1	3
10 : 1	3.5

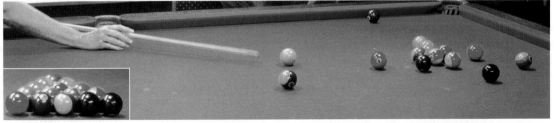

kV - Power behind the cue stick

Whenever a ball hits the side of the table it loses energy in the impact

Balls racked ready to play

mA - Number of balls in play

FIG. 5.3 The game of pool can be used as an analogy of the technical factors of radiation exposure. The kilovoltage (kV) is the power behind the cue stick; milliamperage (mA) is the number of balls on the table.

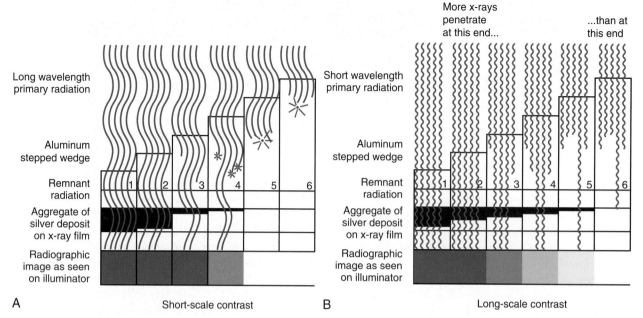

FIG. 5.4 An aluminum wedge with a series of graduated steps is used in this model. How contrast affects the image: **A,** Low kilovoltage = short-scale contrast. **B,** High kilovoltage = long-scale contrast; with very high kilovoltage, the entire wedge is penetrated and there is no contrast.

radiation or not visualized because it is absorbed by another interaction within the animal.

Nonuseful radiation contributes to either the radiation dose to the patient or technician or appears as film fog. When the technique chart is developed, the kilovoltage must be set as low as possible in order to have enough energy to penetrate the body part, as well as keeping the scattered/secondary radiation to a minimum. The kilovoltage is responsible for the penetrating power of the x-ray beam. In our analogy, it is the power behind the cue stick. The energy (the kV) of the x-ray beam affects contrast. If the energy is set so high that it penetrates every tissue evenly, there will be no contrast and the image will be black. Similarly, if it is set so low that it penetrates nothing and never arrives at the film, there will be no contrast on the image, as there will be no image. Thus in that way the extremes of kV also affect density, but that is not the effect when we have an acceptable exposure on our image.

Fig. 5.4A illustrates that kilovoltage greatly affects contrast (Tables 5.3 and 5.4). With a low kilovoltage the x-ray beam has longer wavelength primary radiation and penetrates fewer structures, producing a shorter scale of contrast (black and white), which is demonstrated as a larger density difference between steps. It does not take long to read the image from black to white. Fig. 5.4B has long-scale contrast (black, gray, gray, white), is produced by increasing the kV, and represents a greater number of steps between black and white less of a density difference between steps. When the veterinarian states that he or she would like to see more contrast, this needs to be clarified.

- More contrast = higher contrast = fewer shades of gray = fewer steps from black to clear
- Less contrast = lower contrast = more shades of gray = more steps from black to clear

TABLE 5.3	Relationship Between Kilovoltage and Contrast
HIGH KV PRODUCES	**LOW KV PRODUCES**
Long scale (more grays)	Short scale (fewer grays)
Low contrast	High contrast
Less contrast (fewer "clear" areas)	More contrast (more "clear" areas on the film)

TABLE 5.4	Technical Factors Affecting Contrast
INCREASING THIS FACTOR	**RESULTS OF INCREASE**
Kilovoltage	Decrease in contrast (more grays)
mAs (milliampere-seconds)	Decrease in contrast (at very high mAs, image is black)
Collimation (narrowing the x-ray beam)	Increase in contrast (reduction in secondary radiation)

◆ APPLICATION INFORMATION

Contrast is the key word on any radiographic image. If the veterinarian requests more contrast, it is always wise to clarify whether he or she wants to see more shades of gray (long scale) or a shorter-scale, high-contrast, black-and-white image. Sometimes that is not clear.

A veterinary radiologist called the consultant in to discuss the x-ray images and said he wanted more contrast. The consultant changed the chart and then also changed the film/screen combination to give him more short-scale contrast (black-and-white images). The veterinary radiologist called the consultant back and

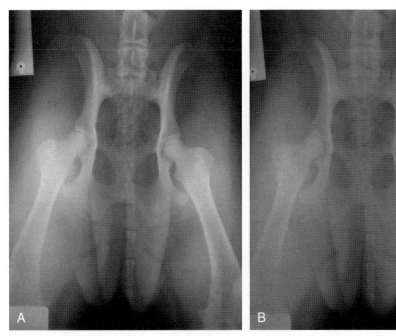

FIG. 5.5 Optimized kilovoltage versus high kilovoltage. **A,** Optimized kilovoltage. The bony structures are visible and trabecular patterns are well visualized. **B,** High kilovoltage. The bony structures are overpenetrated and now blend in with the muscle tissue. Trabecular patterns are no longer visualized.

explained that what he wanted was more contrast—more shades of gray! She had done everything to produce fewer shades of gray. The problem was quickly resolved by increasing the kV and reducing the mAs. It is always best to clarify what is being requested.

Optimizing Kilovoltage

The normal range of use of kilovoltages on a general radiography unit is usually between 40 and 90 kV. When the technique chart is developed for the facility, it must be fine-tuned to consider all of the variables inherent in the production of the final image (Fig. 5.5). The main objective in optimizing the technique chart is to use the lowest kV value that will penetrate the region of interest within the body and enhance the tissue contrast surrounding it. Each body part or component can be penetrated by an optimum kilovoltage. Table 5.5 is provided as a starting point to develop a technique chart for an average-sized animal.

For larger animals or for pocket pets and smaller animals, the kilovoltage is adjusted on the final chart. Because kilovoltage is the energy with which the x-ray beam passes through the body, a change in kilovoltage is not in direct proportion with the increase or decrease in tissue. This difference is due to a variation in tissue absorption (tissue fluence). The radiation that reaches the film is called *remnant radiation.*

The optimum kV is the kilovoltage that penetrates the anatomy so that it is identifiable on the radiographic image. On an abdominal plate, for example, the anatomy has been penetrated if the anatomy is visible on the film after it is processed, the spine is evident, and the intervertebral spaces are clearly defined. The mAs must be altered to optimize the image if it is slightly dark or light. However, if the image is

TABLE 5.5	Optimum Kilovoltage Per Average-Sized Body Part for Film and Digital Imaging	
BODY PART	**OPTIMUM KV FOR FILM/SCREEN IMAGING**	**NOTES**
Extremities	40–55	Techniques in this range work for pocket pets.
Cervical spine/skull	60–75	
Thorax/abdomen/pelvis	64–90	For larger animals, the kV may be increased to a maximum of 95.

far too light or so dark that the anatomy is obscured, the 15% rule may also be used.

The 15% Rule for Changing Kilovoltage

The 15% rule is used to optimize kilovoltage only when a body part has not been imaged satisfactorily. It should not be used to increase or decrease *density* on an image. Density should be increased or decreased only by using mAs

To increase penetration: multiply the original kV by 1.15 (kV + 15%);

for example, $80 \times 1.15 = 92$ kV

To decrease penetration: multiply the original kV by 0.85 (kV − 15%);

for example, $80 \times 0.85 = 68$ kV

Applying this rule will increase or decrease the penetration of the region of interest. This rule will be effective for a kilovoltage between 50 kV and 95 kV, which is the normal range of use in radiography. If the technique chart is optimized and the patient is positioned and measured correctly, the technician will never need to use this formula.

Equipment Purchase

A major point to consider when purchasing a new generator is the number of time stations and mA stations available. Ideally a generator will have a high number of stations, or a high-frequency generator will have anatomical programming. A limited number of stations is workable, but the limitation will be reflected in the choices per centimeter of tissue as the technique chart is prepared. These units will not necessarily produce an optimized image but will take advantage of the forgiveness of the film/screen combination.

The three factors that may be adjusted on the generator are kV, mA, and time. The limits outlined in Table 5.6 are the standard for an average patient. Figs. 5.5 and 5.6 show the result of stepping dramatically outside those limits.

The images in Fig. 5.5 represent changes in kV while adjusting the mA to maintain density 1.0 + base + fog in the ilium of the pelvis. These images demonstrate that an increase in kilovoltage causes a substantial change in contrast as the x-ray beam becomes "harder" or more penetrating.

The images in Fig. 5.6 represent changes in mAs while the kV is adjusted to maintain density 1.0 + base + fog in the ileum of the pelvis. These images show that a decrease in mAs causes a substantial change in density but does not affect the contrast.

Developing Technique Charts

Use of a Phantom

Developing a technique chart for a film/screen system requires a certain amount of experimentation. A phantom (a facsimile of a patient) is used instead of using a live patient; the phantom is always the same size and density with no variations. Using

TABLE 5.6	Standard Factors for Average Patients Using a 400-Speed Film/Screen System (Cat at Low End of Scale, Dog at Upper End of Scale)		
BODY PART	**OPTIMUM KV RANGE**	**OPTIMUM MAS**	**NOTES**
Extremities	40–55	3–8	These are techniques for an **average** patient.
Cervical spine and skull	50–60	4–10	
Thorax	60–90	12–25	
Abdomen/pelvis	60–90	12–25	

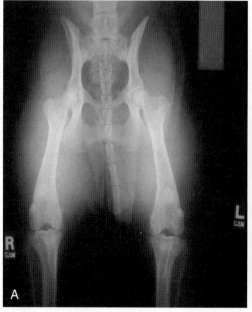 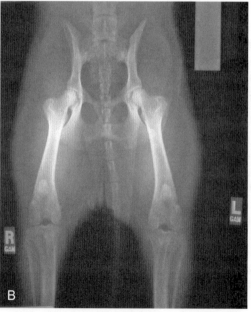

FIG. 5.6 Optimized mA versus low mA. **A,** The density provides a black background with the bony structures well visualized. **B,** The inadequate mAs value provides a flat image with loss of visualization in the bony structures. Note that the contrast is maintained.

an animal as a phantom introduces problems with identical positioning and cooperation on the part of the animal. If the animal is stretched out on one view and not positioned identically for the second view, an unnecessary variable is introduced. In addition, the dose to the animal must be considered if multiple exposures are to be made.

The use of a uniform density phantom eliminates the variables introduced by using an animal. A uniform density phantom consists of water in a container that mimics the thickness of a patient. The body of a mammal is composed of 98% liquid, so a water bucket works well as a standardized patient phantom (Fig. 5.7). The uniform-density phantom creates a density 1.0 + base + fog image from which the rest of the technique chart can be extrapolated.

The best method to replicate patient thickness is the use of a standard flat-bottom bucket with various centimeters of water representing various body parts. It does not need to be repositioned, and it maintains identical measurement throughout the procedure. This is why a water phantom is used throughout the world for dose measurements and technique chart composition. Make sure the bucket is plastic; a metal bucket will act as a filter and reduce the amount of radiation reaching the film.

Procedure

1. Start with tabletop techniques. Check to establish the speed of your system (films/screens, processing temperature). The techniques listed on the charts are for a 400-speed film/screen combination using a correctly calibrated generator and processing on a recently serviced processor.
2. Refer to the technique charts (Fig. 5.8A-B) to find your starting point.
3. Fill the plastic bucket with 5 cm of water.
4. Place a cassette on the tabletop and place the bucket on the cassette.

5. Collimate to the limits of the edges of the bucket; place a marker on cassette #1.
6. Choose the chart that matches your x-ray unit.
7. Set the technical factors found in the charts.
8. Make adjustments if needed using Fig. 5.9.
9. Expose the film and process, ensuring that the processor is clean and well serviced.
10. A density of 1.0 + base + fog is the ideal density (Fig. 5.10). This density is exactly in the midrange of densities as discussed in Chapter 9 (quality control).
11. Go back to the chart and change the water level to correspond with greater or lesser thicknesses of a patient. (Once you have reached a measurement of 10 cm or greater, place the cassette in the grid tray; for any measurement below 10 cm, the cassette will be on the tabletop.)
12. This should now work well for any level of water in the bucket, assuming that a change in technique is accompanied by an appropriate change in water level according to the chart.
13. If the images turn out very light using these techniques, you may have a 200-speed system or the temperature in your processor may be incorrect.
14. Start over and recheck the speed of the system, the calibration of the unit, and the processing parameters. Only then should you increase the mAs.
15. At the end of the experiment, position the patient on the table and correctly measure the patient. Set the technical factors from the chart and process the film. The density of the soft tissue immediately cranial to the iliac crest should be density 1.0 + base + fog.

Sante's Rule

Sante's rule is an alternative method of developing a variable kV technique chart. This chart is useful if the mA and time factors are limited on the radiography unit (Table 5.7). It will only be useful with a single-phase unit. It is not accurate for a three-phase, high-frequency unit. It is also not accurate for a digital system. (See Chapter 8.) This rule estimates kilovoltage in relation to patient thickness. Because it is based on a variable kilovoltage chart, it does not accommodate gradual changes in mAs (or density) as the patient becomes thicker and the tissue becomes less differentiated. The substantial increase in kV will produce scattered/secondary radiation, which will seriously compromise the image if the kV is allowed to exceed 80 kV. mAs totals used are tested for each body part and then preset (Table 5.8).

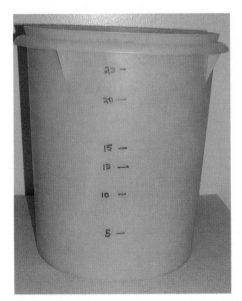

FIG. 5.7 A standard flat-bottomed container. Note the standard measurements on the side. These duplicate extremity, skull, and abdomen equivalents, and the water level can be altered easily.

TABLE 5.7	Sante's Rule for Grid Use	
GRID RATIO	**ADDED KV**	**OR ADDED MAS**
5:1	6–8	×1
8:1	8–10	×2
12:1	10–15	×3

A

Small Animal Technique Chart –Read Chart from left to Right - 400 speed film screen; Single Phase x-ray unit

Chest / Thoracic Sp / Shoulder — Table Top | GRID ▶ | 8:1 Grid Cassette in Grid Tray

CM.	4	5	6	7	8	9		10	11	12	13	14	15	16	17	18	19	20	21	22	23	24	25	26	27	28	29	30	31	32
mAs	2		3		4			12		14		16		18		20		22		24		26		28		30		32		34
kV	48		50		52			60		62		64		66		68		70		72		74		76		78		80		8

Abdomen / Lumbar Sp / Pelvis — Table Top – 100 mA | GRID ▶ | 8:1 grid Cassette in Grid Tray

CM.	6	7	8	9	10	11		10	11	12	13	14	15	16	17	18	19	20	21	22	23	24	25	26	27	28	29	30	31	32
mAs	2		3		4			12		14		16		18		20		22		24		26		28		30		32		34
kV	48		50		52			60		62		64		66		68		70		72		74		76		78		80		82

Skull / Cerv Sp — Table Top | GRID ▶ | 8:1 Grid Cassette in Grid Tray

CM.	4	5	6	7	8	9		10	11	12	13
mAs	2		4		6			12		14	
kV	50		52		54			56		58	

Limbs / Stifles — Table Top | NO Grid | NO GRID All limbs are radiographed table top

CM.	1	2	3	4	5	6		7	8	9
mAs	2		4		6			8	10	
kV	46		48		50	52		52	54	

Read page from left to right – Measurement of the animal correctly is essential
Log all measurements and exposure factors so that any problems may be identified

---

B

Small Animal Technique Chart –Read Chart from left to Right - 400 speed film screen; 3 phase ; Hi Frequency unit

Chest / Thoracic Sp / Shoulder — Table Top | GRID ▶ | 8:1 Grid Cassette in Grid Tray

CM.	4	5	6	7	8	9		10	11	12	13	14	15	16	17	18	19	20	21	22	23	24	25	26	27	28	29	30	31	32
mAs	1		2		3			6		8		10		12		14		16		18		20		22		24		26		28
kV	44		46		48			54		56		58		60		62		64		66		68		70		72		74		7

Abdomen / Lumbar Sp / Pelvis — Table Top | GRID ▶ | 8:1 grid Cassette in Grid Tray

CM.	4	5	6	7	8	9		10	11	12	13	14	15	16	17	18	19	20	21	22	23	24	25	26	27	28	29	30	31	32
mAs	1		2		3			6		8		10		12		14		16		18		20		22		24		26		28
kV	44		46		48			54		56		58		60		62		64		66		68		70		72		74		76

Skull / Cerv Sp — Table Top | GRID ▶ | 8:1 Grid Cassette in Grid Tray

CM.	4	5	6	7	8	9		10	11	12	13
mAs	1		2		3			6		8	
kV	46		48		50			52		56	

Limbs / Stifles — Table Top | NO Grid | NO GRID All limbs are radiographed table top

CM.	1	2	3	4	5	6		7	8	9	10
mAs	0.50		1		2			3		4	
kV	44		46		48	50		50	52	54	

Read page from left to right – Measurement of the animal correctly is essential
Log all measurements and exposure factors so that any problems may be identified

FIG. 5.8 A, The single-phase chart. The completed radiography chart for a small-animal clinic using a single-phase unit, 400-speed system, and correct processing. **B,** Three-phase, high-frequency chart to be used with correct processing, correct measurement, and a 400-speed film/screen system on a correctly calibrated unit.

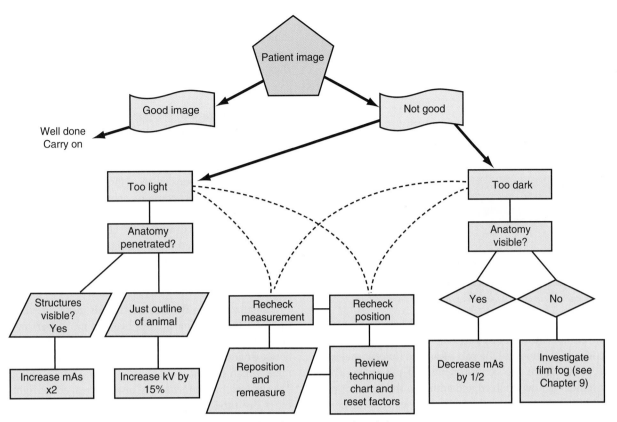

FIG. 5.9 Flowchart demonstrating technical diagnostics.

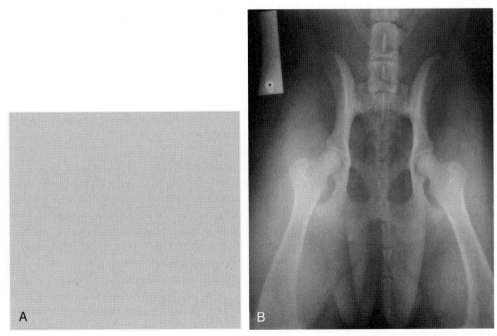

FIG. 5.10 A, An example of a density 1.0 + base + fog image. It is similar to the density at the caudal aspect of the ilium. On the phantom film if this density is matched, then the rest of the technique chart can be filled in according to the rules. **B,** An example of a pelvis image produced using the technique developed by using the water phantom. Note that the density at the caudal ilium is density 1.0 + base + fog.

TABLE 5.8	Sante's Rule for Variable mAs
BODY PART	SUGGESTED BEGINNING MAS
Extremity	5
Thorax (no grid)	7.5
Abdomen (grid)	10
Pelvis/spine	12.5

TABLE 5.9	Effect of Grid Ratio on mAs	
GRID RATIO	LINES/MM	AVERAGE GRID FACTOR
8:1	103	mAs × 1.5
10:1	103	mAs × 2.0
12:1	143	mAs × 3.0

Note: This table gives the information for the most common grid ratios.

With Sante's rule the body part is measured correctly, with the patient in position and the part measured (in centimeters) at the point where the central x-ray will penetrate. This measurement is now doubled and added to the distance (in inches) of the x-ray tube to the tabletop (usually 40 inches). Therefore if a body part measures 4 cm,

$$4\,cm \times 2 = 8 + 40\,inches = 48\,kV$$

If a body part measures 16 cm,

$$16\,cm \times 2 = 32 + 40\,inches = 72\,kV$$

A body part of 16 cm will require a grid. The grid factor for an 8:1 grid will increase the kV to 82 kV *or* the mAs should be doubled (×2) (see Table 5.9).

Grids and Grid Trays

Grids were developed to absorb scattered and secondary radiation. They also absorb a certain amount of primary radiation. They are positioned normally under the tabletop between the patient and the film. Digital imaging often does not use a grid, so the following paragraphs assume a film/screen system. Chapter 6 describes the manufacture of the grid and the different uses for various grids. Here we will discuss it as a factor in the preparation of the technique chart.

When a grid is used, the technical factors must be increased as outlined in Table 5.9. A grid with a ratio higher than 12:1 should be replaced because it requires a considerable increase in technical factors and therefore a considerable increase in dose to the patient. This is hard on the x-ray tube and produces more scattered radiation, which is not necessarily absorbed by the grid. It also "hardens" the remnant x-ray beam, which reduces contrast.

Tabletop vs. Grid Tray in Film/Screen Imaging

Any body part that measures less than 10 cm will be radiographed on the tabletop. Any body part that measures 10 cm or greater will be imaged with the cassette either beneath the tabletop in the grid tray (with a grid installed beneath the tabletop) or using a grid taped to the cassette. The use of the grid and precautions are covered in Chapter 6.

Producing a Working Technique Chart

It is now vital that we review the objective of any radiograph produced by any imaging system. The objective is to optimize the differences in tissue density of the anatomy being examined. A basic knowledge of veterinary anatomy is essential to setting up a technique chart. Historically, veterinary technique charts were based on human technique charts. A lot of early x-ray units were purchased from hospitals and clinics that were upgrading from their single-phase generators. There are still many human radiography units installed in veterinary clinics.

The anatomy of the animal chest is quite different from that of a human. The human heart is much narrower and takes up far less space in the chest cavity. This is mainly because of our upright stance and greater overall heart-to-lung ratio, which produces maximum contrast on a radiograph. The typical human chest is always imaged upright with the x-ray tube at 6 feet (180 cm) or more from the grid tray. Because of these differences, human technique charts do not transfer well to veterinary charts, which normally use a consistent distance of 40 inches (100 cm) with a prone (DV [dorsoventral]) or supine (VD [ventrodorsal]) animal.

In technical terms, the tissue density of the animal chest is very similar to the animal's abdominal density; the heart occupies a large proportion of the chest, and there is a fairly even mix of muscle tissue, air cavities, and bone. Therefore the techniques for chest and abdomen can be virtually the same.

The Three "Rules"

Three rules must be followed before attempting to develop a technique chart for any medical, veterinary, or research facility.

Rule #1

The x-ray unit must be calibrated by a qualified x-ray service engineer. Quality control tests must be carried out on every station that will be "within normal range of use" to ensure that what is being set exactly conforms to the output of the x-ray unit. There is no point in setting up a chart only to find that a setting of 70 kV is actually 76 kV on one mA station and 68 kV on a second mA station.

This rule cannot be emphasized enough. There are countless examples of major frustration within the x-ray room because the service engineer did not bother to calibrate the mA stations correctly or because a unit has "drifted" over the 20 years since it was last calibrated. Every x-ray unit should be calibrated a minimum of once every 2 years. As the unit ages, it should be recalibrated annually.

◆ APPLICATION INFORMATION

When the mA stations are tested, they must be linear. Because the output of the mA station is directly proportional to the increase or decrease, 200 mA must produce double the radiation of 100 mA. In addition, each kV station must be matched so that the output of 70 kV at 100 mA is double the output of 70 kV at 50 mA, and so on.

This can be determined on the engineer's test tools and should be checked by the veterinary technician before the service person leaves the facility. If the service engineer does not calibrate the unit correctly or does not match the unit to the incoming electricity, it will be impossible to set up and follow a technique chart.

Rule #2

The technique chart is set up to reflect the thickness of the body part that is being radiographed. It is not intuitive! The animal must be placed in the correct position on the x-ray table before being measured. Fig. 5.11 demonstrates a possible difference in measurement of 8 cm between when Microchip (the patient) was not measured correctly and when he was in the correct position and measured accurately. This represents a huge difference in technical factors.

? POINTS TO PONDER

Measuring correctly cannot be stressed enough. The x-ray unit is not intuitive. It will produce the radiation that is requested for the measurement that is set. The difference in measurement at one clinic for one dog measured separately by seven people was 17 cm! (Incidentally, every person obtained a different measurement, depending on how the dog accepted the person with the calipers. Because the staff measured the dog standing either on the tabletop or on the floor, it could either shrink away from the technician or stand quietly. Once the dog was in VD position with legs extended, the measurement was entirely different again. Training the staff to measure uniformly with the animal in position resulted in consistently optimized radiography.

Rule #3

The measurement must be made at the area of particular interest. The central x-ray must enter the body part that was measured. If the area of interest on a greyhound or a whippet is the bladder (8 cm) and the dog is measured at the level of the kidneys (17 cm), the image will be far too dark in the area of interest.

If the area of interest is on a dog with a very high chest-to-abdomen measurement ratio, then the widest part and the narrowest part should be measured and the technique set at the midrange (e.g., 20 cm for a chest measurement and 10 cm for a pelvis measurement, with the technique set for 15 cm). The central ray would then enter the midrange of the abdomen (see Chapter 16). The anode heel effect can be used in this instance (see Chapter 2).

? POINTS TO PONDER

The x-ray generator will deliver only the amount of radiation requested by the operator, and it will not take operator error into account when the exposure is made. Measuring patients correctly is fundamental to the use of a technique chart. The amount of tissue to be penetrated is finite. It is not a guessing game and has no relation whatsoever to the weight or species of the animal.

Manipulating Technical Factors: The 15% Rule

Earlier in this chapter we discussed the codependency of kV, mA, time, and distance. The following example helps illustrate how to manipulate a factor for a particular result.

You have produced a good image, but the veterinarian now requests that you increase the contrast to image an obscure bladder stone. All other factors taken into consideration, the optimum kV for the abdomen was 70 kV at 22 mAs.

70 kV will penetrate the bladder, but what do you do with the mAs, because the density on the first film was fine?

When **decreasing** kV, multiply by 15% ($70 \times 15\% = 10.5$). Subtract that from your original kV (59 kV) with the .5 kV rounded off.

To maintain the same density, multiply the original mAs by 2 (44 mAs in this example)

When **increasing** kV, multiply by 15% ($70 \times 15\% = 10.5$). Add that to your original kV (80 kV) with the .5 kV rounded off.

To maintain the same density, divide the original mAs by 2 = (11 mAs in the example).

It is important to understand that the 15% rule applies only to kV values of 50 kV to 90 kV, which is the usual range of kVs in veterinary medicine. Outside these parameters the characteristics of the x-ray beam are completely different, and different rules apply.

Technical Rules

- **Rule 1.** When you are having difficulty with your images and you request a calibration by a service engineer, *always* make sure that a staff member at the clinic meets with him or her in the x-ray room and verifies the numbers on the meters. The kVs *must* be verified on each mA station individually. Unfortunately, many service engineers are not as conscientious as they should be; hence this is the first technical rule:
  - 70 kV must be 70 kV (±1 or 2 kV either way is not a problem; ±5 to 10 kV is a problem). The output of 100 mA *must* be 50% of the output of 200 mA. The output of 300 mA *must* be three times that of 100 mA.
- **Rule 2.** Review the three "rules" of calibration, positioning, and measuring. A technique chart cannot be optimized unless these rules are followed.

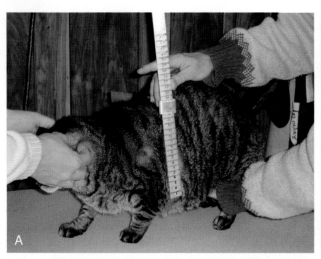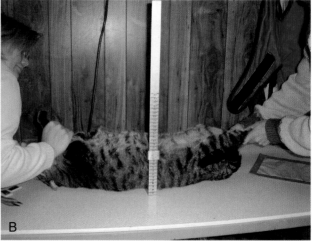

FIG. 5.11 Microchip being incorrectly measured (16 cm) **(A)** and then correctly measured (8 cm) **(B)**. The staff will immobilize Microchip, the cat, and step away from the table for the exposure.

- **Rule 3.** If the region of interest is not demonstrated and the technique chart is usually accurate, reposition and remeasure.
- **Rule 4.** When you have an image that is unsatisfactory, always adjust the mAs first, assuming that you have penetrated the region of interest, but not before you have reviewed Rule #3. A change in density on the image is directly proportional to a change in mAs. 20 mAs is half as dense as 40 mAs and two times as dense as 10 mAs. Changes in kV are semilogarithmic, and therefore the end result is not easy to predict or calculate.
- **Rule 5.** If the film is very light and it is usually satisfactory, check the temperature of the chemicals, either in the tank or in the developer of the processor (see Chapter 7).
- **Rule 6.** If the image is dull gray and does not improve with a change in technique, assume that the film has been fogged and look for light leaks in the darkroom or an opened or broken cassette (see Chapters 4 and 7).

Anatomical Considerations

Skull and Cervical Spine

Both the skull and cervical spine represent bone and tissue with high-contrast tissue densities. They do not require high kilovoltage or mAs.

Chest, Thorax, Abdomen, Lumbar Spine, and Pelvis

The chest, thorax, abdomen, lumbar spine, and pelvis are similar in the differences in tissue density and are a mix of air, fat, tissue, muscle, and bone. These body parts will be difficult to image if very high kilovoltage is used because the potential for photons producing secondary/scattered radiation increases as the thickness of the animal increases. It is important to keep the kilovoltage as low as possible and to increase the mAs proportionally as the tissue thickness increases.

Extremities

The tissue-to-bone ratio in extremities is high, and because the body parts are thin, a low kilovoltage is indicated. This will emphasize the contrast between the bone and the small amount of soft tissue.

Pocket pets and birds should be radiographed with technical factors similar to the extremities of cats and dogs unless a special film/screen combination is used. In addition, mAs will be proportionally low.

Completing the Technique Chart

Provided that the densities on the test images were satisfactory, each of the techniques may be extrapolated. Fill in the blanks on your chart. Increase 2 mAs for every 2-cm increase in density, and increase 2 kV for every 2-cm increase.

Take careful measurements, and record the results in your clinic log book. Always make sure that the patient is measured correctly and that the techniques are logged correctly. The only way to optimize the chart is to monitor it carefully, correctly, and consistently.

Small-Animal Technique Charts

The charts shown in Fig. 5.8 are in use in many clinics in North America. They are set up to be used on the specific units identified in the legends. These units must be correctly calibrated, and the patients must be correctly measured and correctly positioned, with obedience to the rules outlined previously.

The use of a large-animal portable unit in a small animal radiography clinic can produce acceptable images; however, the lack of technique selection and the limited mA values (usually a maximum of 30 or 50) can be frustrating.

Nonstandard Radiography Units (Alternative Charts)

If the radiography unit is limited in the number of mA stations or time stations, then adjustments need to be made within the chart to compensate for the lack of variables.

If a 200-speed system is used in the hospital/clinic, the mAs should be doubled and the kV left at the same settings. With a 200-speed system it is important to compare system speeds to ensure that the system is actually 200 using the procedure outlined in Chapter 4. (These screens would be quite old and therefore may have deteriorated dramatically.)

Non–rare earth systems are not normally available for sale at this time. They can be specially ordered at a premium price.

Equine Radiography

Equine radiography is typically carried out on location using a large-animal portable radiography unit that is specially adapted to be transported from location to location.

The technique chart shown in Fig. 5.12 will work well with standard units. This chart is typical for a typical large-animal unit. The film/screen system speed is 400-speed class, and the films were processed in an automatic processor.

The unit must be calibrated correctly, and it is essential that any personnel in the vicinity wear leaded aprons, thyroid collars, and gloves while the examination is in progress. Each unit is equipped with a measuring device that must be used to ensure that a consistent distance is used for each view. The cassettes must be protected both before and after the exposure is made, and a method of separating exposed cassettes and unexposed cassettes must be used consistently so there is never a question as to whether a cassette has been used or is available for an exposure.

The Radiography Log Book

Legally, the clinic must keep a record of every patient radiographed (Fig. 5.13). The log book must include the patient's name, identifiers, the views taken, the measurements, and the technical factors. Leaving a space for a comment is often useful. The log book must be completed every time a patient is radiographed.

**All these techniques are set up for 30" distance
All views are full size horse unless otherwise noted

Body part	Size/view	kV	mAs	Grid (if used)
Navicular	**AP**	**74**	**2.5-2.8**	**4.0-5.0**
Coffin	A.P.	74	.8	
Coffin Jt/foot	Lat	74	.5	3.2
Coffin Jt./foot	Obl.	74	.5	3.2
Fetlocks and	**A.P.**	**74**	**.5**	**2.5-4.0**
splint bone	lat	74	.6	
	Obl	74	.5	
	Flexed lat	74	.5	
Knees	**A.P/Lat/Obl**	**74**	**.5**	
	Flexed lat	74	.5	
	Skyline	74	.5	
Hock	**A.P.**	**74**	**.8**	
	Lat/Obl.	74	.6	
	Flexed lat	74	.6	
	S1 talus	74	.5	
Stifle	**Lat Jt.**	**76**	**1.2**	**4.0-5.0**
	Lat patella	76	1.0	
	A.P.	80	3.2-5.0	8.0-10
Elbow	**Lat**	**74**	**.8**	
	A.P.	74	1.0-1.2	
Shoulder		**80**	**6.2-8.0**	
Thoracic sp./	**T 1-3**	**76**	**.5-.8**	
withers	**T 4-6**	**80**	**.8-1.8**	
Cerv. sp.	**Foal C1-C2**	**76**	**.6**	
	Foal C3-C4	76	.8	
	Foal C4- C6	78	.8	
Skull	**Incisors/Wolf**			
	teeth	**74**	**.5**	
	Malaise	74	.8	
	A.P.	76	1.0-1.6	
	Jowl	74	1.2	

FIG. 5.12 The large-animal portable chart. Note that the time stations and kV stations are limited; therefore the images will not always be optimized but they will be diagnostic.

Date	Film #	Client	Breed	Area of body	Measure-ment Cm	kV	mA mAs	Time	Comment

FIG. 5.13 A radiography sample log book page.

The technical factors and measurements are critical to maintaining a working technique chart. If a problem arises and the technical factors are completed correctly, it is much easier to diagnose. The technical factors must be entered as the images are completed. Guessing techniques based on past images is not an option.

Summary

The technical factors introduced and discussed in Chapters 2 and 4 have now been explored and put to use.

In this chapter we have examined the variables of kV and mA and how each of these factors affects the overall image. It is vitally important to approach the technique chart with a scientific mind. The settings on the unit indicate the correct settings in order to produce an optimized image. If a service consultant is on site, the first place he or she will look is the log book to see if any inconsistencies of exposures have been occurring.

Each facility is unique, but the universal truth is that 70 kV is 70 kV, and the generator and the technical factors set on the generator must be accurate and reproducible.

REVIEW QUESTIONS

1. The main objective of all imaging systems is to:
   a. Produce a radiograph with a recognizable image
   b. Demonstrate differences in tissue density
   c. Demonstrate the image with no movement
   d. Show how much contrast and density are alike
2. Every radiography generator has kV, mAs, and time; the following statement is true:
   a. These may vary from unit to unit.
   b. These must be calibrated correctly so that 70 kV is 70 kV on every unit.
   c. The factors are variable and should be adjusted when the chart is set up.
   d. The factors do not matter as long as you follow the chart.

3. Film fog is a plus density artifact on an image; the following statement is true:
   a. It may be caused by light leaks in the darkroom.
   b. Film is not sensitive to light, only to x-rays.
   c. Film fog shows as a minus density after development.
   d. It may be caused by dropping a cassette after exposure.
4. Base + fog, which is an inherent part of the exposure:
   a. Does not appear on the processed film
   b. Appears only on reflected images
   c. Must always be included as part of the exposure
   d. Is a part of the manufacturing process and not important
5. The expiration date on the film box:
   a. Is not important because it has to do with the manufacturer
   b. Is important because it affects the processing of the film
   c. Is a critical piece of information when the box of film is used
   d. Has to do with the purchasing of film and not with its use
6. Radiographic contrast is part of the image controlled by:
   a. Patient thickness, density, and grid ratio
   b. The body part being examined and the bone-to-muscle ratio
   c. Grids, anode heel effect, and technical factors
   d. Collimation, distance, and patient thickness
7. Subject contrast is part of the image controlled by the patient thickness.
   a. True
   b. False
8. The inverse square law is particularly important in:
   a. Measuring the distance from the top of the patient to the grid tray
   b. Adjusting the technical factors between kV and mAs
   c. The distance between the table and the grid tray
   d. The distance measured in equine radiography

9. Kilovoltage is primarily responsible for:
   a. The hardness of the x-ray beam and its penetration
   b. The amount of density on the radiograph
   c. The intensity of the radiation and the density
   d. The blackness of the perimeter surrounding the image
10. The 15% rule is primarily used:
    a. When the image is far too dark or too light
    b. When the density on the image needs to be a little darker
    c. When the contrast on the image needs to be enhanced
    d. To reset the technical factors because of fogged film
11. If the original kV is 80 (we will increase the kV), the 15% rule calculation yields the following value:
    a. 87
    b. 92
    c. 97
    d. 79
12. Milliamperage is responsible for the intensity of the radiation, which:
    a. Translates to the density on the image
    b. Translates to the contrast on the image
    c. Relates only to the time of the exposure
    d. Does not concern the blackness of the background.
13. The three rules of using a technique chart correctly include:
    a. Positioning on the table, measuring, and centering the central ray
    b. Positioning the animal on the floor and centering to the film
    c. Measuring the animal in the cage and then setting the technical factors
    d. Measuring the animal upright, setting the techniques before measuring, and then centering to the grid tray

14. If the images are consistently dull and gray, the first check should be made in the:
    a. Processing to see whether the fluids are still fresh
    b. The cassettes to make sure they have not changed
    c. The darkroom to ensure that there are no light leaks
    d. The generator to ensure that the techniques did not change
15. The radiography log book is a record of exposures; the following statement is true:
    a. It is also a legal necessity and maintains a record of technical factors.
    b. It is not necessary because we always remember the techniques.
    c. It is not necessary because the animal always measures the same.
    d. It is necessary only to write down the animal's name for accounting purposes.

Answers to Review Questions can be found on the Evolve website.

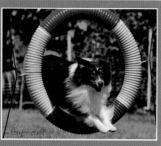

CHAPTER 6
Optimizing the Image

Lois C. Brown, RTR (Can/USA), ACR, MSc., P.Phys

Good, better, best. Never let it rest. 'Til your good is better and your better is best.

—St. Jerome, Biblical saint, 347–420

Sometimes you need to "jump through hoops" to obtain a good image.

OUTLINE

LEARNING OBJECTIVES

When you have finished this chapter, you will be able to:

1. Define motion, distortion, magnification, and blur.
2. Understand the purpose of filters.
3. Define collimation.
4. Understand the purpose of illuminators.
5. Know when to use a grid.
6. Understand the grid ratio and the difference between various grids.
7. Determine the importance of line pairs in relation to the grid ratio.

APPLICATIONS

The application of the information in this chapter is relevant to the following area:

1. Optimizing the images (radiographs) to aid in diagnoses

KEY TERMS

Key terms are defined in the Glossary on the Evolve website.

Blur
Central ray
Coincidence
Collimation shutters/leaves
Collimator
Collimator indicator
Compensating filters
Diffusion
Distortion

Filtration
Grid
Grid deterioration
Grid ratio
Grid tray
Heterogeneous beam
Illuminator
Illuminator mask
Inherent filtration

Line pairs/inch (grids)
Line pairs/mm (resolution)
Magnification
Motion
Object image receptor distance (OID)
Off-focus radiation
Region of interest (ROI)
Resolution

Scattered radiation
Secondary radiation
Source image distance (SID)
Source object distance (SOD)
Umbra/penumbra

This chapter is the compilation of all of the technology introduced thus far and introduces the tools necessary to optimize the image. This chapter refers to the central ray, which is the x-ray beam produced off the central point of the focal spot of the anode and directed at 90 degrees to the image receptor (Fig. 6.1). The ROI (region of interest) is the area of the patient through which the central ray must pass to obtain a correctly positioned radiograph.

It is essential to ensure that as much cooperation as possible is obtained from the patient. If an animal is so ill or terrified that it tremors continuously, obtaining an optimized radiograph will be very difficult unless the animal can be reassured or sedated to the point at which it will be cooperative and remain motionless throughout the x-ray examination. Many veterinary facilities are limited to $\frac{1}{120}$ of a second on their radiography units, and at times this is not fast enough to arrest involuntary motion such as tremor or panting.

Other factors, such as magnification, distortion, and blur, can be minimized by understanding the principles behind these factors. The use of collimation and grids reduces the scattered/secondary radiation. Understanding the principles of grids, the limitations of various grid ratios, and how to position the grid correctly is vitally important to obtaining a good, clean image. Filtration eliminates a certain amount of secondary radiation and prevents most of the scattered radiation. Illuminators are vitally important to film/screen radiography, and the correct placement of the illuminator and the correct lighting tubes within the illuminator will optimize viewing of the x-ray film image.

Motion, Distortion, and Magnification

Motion

Resolution is the ability to differentiate fine details within the x-ray image (Fig. 6.2). Motion will destroy resolution. Unsharpness resulting from patient motion may be voluntary or involuntary. Reducing involuntary motion or waiting a few extra seconds until the patient settles is very important to good radiography.

Diagnosis is impossible if the patient appears to be leaving the table as the exposure is made. This is also true if a wagging tail is moving across the image. The use of sandbags and rolled towels can support body parts that are unstable and out of the region of interest (ROI). Sandbags can be obtained commercially or, if someone in the facility can sew, can be made quite easily. Be aware that sandbags are not radiolucent and should never be placed where they will obscure the ROI. For all other methods of nonmanual restraint, please review Chapter 15 and each of the views in Part Two.

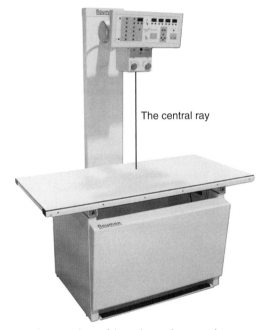

The central ray

FIG. 6.1 The central ray of the radiography unit is the point at which the x-ray beam enters the patient.

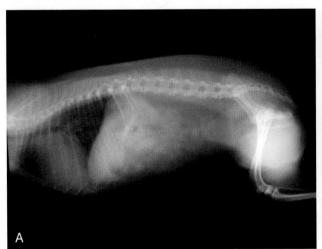
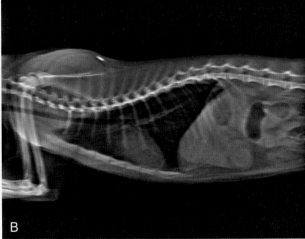

FIG. 6.2 A, An example of involuntary motion (tremor); the abdominal contents are no longer distinct. **B,** Blur can be very subtle. Here the patient is in tremor; the image almost looks like a double exposure except for the trachea and the heart, which are clear.

Colorful slipcovers can be sewn and secured at the top with hook-and-loop (Velcro) strips to make a standard-size sandbag. Larger or smaller sizes are also useful. If no one at the facility can sew, sandbags and foam blocks for positioning can be purchased from commercial suppliers.

Blur

Blur is another factor in patient motion, which in some cases may be useful when imaging a particular body part that is obscured by overlying anatomical structures. Blur is the principle of computerized tomography; we investigate this principle in depth in Chapter 12.

Blur can be dramatic, with the structures completely obscured and the image appearing as if the patient is leaving the table. It can also be subtle, such as in Fig. 6.2B, in which the patient is in tremor and every body part uniformly appears as if it is a double exposure. In this case the large organs appear in focus but resolution is lost in the extremities and spine.

Distortion

Distortion is the foreshortening or elongation of a body part due to angulation of the body part, x-ray receptor, or x-ray tube (Fig. 6.3). Distortion can be useful when one body part obscures the area of interest. For example, if the left (upper) shoulder obscures pathology of the right (lower) humerus on an upper-right lateral thorax view, the x-ray tube may be angled obliquely so the left shoulder is projected away from the right humerus. The patient may also be rotated slightly to demonstrate pathology. Useful distortion is practiced regularly in dental radiography and is discussed in Chapter 22.

◆ **APPLICATION INFORMATION**

It is due to these factors that when a patient's spine is radiographed, the patient is positioned in the ventrodoral (VD) position. If the left side of the chest is of concern, then the patient must be turned onto the left side for the lateral view.

Distortion is not useful if it results in elongation or foreshortening of the ROI. Shape distortion can occur from inaccurate positioning of the central ray. For example, if the ROI is the thorax and the central ray is directed to the abdomen, the anterior ribs will be projected cranially and the shape of the thorax will be distorted. It is important that the ROI is centered beneath the central ray of the x-ray tube.

? **POINTS TO PONDER**

Elongation and foreshortening are eliminated by ensuring the correct alignment of the x-ray tube, body part, and image receptor and central ray.

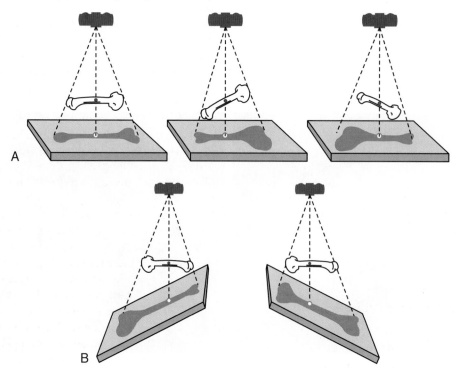

FIG. 6.3 Distortion. **A,** Body part not parallel to the image receptor. **B,** Image receptor not parallel to the body part. (From Fauber TL. *Radiographic Imaging and Exposure,* 4th ed. St. Louis: Mosby, 2013.)

Magnification

Magnification of a body part is reduced if the body part is placed as close as possible to the image receptor (Fig. 6.4). The source image distance (SID) on most veterinary radiography units is 40 inches (100 cm). If the object of interest is raised or anatomically positioned above the image receptor, the object will be magnified. In everyday practice the actual measurement of an object in question is not an issue.

Magnification Calculation

To calculate the size of an object (e.g., a kidney stone), the source-to-object distance (SOD) first needs to be calculated by using the following formula:

$$SID - OID = SOD$$

Measure the distance of the object from the image receptor (object-to-image receptor distance; OID) by measuring on the lateral view. To do this, position the film on the illuminator and measure the distance (in centimeters) from the dorsal surface of the abdomen to the object in question. (For a kidney stone, this measurement is typically one third of the measurement from the dorsal surface to the ventral surface.) The source-to-image receptor distance (SID) on most veterinary radiography units is 100 cm.

If the OID is 12 cm, then the SOD will be:

$$100 \, cm - 12 \, cm = 88 \, cm$$

The magnification factor (MF) is calculated by using the following formula:

$$SID/SOD = MF$$

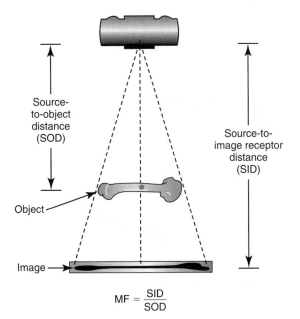

FIG. 6.4 Example of magnification of an image structure. *MF,* Magnification factor. (From Fauber TL. *Radiographic Imaging and Exposure,* 5th ed. St. Louis: Mosby, 2017.)

If the SID is 100 cm, then the MF will be:

$$100/88 = 1.13$$

Actual object size is calculated by using the following formula:

$$\frac{\text{Measurement on a radiograph}}{\text{Magnification factor}} = \text{Object size}$$

From our previous calculation, we know that the MF is 1.13. If the object size on the radiograph is 1.5 cm, then the object size will be:

$$\frac{1.5 \, cm}{1.13} = 1.327 \, cm$$

Geometrical Unsharpness

Every feature in the image is best viewed in its natural size unaffected by unsharpness caused by geometrical factors. Therefore both the SID and OID are vitally important. The source of the radiation is the x-ray tube. The collimator ensures that the beam is focused directly on the ROI. Together the SID and the OID, along with the size of the focal spot, determine the sharpness of the image.

Unsharpness Due to Increased Focal Spot Size

In very rare cases the focal spot of the x-ray tube can become enlarged due to overheating or age. In this case the bony structures appear to be double-exposed, with a second image exactly superimposed on the original image but offset by approximately $\frac{1}{8}$ of an inch (0.32 cm). There is no way to remedy this problem, and the x-ray tube must be replaced.

Filters and Filtration

Once radiation became useful in general radiography, the problem of scattered/secondary radiation had to be addressed. As the body parts being examined become thicker, the technical factors need to be increased, and there is even greater scattered/secondary radiation, particularly as the kV is increased.

The standard reaction to increased body size is to increase the kilovoltage (kV). 2 kV per centimeter is usually the norm, starting around 40 or 50 kV. A proportionate increase in kV along with an increase in patient thickness causes two factors to enter the equation:
1. There is less difference in tissue density because fat and flabby muscle tissue become more prevalent.
2. The production of scattered/secondary radiation is greater because the kilovoltage controls the penetrating power of the x-ray beam. An increase in the penetrating power of the x-ray beam (obtained by increasing the kV) will produce higher levels of secondary radiation and then more scattered radiation, which will fog the film and reduce contrast considerably.

Chapter 5 explains how to control the technical factors to reduce secondary radiation. It also explains *kilovoltage, milliamperage,* and *time* and how kV affects the image.

When radiation enters the patient, it does so as a heterogeneous beam. When 70 kV is set on the x-ray unit, only a portion of the actual radiation produced will actually be 70 kV. This is the *effective kV*. Diagnostic x-ray tubes produce an x-ray beam with various different energies. Therefore a 70 kV beam contains radiation representing 70 kV but also contains photons of varying amounts of energy that are both absorbed within the patient and scatter from the patient as scattered/secondary radiation. Because this radiation is not useful, it must be filtered out either before it enters the patient or after it exits the patient. The first method to filter out the soft or lower-energy radiation before it reaches the patient is through inherent filtration within the collimator.

Inherent Filtration

The collimator of the radiography unit is equipped with inherent filtration when it is installed (Fig. 6.5). Before the x-ray beam exits the port of the x-ray tube, it is attenuated by the glass envelope of the tube, the oil surrounding the tube, the mirror, and an added filter made of aluminum just inside the port of the collimator (the beam restrictor located just below the x-ray tube). This is inherent filtration—the filtration that is part of the x-ray tube assembly that includes the collimator. This filtration cannot be changed in the radiography room.

Added Filtration

The beam is further attenuated by the added filtration installed by the manufacturer. Federal guidelines are very clear regarding the amount of filtration that must be installed in each radiography unit. This added filtration may be adjusted according to the typical procedure in the radiography room. Canadian and U.S. federal guidelines specify a minimum of 2.1 mm of aluminum for x-ray units operating above 70 kV (National Council on Radiation Protection & Measurements, 1988).

Most installations include a label on the back of the x-ray tube. This is a legal requirement in most countries. The label must include the date and country of manufacture, the amount of inherent filtration of the x-ray tube, model number, and serial number.

Special Filters

Other filters known as *compensating filters* may be added to the primary beam to enhance the imaging process. For example, a wedge filter may be added to the collimator, with the thicker part of the wedge over the thinner area of the abdomen if the ROI is the upper abdomen of a dog with a large discrepancy between the measurement of the pelvis and the area of the diaphragm (Fig. 6.6). The technique would be set for the caudal rib measurement, with the x-ray tube positioned over the ROI at the level of the spleen and kidneys.

Many other filters are available, both to even out the discrepancy between different areas of the body and to absorb scattered/secondary radiation.

Blockers

Filtration to eliminate scattered radiation on the image is as simple as laying a mask of leaded rubber on the tabletop along the lumbar spine for a lateral exposure (Fig. 6.7). (This is particularly useful if the suspected pathology is within the dorsal aspect of the spine.) The leaded rubber absorbs the scattered radiation and prevents it from reaching the image receptor. Other effective blockers and filters are large intravenous saline bags and plastic bags filled with flour or rice. The advantage of the saline bags and flour bags is that they are radiolucent and do not produce an artifact. Leaded blockers may also be used to reduce or eliminate the effect of scattered/secondary radiation, which will "splash" onto the image and blacken areas of interest. Leaded gloves are particularly useful, as the curve on the glove can lie along the abdomen and not encroach on the anatomy. It is important that these blockers lie beside the patient and not beneath the area of interest.

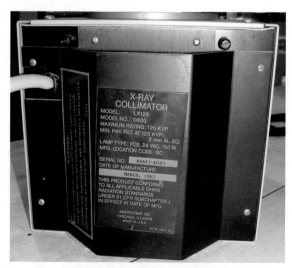

FIG. 6.5 The back plate of a collimator showing the amount of inherent filtration within it.

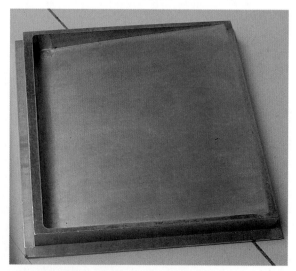

FIG. 6.6 A wedge filter will even out the difference in tissue measurement. It is attached to the collimator with the thickest end at the thinner part of the patient. The technique set is the measurement of the thicker body part.

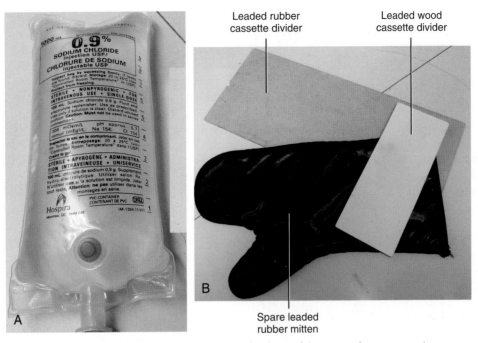

Leaded rubber cassette divider

Leaded wood cassette divider

Spare leaded rubber mitten

FIG. 6.7 A, Simple intravenous saline bags absorb scattered radiation if the region of interest is on the outer aspect of the anatomy. **B,** Special lead blockers also work well as long as they are not pushed under the patient, which would block primary radiation. Leaded rubber gloves and cut-up pieces of lead apron also serve this purpose.

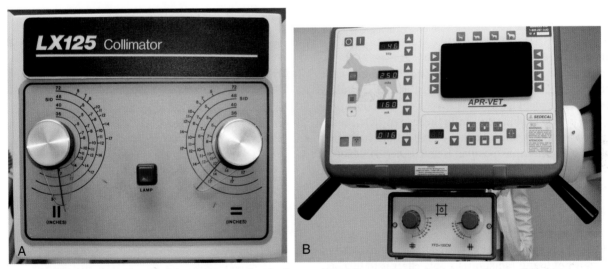

FIG. 6.8 Two different collimators. **A,** Collimator for Raymax LX125 (Raymax Medical, Brampton, Ontario, CA). Note the indicators for height of the x-ray tube and film size on the front. **B,** The collimator for Sedecal APR VET (Sedecal USA, Inc., Arlington Heights, Illinois) is mounted directly below the generator control panel.

Collimators and Coincidence

The unit immediately beneath the x-ray tube is the collimator (Fig. 6.8). There are many varieties of collimators, but they all have one main function—to produce a light beam that is coincident with the x-ray beam and covers the ROI. It is very important that the light beam be centered and coincident within 0.50 inch (1 cm) of the area of the x-ray beam. In addition, the x-ray beam and the light beam should completely match each other in position and size. If the collimator light and the x-ray beam overlap each other completely, they are said to be "in coincidence." Chapter 9 discusses quality control tests regarding collimators and collimation.

? POINTS TO PONDER

As the collimation increases, the area covered becomes smaller, the beam size becomes smaller, and the amount of scattered radiation is reduced. As the collimation decreases, the area radiographed becomes larger, the field size increases, and the potential for scattered radiation is increased.

Scattered/Secondary Radiation

Scattered/secondary radiation produced has much lower energy than the usable x-ray beam and does not have the capability

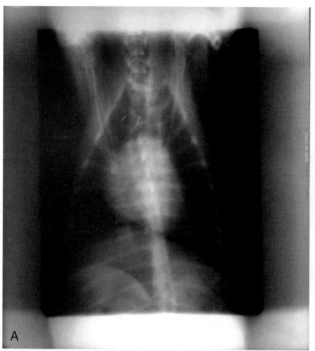

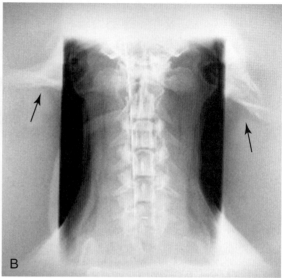

A

B

FIG. 6.9 A, An example of scattered radiation. The collimated field is visible, but the radiation is strong enough to scatter to the outer edges of the image receptor. In this case it is caused by high exposure. The kilovoltage should be reduced so that the lung markings are visible and the spinous processes of the thoracic spine fade as the spine descends caudally to the abdomen. **B,** Evidence of extrafocal radiation *(arrows).* Note that this is different from scattered radiation because the folds of the dog's ears are also evident along with the much thicker shoulder area.

of producing an organized image beyond the limits of the collimator (Fig. 6.9). The presence of scattered/secondary radiation is the main reason that anyone in the room at the time of exposure should never be in the field of view, should be appropriately gowned and gloved, and should stay as far from the x-ray beam as possible (see Chapter 3). Refer to Chapter 5 to learn how to evaluate technical factors on a radiograph.

Collimation and Contrast

As the radiation area decreases, the amount of radiation scattered from the ROI decreases. Scattered radiation that reaches the film is not useful radiation. Its only effect is to increase the base density and reduce the contrast between the base density and the imaged structures. If collimation restricts the beam size dramatically, the technical factors may need to be increased slightly to accommodate for the restriction of some of the useful radiation (Table 6.1). To change the density on a radiograph, only the mAs should be increased, not the kV.

Collimator Problems or Scatter From the Patient?

The collimator is the last filtration system of the x-ray beam before it reaches the patient. In some cases, when the beam is collimated, there is a shadow of the patient's anatomy on the image beyond the edges of the collimator (see Fig. 6.9A). This may be caused by scatter from the patient itself. If the "splash" of radiation is larger when the patient being radiographed is large and is not visible when the patient is quite

TABLE 6.1	Effect of Changing Collimation*
COLLIMATION	**RESULT**
Decrease field size	Patient dose decreases
	Scattered radiation decreases
	Radiographic contrast increases
	Radiographic density decreases
Increase field size	Patient dose increases
	Scattered radiation increases
	Radiographic contrast decreases (due to increased scattered/secondary radiation)
	Radiographic density increases

*Increasing the collimation narrows the field of view. Increasing the field size is the same as opening the collimator shutters.

small, the problem is most likely scattered/secondary radiation from the patient. Placing a lead strip along the side of the patient prevents this scatter from affecting the image.

? POINTS TO PONDER

When placing any blocker alongside the patient to absorb scatter, it is very important that the blocker does not overlap the anatomy being imaged.

Extrafocal Radiation

If parts of the patient's anatomy are clearly visible, such as a leg or the spinous processes in an otherwise collimated spine, then the fault is most likely *extrafocal radiation* (see Chapter 2) or *off-focus radiation* (see Fig. 6.9B). This is radiation that is created by the photon stream outside the actual focal spot. It may be due to a defect in the design and manufacture of the x-ray tube and shielding system or the collimator filtration, or the kV may be set too high, causing excessively active photons in the thermionic cloud.

Umbra and Penumbra

The umbra is the portion of the x-ray image that is sharp and clearly collimated. The penumbra is the outside edge or shadow where the film has been imperfectly collimated. This image is not magnified or distorted. Most modern collimators are efficient enough that penumbra is eliminated.

Changing the Collimator Light Bulb

When the light bulb inside the collimator burns out, it may be replaced by veterinary staff, but a service person should be called the first time to demonstrate the correct method of changing the light bulb. The installing engineer of a new unit should demonstrate how to change the light bulb before turning over the unit to the veterinarian.

New radiography units should be supplied with a spare collimator light bulb. The replacement bulb should be kept in a specific place and its location noted on the x-ray generator. Whenever the light bulb is changed, a new one should be ordered right away so that there is always a spare on "hot stand-by." Collimator bulbs are usually supplied by x-ray service companies or can be ordered online (just type in the alphanumeric code of the bulb followed by the words "light bulb" in your search engine). Always make sure that the voltage of the bulb you are ordering is the same as the one you are replacing. The wattage should also be the same, but the voltage is more important. If you are not sure which bulb to order, check the back of the collimator. There is usually a label specifying voltage and wattage (Fig. 6.10). If there is no label, then carefully follow these instructions:

- Make sure the generator is turned off at the wall switch. Have a multiple-tip screwdriver handy to remove the cover of the collimator.
- Search for a cover plate on the collimator. It is usually on the back or on the side. Remove the cover plate. Typically, the light bulb is now visible. On some collimators, the shutters must be closed to expose the bulb, and other collimators have a small black box that must be removed. Carefully note the position of the box before you remove it.
- Once the light bulb is exposed, remove it, noting whether it requires turning or just a gentle tug to do so. **This is very important.** Some light bulbs are mounted between

what appears to be two steel plates. If you look very closely you will see a slight opening for the end of the new bulb. Some light bulbs have a bayonet mount and require turning as well as pulling to remove them. ***Be very gentle; these bulbs are often small and fragile!***

- Check to ensure that the bulb you are replacing is identical to the new bulb. The code numbers or letters may differ, but the wattage and, particularly, the voltage must be the same.
- The new light bulb will probably be a halogen bulb, so it is important not to touch it with bare hands or fingers. The bulb usually comes wrapped in a plastic cover from which the bottom may be cut away to reveal the insertion end of the bulb. Using the cover, gently and firmly insert the bulb in the exact spot from which you removed the old bulb, then slide off the plastic cover.
- Once the bulb is firmly in place, turn on the main power to test that the bulb is working.
- Turn off the power again and reaffix the collimator cover plate.

Illuminators

Illuminators transmit light evenly through a specially produced glass in order to visualize and interpret radiographic images (Fig. 6.11). This is the means by which the veterinarian and often the client view and discuss the results of the radiographic examination. It is very important that the conditions under which the radiographs are interpreted are of the highest possible quality; therefore it is vital that the illuminators be checked regularly for optimum brightness.

Illuminator Specifications

The inside of the illuminator must be painted a bright white to reflect as much light as possible toward the diffusion glass. Illuminators with the light tubes mounted in unpainted wooden or stainless steel boxes are not suitable because they absorb the light and diminish the amount projected toward the diffusion glass. The luminance across the entire face of the illuminator should be the same. The illuminator must be equipped with a diffusing glass or Plexiglas so the corners of the illuminator are the same brightness as the central portion.

Commercially available bulbs may be purchased at a hardware store. The light tubes must be labeled "daylight" or "blue/white" light to match the color spectrum of radiographic film. Bulbs with a green, yellow, or pink tone are not suitable for viewing radiographs. If one light tube becomes faulty, all light tubes within that illuminator should be replaced so the brightness is uniform across the width of the illuminator. The face of the illuminator should be cleaned regularly using a commercial glass cleaner whenever the countertops and shelves are dusted. The switch must be a safety switch and must be checked to ensure that it is not worn, loose, or faulty. At least once per year, the glass panel should be removed so the illuminator box can be dusted and cleaned and the bulbs checked for brightness and consistency.

2 mm AL. EQ.
LAMP TYPE: FCS, 24 VAC, 150 W

FIG. 6.10 Cover plate on the back of a collimator. Note the lamp type information. This collimator label also includes the amount of filtration inherent in the components of the collimator.

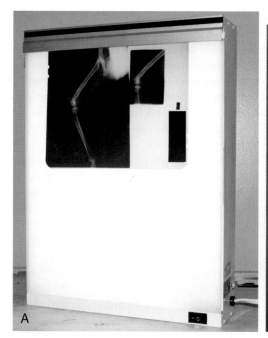
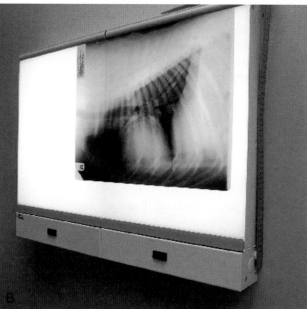

FIG. 6.11 A, A typical stand-alone illuminator. This illuminator may be placed on a table, mounted on a wall, or inserted into the wall between the upright joists. **B,** This two-bank illuminator is mounted on the wall of the x-ray room. A mask would direct the intensity of the light through the image and prevent glare from the areas surrounding the radiograph. **(B** courtesy of Westbridge Veterinary Hospital, Mississauga, Ontario.)

FIG. 6.12 Illuminator mask. Keep the piece that is cut out and use it to cover that hole. Then you can cut out similar areas to fit the various sizes of film that are used in the facility. Make the cutout close to the middle of the illuminator to ensure you have the brightest light.

✓ CHECK IT OUT

- A combination of correct color and brightness enhances the contrast of the radiographs. As a quick test to reveal whether the color of the illuminator bulbs in the facility is correct, review a correctly exposed radiograph on the clinic illuminator.
- Now go to a window on a cloudy, bright day and review the same radiograph (this light is the same color as the daylight light tube).
- If the image looks the same, then the light tubes are most likely daylight.
- Most fluorescent tubes are labeled at one end with the manufacturer and the color.
- An illuminator that is not working correctly or does not transmit the light effectively can seriously compromise the reading of a radiograph and can actually affect the technical factors used to produce the image.

Illuminator Position

An illuminator may be mounted on the wall or positioned within the wall so that the front is flush with the wall. The films are hung from holders at the top of the illuminator, and these should be checked regularly to ensure that they do not catch and hold the film so firmly that it cannot be removed without incident.

The illuminator should be positioned in the room so that the overhead light may be switched off. This way there will be no backlighting to reduce the brightness of the light transmitted from the illuminator.

Illuminator Masks

Illuminator masks (Fig. 6.12) should be available to cover any part of the illuminator panel not covered by the film so that all available light reaching the eye of the clinician is directed through the radiograph.

Grids and Grid Trays

Scattered/secondary radiation is a problem as the body parts to be x-rayed become larger. Any body part more than 10 cm will produce enough scattered/secondary radiation to seriously compromise the contrast on an x-ray image.

In 1913 Gustave Bucky invented the radiographic grid (Fig. 6.13). This consisted of vertical, very fine strips of metal interspaced with radiolucent interspaces. The strips are positioned vertically to the axis of the table, and the entire "grid" is positioned between the patient and the cassette. The original grid was positioned with a spring that had to be set (or cocked) before each exposure; when the exposure was made, the lock released and the grid moved across the face of the cassette to absorb scattered/secondary radiation. This somewhat complicated contraption worked on the principle of the windshield wiper moving across the car windshield—your eyes do not focus on the windshield wiper but rather through the window to the road outside.

A couple of problems arose when this technology was transferred to the veterinary market. The grid oscillating device made a fairly loud noise as it was released. Once the spring was converted to a motor, the whirring noise of the motor was bothersome to some animals. The other problem was the timing of the original units, which needed an exposure time of at least $\frac{1}{10}$ of a second for the strips to move rapidly enough to blur out the image of the individual strips. Most veterinary exposures must be far less than $\frac{1}{10}$ of a second, so grid lines are a problem. These units have occasionally been installed in veterinary hospitals, and the motorized mechanism should be removed and the ancient grids replaced by newer stationary grids.

Grid Nomenclature

Every grid manufactured throughout the world is imprinted or labeled with the grid ratio, the lines per inch, and the manufacturer.

Grid Ratios and Line Pairs per Inch

A ratio is expressed as a number with a relationship to a second number; for example, the ratio of 25 apples to 5 apples is 5:1. It is always expressed with a colon (:) in between the two numbers.

Grid ratio = Height of the lead strips : Distance between the lead strips.

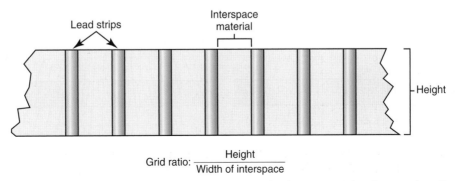

$$\text{Grid ratio:} \frac{\text{Height}}{\text{Width of interspace}}$$

FIG. 6.13 Grid ratio is the ratio of the height of the lead strips to the distance (interspace) between them. (From Fauber TL. *Radiographic Imaging and Exposure*, 5th ed. St. Louis: Mosby; 2017.)

As grids were used in various procedures, the manufacturers made them more sophisticated. The best way to identify them was by expressing a ratio of lines of the material used to "clean up" the scatter: 5:1, 6:1, 8:1, 10:1, 12:1, and 16:1. It was soon discovered that grids with lower ratios (5:1 and 6:1) did not work as well as grids with higher ratios because they did not clean up enough scattered/secondary radiation. Introducing more leaded strips and a higher ratio cleaned up much better. Also, the grids with very high ratios—16:1 and higher—were useful only for specific applications and not for general radiography. The higher ratio grids required much more radiation because they were so efficient that they absorbed much of the primary beam as well as the scattered/secondary radiation, thereby increasing patient radiation dose. (If some of the useful beam is eliminated, then technical factors would have to be increased, thereby increasing patient dose.)

The problem with expressing the grid ratio alone is that it does not specify the number of line pairs (lp) per inch. One line pair is one vertical strip and one interspace strip. A grid may have an 8:1 grid ratio, but if the lines are spread too far apart, they will show up on a radiograph.

Because the ratio numbers identify the height of lines or strips compared with the space between them, the number of line pairs is as important as the grid ratio.

In the medical and veterinary general radiography field, grids with ratios of 8:1 and 10:1 with 103 lp/inch work the best. The scatter control is good without the need to increase the radiation dose by too much to overcome the clean-up of the grid.

Parallel vs. Focused Grids

The original grids were manufactured with parallel lines running in the vertical direction of the table (Fig. 6.14A). A problem arose when larger cassette sizes became available and the collimators opened to a 17-inch lateral width. The parallel grid strips cut off the radiation at the edges of the image so that the edges of the films were exposed to little or no radiation.

The solution to this problem was to "focus" the grid (Fig. 6.14B). As grid manufacturing techniques became more sophisticated, newer grids were manufactured with the lines vertical strips tilted slightly to match the divergent x-rays of the primary beam (Fig. 6.15). These focused grids allowed more primary radiation to reach the film edges than did the older parallel grids, but they also introduced another variable that had to be addressed—focal length.

Grid Focus and Focal Length

Grid focal length is the distance from the focal spot of the x-ray tube to the grid. The focused grids assumed a 34- to

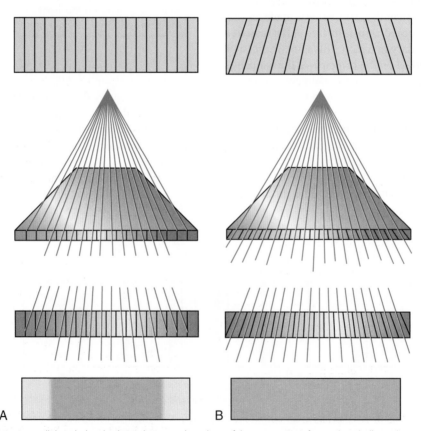

FIG. 6.14 A, A parallel grid absorbs the radiation at the edges of the image. B, A focused grid allows the x-rays to pass through to the outer edges of the image. (From Fauber TL. *Radiographic Imaging and Exposure*, 5th ed. St. Louis: Mosby; 2017.)

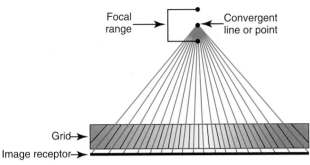

FIG. 6.15 A focused grid. The lead lines are angled coincident with the divergent primary rays. The focal length is now preset, and the focal range is slightly above and slightly below the convergent point. Typically, a 40-inch focal length grid has a focal range of 34 to 44 inches. (From Fauber TL. *Radiographic Imaging and Exposure*, 5th ed. St. Louis: Mosby; 2017.)

TABLE 6.2	Common Grid Focal Lengths	
SIZE	INCHES	CENTIMETERS
Small	26–32	66–81
Medium	34–44	86–111
Large	48–72	122–183

44-in (86- to 112-cm) focal length. The divergent rays of the x-ray beam exit at a prescribed distance from the grid (40 in or 100 cm). If the primary beam is changed to a shorter or longer focal length (distance from the focal spot of the x-ray tube), a grid of a different focal length is needed to correspond to the new distance. Another problem occurs with equine radiography when the x-ray unit is held too close to the grid.

Various focal lengths are now available, and the most common are listed in Table 6.2. The following factors must be included when a grid is purchased for a veterinary hospital:

- **Grid ratio**: Usually 10 : 1
- **Number of line pairs**: Usually 103 lp/inch
- **Focal length**: Usually 34 to 44 inches (86 to 111 cm)

Grid Installation

The grid is installed beneath the tabletop and above the cassette. A grid tray is usually in place below the grid, and the folded metal edges of the grid tray holder will support the grid. It is important that the grid is centered correctly and maintained in the correct position. An older installed grid may be screwed in place, glued in place, or held in place by hook-and-loop tape (Velcro). Strips of adhesive-backed Velcro tape work well to attach the grid to the grid tray holder. It may be necessary to cut the strips to a width of 0.5 in (1.27 cm) lengthwise so there is no chance that they will catch on the cassette as it is drawn in and out of the tray.

When replacing a grid, the size of the grid tray is important. The grid should overhang the edges of the cassette slightly to effectively absorb the scattered radiation and not be visible on the image. For example, an 18 in × 18 in (46 cm × 46 cm) grid will cover a 14 in × 17 in (35 cm × 43 cm) cassette effectively both vertically and longitudinally.

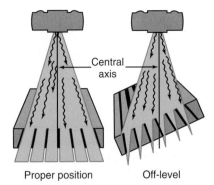

FIG. 6.16 A focused grid raised on one side of the table. One side of the grid acts as a parallel grid; the other side absorbs the primary and secondary radiation. (From Fauber TL. *Radiographic Imaging and Exposure*, 5th ed. St. Louis: Mosby; 2017.)

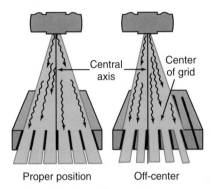

FIG. 6.17 A focused grid set off-center does not allow the radiation to penetrate the grid correctly, causing off-center cutoff. (From Fauber TL. *Radiographic Imaging and Exposure*, 5th ed. St. Louis: Mosby; 2017.)

Grid Positioning

Positioning the grid is critical because it must be exactly in the center of the table or, in equine radiography, the central ray must be centered exactly on the center line of the grid. The grid must also be installed flat on the grid tray, exactly parallel to the port of the x-ray tube. If it is tilted slightly from one side to the other, it will allow the radiation on one side to pass through but will cut off the radiation prematurely on the raised side (Figs. 6.16 and 6.17).

If the grid is installed upside down, an image such as that shown in Fig. 6.20AB will result. The x-ray beam will pass through the vertical strips in the center and will be cut off on both sides evenly toward the edges.

◆ **APPLICATION INFORMATION**

The consultant was called into a clinic with a problem that the hospital had finally identified as an equipment problem but they had no idea what caused it. The images were all slightly lighter on one side than on the other. The problem worsened on the lateral edges of the film. So on a large dog VD chest the right lung was considerably lighter than the left. It appeared that every dog that they x-rayed had pneumonia on the right lung, whereas the left lung appeared to have overinflated lungs.

The x-ray unit had been serviced just weeks before, and the hospital hadn't had any need for grid radiographs for about 2 weeks. That was when a patient who had suspected pneumonia came in, and the image appeared to be what the veterinarian suspected. But when the next dog came in with suspected left-side pathology and the right side was as bad as or worse than the left, they began to suspect there was a problem with the x-ray unit.

After the tabletop was removed, the consultant lifted the grid and discovered a screw had been left on the track of the grid unit. The grid was lifted about ¼ inch on the right side. This was enough to cause the left side to assume a parallel grid configuration, producing an image of overinflation in the lungs on the left. The right side of the grid with this tilt would filter the radiation, causing a light image appearance that would look like pathology on the right. The images showed poor aeration of the lungs on the left and overinflation on the right.

See Figs. 6.16 and 6.17 for off-level and off-center grid examples.

The Effect of a Grid on Technical Factors

The grid absorbs some of the primary beam as it impacts directly on the lead strips. The grid conversion factor is the formula that determines the increase in technical factors to compensate for this absorption. As the grid ratio increases, the radiographic density decreases, and vice versa. The mAs value changes according to Table 6.3. This table should not be necessary if the technique chart is set up correctly at the original installation.

TABLE 6.3	Grid Conversion Factors*
GRID RATIO	**CONVERSION FACTOR NUMBER**
5 : 1	1
6 : 1	2
8 : 1 and 10 : 1	3
12 : 1	4
16 : 1	5

*To calculate the grid conversion factor, multiply the mAs by the grid conversion factor number for each grid ratio.

Summary

The options discussed in this chapter are essential for producing the best images possible, no matter which radiography unit and technique chart are used. Motion, blur, distortion, and magnification have been discussed. This chapter also contains the basics of optimizing radiographic images, including the use of an optimized illuminator. The installation of a grid is necessary for reducing the scattered radiation that affects the image.

Image Gallery

Figs. 6.18 to 6.21 illustrate some of the problems that occur with grids. Because grids are located beneath the tabletop, they are out of sight and are often not included in a routine quality control protocol.

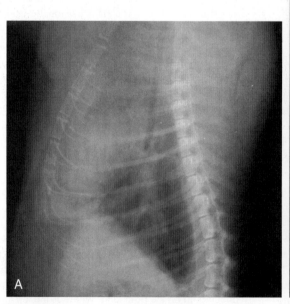
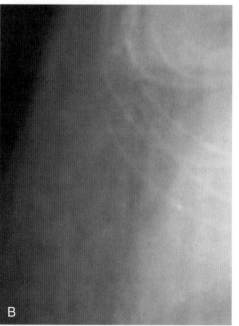

FIG. 6.18 A, The grid ratio in this image was 6 : 1, 85 lines. The grid lines are obvious on the radiograph, and the grid has started to deteriorate, placing a pattern on every image and obscuring a correct reading of pathology. **B,** Grid deterioration up close. The mottled pattern is the absence of the interspace material. Newsprint was frequently used as interspace material. Over time it would disintegrate.

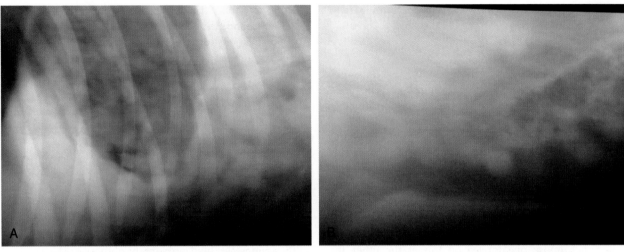

FIG. 6.19 A, Another example of grid deterioration. In this case a window screen was encased in plastic and used as a grid. The window screen was slowly deteriorating and leaving areas of the image produced with no grid. **B,** A close-up of a portion of **A.**

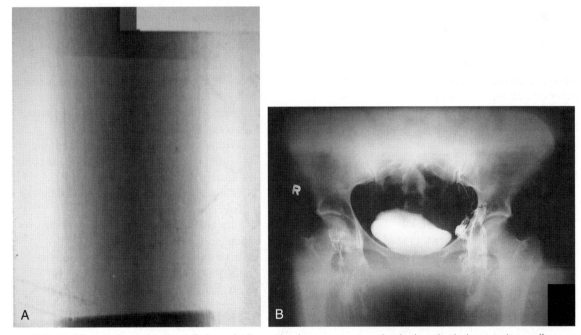

FIG. 6.20 A, A focused grid installed upside down. The divergent rays are absorbed, and only the central rays affect the film. **B,** The grid has been installed upside down and rotated 90 degrees. The grid lines should run parallel to the tabletop.

REVIEW QUESTIONS

1. The description of the central ray includes:
   a. A primary beam projected at 90 degrees to the angle of the anode
   b. A primary beam projected at 90 degrees to the photons affecting the anode
   c. The photon array projected from the cathode
   d. The number of photons affecting the anode

2. Distortion concerns the angulation of the patient:
   a. Because it is uncomfortable on the radiography table
   b. Due to anatomy that is unnecessary on the image
   c. In order to foreshorten or elongate a body part
   d. In order to project one body part away from obscuring the region of interest

3. Blur is the intentional movement of one body part to allow the underlying anatomy to be visible.
   a. True
   b. False
4. Motion degrades the image:
   a. Because it detracts from resolution
   b. Because the image becomes darker and indistinct
   c. By arresting the movement of a wagging tail
   d. By causing the density of the image to be reduced
5. Useful distortion is used to:
   a. Prevent any body parts from superimposing on any other anatomy
   b. Project one body part out of the way of the region of interest
   c. Rotate the x-ray tube to distort the final image
   d. Superimpose one foreleg on top of the other for measurement
6. Magnification is _____ if the body part is moved _____ the image receptor.
   a. decreased, closer to
   b. decreased, farther from
   c. increased, at an angle to
   d. increased, closer to
7. The source image distance (SID) is the measurement:
   a. From the patient to the image receptor
   b. From the patient to the x-ray tube
   c. From the tube to the image receptor
   d. Including the tube and the tabletop
8. The object image distance is a factor in:
   a. Blur
   b. Distortion
   c. Magnification
   d. Rotation
9. To determine the size of an object within the patient, one must measure:
   a. The area of the region of interest
   b. The distance of the object from the tabletop using the lateral view
   c. The distance from the patient to the tabletop
   d. The size of the original collimation
10. Inherent filtration includes the:
    a. Added aluminum from the installation
    b. Distance from the tube to the patient
    c. Glass envelope of the x-ray tube and the oil within the tube
    d. Thickness and weight of the patient
11. Federal law dictates that filtration must be added to equal:
    a. 2.5 mm at 70 kV
    b. 3.5 mm at 70 kV
    c. 2.5 mm at 80 kV
    d. 3.4 mm at 80 kV
12. A collimator is located beneath the x-ray tube to:
    a. Indicate that the x-ray unit is ready to be activated
    b. Outline the size and shape of the cassette in the grid tray
    c. Provide a light source so that the patient is more visible
    d. Provide a light source outlining the area of interest

13. A secondary function of the collimator is to:
    a. Change the radiation to light coincidence
    b. Demonstrate the size of the field of view and change the focus
    c. Narrow the size of the field of view and reduce scattered radiation
    d. Narrow the size of the field of view but elongate it
14. Collimation correctly applied will _____ contrast _____.
    a. degrade, by decreasing brightness
    b. degrade, by increasing brightness
    c. enhance, by decreasing scatter
    d. enhance, by increasing scatter
15. Collimation correctly applied will _____ patient dose _____.
    a. increase, by decreasing brightness
    b. increase, by increasing scatter
    c. reduce, by decreasing scatter
    d. reduce, by increasing brightness
16. Collimation correctly applied will _____ density _____.
    a. decrease, by decreasing scatter
    b. decrease, by increasing brightness
    c. increase, by increasing scatter
    d. increase, by decreasing brightness
17. Off-focus radiation is produced:
    a. By the photon stream outside of the actual focal spot
    b. Outside the area of the focal spot and has low energy
    c. Within the patient and is not harmful to staff
    d. Within the x-ray tube but outside the collimator
18. An illuminator should be mounted:
    a. In a dimly lit area so that the illuminator does not have to be so bright
    b. In a well-lit area in the treatment area so everyone can see the image
    c. In an area where the lights may be dimmed to enhance the image
    d. So that a darker image is projected in a brightly lit area
19. The fluorescent tubes within the illuminator must be:
    a. A green tone if you are using green-receiving film
    b. Daylight or a very pale blue tone
    c. Soft light or a very pale mauve tone
    d. A light pinkish tone to match the color of green-receiving film
20. The main purpose of a grid is to:
    a. Absorb scattered radiation and enhance density
    b. Reduce scattered radiation and decrease dose
    c. Reduce scattered radiation and enhance contrast
    d. Reduce scattered radiation and reduce contrast

21. Grid ratio describes:
    a. The height of the lead strips compared with how many there are to the inch
    b. The height of the lead strips compared with the distance between them
    c. The width between the lead strips and their interspace material
    d. The width of the lead strips compared with their height
22. An installed grid is positioned beneath the patient:
    a. Above the cassette and beneath the grid tray
    b. Above the cassette and beneath the tabletop
    c. Beneath the cassette in the grid tray
    d. Beneath the patient and above the tabletop
23. The focused grid is positioned _____ and at a _____ distance from the tube.
    a. beneath the cassette, any
    b. beneath the cassette, prescribed
    c. in the center of the table, prescribed
    d. in the grid tray, any
24. A grid whose focal length is 34 to 44 inches will cause:
    a. Grid cutoff if the tube is set at 44 inches
    b. Grid cutoff if the tube is set at 72 inches
    c. Scattered radiation if the tube is moved to 56 inches
    d. The grid ratio to shift if the tube is not centered

Answers to Review Questions can be found on the Evolve website.

Bibliography

American Society for Testing in Medicine: *ASTM E1390-90(2000), Standard Guide for Illuminators used for Viewing Industrial Radiographs*, West Conshohocken, PA, 2000, ASTM, www.astm.org.

Bushong SC. *Radiological Science for Technologists*. 10th ed. St Louis: Elsevier; 2013.

International Commission on Radiation Protection: www.icrp.org.

National Council on Radiation Protection & Measurements, United States: http://www.ncrponline.org.

National Council on Radiation Protection & Measurements. *Quality Assurance for Diagnostic Imaging, NCRP Report No. 099*. Bethesda, MD: NCRP Publications; 1988.

Radiation Emitting Devices Act, Radiation Emitting Devices Act, RSC: 1985. c R-1, Canada. http://canlii.ca/t/hzzs. www.hc-sc.gc.ca/ewh-semt/pubs/radiation/safety-code_20-securite/index-eng.php.

Terri L. *Radiographic Imaging and Exposure*. 4th ed. St Louis: Elsevier; 2013.

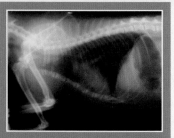

A perfectly exposed and processed x-ray film will demonstrate superior imaging.

CHAPTER 7
Processing the Image

Lois C. Brown, RTR (Can/USA), ACR, MSc., P.Phys

It is an old maxim of mine that when you have eliminated the impossible, whatever remains, however improbable, must be the truth. *

—Sherlock Holmes, Character of Sir Arthur Conan Doyle, 1859–1930

OUTLINE

LEARNING OBJECTIVES

When you have finished this chapter, you will be able to:

1. Understand darkroom specifications.
2. Understand the purpose of developer and fixer.
3. Understand processor construction.
4. Discuss the sequence of the production of the image in the processor.
5. Explain the process of washing and drying.
6. Describe the sequence of successful processing of x-ray film.
7. Discuss the causes of darkroom fog.
8. List some causes of artifacts.

APPLICATIONS

The application of the information in this chapter is relevant to the following areas:

1. Optimizing images (radiographs) to aid in diagnoses
2. Processing film images in a manual tank
3. Processing film images in an automatic processor

KEY TERMS

Key terms are defined in the Glossary on the Evolve website.

Activator	Diffusion	Main drive	Rollers
Ammonium thiosulfate	Electrolysis	Odor masks	Safelight
Antifroth	Feed tray	Phenidone	Solvent
Antisludge	Fixer	Preservative	Stir rods
Artifacts	Fixing agent	Processing	Thermostat
Crossover rollers	Fixing agent	Recirculation	Wash
Darkroom integrity	Guide shoes	Replenishment	
Developer	Hardener	Restrainer	
	Hydroquinone		

*Sherlock Holmes could have been referring to film artifacts!

The final phase of image production is processing. Film processing in the radiography department is very similar to any photographic processing. It occurs either manually with the use of wet tanks and hangers or through an automatic processor. Ninety-five percent of all imaging artifacts occur during the imaging process. Examples of some of these artifacts are listed in the image gallery at the end of this chapter.

This chapter also discusses the architecture and layout of a suitable darkroom in which to carry out the procedures. Suggestions for new facilities are also included.

A Word About Chemicals

As human hospitals and veterinary clinics convert to digital radiography and cancel their chemical contracts, chemical suppliers have been challenged to support their business by switching to the sale of other products. As a result, the production of processing chemicals has reduced considerably. In addition, the developer and fixer components have been altered to remove any product that does not directly involve actually processing the films.

Along with the antisludge and antifrothing components, some manufacturers have removed most of the odor masks. As a result, the smell of the chemicals has emerged to a point at which it is objectionable to stay in the darkroom for any length of time. One way to address this problem is to search for a brand of chemicals that has not removed the odor mask; such brands are quite easy to find. The fixer is the worst culprit, and sampling various brands of fixer is quite straightforward as long as the chemicals from two different companies are never mixed together in one tank.

Another solution to the odor problem is to increase the ventilation in the darkroom. Adding a fan and keeping the darkroom door open when it is not in use is helpful. A light-tight air vent window is also available. This mesh window, which is installed in the darkroom door at eye level, allows air but not light to pass through. Known as darkroom light-tight airflow pass-throughs, these windows are available from any supplier of photography equipment or radiography accessories.

TABLE 7.1	Acidity/Alkalinity of Processing Solutions	
COMPONENT	**ACID/ALKALINE**	**pH**
Developer	Alkaline	9.8–11.4
Fixer	Acidic	4.0–4.5
Water	Neutral	6.5–7.5*

*Ideally the pH of water is 7.0. Most tap water is either slightly acidic or slightly alkaline.

Automatic processing also helps reduce the odor to a degree because the chemical containers remain covered during processing.

One other problem that has resulted from the changes in chemistry concerns the mixing of the chemicals. In manual processing, it is very important to stir the chemicals with an up-and-down motion before processing a film. If the chemicals stratify, the hardener will sink to the bottom of the tank and will not affect the film. A stainless steel stir rod with a flat bottom plate is ideal for stirring the chemistry.

Developer Components

The developer is an alkaline solution with a pH of 9.8 to 11.0. The two main components in the developer are phenidone and hydroquinone. Their function is to reduce the silver halide in the film emulsion to metallic silver by donating additional electrons to the sensitivity specks in the latent image center. The other and equally important function is to amplify the amount of metallic silver on the film by increasing the number of silver atoms deposited in each latent image center. Unexposed silver halide in the film emulsion does not react to the developer chemicals because it has not been ionized and therefore will not accept electrons from the solution. Table 7.2 lists the developer components and their functions.

> ### ✎ TECHNICIAN NOTE
>
> **Safety Alert!**
> The Workplace Hazardous Materials Information System (WHMIS) and the Occupational Safety and Health Administration (OSHA) require that safety glasses and gloves be used whenever chemicals are handled.
>
> The developer is highly alkaline, and the fixer is highly acidic (Table 7.1). Both chemicals must be treated with great respect. A drop of fixer concentrate can melt the lens of the eye in seconds. An eyewash station must be positioned close to the processing area and must be checked regularly by the clinic's quality assurance officer. When handling chemicals, it is essential that personnel are equipped with protective safety goggles and rubber gloves. These are inexpensive are available for purchase at any hardware or department store.

> ### ? POINTS TO PONDER
>
> The components of the developer and fixer have changed dramatically over the years. The chemical manufacturers have developed products that mix together and meet most municipal hazardous waste standards. Therefore in most communities it is safe to dispose of the chemicals down the drain in small effluent quantities with the other waste products from the facility.
>
> Each facility should review the chemical waste guidelines with its municipality and must always have the component sheets from the chemical manufacturer on hand. The hazardous waste sheets for most chemicals are available online and are always available from the manufacturer.
>
> It is important to note that clear water makes up 98% to 99% of the liquid in the chemical bottles that are then diluted again when mixed for use.

TABLE 7.2	Developer Components and Their Functions			
AGENT	**CHEMICAL**	**FUNCTION**		**KEY TO REMEMBERING**
Developing agent	Phenidone	Fast—produces the gray densities, stable, and long lived		**Ph**enidone—**ph**ast—mainly grays
Developing agent	Hydroquinone	Slow—produces blacks; increases contrast on the image; sensitive to temperature, oxygen, and aging		**Longer** name—**longer** time—mainly blacks The sensitive one, reacts to time, temperature, gases, and air and will be the first to become exhausted
Activator	Sodium carbonate	Stabilizes the pH; maintains acidity		**Bi**carbonate of soda stabilizes the acidity in your stomach if you have eaten rich food
Restrainer	Potassium bromide	Decreases the reduction of the unexposed silver halide		This is the stopper—**POTAS**sium (read it backward)
Preservative	Sodium sulfite	Decreases sensitivity to oxidation		
Hardener		"Glues" the emulsion to the base to reduce scratches from the processor		
Solvent	Water	Makes up about 98%–99% of the solution		

TABLE 7.3	Fixer Components and Their Functions			
AGENT	**CHEMICAL**	**FUNCTION**		**KEY TO REMEMBERING**
Fixing agent	Ammonium thiosulfate	Clears away unexposed silver halide		This causes the rotten egg smell
Acidifier	Acetic acid	Stops development		Vinegar
Preservative	Sodium sulfite	Prevents a reaction between fixing agent and acidifier		Same as developer
Hardener	Chrome alum, potassium aluminum sulfate, or aluminum chloride	Hardens the emulsion		Similar to what is in your deodorant—a drying agent
Solvent	Water	Makes up about 98%–99% of the solution		

Fixer Components

The main ingredient in the fixer is sodium thiosulfate. Sulfur is another component, and if the fixer breaks down for any reason, the sulfur precipitates and a rotten egg smell pervades the area (a process known as *sulfiding*).

Another important ingredient is the hardener, which can be one of three types (Table 7.3) The function of the hardener is to ensure that the emulsion stays attached to the base. The chemicals in a manual tank must be stirred with an up-and-down motion or the hardener will remain at the bottom of the tank. If the film is then left in the wash for an extended period, the emulsion will slide off the base.

Darkroom Layout

In a new clinic, it is useful to make the radiography room light-tight and to place the processor in one corner of the room. The patient can be removed during film processing or can stay on the table as long as the room is lit with two safelights so the patient can be monitored. Using the radiography suite as a darkroom makes better use of space than a very small, cramped darkroom with the risk of chemicals splashing onto the cassettes and screens during processing. In addition, many new clinics are setting up temporary darkrooms until they can afford to purchase a digital imaging system. In such cases, when the cost of square footage is an issue, many veterinarians are prompted to use the radiography suite as a temporary darkroom.

If a darkroom is set up as a stand-alone room, it must be large enough that a person can enter, open a cassette on a counter, and place it either on a hanger or in the processor without the risk of spilling chemicals on himself or herself or the cassette (Fig. 7.1). The darkroom should have a countertop large enough to open a 14 inch × 17 inch (35 cm × 43 cm) cassette, and the processing area should be removed from the dry film area so there is no chance of chemicals being transferred to the cassettes and screens. The technician must be able to walk into the darkroom, close the door, and fit inside without any possibility of bumping into the processor or wet tanks. Once the processor is in position and the tanks are filled, it is very easy to jostle the processor and cause chemicals to overflow from one tank to another or, worse still, to splash onto the control boards, destroying them completely and causing the processor to malfunction (Fig. 7.2). A minimum darkroom size of 5 feet (1.5 m) by 7 feet (2.13 m) is sufficient to position the processor or wet tanks. One extra foot (30 cm) in both directions would be an ideal minimum.

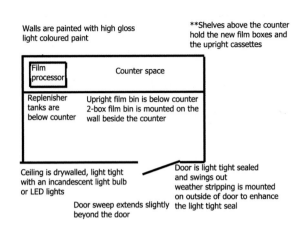

Walls are painted with high gloss light coloured paint

**Shelves above the counter hold the new film boxes and the upright cassettes

Film processor	Counter space
Replenisher tanks are below counter	Upright film bin is below counter 2-box film bin is mounted on the wall beside the counter

Ceiling is drywalled, light tight with an incandescent light bulb or LED lights

Door is light tight sealed and swings out weather stripping is mounted on outside of door to enhance the light tight seal

Door sweep extends slightly beyond the door

FIG. 7.1 A typical ideal darkroom layout. The wet side is on the left and the dry side on the right. Ventilation is achieved through a door vent and a ceiling exhaust fan that is light-tight.

FIG. 7.2 Chemicals spilled on the processor between the feed tray and the developer. This chemical could easily seep down onto the processing boards, causing a malfunction and an expensive repair.

◆ **APPLICATION INFORMATION**

A large-animal veterinarian installed an automatic processor in a darkroom in his basement. He did not bother with a safelight because he felt he could work quite well in the darkened room.

Then he called the consultant with a problem. Every time he turned on the processor, the replenishment pumps started to run and did not stop until he turned the processor off. The consultant told him to check the switches that the film contacts when exiting the feed tray (see Fig. 7.8C); the contacts were clean.

The consultant found that chemicals had spilled out of the developer tank and onto the main circuitry board at the front of the processor (see Fig. 7.2). This short-circuited the replenishment circuit, and the board was ruined and had to be replaced.

The veterinarian admitted that he had bumped into the processor a few times in the dark. The chemistry tanks are full when the processor is running and the racks are in place, so chemicals had spilled out of the developer and into the main circuitry. This was a large price to pay for having a small darkroom and no safelight.

The darkroom door should be hung to swing out from the darkroom. An inward-swinging door is not an option in a minimum-sized darkroom. Weather stripping around the entire frame of the door is essential to prevent light leaks. Placing the weather stripping on the outside of the door prevents it from being rubbed and worn by the door opening and closing over time. Weather stripping that overlaps the edge of the door by 1 inch (2.14 cm) creates a light seal that will last as long as the room is used as a darkroom. If the floor is uneven, a light-eliminating door sweep is essential.

The temperature in the darkroom should be maintained at 68° F (20° C), and the humidity should be maintained at 40% to 60%. The door to the darkroom should be left open when not in use. This practice will maintain the temperature

and humidity and will also ensure good airflow. If the darkroom is sealed too tightly, it may be difficult to close the door. A light-tight airflow pass-through is available.

The walls should be painted a light reflective color to take advantage of as much light as possible from the safelight. The countertop should be positioned between 29 inches (74 cm) and 33 inches (84 cm) above the floor.

The cassettes and film boxes must be stored upright and well away from the chemical storage (Fig. 7.3A). Ideally, a film bin will be mounted on the wall (Fig. 7.3B) to store the film out of the light and prevent accidental exposure. A metal film bin must be used if the processor and film are located in the radiography room (Fig. 7.3C). Scattered/secondary radiation will penetrate a plastic film bin unless the bin is located a minimum of 10 feet from the source of the scatter. Film should be used on a first in/first out basis so that the boxes are rotated systematically and the film does not become stale-dated.

Ideally, the replenishment tanks are positioned beneath the tabletop processor. If this is not possible, they should be accessible both for cleaning and for "topping up" chemicals. Chemicals should be stored in their original containers until they are used. Extra chemicals should not be stored in the darkroom but rather in an appropriate storage place in the facility.

The darkroom should be cleaned regularly as part of the quality assurance program in the clinic. Dust and dirt that accumulate on the processing tray will affect the film emulsion as it is being processed. The darkroom is not a cloakroom, and coats and linens should be stored elsewhere.

Darkroom Integrity

Light is very pervasive, and it is vital that all light is eliminated in the darkroom. The door of the darkroom must be light-tight, and the darkroom must be completely dark. **This is non-negotiable.** Even if the human eye does not readily see the light, the film will "see" it instantly and record it as fog.

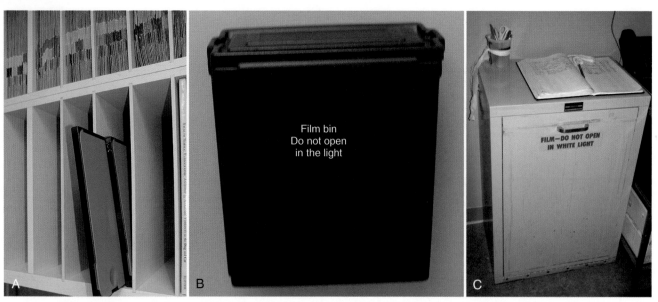

FIG. 7.3 A, Cassettes are stored upright above the processor. The films are filed above the cassettes. **B,** A plastic film bin for use in the darkroom is hung on the wall. **C,** A full-sized steel bin sits on the floor and is positioned in the dual-purpose radiography/processing room.

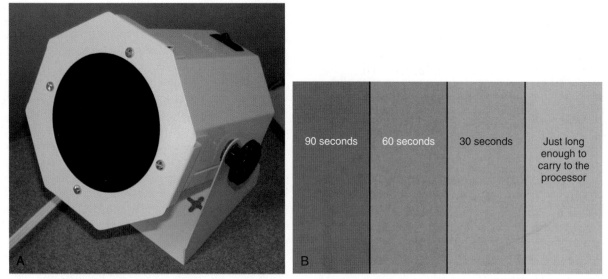

FIG. 7.4 A, A red light–emitting safelight. The filter is very important and must match the spectral sensitivity of the film. **B,** Safelight test. The film has been preexposed and placed beneath a cassette in the darkroom. The exposure time has allowed the film to fog. The safelight should be checked and altered, and then the test should be repeated.

The human eye requires about 5 to 8 minutes to adjust to darkness after being exposed to a lighted room. If the door is closed and the technician sees no visible light leaks after 5 to 8 minutes of moving about in the pitch-black dark, the integrity of the darkroom is confirmed. Complete instructions for the darkroom integrity test are included in Chapter 9.

Safelight Specifications

Film responds to color at the ultraviolet/blue-green side of the spectrum. Safelights manufactured before 1981 were Wratten series 2B red-brown. Once green light–receiving films appeared on the market, the safelight color had to change because the red-brown tint had a yellow component and the color green is made up of blue and yellow. The most common film in use today is the green-receiving film; blue-receiving film is being phased out. Therefore when a facility purchases or replaces a safelight, the light emitted from the safelight should be dark red, with no orange or yellow (Fig. 7.4A). The safelight should be mounted on the wall a minimum of 4 feet (1.22 m) above the working surface where cassettes are loaded and unloaded.

Properly processed film will be completely clear, with only the base + fog on it. The optical density will be less than 0.10. Fig. 7.4B shows the results of a safelight test in which there was a definite problem with the positioning or wattage of the safelight. For complete instructions for performing a safelight test, see Chapter 9.

Film Identifiers

The traditional veterinary identification (ID) labels and labeling tape are slowly being phased out because they are not as efficient now that a lead replacement material is being used to produce the labeling tape (Fig. 7.5A). Individual lead lettering is certainly sharper but very time consuming because each patient's information must be set up one letter at a time (Fig. 7.5B).

An electric or battery-operated photoidentifier is preferable, and the information is much clearer on the images than those produced by the older method. An electric or battery-operated photoidentifier works in conjunction with the cassettes (Fig. 7.5C). A light cardstock or standard typing paper is used with a template to write or type the information. Fig. 7.5D is an example of a label that has been typed. A black marker fine-point pen can also be used.

The following steps must be taken before using the labeler:

1. Choose a corner of every cassette, and put a black label over each screen in the appropriate corner inside the cassette. The label material can be black cardstock or even blackened x-ray film held in place with double-sided sticky tape. These blockers will prevent the radiation from affecting the screen in that area. Use the same label position on every cassette in the facility.
2. Label the cassettes on the outside over the blocked-off portion so that patient anatomy and identifying markers are not positioned over the blocker.
3. ID labels must be printed and include the patient's name, date, ID number, and the name and address of the veterinary facility. This is required legal information in most countries and must be visible on each film.
4. Once the film is exposed, take it to the darkroom and remove it from the cassette. Place the film in the photoidentifier and press down on the lid of the identifier. This will turn on a timed light flash, which exposes the film through the printed label and imprints the label information onto the film.
5. The film is now processed normally.

With this method, each film is identified before processing. This is by far the most efficient method of identifying individual films.

Secondary film identifiers such as right and left markers, positioning markers (VD, DV, upright), and time of day must all be positioned within the radiation area and must be clearly identifiable (Fig. 7.5E).

Manual (Nonautomatic) Processing

Some low-volume sites still process film manually. The chemicals used in manual processing are the same as for automatic processing, except that the temperature and time are very different (Fig. 7.6A and Table 7.4).

Safety and Protocols

Cleanliness is essential during film processing because it is very easy to splash chemicals onto the cassettes and screens. In the manual processing area, the cassettes must never be left open on the counter.

Chemical fumes can be irritating, and the chemicals are dangerous to ingest or splash into one's eyes. Safety glasses must be worn by anyone processing film or replenishing chemicals (see WHMIS/OSHA guidelines). A 14 inch × 17 inch (35 cm × 43 cm) film is lifted almost parallel with the eyes when the hangers are moved from tank to tank. It is very important that the technician is careful not to splash chemicals during this procedure.

The wet tanks are always checked for the correct temperature (68° F [20° C]), and the chemicals are agitated immediately before processing the films. This is the only time the chemicals are agitated. Agitating the chemicals before radiography is premature, and the chemicals will have settled by the time the film is introduced into the tanks.

Equipment

Wet Tanks

The welds on a stainless steel tank must also be stainless steel. If the tanks are not welded correctly, the welding material will corrode in the first few weeks. The chemistry will be contaminated, and the wash water will always be cloudy and rust colored. After that the tank will start to leak through pinpoint holes in the welding material.

An alternative tank construction is heavy plastic. After about 10 to 15 years the plastic will absorb chemicals and leach out into fresh developer. This eventually will contaminate the fresh chemicals within days or even hours.

◆ APPLICATION INFORMATION

A consultant received a frantic call from a veterinarian who had changed the chemicals in the developer before radiographing a dog that had swallowed a peach pit. The dog had not eaten for several days and was in distress, and the veterinarian needed to know the location of the peach pit. When he took the films out of the developer, there was a very faint image—not nearly diagnostic. Overlying the image was a "watercolor" artifact of every color of the rainbow. Reds, yellows, blues, purples, and blacks were running down the film. He took several more films and then searched for help.

The consultant was driving near the hospital when she received the call and by total coincidence had a stainless steel, 5-gallon processing tank in her car. She drove to the hospital and, together with the veterinary staff, mixed new chemistry in the darkroom. The images were perfect, the peach pit was located, and the patient did well.

The developer drained out of the old tank was severely contaminated. They switched out the stainless steel tank and placed it in the plastic main tank, and the next day they did the same thing with the fixer tank. The hospital never again had a problem with contaminated chemistry.

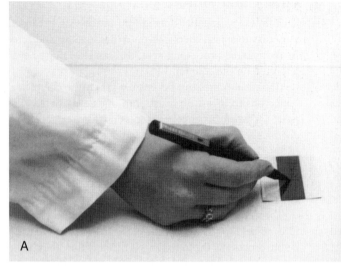

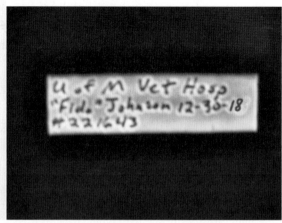

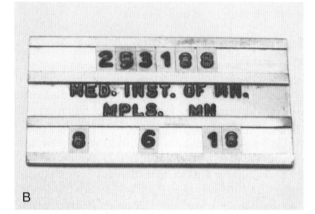

Eastern Veterinary Hospital

1234 Pet Hospital Way, Akron, Ohio, 46777

Name:	Weasily Whiskas Brown	
Views:	VD Chest, Lateral Chest	
Date:	December 21, 2017	DVM: Dr McHappy

Printed ID Label with two different labels
used for two different patients

Eastern Veterinary Hospital

1234 Pet Hospital Way, Akron, Ohio 46777

Name:	I Curious Tiberius Brown	
Views:	VD Abdomen, Lateral Abdomen	
Date:	December 21, 2017	DVM: DR McNice

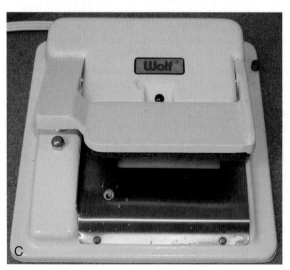

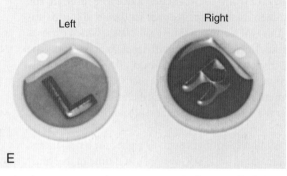

Left   Right

FIG. 7.5 A, A leaded tape labeler. After the identification details are written on the tape, it is attached to a small plastic and aluminum filter that is color-graded according to the kilovoltage that is used. It is then placed on the table within the collimated area. **B,** A metal marker. The metal is usually aluminum, and the individual letters are lead. The identifying letters are loaded into the guide for each individual patient. The marker is then placed on the tabletop within the collimated area. **C,** An electric ID labeler ready to be used. An ID card is written up and placed in the unit. The film is placed in the unit and the top is pressed down, which turns on a light. The image of the marker is imprinted onto the film. The film is then processed normally. **D,** An example of an ID label to be cut apart and used with the ID labeler in **C. E,** Left and right markers. The shape is less important than the thickness of the lead. They must be visible on every image.

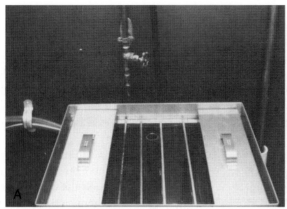
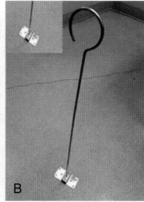

FIG. 7.6 A, Manual processing tank. Lids cover the developer tank *(left)* and the fixer tank *(right)*. The common wash tank is in the middle. Temperature is maintained by circulating water in the wash at the correct temperature. **B,** A stainless steel stir rod. Note the flat plate at the bottom with holes *(see inset)*. The stir rod is used in an up-and-down motion to bring the chemicals up from the bottom of the tank.

TABLE 7.4	Development/Fixer/Washing Guidelines*		
PROCESS	**TIME**		**TEMPERATURE**
Developer	4 minutes with agitation		68°F (20°C)
Rinse*	15–30 sec with agitation		68°F (20°C)
Fixing	8 minutes with agitation		68°F (20°C)
Washing	12 minutes with agitation		68°F (20°C)

*Applies to manual processing only.

Stir Rods

One stir rod is all that is necessary, provided that it is used in the correct order: developer first, then fixer, then wash (Fig. 7.6B). The stir stick may be rinsed between the developer and the fixer, but it is not essential. The stir stick must move sequentially through the developer →fixer → wash—not the other way around—otherwise fixer will be brought back into the developer on the stir rod. This can cause an artifact called *dichroic fog.*

The stir stick must be made of stainless steel. Wooden paddles, stir rods, and broom handles will all absorb chemicals

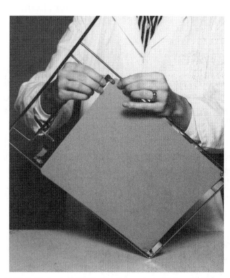

FIG. 7.7 The film is placed in a hanger for manual processing. The bottom clips are loaded first and then the spring clips are attached.

that will be leached out when used to stir fresh chemicals. The end of the stir rod is a flat plate with holes punched through it. The technician stirs the chemicals using an up-and-down motion. This up-and-down motion reduces the tendency for the chemicals to overflow the tanks, but it also brings the stratified liquids up from the bottom of the tank to mix thoroughly. Ten to 15 vertical motions are all that is necessary to completely mix the chemicals.

Film Hangers

Once the film is removed from the cassette and identified (if a photo ID labeler is used), it is then hung on a film hanger (Fig. 7.7) in preparation for processing. Film hangers have flexible clips at the top and stationary clips at the bottom. The film is hung on the stationary clips first and then on the flexible (spring-equipped) clips at the top. Some hangers have channels into which the film is slid. These are rare, however, and are also difficult to keep clean.

Developing the Image

Developing the image is the first step in processing the film. The purpose of the developer is to cause the latent image to become a manifest image. This change is achieved by immersing the film in a chemical solution. The developer has two main components and several other auxiliary components (see Table 7.2).

The unexposed areas of the film are not affected unless the film is left in the developer for too long. If this occurs, the unexposed areas will start to react to the developer, and the film will increase in overall density (developer fog).

The hanger is held by the top (handle), and the film is introduced into the chemicals slowly and steadily. Once the film is completely immersed, it is agitated slowly in an up-and-down motion several times to ensure that any air bubbles that have entered with the film are removed. The timer is set for *4 minutes.* At 2 minutes the film is agitated up and down once again. This moves away the used chemicals directly next to the film and places fresher chemicals against the film.

◆ APPLICATION INFORMATION

With manual processing, it is very important that the technical factors used to produce the image are correct. The film must take the correct length of time to process because the hydroquinone takes longer to start affecting the emulsion than does the phenidone. Therefore if the film is removed too early, the full effect of blackening the image will not occur. "Overexposing and underdeveloping" is not a good practice; safe exposure factors must be practiced in all facilities.

Rinsing the Film

At 4 minutes, the film is agitated up and down two to four times and then moved to the intermediary wash tank. It is agitated two to four times in the wash tank to arrest the development and remove some of the developer, and then it is placed in the fixer tank.

Fixing the Film

Fixing the image to the film is the third step in manual processing. Here the image is made visible by removing all of the emulsion that has not been affected by radiation and subsequent developing.

The film is placed into the fixer tank using the same method: introduced slowly and steadily and then agitated up and down. This agitation will remove air bubbles that have been carried into the fixer and remain on the film.

The timer is set for *8 minutes.* At 2 minutes the light may be turned on and the film may be checked. If there is still unexposed emulsion on the film, the fixer is no longer fresh and should be changed once the films are processed. At 4 minutes, the film should have cleared completely and may be viewed momentarily on an illuminator by the staff.

Once the film is reviewed, it must be put back into the fixer to complete the fixing process. It is essential that the fixing process be completed to ensure the archival quality of the image.

Washing the Film

The film is removed from the fixer and lowered into the wash tank. It is preferable for the wash tank to have flowing water. Ideally, the water should enter from the bottom of the tank and exit from the top through a stand pipe placed in the drain.

The entire film, including the hangers, must be immersed in each solution. The fixer cleans the developer out of the clips of the hangers, and the wash removes the fixer from the hangers and leaves them clean for the next film.

As the clean water flows over the film, it is washed by a diffusion process. The chemicals in the fixer are diffused into the wash water. The water must move around the film so that a concentration of fixer does not remain within the emulsion of the film.

Hanging the films in static clean water will work only if the films are agitated frequently during the wash time. The wash time is *12 minutes* with flowing water. Once again, it is important to wash the films to ensure archival quality. If the used fixer is not removed, the films will turn yellow-brown within weeks (see Fig. 7.26 in the image gallery at the end of the chapter).

Running a hose over the films for 2 to 3 minutes in a bathtub is not sufficient to wash the films thoroughly. This problem is evident on a film reviewed several weeks after it has been dried and stored. Sulfiding and staining are the result of poor washing.

It is vitally important to remove the films from the wash water and place them on the drying rack within a maximum 2 to 3 hours of washing (see the Application Information box).

◆ APPLICATION INFORMATION

The consultant received a phone call from a very worried client. A cat had been brought into the clinic late the night before, and the radiographs showed a fractured leg, which the veterinarian set and immobilized in a cast. Postreduction films were taken, and the fractured bones were in perfect alignment.

The cat was stabilized, and the veterinary staff went home. The next morning the veterinary technician realized that she had forgotten to take the films out of the wash tank the previous night. The images were completely gone, and the film base was completely clear.

The problem was that in the rush to process the films, the fixer had not been stirred correctly and the hardener had not affected the emulsion. The emulsion just slid off the film base overnight.

Drying the Film

If the processing is completed correctly, there are no artifacts on the films. The drying process takes several hours because even though the films feel dry to the touch, the emulsion takes longer to dry completely. If the films are placed in the envelopes too soon, they will stick together and will be impossible to separate.

The film must be dried either by hanging the films in a dryer cabinet or by allowing them to dry naturally in the air of the clinic. Drying removes 85% to 90% of the moisture in the film emulsion. If too much moisture is removed, the emulsion will crack, compromising the quality of the image.

The film is now ready to be reviewed and stored permanently.

Further Notes

Timing the exposure of the films to the chemicals and maintaining the temperature of the chemicals is very important, particularly in manual (nonautomatic) processing. If the developer solution is overheated or the film is left in the solution for an extended time, the unexposed crystals start to react to the solution and "developer fog" occurs.

Chemical manufacturers produce a solution that is optimized for manual processing at 68°F (20°C). It is not a coincidence that this is also the average room temperature in a veterinary clinic. The chemicals do not need to be heated or cooled before use.

The technique chart should be optimized so the film is processed at 4 minutes in the manual developer at 68°F (20°C). If the image appears too quickly or too slowly, the technical factors should be adjusted, not the temperature of the chemicals. The hydroquinone works slowly to build up the blacks and therefore enhance the contrast of the image. If the solution is either too hot or too cold, the hydroquinone does not function correctly and the image is compromised.

Automatic Processing

Equipment

The automatic processor facilitates the routine of producing a manifest image on the film. It must do so quickly, efficiently, and without imprinting an artifact or scratching the emulsion off the film during the process. Most automatic processors now are sold as "90-second" processors, which means that the film enters the processor and exits within 90 seconds (Fig. 7.8A).

Because processors are smaller and fit nicely on a table or countertop, this arrangement works very nicely for veterinary hospitals.

Feed Tray

The feed tray is situated at the entrance of the processor (Fig. 7.8B). The film is placed either horizontally or vertically on this tray, and from there it is accepted into the processor by means of the motor drive. It is essential that the film is placed squarely on the tray. When a film enters the feed tray, it is within 1 to 2 inches (2.5 to 5 cm) of the developer.

Once the film enters the processor, it *must not, under any circumstances,* be drawn back onto the tray:

- Typically, the replenishment switches are situated just at the edge of the entrance to the processor (Fig. 7.8C). If the film is drawn back, it will deposit developer onto these switches. Developer becomes very sticky when it dries. If even one of the replenishment switches sticks open, it will pump the replenishment chemicals continuously through the processor until the tanks are empty. If this problem is not noticed in time, the pump will burn out because there are no chemicals flowing through it.
- If the film is pulled backward after it has entered the developer rack, it may lift the rack off the gears and not only damage the gears but also compromise the position of the rack for the next film.
- If the film has entered the developer and is drawn backward onto the tray, the developer solution is then smeared on the tray. There it will adversely affect the next film that is placed on the feed tray.

The feed tray may be stainless steel or plastic. Either way, if the air in the darkroom is dry, static may build up on the tray and discharge when a film is placed on it. The feed tray should be wiped with a fabric softener cloth at the beginning of the day to prevent static buildup (see Fig. 7.27 in the image gallery at the end of the chapter).

The processor is essentially an assembly line in which the film is drawn across a series of rollers through the developer, fixer, and wash tanks. The rollers in series from a typical processor are shown in Fig. 7.8D.

The film is affected by several systems once it enters the processor. Each system is vital to the production of the final image (Table 7.5).

TABLE 7.5	Automatic Processor Systems
SYSTEM	**FUNCTION**
Transport system	Chain or gear mechanism moves the rollers by a process of gears and drive shaft in order to transport the film through the processor (see Fig. 7.9).
Replenishment	Two pumps are set to replenish the chemicals (developer and fixer) so that it maintains consistent pH and solution concentration throughout the day.
Recirculation	Mixes the fresh chemicals with the working solutions so that the films are processed evenly.
Thermostats	Two—maintain a consistent temperature in the working solution and in the dryer.
Silver recovery	Not part of the processor, but an essential unit placed in the outgoing fixer line.

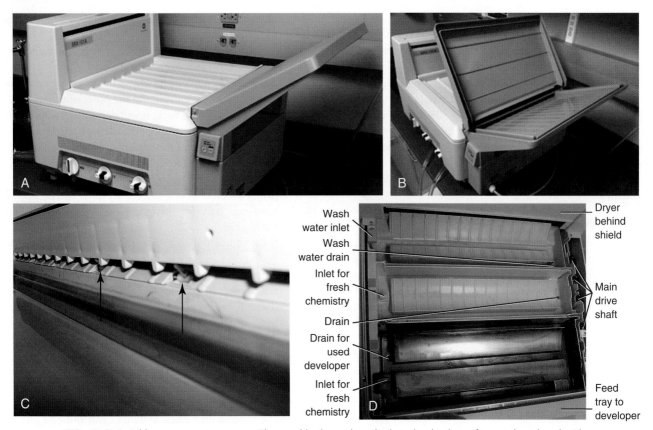

FIG. 7.8 A, Tabletop automatic processor. The round knobs on the side drain the developer, fixer, and wash tanks. The feed tray is to the right. The processed film will drop out of the dryer slot on the left onto the top of the processor. **B,** Automatic processor feed tray. The film to be processed is placed on the tray and the lid is closed, providing a light-tight seal. **C,** On this processor, four small fingers *(arrows point to two of them)* are pressed down when the film slides through the feed tray into the developer. The replenishment pumps stay activated while these fingers are depressed. **D,** The Konica SRX-101A Processor *(top view)* with the lid and racks removed.

Film Transport

The processor must be built so all rollers move at the same speed and are positioned to transport the film evenly and continuously with no hesitation through the developer, fixer, and wash and then into the dryer (Fig. 7.9). The rollers that transport the film must be close enough together to move the film but far enough apart that they transport the film without imprinting a pressure artifact or otherwise scratching the emulsion. The rollers must be made of the right material so they are firm enough to transport the film without absorbing chemicals and imprinting the stale chemicals onto films processed later in the day. In addition, they must be soft enough that they do not damage the fragile wet emulsion.

Every time a roller touches the film, there is the possibility of an artifact or damage to the fragile emulsion. The main drive motor must be high quality to ensure that it runs evenly and consistently for many years. The Teflon gears must be solid and resist cracking or breaking (see Fig. 7.9B).

There are several varieties of film processor on the market. The unit used to demonstrate the internal workings in this text is a Konica model SRX 101A. The film is guided by the rollers, and the curves and turns it must make are guided mostly by sheets of high-grade stainless steel or high-grade smooth plastic. These "guide shoes" have raised ridges that hold the film away from the turnarounds as it is transported

through the processor (see Fig. 7.9A). This particular method of travel is called *undulating* because the film is guided in a wavelike path (Fig. 7.10).

Larger processors use a system of offset rollers and a vertical transport system. The film enters the processor and is transported by means of the entrance roller assembly into the developer tank (Fig. 7.11). At the bottom and top of each turn, a large roller (called a *sun roller*) turns the film 180 degrees and sends it back up the assembly to meet a guide shoe at the top, which then turns it back down through the fixer. A unit of this size is most efficient when it is processing 150 films per hour. A typical veterinary clinic, even a busy clinic, does not handle that volume of films, and so a tabletop processor is quite adequate.

The most efficient and easiest processor to maintain is one with very few rollers and an efficient and reliable transport system. The Konica SRX model (see Fig. 7.8D) is an example of this type of processor. There are few rollers, and each one is easy to see and access if there is a problem. The roller assembly is fairly easy to take apart and service because each rack assembly is easily lifted out of the processor and washed. Daily maintenance is quite simple.

The main drive motor on a tabletop processor is connected to a simple geared shaft that fits to the gears on the roller assembly (see Fig. 7.9). This arrangement ensures that all

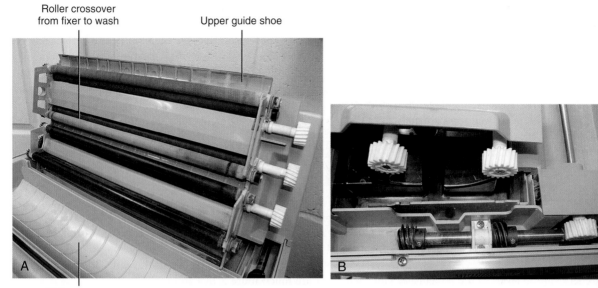

Roller crossover
from fixer to wash　　　　Upper guide shoe

This acts as a
lower guide shoe

FIG. 7.9 A, The transport system. This figure shows the developer fixer rack tilted out of the processor to show the gears—which will mesh with the drive shaft when it is put in place—and the rollers. **B,** A closeup of the main drive shaft. The gears will mesh with the windings on the shaft, allowing each roller to move steadily and consistently without hesitation. The gears are lifted on the left and are in place on the right.

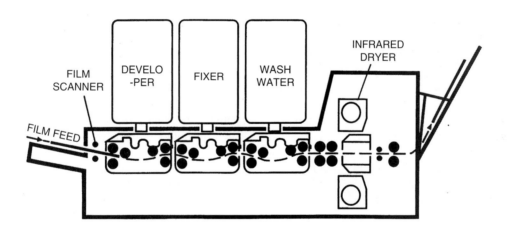

FIG. 7.10 A tabletop processor showing undulating film travel. The line drawing is of an Agfa tabletop processor. The large jugs behind the processor are the replenishment tanks.

rollers turn at exactly the same speed. A broken or worn gear may cause an inconsistency in the rotation of the gears. This problem is easily identified by lifting the lid of the processor and watching for a hesitation or "bumping" of the rack assembly.

? POINTS TO PONDER

Every time a roller comes into contact with the film, it has the potential to damage the emulsion and imprint an artifact on the film. The more rollers there are, the easier it is for them to damage films. Cleanliness and quality control of the processor are vital, especially if the processor has many rollers. In most veterinary facilities, tabletop processors work well. It is best to purchase a processor with as few rollers as possible.

Chemical Replenishment

The chemicals in the working tanks become exhausted as the chemicals interact with the silver halides in the emulsion of the film. The developer also interacts with air, which reduces its effectiveness. The fixer is weakened from the silver halides that it removes from the film base and by the introduction of developer carried over in the film emulsion.

The film is processed by the chemicals in the individual tanks. It is important that fresh chemicals are introduced as the old, used chemicals are removed. The dimensions of the film and the method by which they are fed into the feed tray determine the amount of replenishment. The switches for replenishment are situated at the back end of the processor, immediately below the feed tray (Fig. 7.12A). Every processor built after 2000 will have a method of monitoring the replenishment, whether it is inside the processor itself or outside, as is the case with the Konica.

The tanks that hold the fresh chemicals are situated close to the processor and are joined by tubing and a pump within the processor that supplies the fresh chemicals when needed (Fig. 7.12B). There are two replenishment pumps. One pump for the developer is set to deliver approximately 60 mL of chemicals for every 14 inches (35 cm) of film. The second pump for the fixer is set to deliver approximately 110 mL of chemicals for every 14 inches (35 cm) of film. The amounts of chemicals are different because the film entering the developer is dry and is affected only by the developer. The film then carries contaminant (developer) into the fixer and also removes fixer when it leaves. Therefore the fixer requires more replenishment to keep it fresh and to replenish what is removed.

A quick check on the levels in the replenisher tanks will show that the fixer level drops almost twice as fast as the developer level. If this is not occurring, the lines and pumps should be checked for kinks or bends that are preventing the chemicals from flowing correctly.

A second form of replenishment is called *"flood replenishing"* in which the chemicals are replenished at timed intervals independent of the amount of film used. This arrangement works well if a low amount of film is being processed through a large processor. Because the volume of chemicals is great and the film volume is low, it is much more difficult to maintain stability and concentration of the chemicals. This system is not available on many tabletop processors but it is available on most free-standing processors.

The replenishment tanks are normally positioned beneath the counter that holds the processor (see Fig. 7.12B). The developer and fixer tanks must be monitored continually so the chemicals do not reach abnormally low levels or empty completely.

Chemical Recirculation

When fresh chemicals are delivered to the working tank, they must be introduced gradually and in a portion of the processor separate from where the film is traveling. The fresh chemicals are much more active and will react more quickly with the emulsion on the film. This can cause a plus-density artifact on the film—a pattern of the spray of the new chemicals across the film (see Fig. 7.25 in the image gallery at the end of the chapter).

In some tabletop processors, the working chemicals in the processing tanks are directed into an auxiliary tank within the processor. It is here that the fresh chemicals are introduced to the working chemicals, and together they enter the working tank. Some processors have a baffle system so the chemicals are introduced and immediately directed away from the film being processed.

Thermostat

There are two main thermostats in the processor. One maintains the temperature of the chemicals, and the other maintains the temperature of the dryer:

- The typical temperature of the developer and fixer solutions is 93°F (34°C).
- The typical dryer temperature is 131°F (55°C).

It must be noted that the thermostat does not have a cooling function. If the temperature in the darkroom is very hot, the thermostat will not cool the chemicals.

Heating coils may be placed in the bottom of the developer and fixer tanks, or the heaters may be placed in the

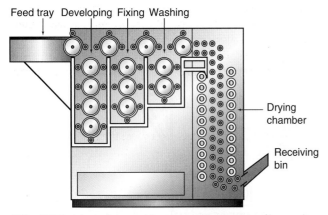

Feed tray Developing Fixing Washing

Drying chamber

Receiving bin

FIG. 7.11 A large floor-model processor demonstrating film traveling through the three tanks and into a long dryer on the right. The film exits into a bin almost at floor level. (From Fauber TL. *Radiographic Imaging and Exposure*, 5th ed. St. Louis: Mosby; 2017.)

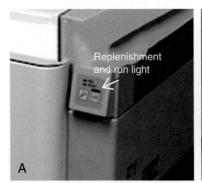

Replenishment and run light

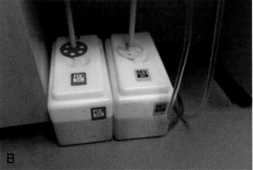

FIG. 7.12 **A**, The replenishment and run lights on this processor are at the front and easily accessed. **B**, The developer *(left)* and fixer *(right)* replenishment tanks are stored beneath the processor.

recirculation system. It is essential to maintain a constant temperature in the developer and fixer tanks because the activity of the processing solutions depends directly on the temperature.

The dryer temperature is important to ensure that the films exiting the dryer are dry and not sticky to the touch. They must not be overheated or the emulsion may crack and split.

Dryer System

The rollers in the dryer must be suitable to transport the film while it dries, and the temperature must be hot enough to dry out about 80% of the moisture. If the film is dried too much, the emulsion will crack and degrade the image. If the film is not dried sufficiently, it will be sticky to the touch, and if several films are laid on top of each other, they will stick together and be impossible to break apart.

The ideal dryer temperature depends very much on how long the film will be traveling through the dryer. The temperature will be noted in the instruction manual of each processor or can be found online by searching for the make and model of the processor.

Developing the Image

The chemistry used in the automatic processor is the same as the chemistry used in manual processing. The typical temperature is 34°C (93°F). The length of time that the film is in the developer solution is set up for every individual processor and programmed so the chemicals have time to react sufficiently to optimize the image. As noted in the replenishment section, the rates of replenishment are preset to preserve the correct concentrations of developer and fixer.

The image is in the formation stage while in the developer, and many problems can occur during this process. In fact, approximately 80% of processing artifacts occur during the development stage. The image may be deleted in places where the latent image undergoes pressure from a swollen roller, or it may acquire density from other factors. The image gallery at the end of this chapter illustrates developer artifacts.

Fixing the Film

The main purpose of the fixer (see Table 7.3) is to remove the unexposed silver halide from the film base and ensure that the image that has been developed remains intact and permanent. The fixer also stops the development of any unexposed crystals of silver halide (by removing them from the film base) and it hardens the image to the base. The image is "fixed" onto the base by a two-stage process:

1. Clearing—the unexposed emulsion is cleared from the film base.
2. Fixing—the remaining emulsion is stabilized onto the base.

Fixing occurs after developing and stabilizes the emulsion to the base. The emulsion before this stage is very thin and easily marked or scratched off the base. If the film is not fixed correctly, it exits the processor with a milky or even pink appearances. (See Fig. 7.23 and other fixer artifacts in the image gallery at the end of the chapter).

Washing the Film

The film travels through the fixer and into the wash tank. It must be thoroughly washed to preserve its archival quality. Staining or sulfiding results if the film is not washed with flowing water. (See Fig. 7.26 in the image gallery at the end of this chapter.)

The wash should provide clean water that flows through the processor as the films are being washed. Washing takes place by a process called *diffusion*. The wash water contains less thiosulfate than the fixer, and so the chemicals in the fixer are diffused into the wash water. The water must move about the film so a concentration of fixer does not build up next to the film. This is achieved by the action of the rollers and fresh water running through the processor.

If the wash water is not turned on, the film will appear "dirty" in reflected light. It may be "sticky" when touched. Sulfiding and staining are the result of poor washing and are also evident on a film that is reviewed several weeks after it has been dried and stored. To review artifacts connected with washing the film, please review the image gallery at the end of this chapter.

Drying the Film

As noted, earlier, the dryer temperature should be set to ensure that the films are not tacky or sticky. Approximately 85% to 95% of the moisture should be removed from the films as they travel through the dryer. If they are too hot when they emerge, the film base may become fragile and crack.

If the dryer temperature is optimized and the films are still slightly damp, adjusting the replenishment rates in the processor may solve the issue.

Silver Recovery

It is the function of the fixer to remove the unexposed silver halides from the film base (Fig. 7.13), resulting in a high

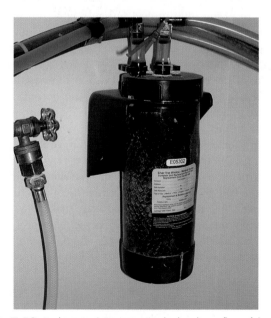

FIG. 7.13 A silver recovery unit is attached to the outflow of the fixer tank.

concentration of silver halides floating in the fixer. If this silver is not removed from the fixer and the fixer is not correctly replenished, the silver may plate out onto the film. (See Fig. 7.22 in the image gallery at the end of the chapter.) A silver recovery unit removes the silver from the effluent of the processor as it exits the fixer tank.

◆ **APPLICATION INFORMATION**

A good method to test whether the silver recovery unit needs to be replaced is to place a copper penny or a piece of copper pipe in its outflow. The copper penny is electrolytic and attracts the silver ions, which plate onto the copper. If the copper turns silver, it is time to replace the cartridge.

Metallic Replacement

The silver recovery unit typically used in veterinary clinics consists of a glass jar containing steel wool. The effluent from the fixer tank enters the jar on one side and is directed through the steel wool. The acidic fixer breaks down the the iron in steel wool and replaces it with silver. The iron oxides are replaced by silver as it precipitates onto the remaining steel.

Electrolysis

A second method of silver recovery is an electrolytic process that is used mainly for large-volume units. A very low current flows through a unit equipped with metal plates, and the negatively charged silver ions bind to the plates. This method is the easiest way to collect the metallic silver, but if the current is flowing and there is no silver, the fixer may start to break down. Because the main component of fixer is sulfur, a terrible odor may result as it starts to break down. This process is called *sulfiding*, and the smell is exactly the same as rotten eggs.

Film Storage

After processing, the finished image is now available for viewing and storage. Films should be stored in individual envelopes specific to each patient. They should be stored upright in slotted shelves (Fig. 7.14). Films contain a fair amount of silver and are very heavy to sort through if they are stored in a pile. Because the envelopes rarely contain only one size of film, the piles become unwieldy if they are not stored correctly.

Film should be stored in a temperature-controlled area (68° F [20° C]). Ideal humidity in the storage room is 40% to 60%. If the humidity is too high, the emulsion absorbs the moisture and the films stick together. They are virtually impossible to separate unless they are soaked in water. However, if there was insufficient hardener in the processing chemicals, soaking the films in water will only serve to lift the emulsion off the base.

Image Artifacts

Artifacts may be categorized into three groups: equipment artifacts, processing artifacts, and handling artifacts.

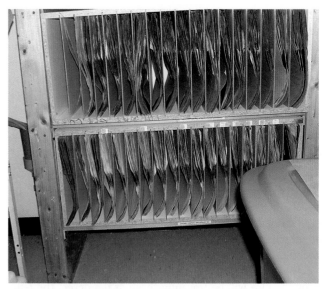

FIG. 7.14 These films are stored alphabetically in a solid wood cabinet in the darkroom.

Processing is the single greatest cause of artifacts on the films. As already stated, 98% of all film artifacts are due to problems with processing. With automatic processing, the emulsion is softened and the rollers must touch the film as they transport it from tank to tank. The distance between the rollers is very narrow, and if a roller should swell, it will place a plus-density or minus-density mark on the film.

Artifacts are categorized as visible by reflected light (looking at the film as a page out of a book) or by transmitted light (reviewing a film hung on an illuminator). Most artifacts are visible by transmitted light. Artifacts that are visible by reflected light are very difficult to illustrate in a textbook and consist mainly of the following:

◆ **APPLICATION INFORMATION**

The darkroom of a brand-new veterinary hospital was equipped with an automatic processor, cassettes, and film. Business was slow at first, and even though the processor had been set up correctly, it was 6 weeks before a patient arrived and radiographs were taken.

The films turned out gray and washed out, and subsequent films showed only a brief outline. A consultant was called, and she checked the x-ray unit and found that exposures were producing x-rays and the calibration was in order.

Next she checked the chemistry. The developer was dark brown, almost black. The processor had been used on the day the hospital opened to confirm the settings on the technique chart. The chemistry was heated and produced excellent images the first day but then sat and oxidized slowly over the next 6 weeks. As a result, the developer in the processor was completely contaminated and had to be cleared out from both the working tank and the replenishment tank.

New fresh chemistry was installed, and the resulting images were excellent.

- Smear artifacts from water drips after the film is processed
- Dichroic fog from fixer that has leaked into the developer; the fixer will eventually contaminate the developer but, initially, the films will come out of the automatic processor with an array of colors visible by reflected light

Summary

This chapter has discussed image processing and all of the protocols and problems associated with chemicals, films, screens, and cassettes. We also discussed artifacts and the situations that cause them. The artifacts are well represented by the quotation at the very beginning of this chapter.

Image Gallery

Figs. 7.15 to 7.30 have been collected over many years but are all possible with today's technology.

Equipment Artifacts

The following equipment malfunctions create artifacts:
- Collimator parts on the window (Fig. 7.15)
- Grid artifacts (see Chapter 6)
- Spilled chemicals (Fig. 7.16)

Processing Artifacts

Artifacts are possible throughout the entire processing cycle. Occasionally several overlapping artifacts make a diagnosis impossible. Fig. 7.17 displays handling, pickoff, and darkroom fog artifacts along with incorrect technical factors.

Transport Artifacts

- *Plus density.* These marks are darker than the surrounding emulsion.
- *Minus density.* These marks are lighter than the surrounding emulsion but still maintain emulsion (see Fig. 7.19).
- *Scratch marks.* The emulsion is removed from the base either before processing or within the processor.
- *Pick-off.* The emulsion is picked off (removed from) the film base and redeposited on another area of the film, leaving a tiny hole in the emulsion and therefore in the image. This problem is not as evident on double-emulsion film as on single-emulsion film (Fig. 7.18).

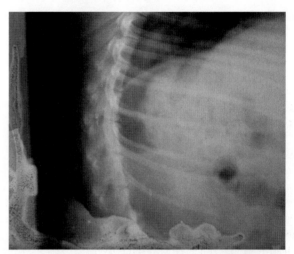

FIG. 7.16 Spilled barium seeped beneath the front screen, and its shape was superimposed on the image. This artifact was visible on every image taken using this cassette.

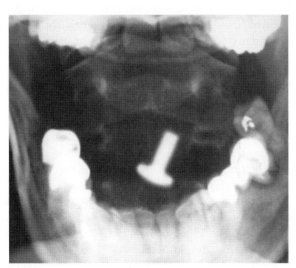

FIG. 7.15 An example of an equipment artifact. A collimator screw on the Plexiglas cover appears superimposed on a radiograph. The small screw fell out of the collimator shutter onto the collimator window. It was not noticed until the image was processed. Because of the distance to the patient, it is also magnified.

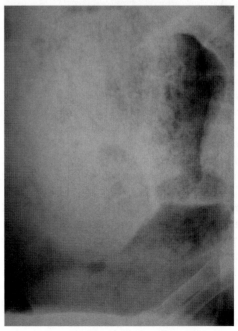

FIG. 7.17 A radiograph of a goat abdomen. This image has many artifacts: technique, handling, and processing.

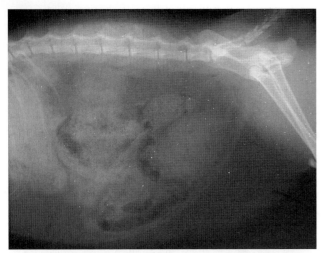

FIG. 7.18 Pickoff (visible as very small, clear "dots" on the film) occurs when the processor rollers are not clean. The emulsion is picked off by the dirt on the rollers and usually deposited somewhere else on the film.

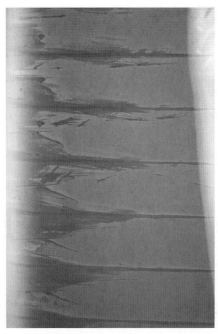

FIG. 7.20 Pi lines caused by wet entrance rollers, which were washed but not dried and therefore imprinted their dampness onto this image.

FIG. 7.19 Pi lines are caused by a swelling of the processor roller. They may be either plus-density or minus-density lines. The roller is easily identified from the measurement of the circumference of the roller; hence the name "pi."

- *Chatter.* This artifact occurs when two or more gears need to be replaced. The plus-density or minus-density marks are not deposited in a specific pattern. They may be similar to pi lines but are randomly spaced.
- *Pi lines.* These plus-density marks are specific to the circumference of the roller that caused the artifact (hence the term *pi*, the mathematical constant related to a circle's circumference) (Fig. 7.19). Pi lines are not a diagnosis of the problem but are rather the result of a problem that must be identified, such as the following:
  - *Hesitation marks.* These can occur when the rollers move unevenly and the film hesitates slightly. These marks can be mild (plus-density or minus-density lines) or severe (the emulsion is removed from the base).
  - *Wet entrance rollers.* Pi lines can occur when the entrance rollers are not dried after cleaning and before a film is

processed (Fig. 7.20). The image of the wet roller is imprinted on the film.
- *Guide shoe marks.* These artifacts appear as fine lines on either the leading edge or trailing edge of the film and are caused by the "snapping" of the film against the film guides as it travels from one tank to the next. They can be matched against the guide shoe ridges in the processor.

Chemical Artifacts

- *Dichroic fog.* The film appears to have an oily pattern of color in reflected light. This is caused by of fixer leaking or dripping back into the developer (a reflected light artifact).
- *Underreplenishment (exhausted developer).* The films are often damp when they exit the processor, and the film is flat and has poor contrast (Fig. 7.21).
- *Temperature too cool.* The hydroquinone is too cool to function correctly, and the images are dull and lack contrast.
- *Temperature too warm.* The developer will exhaust quickly and turn dark brown, and images are dark and dull and lack contrast.
- *Fixer not replenishing correctly.* Silver plating appears on the images (Fig. 7.22).
- *Fixer overconcentrated.* Fixer precipitates as a white, grainy material on the rollers and in the gears, causing scratches.
- *Fixer exhausted.* Films are milky white or pinkish and feel grainy and rough (Fig. 7.23).
- *Fixer tank empty.* Films are either green (blue-receiving film) or mauve/pink (green-receiving film). There is an image, but it blackens quickly.
- *Incorrect mixing (manual).* The film has a blur pattern of minus densities and plus densities (Fig. 7.24).

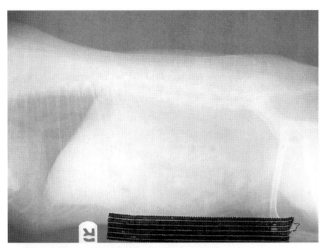

FIG. 7.21 Film processed with exhausted developer. The overall image lacks correct density and contrast; it has a washed-out appearance and is nondiagnostic.

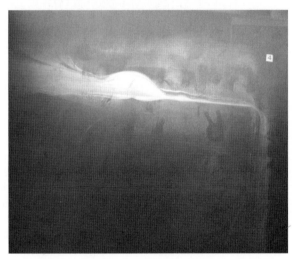

FIG. 7.22 Silver has plated out onto the film as the fixer lines were crimped and replenishment had ceased.

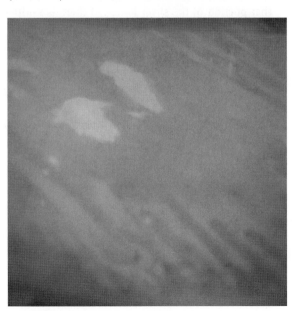

FIG. 7.23 Film processed with exhausted fixer. The film has a milky appearance and may even appear to be pink from the dye used in the green-receiving film.

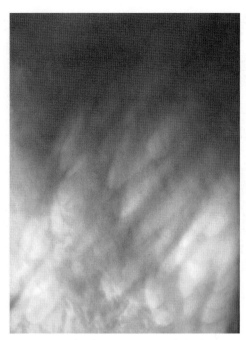

FIG. 7.24 An example of incorrect mixing of developer in a manual tank. The image of the anatomy is completely overshadowed by the uneven chemistry.

FIG. 7.25 A treelike shadow overlays the entire film. This occurred because the developer replenisher was introduced into the developing tank, bypassing the recirculation tank. The fresh developer affected the film and activated the developing process, but the older chemicals took longer to accomplish development. The solution to this problem was to install a diversion baffle for the new chemicals so they mixed with the old chemicals before reaching the film.

- *Incorrect mixing (automatic).* A treelike spray pattern appears across the film when the recirculation tank has not mixed the old chemicals with the new chemicals. The fresh chemistry is more active, darkening the image as it travels across the film. The image in Fig. 7.25 was caused because a service person forgot to replace the diversion baffle in the recirculation tank, which prevented the chemicals from mixing correctly before entering the working tank.
- *Wash water tank empty.* The films are milky and look streaky in reflected light.

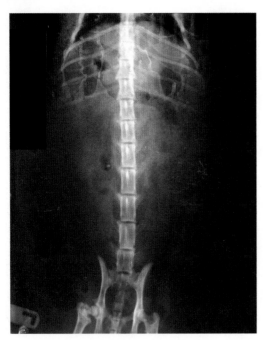

FIG. 7.26 Sulfiding from the residual thiosulfate is very evident on this image as the result of inadequate washing.

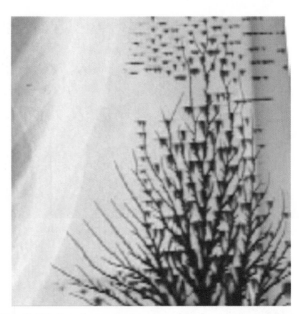

FIG. 7.27 Static from a feed tray. Note the flat lines produced when the film was placed onto the feed tray.

- *Wash water tank not circulating.* The films appear dirty and streaky. Archival quality is compromised, and the films turn yellow within 2 or 3 weeks (Fig. 7.26).

Handling Artifacts

Determining the causes of artifacts on film may turn into a Sherlock Holmes–type adventure. This is where good record-keeping and good darkroom practices pay off. The following are some of the causes of handling artifacts:

- Foreign objects in the cassette
- Dust on the feed tray (particularly common with large-animal radiography in a barn)
- Double exposure caused by not keeping track of which cassettes are already exposed and which are unexposed
- Film fog from heat, age, or other factors
- Scattered radiation fog
- Secondary radiation fog
- Extrafocal radiation
- Static—smudge, spot, or tree static (Fig. 7.27)
- Sweaty fingerprints
  - Identical to the fingerprints of whoever processed the film
  - Particularly common with single-emulsion film
  - Salts in sweat dissolve the emulsion so it does not develop when processed
- Film creases
  - Caused by bending the film when it is taken out of the film box, roughly placed in the cassette, or roughly removed from the cassette before processing
  - May be dark (caused by concentrating the ions in the silver lattice) (Fig. 7.28A) or light (caused by destroying that portion of the silver lattice so there is no longer an image beneath the crease) (Fig. 7.28B)
- Incorrect darkroom conditions:
  - Safelight filter (Fig. 7.29)
  - Safelight wattage
  - Safelight color
  - Safelight distance from countertop
  - Chemical odor (a highly concentrated odor can cause film fog)
  - Darkroom integrity (Fig. 7.30).

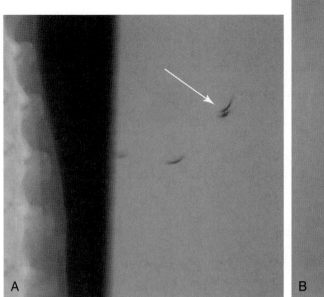

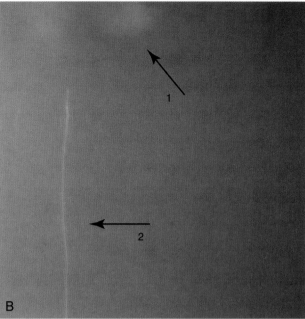

FIG. 7.28 A, Fingerprint creases are caused by flexing the film roughly; they may be plus density or minus density. B, *(1)* Minus-density artifact from fingers pressing too hard on film emulsion. *(2)* Minus-density artifact from rough handling of film.

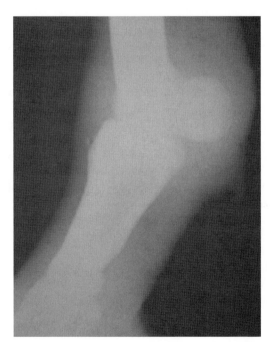

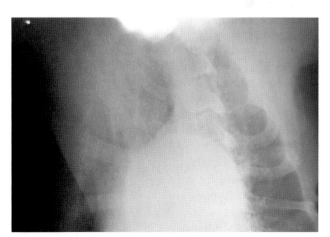

FIG. 7.29 An incorrect safelight filter fogged this film from a large-animal darkroom. Film fog usually lays a gray film over the image. In this case it caused total lack of contrast, rendering the image nondiagnostic.

FIG. 7.30 Film fog on an image caused by a light leak around the door of a darkroom. The fingers holding the film at the top protect the film from the light, and the balance of the image has a fog overlay.

REVIEW QUESTIONS

1. The temperature of the darkroom should be _____; the humidity should be _____.
   a. 40°F (4°C), 40% to 60%
   b. 60°F (15.5°C), 50% to 70%
   c. 68°F (20°C), 40% to 60%
   d. 75°F (24°C), 50% to 70%

2. If the radiography room doubles as a darkroom, cassettes and film should be stored:
   a. In a metal film bin out of the way of scattered radiation
   b. In the darkroom, on shelves, and lying flat
   c. In the x-ray room in a plastic film bin in a far corner
   d. In the x-ray room on shelves, in an upright position

3. The darkroom should be painted using _____. The safelight should be mounted _____ feet (_____ meters) above the counter.
   a. black-absorbing paint, 6, 1.82
   b. dark, light-absorbing paint, 4, 1.22
   c. light-reflective paint, 4, 1.22
   d. light-reflective paint, 6, 1.82

4. The information on the ID label must include which of the following?
   a. Clinic address, date, and time of examination
   b. Patient's name, clinic address, and date
   c. Patient's name, clinic name, and location of the clinic
   d. Patient's name, clinic name, and right or left view

5. Automatic processing a film requires four separate steps. Which of the following lists the correct order?
   a. Develop, fix, wash, dry
   b. Develop, wash, fix, dry
   c. Fix, develop, wash, dry
   d. Wash, develop, fix, dry

6. The two main components of the developer are:
   a. Hydroquinone and phenidone
   b. Hydroquinone and sodium carbonate
   c. Phenidone and potassium bromide
   d. Sodium sulfite and sodium carbonate

7. The purpose of the developer is to:
   a. Alter the chemical makeup of the film to accept the fixer
   b. Reduce the potassium bromide in the film to metallic bromide
   c. Reduce the silver halide in the film base to metallic silver
   d. Reduce the silver halide in the film emulsion to metallic silver

8. A second purpose of the developer is to:
   a. Amplify the amount of metallic silver on the film
   b. Decrease the amount of silver left on the base
   c. Increase the number of silver atoms in each sensitivity speck
   d. Reduce the number of silver halide atoms to enhance the image

9. One of the components of the developer is to reduce its activity; this is:
   a. Potassium bromide
   b. Sodium carbonate
   c. Sodium sulfite
   d. Water

10. The main function of the hydroquinone is to:
    a. Build up the blacks and enhance the contrast
    b. Slowly build up grays to enhance contrast
    c. Start to work immediately to build up the blacks in the image
    d. Steadily enhance the gray tones of the image

11. The main function of the fixer is to:
    a. Fix the contrast problems left by the developer
    b. Harden the image and fix it to the base
    c. Remove unexposed silver halide from the film base
    d. Solidify the image to the base

12. The main component of the fixer is:
    a. Acetic acid
    b. Aluminum sulfate
    c. Ammonium thiosulfate
    d. Chrome alum

13. Developer is chemically _____; fixer is highly _____.
    a. acidic, alkaline
    b. alkaline, acidic
    c. alkaline, neutral
    d. neutral, acidic

14. The main purpose of the wash water is to:
    a. Remove the leftover chemicals from the film to preserve archival quality
    b. Remove the soapy residue of the precipitate from the fixer
    c. Stop the developer from developing the unexposed silver halides
    d. Stop the fixer from removing the image from the film

15. Drying should remove about _____ of the moisture from the film.
    a. 60% to 70%
    b. 70% to 80%
    c. 85% to 90%
    d. 90% to 100%

16. Two of the systems of the automatic processor are _____ and _____.
    a. cooling anode, replenishment
    b. replenishment, recirculation
    c. thermostat, heating coils
    d. transport, cooling system

17. Every time a roller comes into contact with the film emulsion:
    a. It has the potential to imprint an artifact on the image
    b. It has the potential to stop the film from developing
    c. It is started and stopped by the action of the film
    d. The roller assists the fixer to fix the image on the film

18. Once the film is placed on the feed tray and enters the rollers:
    a. It is affecting the replenishment, so it must not be drawn back
    b. It must not be drawn back onto the feed tray
    c. It will enter the fixer and must not be pulled back
    d. The developer will arrest the motion of the film so it will be fixed

19. The transport system of the processor:
    a. Carries the films through the tanks by a series of rollers and gears
    b. Slides the film along the rollers using the guide shoes to bend it
    c. Transports the chemicals to the developer tanks by means of pumps
    d. Transports the replenisher into the processor without any air gaps

20. The developer chemicals are replenished with _____ chemicals in comparison with the fixer.
    a. less
    b. less (but diluted)
    c. more
    d. the same amount of (but diluted)

21. The fixer requires _____ replenisher because it contains _____.
    a. less, bromines
    b. less, water
    c. more, developer
    d. more, water

22. The most typical silver recovery unit in a veterinary clinic is the:
    a. Copper replacement model
    b. Electrolytic model
    c. Ionic attachment model
    d. Metallic replacement model

23. A test to determine whether the silver recovery unit needs to be replaced is:
    a. Checking the inside of the unit for fixer precipitate and smelling the outflow
    b. Checking the inside of the unit for metallic silver and absence of steel wool
    c. Placing a 5-cent piece in the outflow, which will polish the nickel
    d. Placing copper in the outflow; silver will plate out on the copper

24. A large percentage of artifacts are caused by which of the following reasons when processing the film?
    a. Most of them are caused by rough handling.
    b. Most of them are caused in the developer tank.
    c. Mostly they arise in the darkroom before processing.
    d. The majority are caused by incorrect concentration of chemicals.

25. Dichroic fog is caused by:
    a. Developer contaminating the fixer
    b. Fixer leaking back into the developer
    c. Fixer leaking into the wash water
    d. Wash water staining the films after drying

26. Pi lines are caused in the processor by a swelling of a roller. They are:
    a. Called this because the separation of the artifact is the circumference of the rollers
    b. Named after the art of pi; they compromise the image
    c. Usually minus-density lines at random intervals along the film
    d. Usually plus-density artifacts along the edges of the film

27. Developer under replenishment causes the film:
    a. To appear as if it had been smeared with chemicals after it was processed
    b. To have a gray, washed-out appearance due to exhaustion of hydroquinone
    c. To have a gray, washed-out appearance due to exhaustion of phenidone
    d. To look very colorful under reflected light with green and blue colors

28. Overheating the developer will cause it to _____ and turn _____.
    a. exhaust quickly, dark brown
    b. exhaust quickly, light yellow
    c. remain stable, dull gold
    d. remain stable, light yellow

29. If the fixer is overconcentrated, it will:
    a. Precipitate onto the tank and cause grainy images
    b. Precipitate out onto the gears and rollers
    c. Remain in solution and enhance the contrast
    d. Remain in solution and fix faster

30. Crease artifacts on the film are the result of:
    a. Incorrect handling before or after exposure
    b. Incorrect placement of the film on the feed tray
    c. Not maintaining good darkroom cleanliness
    d. Static electricity affecting the film transport

Answers to Review Questions can be found on the Evolve website.

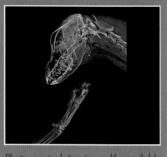

Photo manipulation is readily available with digital imaging.

CHAPTER **8**
Computed Radiography and Digital Imaging

Lois C. Brown, RTR (Can/USA), ACR, MSc., P.Phys

The digital camera is a great invention because it allows us to reminisce. Instantly.

—Demetri Martin, American comedian, b. 1973

OUTLINE

LEARNING OBJECTIVES

When you have finished this chapter, you will be able to:

1. Know the difference between computed radiography and digital imaging.
2. Understand the fundamentals of computed radiography.
3. List the basics of direct digital imaging.
4. Understand the purpose of the charge-coupled device camera.
5. Understand digital technique charts.
6. Know the difference between windowing and leveling and between contrast and density.
7. Know the rules to follow when purchasing a digital system.
8. Understand the software variables.
9. Understand picture archiving and communications systems.
10. Know how to look for artifacts in the images.

APPLICATIONS

The application of the information in this chapter is relevant to the following area:

1. Producing digitized x-ray images (radiographs) for evaluation and diagnosis.

KEY TERMS

Key terms are defined in the Glossary on the Evolve website.

Charge-coupled device
Imaging plate
Photodiode

Photomultiplier tube
Photostimulable luminescence

Photostimulable phosphor
Storage phosphor screen

Storage plate
Thin film transistor

Caveat Emptor: Let the Buyer Beware

The current conversion to digital imaging emphasizes the appropriateness of the Latin phrase *caveat emptor* ("Let the buyer beware"). This chapter discusses how these systems function and the reasoning behind their development. This discussion will hopefully emphasize the importance of researching computed radiography and/or digital imaging systems and their images before making a purchase.

After several years of consultation with vendors and purchasers, we have compiled the following "10 commandments" of digital imaging purchase. Caveat emptor!

1. **First reviews.** Researching digital imaging is a fascinating look into the possibilities. However, just as with everything else, it is vital to remain grounded in reality. The vendors will be very pleasant and agreeable and will have a vested interest in your clinic. It is important not to allow emotions to cloud objectivity but to make a decision based on the best interests of the clinic and staff.

2. **Narrowing the possibilities.** Search the Internet to find out what is available and where the vendors are located. If you decide to purchase a digital system, you will be committed to your vendor, and your happiness with your images will depend on the system and the vendor's expertise. You will also depend on the commitment of the service person that the vendor provides and will, initially, interact with that person daily.

3. **Site visits.** It is worth the trip to see the system in which you are interested. Ask the purchaser why this system was chosen over the others. Ask to see images—a lot of images. Request extremity and bony anatomy views. (Abdomen images are always impressive unless the system is very bad.) Check out the contrast on chest images, and play with the brightness, contrast, and all the postprocessing options. Decide whether a hairline fracture would be visible. It is a rare veterinary digital system that demonstrates a hairline fracture in bony anatomy.

4. **Service, cost, and location.** An assurance from the vendor to "look after you" is not enough. Does the vendor have a nearby service department or company? Are they even in the same country? If the head office is in a different country or across the continent, is there a local qualified service engineer who can service not only the digital system but also the x-ray generator? If the system breaks down (and they all do), what is the guaranteed "down time"? How will they service the unit? Will they supply a replacement product while yours is being serviced? Is there any warranty on the part that is being serviced or on the replacement part? Ask to speak with a client who has had his or her unit serviced. Discuss holidays and weekends. Is the service department available "24/7"?

5. **Warranties.** Discuss the warranties in depth. Most systems are very reliable, but no system is infallible. If the system breaks down or if the image is unsatisfactory from the start, only a company with a good service record can help restore it. The price of a digital system is too high to use as a backup computer if the images are pixilated from the first day and there is no one to service it. Again, is there a warranty on any part that needs to be returned to the manufacturer for service? This issue is vital and worth repeating.

6. **Software licenses and upgrades.** Licenses and upgrades are the areas in which a number of digital system vendors add on to the cost of the original system. What is the cost of licensing two, three, or four computers within the same hospital? Extra work stations should be billed only for the price of the computer. These separate computers are not separate systems; they are piggybacked to the main system. There is no reason for the clinic to be invoiced for an auxiliary system when all computers feed from the same software. Upgrades should be added automatically during the warranty period. Once the warranty is finished, an agreement may be reached regarding the price of future software upgrades.

7. **Service contracts.** After selling you the digital equipment, the only way the vendor can make more money is through service contracts. A service contract with any x-ray company is designed to cover the most expensive piece of equipment that will need to be replaced during the time of the contract. Typically, service contracts do not cover glassware (the x-ray tube). Any service contract that covers the digital imaging plate is going to be prohibitive costwise and probably unnecessary. Read and discuss any service contract very thoroughly. Make very sure you are aware of what is, and is not, covered.

8. **Lease-to-own or time payment plans.** Technology moves forward quickly, and imaging is improving because the competition in this field is fierce. The medical market drives the technology, and the veterinary market benefits from the research. It is important that the digital unit pay for itself in a timely manner. By the time a 5-year loan is paid off, the veterinary clinic is left with a paid-for technological dinosaur. Speak to your potential vendor about trade-ins or upgrades to your unit.

9. **The digital unit is the image receptor.** The digital system replaces only the detector portion of the radiography system. A correctly calibrated radiography unit of any age is quite capable of delivering the radiation necessary to produce digital images. The clinic does not need to upgrade the radiography unit if it is correctly calibrated and serviceable.

10. **The golden rule of business.** Make sure the unit you purchase is a good business decision for the clinic or hospital. Does it make good business sense to purchase a unit, and can the number of radiographs produced each month pay for the monthly payment on the equipment? It is unwise to expect the other areas of the hospital to contribute to the purchase of a digital imaging unit.

Introduction to Computed Radiography and Digital Imaging

The imaging process has traditionally involved several steps: positioning the patient, measuring the patient, setting the technical factors, making the exposure, processing the film, and reading and archiving the images.

Computers started to change these traditional steps, and quite slowly at first. The changes came first in fluoroscopy and the related modalities of nuclear medicine and ultrasound. These modalities already used a closed system for viewing images. It was possible to print the images (usually on special single-emulsion film) to archive them, but storing the images in the system was more efficient and economical. The original storage devices were enormous and worked very much like the jukebox that was familiar in those days. The files were stored on discs or tape and retrieved by an arm moving to a tape and placing it in the correct position to be played.

As technology progresses and data become larger, everything needs to be scaled down. The images and data used in hospitals and clinics today can be stored on a personal computer with exchangeable hard drives. The backup images are often stored in data banks anywhere in the world.

With technology, the future of imaging is limitless. One thing that remains consistent with any system is the x-ray unit itself. Any correctly calibrated unit can be joined with any digital imaging system. The two systems are completely separate. As long as the system has a grid tray and is consistent, it will work just fine.

Computed Radiography

Computed radiography (CR) was the first step toward digital imaging in veterinary medicine (Fig. 8.1). There are many similarities between CR and traditional imaging (Table 8.1). Both use a cassette that must be processed in a separate unit. Both have imaging plates coated with photostimulable phosphors (PSPs), and the cassettes protect the PSPs from light and abuse. Both modalities require processing to archive the images.

The only step that CR eliminates from the traditional imaging protocol is reloading film into the cassette. This is done by the CR reader if that option is supplied. In some cases the operator will remove the screen from the cassette, wait for it to be "read" and erased, and then replace it in the cassette (Fig. 8.2).

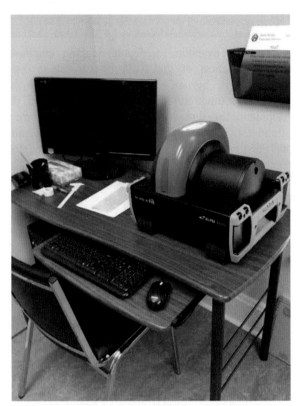

FIG. 8.1 The Scanx unit set up in a small-animal hospital. A more robust unit is available for the equine veterinarian. A smaller unit will process dental images.

TABLE 8.1	A Comparison of Protocols*		
TRADITIONAL FILM/ SCREEN IMAGING	**COMPUTED RADIOGRAPHY (CR)**	**DIRECT DIGITAL IMAGING (DDI)**	
Load cassette	Prepare the cassette	This step is eliminated	
Prepare photoidentifier	**Enter patient's data**	**Enter patient's data**	
Position patient	**Position patient**	**Position patient**	
Measure patient	**Measure patient**	**Measure patient**	
Set technique/ make exposure	**Set technique/ make exposure**	**Set technique/make exposure**	
Process film	Process the image	This step is performed by computer	
Reload cassette	**This step is eliminated**	This step is performed by computer	
Hang the film	Post the image	This step is performed by computer	
Read the film	**Read the image**	**Read the image**	
Postprocessing not available	Postprocess the image	Postprocess the image	
Archive the film	**Archive the image**	**Archive the image**	

*_**Bold**_ type indicates similar processes across imaging types; red type indicates differences across imaging types.

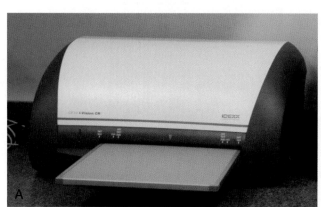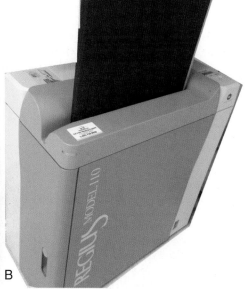

FIG. 8.2 A, This Idexx model has the cassette entering from the side and sits easily on a countertop. The IP is drawn out and wrapped around a drum in a similar fashion to the Scanx model and then returned to the cassette after the original image is erased. **B,** The Konica system is a stand-alone model. The cassette is placed in the top, and the IP is drawn straight out and inserted back into the cassette, which is then lifted out of the unit.

A single imaging plate (IP) in the CR cassette acquires and stores the image (ready for processing), thereby eliminating the need for film. The function is the same as in film/screen imaging except that the screen retains the image instead of transferring it to film.

The similarities between traditional imaging and CR end when we compare how the images are acquired, processed, and viewed. In addition, postprocessing is available with CR but not with traditional imaging.

The Imaging Plate and Identifiers

Inside the CR cassette is a single intensifying screen that traps the image by means of a PSP. In this form the screen is referred to as an *imaging plate (IP)*. This is a distinct advantage to CR. With a Scanx unit, the cassettes can be easily substituted from film/screen imaging and used as holder/protective coverings for the IP. Specialized cassettes must be purchased specific to the type of CR unit if the cassette is handled by a reader unit (Fig. 8.3A). Tabletop exposures are possible, so radiation doses may be kept low. The back of the cassette contains a small identifier that contains the patient data. It must be read by the CR unit before the IP enters the reader (Fig. 8.3B).

The front of the IP is coated with a PSP, usually barium fluorohalide, which reacts instantly to the x-ray beam and to light. The electrons within the PSP become metastable when stimulated by the x-ray beam. Approximately 50% of the electrons return immediately to their stable state and give off a prompt emission of light. The other 50% remain unstable and give up their unstable state over time. This feature is important because it is this 50% that holds the patient's image

on the IP until stimulated by an infrared (laser) light (Fig. 8.4).

If the IP is not placed in a reader unit, the image will fade within 6 to 8 hours as the electrons return to their original state. When the IP is placed in a reader unit, the laser (which is 50 to 100 nanometers wide and covers the plate side to side) passes over the plate as it is drawn out of the cassette. The laser causes the remaining unstable electrons to return to their original state with the emission of a shorter wavelength light in the blue area of the spectrum. At this point, the latent image becomes visible on the computer monitor.

The spatial resolution on the image depends entirely on the cross-sectional diameter of the laser. The laser beam tends to spread as it leaves the source, so it is collimated by a lens system that keeps it to a 100-μm diameter.

Once the image has been read, the IP is flashed with an intense white light. This light returns all the unstable electrons to their ground state, preparing the IP to be used again immediately. IPs work best if they are used immediately after processing.

IPs should always be "flashed" every morning because they may retain a previous image or may be "fogged" by background radiation from fluorescent lights or concrete walls. Fogging of the PSP is possible from direct or scattered radiation, heat stimulation of the IP, or light leaks within the cassette.

Sources of Image Noise

Noise is greatest in CR at the lower level of exposure as a result of background fog and scattered radiation. Table 8.2 lists sources of noise in the CR system.

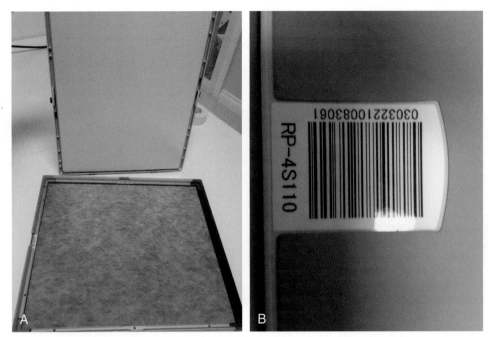

FIG. 8.3 A computed radiography cassette looks similar to a traditional radiography cassette. In this view it has been opened to show the IP on the back of the cassette, and the protective front of the cassette is lying on the table (**A**). It opens at the top to allow the IP to be drawn out to be scanned, and the cassette identifier is imprinted in a window at the back of the cassette (**B**). This identifier links the patient acquisition numbers to the cassette.

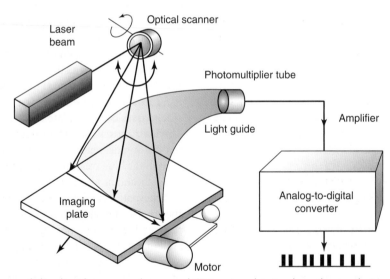

FIG. 8.4 The neon-helium laser beam scans the exposed CR imaging plate to release the stored energy as visible light. The photomultiplier tube "sees" the light, amplifies it, and converts it to an electrical signal. The electrical signal is picked up by the analog-to-digital converter, which converts the analog data to digital data and displays it on the hospital monitor. (Courtesy Fujifilm Medical Systems, USA, Incs, Stamford, Connecticut.)

The principal source of noise on the image is scattered radiation. The dose curve in CR radiography is directly linked to technique. This means that as the IP is stimulated, the response of the plate is immediate. The output of the CR image is constant throughout the diagnostic imaging range of technical factors. This may easily lead to overexposure, because technique charts are supplied by vendors who are unfamiliar with the ALARA (as low as reasonably achievable) principle. It is very important to maintain a technique chart

that sets the technical factors and therefore the dose to an ALARA level. Typically, traditional technique charts at a 400-speed system are acceptable for CR.

Advantages of Computed Radiography

The elimination of the wet processor and the chemicals associated with traditional film processing is a distinct environmental advantage with any type of digitized imaging. Two further advantages are the wide latitude regarding

TABLE 8.2	Sources of Noise Within the Computed Radiography System
SOURCES OF NOISE	**CAUSES**
Mechanical defects	Slow scan driver
	Fast scan driver
Optical defects	Laser intensity control
	Scatter of stimulating laser
	Light quanta emitted by the screen
	Light quanta collected by the optics
Computer defects	Electronic noise
	Inadequate sampling
	Inadequate quantization
Computer defects	Electronic noise
	Inadequate sampling
	Inadequate quantization

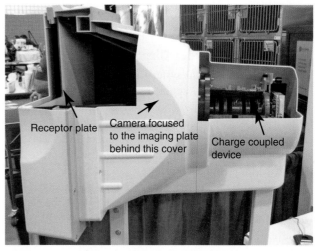

FIG. 8.5 A charge-coupled device (CCD) camera cut away to show the grid, automatic exposure control, and cesium iodide screen. The scintillation light from the cesium iodide phosphor is efficiently transmitted through fiber-optic bundles to the CCD array, camera chip, and computer boards at the back. The result is high x-ray capture and good resolution of up to 5 line pairs per millimeter (lp/mm).

technical factors and the short wait for the image display. The cassettes are replaceable at a reasonable cost.

Disadvantages of Computed Radiography

IPs are consumables and therefore need to be serviced and replaced when they become worn or when the "ghosting" of previous images cannot be erased. They are prone to the effects of scattered radiation and should be flashed before each use if radiography in the clinic or hospital is limited. Noise at low levels of radiation is bothersome, but newer technology promises to reduce this factor.

The readers can be a source of artifacts as the IP is drawn out of the cassette, especially in veterinary clinics, where animal hair and fur are drawn into the unit by fans or a vacuum. *Horizontal plus-density or minus-density artifacts* can be a problem as the IP is drawn out of the cassette if there is hesitation or uneven motion. *Vertical plus-density or minus-density artifacts* can be caused by dust or dirt on the rollers of the unit. These marks appear as long scratches down the length of the image.

Another disadvantage is the intermediate step of needing to process the image in a laser reader. This step delays the viewing process and requires one more piece of (expensive) equipment that must be maintained and serviced.

Digital Imaging

There are two types of digital imaging: indirect and direct.

Indirect Digital Imaging (CCD)

Charge-coupled device (CCD) imaging uses an IP that contains a thin-film transistor (TFT). The TFT converts the radiation to an image that is imprinted on a camera that is preset and collects the image off the back of the IP (Fig. 8.5). After the image is collected, it is handled in the same way as with direct digital imaging.

The response of the CCD is completely linear and therefore can detect far more stimulus than the phosphor in the film/

screen combination; this allows for a much greater range of sensitivity. Another advantage of CCD imaging is that the IP is considerably less expensive than that used for direct digital imaging and the CCD unit is made up of component parts that can be serviced and replaced if necessary.

A disadvantage of CCD imaging is that the image undergoes one extra step in moving from original image to computer image, so there is a chance of data loss. Research into this area has been intense, and the images from CCD units are exceptionally good. The very important aspect is to keep the camera, situated at the back of the unit, focused. The entire unit is mounted beneath the tabletop directly under the central ray. The CCD is not movable, so either the tabletop must move or the animals must be placed in such a way that they are centered on the CCD.

The *sensitivity* of the CCD is its ability to detect very low levels of visible light. This feature makes it valuable in radiography using its sensitivity to detect low patient remnant radiation dose. The *dynamic range* of the CCD is the ability of the detectors to respond to a wide range of light intensity. This system replicates the dynamic range of the 400-speed film/screen system.

Direct Digital Imaging

Direct digital imaging evolved from the CR model. Scientists reasoned that all that was standing in the way of directly reading the image from the input phosphor was an interpretive digital plate. As a result, they developed a system that is stimulated directly within the mechanics of the plate itself so the image can be read directly and immediately from the monitor.

The acquisition of images through direct digital imaging eliminates several steps in the film/screen imaging process: the entire "processing and hanging" steps and the cassette preparation step (see Table 8.1). All that is required is entering the patient's information into the computer and sending the requisition for radiography to the operators. Everything else is carried out by computer.

Mechanics of Direct Digital Imaging

The detector of a digital system is a scintillation phosphor that is spread across a supportive plate that rests on a TFT. The plate transfers the radiation signal to the digital receptor (DR). The DR is fabricated into individual pixels (picture elements) (Fig. 8.6) that convert the radiation into electronic components and transfer the data to the software via the data lines extruding from each pixel.

The end goal of any imaging system is a highly diagnostic radiograph that enhances all the differences in tissue density while achieving the lowest radiation dose possible. Some sophisticated systems achieve approximately a 400-film/screen system speed.

The Thin Film Transistor and Pixel Capture

The acquisition of the image is variable as technology moves forward. Image acquisition is important to manufacturers because it is here that the image is acquired and transferred to the computer. The vendor is always anxious to have the sharpest resolution and the highest-contrast image. It is often the software that allows this to happen.

The limitation of digital imaging is the pixel size, which limits the resolution. The capture element affects 80% of the pixel; the other 20% contains the TFT and the data lines. The 20% of the pixel element that does not contribute to the actual image must be filled in by the computer. Spatial resolution improves as pixel size is reduced, but the patient dose must be increased to maintain signal strength and to compensate for a reduction in fill factor.

A solution to the problem of TFTs and the loss of 20% of the pixel came with research into digital mammography on the human side. An amorphous selenium (a-Se) plate was developed (Fig. 8.7) to interact directly with the incoming radiation; there is no intervening scintillation phosphor. The

a-Se plate is sandwiched between two charged electrodes. X-rays that reach the a-Se plate are collected by a storage capacitor and remain there until the signal is read by the switching action of the TFTs. All of this happens very quickly and results in an image within seconds of radiographic exposure to the digital imaging plate.

Although the number of pixels in the digital plate is important, of greater importance is how these pixels are "wired together." In some systems the advertised pixel number is enormous but the images are not ideal. When the image is magnified it "pixilates" and becomes unclear. This is because the pixels are bundled and read as an average. For example, the 16 squares in Fig. 8.8 represent pixels on a digital IP. Each square has a value that represents a percentage of exposure. Bundling these values together and averaging them results in a unique value of 50%. In the digital system this bundle would give a density of 50% even though none of the squares has a 50% density. This bundling gives a noisy (grainy) image because the individual densities in the image are not represented correctly.

There is no possible way to correct the noisy image in the system because this bundling occurs during manufacturing. Therefore it is very important to research the system thoroughly before investing any money in a digital system.

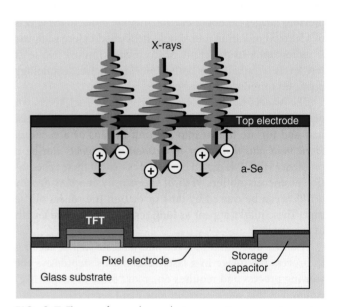

FIG. 8.7 The use of amorphous selenium as an image receptor capture element eliminates the need for a scintillation phosphor. This plate is approximately 200 μm thick and is sandwiched between charged electrodes. (From Bushong SC. *Radiologic Science for Technologists*, 11th ed. St Louis: Elsevier; 2017.)

20	60	60	20
40	80	80	40
40	80	80	40
20	60	60	20

FIG. 8.8 An example of bundled pixels. Each square represents one pixel. The computer program will read all 16 pixels as an average of each value. In this example, average density on the image would appear to be 50% even though none of these values equals 50%.

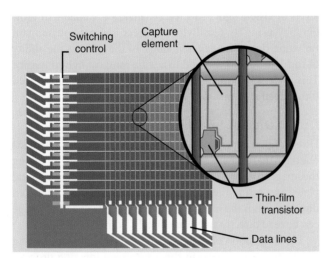

FIG. 8.6 A photomicrograph of an active matrix array showing a thin-film transistor digital imaging image receptor with a single pixel highlighted. (From Bushong SC. *Radiologic Science for Technologists*, 11th ed. St Louis: Elsevier; 2017.)

The Ethical Dilemma: Technique Charts

The technique charts supplied by otherwise reputable vendors can sometimes be worrisome. Setting a technique of 85 kilovolts (kV), 300 milliamperes (mA), and $\frac{1}{120}$ sec (2.50 mAs) for a kitten's paw or a cat's 10-cm abdomen illustrates the vendors' lack of knowledge in creating such charts and the problems encountered by the staff when they trust such charts. Every image must be postprocessed as a result, which adds time to the original examination and causes losses in data. Adjusting windowing and leveling (brightness and contrast) for every image compromises the information on the image. In addition, some of the images will be totally nondiagnostic. In such cases the high kV has penetrated every tissue evenly, eliminating any chance of enhancing contrast. The scattered radiation produced by a 110-kV exposure for a 16-cm abdomen is enough to add to the radiation dose on the technician's dosimeter if the technician is holding the patient and definitely adds unnecessary wear to the x-ray tube.

If the information has not been provided to the image receptor, either because the image is overexposed or underexposed, then no amount of postprocess manipulation will correct it. There is no "do-over," and the images are unreadable. Does the veterinarian order images that he or she knows cannot be read because the digital unit must be paid for? Does he or she have the image postprocessed as best as possible and then revert to the old system of diagnosing clinically because the images are so poor? What about the technicians who have worked at the clinic for 10 to 20 years and are now seeing dose readings on their radiation dosimeters for the very first time because of excess amounts of scattered/secondary radiation? All of these problems are experienced both in the veterinary world and in human medicine.

Technical Factors

Doses, dose creep, and poor technique charts can be a major problem in the radiography department. A technique chart must be developed that is similar to the chart used with the 400-speed film/screen combination in place when the digital unit was purchased. The chart supplied in this chapter is a guide only and can be adjusted to optimize the images after viewing the images produced using this chart (Fig. 8.9A; see also Appendix A on the Evolve website). The best way to adapt a chart that was used before digital imaging is to measure accurately, set the generator to the measurement, and expose the receptor with a patient in place. The computer manipulates the data, but if the image is not perfect, reduce the mAs by a percentage. This will likely follow through for most of the chart.

For example:

16-cm abdomen, 400-speed chart, 62 kV, 12 mAs
= Image dark by about 50%

Decrease technique to 62 kV, 6 mAs
= Image perfect, no postprocessing required

The best diagnostic images in digital imaging are acquired with a technique that is as close as possible to the parameters of the animal being radiographed. The computer will do the rest. Typically, smaller body parts will have a higher technique because the digital plate requires a certain level of radiation to acquire the image. This level will decrease as technology progresses.

kV, mAs, and Distance

Distance is typically not a factor in small-animal imaging because the distance is usually preset, but it is definitely a factor in large-animal imaging. An example of a technique chart is presented in Fig. 8.9 (see also Appendix A on the Evolve website). However, this chart may not work well with every unit. The kV and mAs combine in digital imaging to produce dose, and every system handles the dose slightly differently.

The digital IP requires a radiation dose. It will accept scattered/secondary radiation to add density to the image.

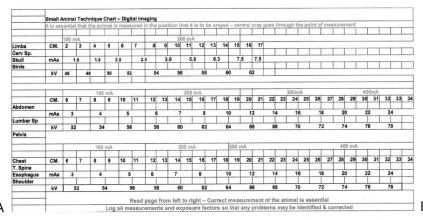

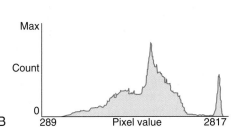

FIG. 8.9 A, An example of a digital technique chart from a unit installed, with no grid, in 2017. This example uses very low doses and the images are excellent. Older digital plates use much higher doses, and the images may still not have the resolution of the newer digital plates. Please see Appendix A on the Evolve website for a chart that compares an older digital plate and a 2017 digital plate. **B,** A histogram showing the number of each of the gray values from left to right (the horizontal axis). The total number (count) of each pixel value is added up vertically. (B from Fauber TL. *Radiographic Imaging and Exposure,* 5th ed. St. Louis: Mosby; 2017.)

Some systems are now sold with a removable grid that will be used only on large dogs (which produce an excessive amount of secondary radiation). The old system of decreasing kV to enhance contrast is no longer an issue. The digital plate looks for dose, and the computer takes care of the rest using two very important systems: histograms and algorithms.

Histograms and Algorithms

Histograms

A histogram is a graphic display of an image (Fig. 8.9B) and is displayed on the software of virtually every digital system. Every pixel is plotted on a graph from lightest to darkest, taking into account the number of all pixels that represent the same dark/light value. Images of extremities are high on the light values and dark values, with very low levels in between. Images of an abdomen peak in the gray areas and are low on both very light and very dark values.

In some cases the operator can manipulate the histogram slightly to enhance some of the features of the image. The histogram is then evaluated on the basis of a known algorithm to enhance the contrast and brightness of the image.

Algorithms

An algorithm is a formula or set of rules used in calculations or data processing. An example of an algorithm is a program that calculates pounds sterling after keying in an American dollar value.

The computer software used in digital imaging contains a series of algorithms that provide a baseline for each type of examination. Each algorithm is based on the histograms obtained from many trials and much research. For example, a dog's foreleg typically consists of bone, muscle, and a little fat, with no internal organs. An algorithm describes what the computer will "see" when a foreleg is radiographed and enhances the contrast and brightness of the image accordingly. This is true for every body part on every animal. A chest image is enhanced as a high-contrast image, and the contrast in the active image is enhanced. An image of an abdomen will be low contrast with many shades of gray.

When a digital unit is purchased and installed, the service engineer who sets up the computers will establish the veterinarian's preferences, such as what level of contrast is acceptable in a chest and what density is preferred for abdomens and spines. Once the algorithms for that hospital are established, the service engineer can go into the computer from any location and correct any problems. The service engineer is usually the only person who has access to the program at the algorithm level, but he or she cannot change anything within the basic programming of the software. He or she may apply filters to adjust the histogram but cannot change the manufacturer's preset algorithms.

Digital Image Processing

Spatial Resolution and Contrast Resolution

Every image is a combination of spatial resolution (the image in space) and contrast resolution. *Spatial resolution* is expressed

---

◆ APPLICATION INFORMATION

On a digital system the algorithm can be fooled with or worked around. For example, a client had a problem with the algorithm programmed for abdominal radiography. The images had no contrast, and the veterinarian wanted more contrast. Until the service person could change the algorithm, the consultant suggested that he request chest imaging when he was radiographing an abdomen. The higher-contrast algorithm worked just fine, and the images were diagnostic with just the right amount of contrast.

---

in line pairs per millimeter. It is the ability to visualize a high-contrast black line that is separated by an interspace of equal width (see Chapter 6). *Contrast resolution* is expressed as the values of black and white. The highest contrast available is an image that is completely black and white with no intervening shades of gray. The descriptor for contrast resolution is *dynamic range*.

The end result of digital imaging should logically be a high-resolution image. However, it is important to note that the limitations of pixel size and monitor output always result in an image that does not have the spatial resolution of film/screen technology (Table 8.3).

Contrast and Brightness (Windowing and Leveling)

The amplification of contrast and brightness enhancement is the most important feature of digital imaging. *Windowing* (Fig. 8.10) refers to the contrast range of densities. Window width controls the range of grayscale images to adjust the contrast on a digital image. *Leveling* (Fig. 8.11) refers to density or brightness. Window level establishes the midpoint of the densities visible on the digital image. This use of windowing and leveling alters the image on the monitor.

Dynamic Range

The question remains: Why do digital images look so much better than film images?

Digital images take advantage of the ability of the digital process to create a greater number of shades of gray in the

TABLE 8.3	Approximate Spatial Resolution for Various Medical Imaging Systems	
IMAGING SYSTEM	**SPATIAL RESOLUTION (line pairs/mm)**
Magnetic resonance imaging	1.5
Computed tomography	1.5
Digital imaging	4–5
Computed radiography	5–6
Film/screen radiography	8–9

From Bushong SC. *Radiologic Science for Technologists*, 11th ed. St Louis: Elsevier; 2017.

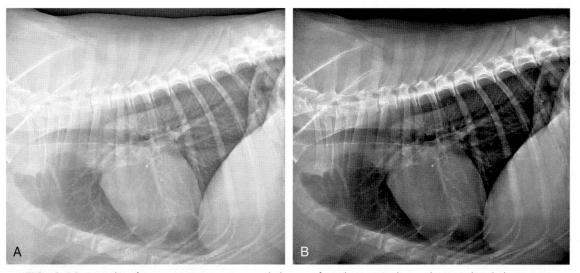

FIG. 8.10 Examples of postprocessing an image with the use of windowing. As the window is reduced, the contrast flattens out so the differences in tissue density become less obvious. **A,** The image lacks contrast in the areas of the lungs and heart. **B,** Windowing the image provides better contrast and demonstrates the vascular areas of the lung tissue.

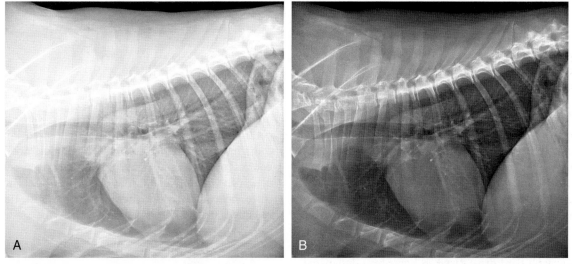

FIG. 8.11 A change in leveling. As the level increases, the overall density of the image becomes greater although the contrast remains the same. **A,** This image has good contrast but is overall too light. **B,** Leveling the image maintains the contrast and enhances the visualization of the anatomy by increasing the density.

image. It remains a fact that no digital image can resolve an object smaller than the pixel size of the image receptor.

Film/screen imaging has a limited dynamic range. The dynamic range of film/screen technology is three orders of magnitude because the density of the image is read from 0 to 3. This represents a dynamic range of 1000; this represents 1000 density variations, or shades of white to black. The viewer can visualize only 30 shades of gray because of the limitations of the human eye.

The dynamic range of digital imaging systems is defined by the bit capacity of each pixel. Typical DR systems have a 14-bit dynamic range ($2^{14} = 16{,}384$ shades of gray). Digital mammography systems and some later digital systems have a 16-bit capacity and therefore image 2^{16} (65,536) shades of gray. The human eye is not equipped to visualize and appreciate

all these features; it is limited to 30 shades of gray. The advantage of the digital systems is that with edge enhancement (a sophisticated computer technique that outlines each edge within the image) and the ability to manipulate the image (which is not available in a film/screen system), the radiograph may be enhanced by the algorithms and computer processing to optimize the contrast and brightness.

Postprocessing and the Service Engineer

If an incorrect exposure is used and the image is compromised because of very low contrast, the operator may alter the contrast and brightness by postprocessing. However, postprocessing is not a substitute for correctly exposing the image using a correct technique chart. It is time consuming, and some information may be inadvertently lost when the image is manipulated. It is also an example of lack of regard for the ALARA principle, which recommends the lowest radiographic technique in order to reduce the dose to both the patient and the operator.

If the correct technical factors are used and the images are still consistently problematic, the system engineer can apply filters to enhance the overall images. This is not true for every system. If the software chosen by the vendor is faulty or lacking in features and does not manipulate the data correctly, the image cannot be enhanced even by the experts. These are the programs that will not last in the marketplace.

Digital Imaging Artifacts

Digital imaging artifacts may be produced by the IP, grid, mechanical system, or software. It is important to identify the cause of the artifact and contact the system engineer to correct it. There are few artifacts in digital imaging, mainly because of the way the systems are installed. Typically, artifacts are caused by human error and can be resolved. A hardware or software problem must be addressed right away. The system engineer can usually resolve most software problems online. Hardware problems may be more difficult to resolve.

Picture Archiving and Communications Systems

Once the image is produced, it must be archived. It is very important to research the archiving of the images carefully. The archive is stored on a computer, and computers fail. All systems must therefore have redundancy, and the data must be stored in more than one place. The intricacies of data storage are beyond the scope of this text and could fill another chapter or even a book.

The simplest means of data storage is the use of inter-changeable external hard drives. Most clinics use three hard drives if they plan to store all the images onsite. Two hard drives store the day's images; the third is traded in at the end of the day, with hard drive #1 taken home by a designated person. The next day's images are stored on drives #2 and #3, and drive #2 is taken home at the end of the day. This system is complicated but inexpensive and secures the images locally.

A second means of data storage is offsite. Several companies offer offsite computer data storage and may be located locally, on the same continent, or on the other side of the world. These companies are efficient and store masses of data from many different modalities. A word of caution: If the company is local, do not assume that the data will be stored locally. Many companies act as intermediaries and store the actual images on the other side of the world. It is wise to know where the data are stored and who controls the storage facility. This is especially true if local politics or turbulent weather damage or destroy storage facilities.

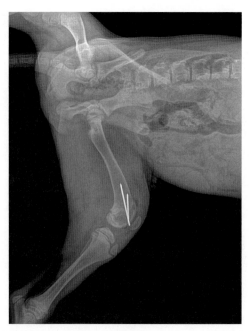

FIG. 8.12 Digital imaging enables the viewer to surround the image with a black background, which eliminates glare from the monitor. Although this image is not ideal from a positioning point of view, the surrounding black background eliminates transmitted glare from the monitor.

Digital Imaging Monitors

The conditions under which the images are viewed must be controlled to take advantage of the optimized image. The room must be darkened so ambient light does not affect the contrast on the monitor screen. Most imaging programs are equipped with automatic collimators that blacken the area surrounding the image on the monitor (Fig. 8.12). This feature reduces glare and viewer fatigue.

Summary

Digital imaging either by means of CR or direct DR is a definite leap forward in radiographic imaging. The future is limitless as research continues to provide imaging applications that use technology to limit radiation exposure and provide high-quality images. Data storage is an ever-expanding area of research, and the sophisticated methods of storage become even smaller and more convenient.

Image Gallery

Figs. 8.13 to 8.18 are images of various body parts of small animals as demonstrated by digital imaging. These figures are not intended to demonstrate correct positioning. Most of these images were taken as a final check before turning the digital unit over to the client.

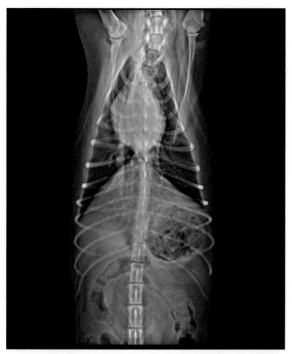

FIG. 8.13 A ventrodoral view of a chest and cranial abdomen.

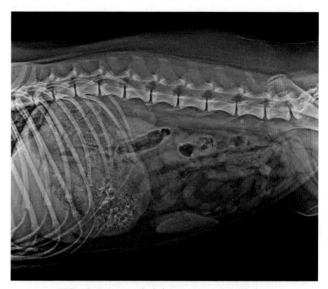

FIG. 8.14 Lateral abdomen on an 18-cm dog.

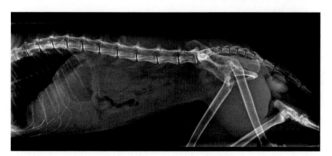

FIG. 8.15 Lateral abdomen on a 6-cm cat.

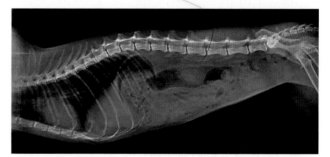

FIG. 8.16 Curiously this cat abdomen contained a small semicalcified fetus, which was not visible on the image because it was a similar density to surrounding tissues.

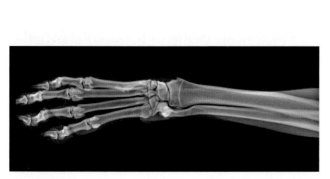

FIG. 8.17 Lower extremity of a large dog who was limping for no apparent reason.

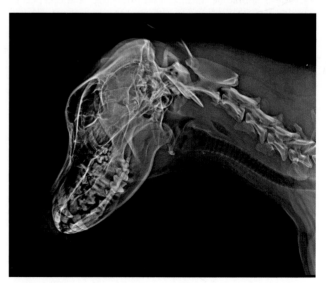

FIG. 8.18 Junction of skull and cervical spine on a large dog. Note the outline and rings of the trachea.

REVIEW QUESTIONS

1. Computed radiography eliminates one step in the imaging process. This is:
   a. Archiving the images
   b. Entering patient data
   c. Processing the image
   d. Reloading the cassette

2. Digital imaging eliminates several steps in the imaging protocol. This is because:
   a. Everything to do with the image is complete when the exposure is made
   b. The technician is not required to enter patient data at the computer
   c. The technician is not required to track the image after the exposure is made
   d. The technician is responsible only for the patient, not the radiography unit

3. Computed radiography is similar to traditional radiography in that:
   a. The cassettes are identical in composition
   b. The methods of processing are similar
   c. They both use cassettes of similar sizes
   d. They both require the technician to open the cassette after the exposure

4. The imaging plate within the CR cassette:
   a. Must be processed immediately because the image will degrade
   b. Can be delayed for processing for 6 to 8 hours
   c. Will hold the image for about 6 to 8 hours after exposure
   d. Will hold the image indefinitely after exposure

5. In CR, in order to read the image, a laser passes across:
   a. The IP after it is removed from the cassette
   b. The cassette after it is put into the reader
   c. The phosphor on the digital plate
   d. The IP after the exposure before it is in the reader

6. The IP should be "flashed" every morning or after a period of nonuse because:
   a. The chemicals start to develop on the plate
   b. It is sensitive to background radiation
   c. The plate is left in the reader
   d. The IP is always fogging after it has been used

7. The speed of the CR system is similar to that of 400-speed film/screen imaging.
   a. True
   b. False

8. Digital imaging is more efficient than computed radiography because:
   a. It eliminates the entire cassette reloading and processing and hanging steps
   b. It is a complete process and does not require separate image processing
   c. It is fast because the cassettes are already under the table
   d. It encourages technicians to use only one technique for every examination

9. Dynamic range is defined as:
   a. The ability to window and level the images
   b. The ability of the detectors to respond to a wide range of light intensity
   c. The latitude of the images once they are postprocessed
   d. The contrast of the images once they are postprocessed

10. A thin film transistor (TFT) is used to:
    a. Transfer the light intensity to the computer components
    b. Convert the signal to sound and then to the electrical system
    c. Transfer the radiation signal to a circuit board within the computer
    d. Transfer a radiation signal directly to the digital receptor

11. Direct digital systems use:
    a. Cesium iodide and an intervening plate
    b. Thin film transistors and cesium iodide
    c. Amorphous selenium to transmit the signal
    d. Amorphous silicon to transmit the signal

12. Windowing is a technique to improve images; it affects the _____.
    a. algorithm
    b. contrast
    c. density
    d. resolution

13. Leveling may enhance the radiographs, but it mainly affects_____.
    a. density
    b. frequency
    c. resolution
    d. spatial contrast

14. Picture archiving and communications systems store the images:
    a. Locally on hard drives or via the Internet anywhere in the world
    b. Locally on several hard drives that must remain in the computer
    c. On several hard drives but only within the facility for safekeeping
    d. Never on the hard drive of the computer because it may fail

Answers to Review Questions can be found on the Evolve website.

CHAPTER 9
Quality Control, Testing, and Artifacts

Lois C. Brown, RTR (Can/USA), ACR, MSc., P.Phys

Quality means doing it right when no one is looking.
—Henry Ford, American industrialist, 1863–1947

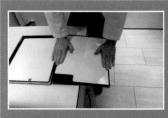

A quality control program ensures that all equipment is functioning correctly.

OUTLINE

LEARNING OBJECTIVES

When you have finished this chapter, you will be able to:

1. Describe the tests necessary to determine the calibration of an x-ray generator.
2. Identify the various problems associated with x-ray generator failure.
3. Test an x-ray unit for compliance.
4. Discuss the various methods to ensure that the collimator is installed and working correctly.
5. Describe the test tools that are used to determine resolution in fluoroscopy and radiography.
6. Identify artifacts caused by films and intensifying screens.
7. Identify artifacts caused by manual and automatic processing.
8. Distinguish between film artifacts and x-ray unit artifacts.
9. Identify artifacts associated with digital imaging.
10. Recognize problems with a digital plate and a computerized screen.

KEY TERMS

Key terms are defined in the Glossary on the Evolve website.

Dosimeter	Milliamperes	Rectifier	Transformer
Generator	Milliampere seconds (mAs)	Reproducibility	Quality assurance
Half-value layer	Patient dose	Timer	Quality control
Kilovoltage			

Throughout the previous chapters we have learned the basic workings of the imaging systems. We have also learned how to protect ourselves from overexposure to radiation. We have reviewed various methods of producing an image and then recording the image to either film or a digital medium.

This chapter is all about when things go wrong and how to identify just what went wrong and what can be done about it. It is divided into sections that reflect the chapters in the text. This chapter will serve to outline all of the quality control tests that may be incorporated into:

- Ensuring the generator is functioning correctly
- Ensuring the film/screen combination is correct and optimized
- Identifying the cause of artifacts on films caused by imperfections in intensifying screens, incorrect cleaning of the processor, or incorrect functioning of the processor
- Conducting virtually all of the tests relevant for confirming the correct functioning of the generator

◆ APPLICATION INFORMATION

- As long as the unit is calibrated correctly and is functioning correctly, the generator make, model, and age have nothing to do with the digital receptor.
- The image galleries within each earlier chapter demonstrate what can go wrong and, for the most part, how to correct deficiencies.
- This chapter strictly outlines the quality control testing procedures linked to the previous chapters.
- The most important density in the testing of films, screens, cassettes, generators, and processing is density 1 + base + fog. Thus we have positioned an image of this density here, at the beginning of the chapter, where it will be easily found during the testing of any equipment (Fig. 9.1).
- Not all facilities have densitometers, and because the human eye is fairly accurate when measuring comparable densities, this figure will be of value.

Quality Control and Quality Assurance

Quality control is the identification of actions that are necessary to ensure, and then verify, the performance of equipment. It is part of quality assurance, which is the documentation of all factors relating to a certain policy or protocol within a field of study. Quality assurance documents quality control and ensures that a facility, system, or administrative component performs safely and satisfactorily in service to a patient. Quality assurance includes scheduling, preparation, and efficiency during an examination or treatment; reporting the results; and conducting quality control.

In short, quality assurance involves the entire hospital or facility—front door to back exit—whereas quality control is the testing of each of the factors (usually the equipment) within the facility or hospital.

Some of the images relevant to quality control are located in this chapter, and some are located in the specific chapters where the particular modalities are described. However, quality control testing procedures are located in this chapter.

What This Chapter Covers and Why

Each piece of equipment within the imaging department must be intact and must perform perfectly in order to optimize every image. First radiography equipment testing is discussed. The x-ray generator and related tests are discussed in depth. It is important to know what these tests are and what they demonstrate, even though few veterinarians and technicians will ever perform these tests. Discussion includes explanation of how each piece of equipment interacts with all the others to produce a perfect image whether film or computers are involved. Next, radiation protection is discussed, including the tests that ensure the leaded products used in the department are safe and intact.

The content and tests in this chapter follow the order of chapters in Sections 1 and 2 and in Fluoroscopy in Chapter 11 of this text. Those earlier chapters covered the subjects for which these tests are required. Those chapters are clearly referred to at the beginning of each section. This chapter explains how the tests are carried out in terms of equipment and identification and the resolution of artifacts. Examples of artifacts that are imaged on the films but are not part of the testing procedures are included in the image galleries at the end of the appropriate chapters.

Radiography Equipment Testing

This section discusses quality control as it relates to Chapter 2, Diagnostic X-Ray Production.

In order to comprehend the radiographic equipment testing discussed, it is critical to understand the concept that the x-ray generator produces the alpha, beta, and gamma rays (x-rays) that are used to radiograph a patient. It is necessary to know when the exposure switch is closed and that what has been set on the generator is actually what is produced, ensuring that the exposure is correct.

The generator, x-ray tube, and transformers are separate components in the imaging system and are not attached specifically to the image detector. They do not need to be. Frequently, an older generator is paired successfully with a new digital x-ray or computer system.

FIG. 9.1 An example of a density 1 + base + fog image. This image will be referred to throughout the chapter and throughout the text.

X-Ray Generator Testing

X-ray generators come in all shapes, sizes, and ages; however, certain characteristics are consistent. Every x-ray generator connects to a power supply. The larger units are wired into facility power sources. The smaller portable units plug into wall outlets or have capacitors (batteries) that hold a charge and provide power when necessary.

Line Voltage

When the x-ray generator is activated, the current and the voltage of the power lines supplying the electricity to the x-ray unit must be stable and consistent. On older x-ray generators there is a needle indicator that must be set to a certain level. The operator can adjust a setting to ensure that the needle falls within the correct boundary (see Fig. 2.14A and B).

Identify a Problem With the Line Voltage

If the images are light or dark when they are normally the correct density and all other factors are consistent, the first place to check is the line voltage meter. Newer models of x-ray generators do not have line voltage compensators, as the correction occurs automatically when the generator is activated.

Fig. 9.2 is a flow chart that indicates what procedures should be taken to ensure that the line voltage is correct. A technician/operator may use this chart to determine if the problem lies with the line voltage on older units.

If the technique is adjusted and the images do not change in density, there is a problem with the line voltage. It is very rare for the line voltage to "drift" upward. It will only do so if there is a "load" on the line for one image and that load is switched off during the next procedure.

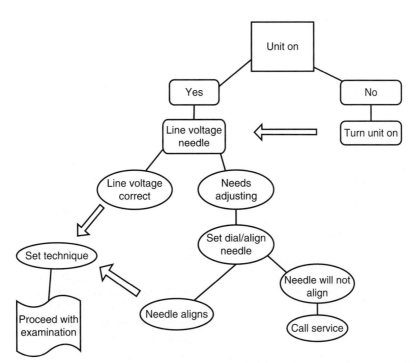

FIG. 9.2 A flow chart illustrating the steps when a manual line voltage compensator is installed.

X-Ray Unit Calibration Testing

The easiest method to identify a problem is to perform external testing using a kV meter, a dosimeter, and a timer test tool (Fig. 9.3). An alternative meter includes all three functions. Because most schools do not include this type of testing, we will simply explain the tests and familiarize the reader with the basic logic of the results.

Generator Compliance Testing

The next few paragraphs will explain how to test for x-ray equipment compliance (Fig. 9.4), will address each test individually, and will explain the procedures. The tests described here are not what is considered "invasive testing," which involves opening up the x-ray unit and attaching meters to various components. The main purpose of outlining these tests is to explain what is involved if a service engineer is called to a facility and uses test meters to determine the calibration of the unit.

Kilovoltage

Testing Techniques

Kilovoltage is tested using a kV meter. The kV stations that are tested are within the normal range of use in graduations of 10 kV. Each station must be tested at every mA setting within the normal range of use.

The kV meter is positioned on the tabletop with the collimator open to the size of the detector. The typical allowance of ±8% is legal in most countries. These parameters are listed in Fig. 9.5. When 70 kV is set on the unit, one expects to receive 70 kV at every mA station in the normal range of use. It is important that the kV does not drift higher or lower than

8% of this total. mA stations and/or kV stations not in the normal range of use should be disconnected and labeled as such on the generator by the service engineer.

Takeaway Tips

Accurate calibration is vital for every kV station at every milliampere (mA) setting. When a service person is in the x-ray room calibrating the x-ray unit, the veterinarian or technician should request a copy of the report to ensure that all of the stations within normal range of use are calibrated correctly. A unit may be installed in an area where the higher stations are not available due to insufficient power coming into the building. These stations must be marked as unavailable, and the technique chart must not include them.

Half-Value Layer

The **half-value layer** (HVL) indicates the thickness of an absorber necessary to reduce the intensity of the x-ray beam to half its original value. In radiography that absorber is aluminum. HVL is a measurement of the amount of filtration between the x-ray tube and the patient.

As the x-ray beam leaves the tube, it goes through three different filters:

1. The glass envelope of the x-ray tube
2. The inherent filtration of the tube port, mirrors, and collimator
3. Added filtration to meet legal requirements

Legally there must be enough filtration to eliminate nonuseful x-rays (which will add to patient dose) and scattered radiation (which is not part of the useful beam).

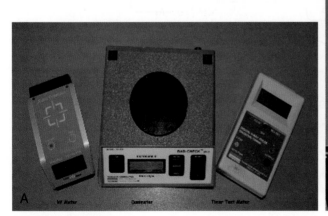
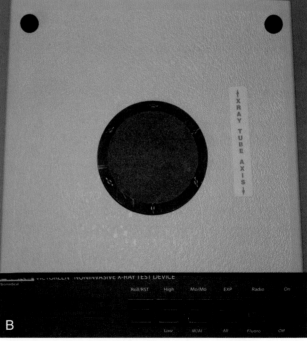

FIG. 9.3 A, Simple component x-ray test meters. A RAd-cal kV meter, a Radcheck dosimeter, a Nuclear Associates Timer Test Tool. **B,** Fluke/Victoreen Non-Invasive All-in-One Test Meter M-4000.

Radiography Technical Services
X-Ray Generator Compliance Testing

Facility Name: _____

Contact Person: _____ Phone # _____

Address: _____

Control Model: _____ Serial # _____ (_Tube)

Kilovoltage (must be accurate to within +/− 8%)   Time Set _____

MA Set	KV Set			
	60	70	80	100
60 or				
120 or				
240 or				
300 or				
360 or				
			Comment	

mA	mAS	Output	mR/mAs
60 or	6	100 mR	16.6
120 or	12	200 mR	16.6
240 or	24	300 mR	16.6
300 or	30	500 mR	16.6
360 or	36	600 mR	16.6

mA Linearity (+/− 10%) __80_ kV _.10_ Time
An example of a perfectly calibrated generator

Timer (+/− 8%) _____ kV_____ mA

Time Set/ Pulses		Output
1/120 or	1	
1/60	2	
1/30	4	
7/120	7	
1/10	12	
3/20	15	

Reproducibility 80kV 10 mAs - +/− 20%
Or___ kV @ ___mAs

	Output
1st	
2nd	
3rd	
4th	
5th	

Filtration 80kV, 10 mAs
or___ kV @ ___ mAs

0 mm Al	
2.3 mm Al	
3.3 mm Al	
HVL= @80kV	

Survey Date_____ Completed by _____ Notes _____

FIG. 9.4 An example of a generator test page for a veterinary clinic. Tests include kV, mA linearity, half-value layer, timer test, and reproducibility.

KILOVOLTAGE ACCURACY TEST

Default kVp	Allowable Range +/− 8% Limits	Actual KvP (Leave blank if default values used)		Small Focus Time ____ mA ____ mAs ____			Large Focus Time ____ mA ____ mAs ____		
				25	50	100	100	200	300
50	46.0–54.0								
60	55.2–64.8								
70	64.4–75.6								
80	73.6–86.4								
90	82.2–97.2								
100	92.0–108.0								

On some units the default kV is not available. Use the middle column for closest values available.

FIG. 9.5 Chart for testing kilovoltage at various mA stations on both large and small focal spots.

HALF-VALUE LAYER TEST

Setup:

1. kVp set at __**__ to deliver 80 or _____ kVp.

2. mA _____ Time _____ (or) mAs _____

3. Focal/meter distance _____ cm Focus _____

4. Filtration: Fixed _____ Variable set at _____

**The kV must be calibrated correctly or the HVL total will be incorrect.
As kV increases, the x-rays emitted by the x-ray tube become progressively harder (i.e., more penetrating). The HVL at 80 kV will be different than the HVL at 90 kV since the beam at 90 kV is "harder" than the beam at 80 kV.

Readings	
0 ____ mm Al added	_____ mR
3 ____ mm Al added	_____ mR
____ mm Al added	_____ mR
____ mm Al added	_____ mR

Actual kVp	HVL
@ 80 kVp	_____ mm Al
@ kVp	_____ mm Al

FIG. 9.6 Chart for testing half-value layer. The half-value layer is a measurement of the amount of filtration necessary to reduce the x-ray beam to half its original intensity at preset factors.

Testing Techniques

The HVL is tested using a **dosimeter**. The kV may have to be adjusted to deliver the specific amount if the x-ray unit is not calibrated correctly. A technique is set (usually 80 kV and 10 mAs), an exposure is completed, and the dose is recorded. Filtration, in the form of aluminum plates, is added to the collimator until the dosimetry reading is half the original value. The plates of aluminum are measured in increments of 1 millimeter. This final reading is the HVL (Fig. 9.6).

Takeaway Tips

Legal filtration is typically 3.4 mm of aluminum at 80 kV. As the kV changes, the penetration value changes, so the HVL will change with an increase or decrease in kV. For example, a higher kV will produce a more penetrating beam, so more aluminum is required to reduce the intensity of the radiation to half its value. The equipment manufacturers arbitrarily set the standard for testing at 80 kV. This way the HVL can be compared uniformly across various x-ray units. The kV reading

mA	Output
60 or	
120 or	
240 or	
300 or	
360 or	

A   mA linearity (+/− 10%) _____kV _____Time

mA	mAs	Output	mR/mAs
60 or	6	100 mR	16.6
120 or	12	200 mR	16.6
240 or	24	300 mR	16.6
300 or	30	500 mR	16.6
360 or	36	600 mR	16.6

B   mA linearity (+/− 10%) __80__ kV __.10__ Time

An example of a perfectly calibrated generator

FIG. 9.7 A, Chart for testing mA linearity. **B,** mA linearity chart filled in. As the mA increases, the dose (output) increases proportionally. This is a 1:1 ratio. Increase the mAs by two times the amount, and the dose will double.

Timer (+/− 8%) _____kV _____mA

Time Set/ Pulses		Output
1/120 or 1		
1/60	2	
1/30	4	
7/120	7	
1/10	12	
3/20	15	

A

Timer (+/− 8%) __80__ kV __100__ mA

Time Set/ Pulses		Output
1/120 or 1		1 or .0083
1/60	2	2 or .016
1/30	4	4 or .033
7/120	7	7 or .058
1/10	12	12 or .100
3/20	15	15 or .150

B

FIG. 9.8 A, Chart for testing time stations. **B,** Timer test chart filled in. Note that the time is read in pulses for a single-phase unit and as decimal time for high-frequency and three-phase units.

may need to be adjusted so that the actual kV output is 80 kV. If the HVL is too low, the "softer" radiation will not be filtered out, adding to the dose to the patient. If the HVL is too high, parts of the useful beam will be filtered out. This puts extra wear on the x-ray tube and decreases contrast in the image ("flattens" the contrast).

mA Linearity Test
The mA linearity test is a measure of the output from each of the mA stations and is done to ensure that the output is consistent from one station to the next.

Testing Techniques
The instrument used for testing is a dosimeter. This test measures the radiation dose to the dosimeter. (kV and time are not changed between exposures.)
- 60 mA must have an output of one-half of 120 mA.
- 120 mA must have an output double that of 60 mA and half that of 240, etc.
- The legal variable is ±10%.

Takeaway Tips
The kV and time are always constant for each exposure and must be accurately calibrated (Fig. 9.7). The source-image distance (SID) must also remain the same. The output will be unique for each x-ray unit, but it must be linear. In an ideal generator, dividing the milliroentgens (mR) dose

value as read on the meter by the milliamperes (mA) value will give the same number for each station. Many meters still read out in the older dose nomenclature and not the SI units.

Timer Testing
The timer on an x-ray generator is set to control the length of time that radiation is produced.

Testing Techniques
A timer test tool is placed on the tabletop. The x-ray beam is collimated to the size of the detector. An exposure is made, and the readout will indicate the time of the exposure as measured by the radiation dose read by the timer test tool. The timer test should include all the stations that are in the normal range of use. Fig. 9.8 shows a selection of stations. Note that even though fractions are set on the generator, the meter reads in decimals only.

Takeaway Tips
Single-phase generators select time by fractions of 120 pulses in North America (100 pulses in other countries). Three-phase generators read actual time, which is in decimals. High-frequency generators read the same as three-phase generators. Three-phase and high-frequency generators have much shorter times available, as they are not limited by pulses per second.

Reproducibility

Reproducibility is a measurement of the generator's ability to produce the same output at the same settings throughout several exposures when the factors have been changed and reset between each recorded exposure (Fig. 9.9).

Testing Techniques

The instrument used is the dosimeter. The dosimeter is placed on the table, and the x-ray beam is limited by the collimator to the size of the detector. The generator is set at 80 kV and 10 mAs. After the exposure is made, the factors on the generator are changed and then reset to 80 kV and 10 mAs. This is repeated a minimum of 5 times but no more than 10 times.

The actual reproducibility mathematics are beyond the scope of this text. It is sufficient to average the output doses and determine whether any individual number is ±15% above or below the average. If any number is beyond the parameter, the service engineer must recalibrate the unit.

Takeaway Tips

Reproducibility is very important in order to produce consistent radiographs. The actual calculations for this test are quite complicated, but it is enough to take 5 to 10 exposures and ensure that they are well within ±15%. The selectors should be changed between each exposure, just as they would be if the x-ray unit was in constant use. If this test demonstrates a greater or lesser 15% flux, it may explain why some images turn out considerably darker or lighter than others at the same setting.

Collimator Tests

The collimator is the final exit point for the radiation from the x-ray tube. It is composed of a metallic outer shield with plates (leaves) installed to widen or narrow the x-ray beam to control the radiation affecting the target (Fig. 9.10).

The collimator must be tested (Fig. 9.11) to ensure that:
- It produces a light field that is perpendicular to the tabletop

Reproducibility 80 kV 10 mAs - +/- 20% Or _____ kV @ _____ mAs	
	Output
1st	
2nd	
3rd	
4th	
5th	

A

Reproducibility 80 kV 10 mAs - +/- 20% Or _____ kV @ _____ mAs	
	Output
1st	243 mR
2nd	246 mR
3rd	244 mR
4th	235 mR
5th	241 mR

B

FIG. 9.9 A, Reproducibility chart. The test is carried out by setting a technique (usually 80 kV and 10 mAs). A dose reading is taken and noted. The dials or light-emitting diode (LED) settings are changed and then changed back to the original, and an exposure is taken. This is done 5 to 10 times. The test ensures that the exposures are reproducible. **B,** Reproducibility chart filled in. Note that the output will vary slightly between exposures. If it varies by more than 15%, the generator should be recalibrated.

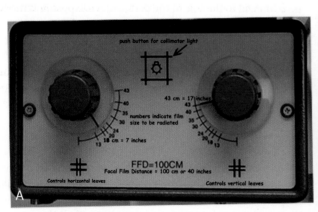
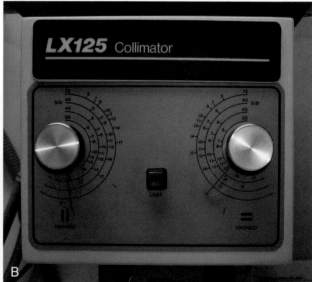

FIG. 9.10 A, Typical collimator without an angulation scale. This particular tube stand has a preset height (100 cm); therefore the dial indicates cassette sizes at that height. **B,** Another collimator that has a variety of SID (source-image distance) settings available. This would be mounted on a variable-height tube stand.

Collimator, Table, and Tube Stand Tests See following procedure charts	Yes	No	Not Available
1. Alignment of the visual field (with the light on) to the x-ray field meets the 2% guideline when the axis of the beam is perpendicular to the plane of the image			These tests are all available with every collimator
2. Minimum collimation does not exceed 5 cm by 5 cm at a target to image receptor distance of 100 cm			
3. Dimensions of light field can be adjusted smaller than the image receptor			
4. Stepless adjustment of field size			
5. Collimator light is visible with room lights on			
6. Perpendicularity of light beam @ 90 degrees to table top			
7. Focus Film Distrance is accurate to +/– 3%			
8. Indicated collimation accurate			
9. Angulation indicator correct			
10. Tube, table, and tube stand stability			

FIG. 9.11 A chart to be completed when testing the collimator.

- The alignment of the visual field (the light field on the table) is not greater or less than 2% of the actual film size when the axis of the x-ray beam is perpendicular to the table
- The minimum collimation does not exceed 5 cm by 5 cm
- The indicated collimation is accurate, if present
- There is a stepless adjustment of the field size
- The dimensions of the field can be adjusted smaller than the field size

Test 1. Collimator Alignment
Objective
To test the alignment of the visual (light) field to the x-ray field.

Equipment
- One cassette loaded with film or a digital imaging plate

Procedure
1. Ensure that the focus film distance (FFD) is 100 cm or 40 inches from the tabletop.
2. Set the control to 50 kV, 100 mA, and a minimum of .03 ($\frac{1}{30}$ sec).
3. Place the cassette on the tabletop so that the central ray will pass through the exact center of the cassette.
4. Place coins on the cassette so that their edges are within the light field but right at the edge of the light field (Fig. 9.12).
5. Place a larger coin on one corner so that you can identify the position of the cassette or plate after processing.
6. Process the exposed film, and place it on the front of the cassette in the exact position it was in before the exposure.
7. Turn on the collimator light.
8. Measure the amount of "shift," or lack of coincidence, between the light field and the radiation field.

Digital Systems
Follow the same procedure, but leave the coins in place while you view the image. Any offset of the x-ray field will be demonstrated on the monitor, which you will compare with the light field on the tabletop.

Conclusion
- The coins mark the edge of the light field.
- If there is a "shift," or lack of coincidence, greater than 2 cm, then an adjustment is necessary.
- Sometimes this adjustment may be made in-house with an adjustable lever mounted above the x-ray tube. More often, a service person will have to make the adjustment.

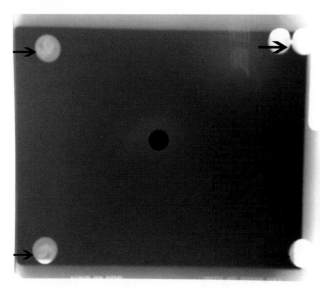

FIG. 9.12 Testing collimator alignment. The coins are placed at the edges (corners) of the light field. An image is generated. In this case the light field and the x-ray field are not coincident. The x-ray field is 1 cm to the left of the coin edges. This is due to a very slight angulation of the x-ray tube.

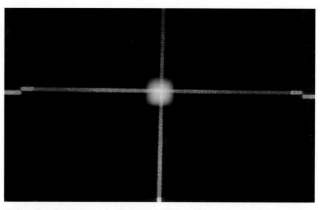

FIG. 9.13 Minimum collimation. This collimator is equipped with a laser light source to assist in viewing. The collimator leaves are closed to less than 5 cm by 5 cm (2 inches by 2 inches).

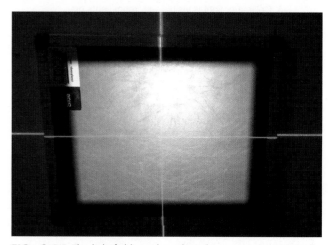

FIG. 9.14 The light field can be adjusted to cover an area smaller than the smallest image receptor.

- Occasionally, on older x-ray tubes the weight of the tube will bend the tube arm and cause a horizontal shift due to the weight of the tube and the length of the tube arm. This is quite common and must be adjusted by an x-ray engineer unless the tube stand is equipped with an adjustment handle.

Test 2. Minimum Collimation
Objective
To ensure the minimum collimation does not exceed 5 cm by 5 cm (2 inches by 2 inches) at a target to the image receptor distance of 100 cm (40 inches).

Equipment
- Ruler with centimeter and/or inch markings

Procedure
1. Position the x-ray tube over the center of the table at 100 cm (40 inches) above the tabletop.
2. Turn on the collimator light
3. Close the collimator leaves to the minimum (Fig. 9.13).
4. Measure the lighted area on the tabletop.

Conclusion
The lighted area should be closed to allow a minimum light field/x-ray field of 5 cm × 5 cm (2 inches × 2 inches).

Test 3. Dimensions of Light Field Can Be Adjusted Smaller Than the Image Receptor
Objective
To ensure that the leaves of the collimator can be adjusted to an area smaller than the smallest image receptor. This will ensure that each image demonstrates collimation.

Equipment
- One cassette (the smallest cassette in the normal range of use in the facility)

Procedure
1. Position the x-ray tube on the center of the table.
2. Position the cassette on the tabletop beneath the collimator.
3. Turn on the collimator light (Fig. 9.14).
4. Adjust the collimator leaves so that they will provide collimation smaller than the outer edges of the cassette.

Conclusion
The leaves of the collimator should close so that the lighted area is smaller (both horizontally and vertically) than the smallest cassette in the facility.

Test 4. Stepless Adjustment of Field Size
This test ensures that the field size can be made larger or smaller by turning the collimator knobs without hesitation or "notching."

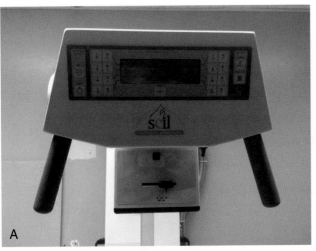
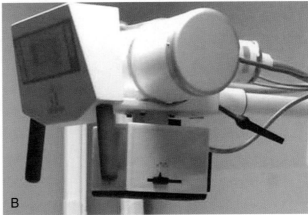

FIG. 9.15 **A,** Stepless adjustment of field size. A sliding bar at the front of the collimator adjusts the horizontal collimation (front to back of the table). **B,** The sliding bar at the side of the collimator adjusts the vertical collimation caudal-cranial.

Equipment
- Collimator

Procedure
1. Position the x-ray tube over the tabletop (Fig. 9.15).
2. Open and close the leaves of the collimator to make sure that they open and close smoothly with no hesitation or "notching."

Conclusion
- This test is essential to ensure that the collimator leaves are not being obstructed by the internal components.
- Collimators are difficult to service in-house, but any difficulties with their movement must be addressed.

Test 5. Collimator Light Visibility
Objective
To ensure that the collimator light is visible with the room lights on.

Equipment
- One x-ray cassette
- One piece of black paper or cardstock with a textured design

Procedure
1. Position the x-ray tube over the center of the table at 100 cm (40 inches) above the tabletop.
2. Turn on the collimator light and open the leaves to 10 cm by 10 cm (4 inches by 4 inches).
3. Slide the piece of black paper into the light field, and observe whether the light is still visible (Fig. 9.16).

Conclusion
- The light should be clearly visible on the black paper.
- The Plexiglas plate covering the collimator light can become stained or burned with age. If the light is a standard

FIG. 9.16 Collimator light visibility. The laser light is visible, but the collimator light is also visible on this textured surface.

(nonhalogen) bulb, it may not be bright enough to penetrate the discolored Plexiglas plate.
- If the light is not visible on the black paper, it will not show up on the black coat of a patient.

Test 6. Perpendicularity of Light Beam at 90 Degrees to Tabletop
Objective
To ensure that the light beam of the collimator is perpendicular to the tabletop.

Equipment
- One carpenter's level

Procedure
1. Position the x-ray tube over the tabletop.
2. Place the level on the x-ray tube (or the front edge of the collimator if possible) so that it rests evenly on both ends.

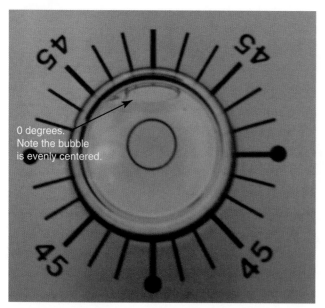

FIG. 9.17 Perpendicularity of light beam at 90 degrees to the tabletop. The bubble in the level on top of the collimator indicates that the tube is not angled and the central ray will be perpendicular to the tabletop. It corresponds to the reading of the level mounted within the collimator.

3. Observe the bubble in the level, and adjust the angle of the x-ray tube if necessary to ensure that the bubble is centered and that the central ray from the x-ray tube is perpendicular to the tabletop (Fig. 9.17).
4. If the x-ray tube has an angulation feature, it may slowly twist into a slight angle just from being moved up and down the table during routine radiography.

Test 7. Focus Film Distance Is Accurate to ±3%
Objective
To ensure that the FFD is correctly marked on the x-ray tube column.

Equipment
- Measuring tape
- Yard stick ruler or meter stick that is at least 1 yard (meter) long

Procedure
1. Position the x-ray tube column in the center of the table longitudinally.
2. Locate the position of the focal spot on the x-ray tube. The focal spot position is usually marked on the x-ray tube with a small indentation about one-third of the way from the bottom of the tube housing. If it is not marked, then mark a spot one-third of the diameter of the tube starting from the bottom of the x-ray tube.
2. Tape the meter (yard) stick to the table so that it extends over the edge of the table and rests against the tube column.
3. Raise the x-ray tube until it is positioned at the 100-cm (40-inch) mark on the tube column (Fig. 9.18).

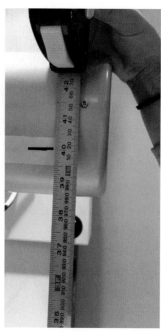

FIG. 9.18 The level of the focal spot is marked on the tube. The measurement is taken at 100 cm (40 inches). This is then compared with the marking on the tube stand.

4. Measure the distance from the meter stick to the focal spot mark on the x-ray tube.

Conclusion
- The focal spot must be within ±2% of 100 cm (40 inches).
- If the focal spot is beyond these parameters, then the measuring point on the tube stand must be corrected.

Test 8. Collimation Indications Are Accurate
Objective
To ensure that the measurements on the collimator indicating the cassette size are accurate both horizontally and vertically.

Note: Keep in mind that not all collimators are equipped with field size indicators (Fig. 9.19). However, the law states that if they are part of the collimator apparatus, they must be correct.

Equipment
- One cassette of each size in the normal range of use in the facility

Procedure
1. Ensure that the focal spot is 100 cm (40 inches) above the tabletop.
2. Place a cassette on the tabletop under the collimator.
3. Adjust the indicators on the collimator to coincide with the size of the cassette both horizontally and vertically.
4. Turn on the collimator light and observe whether the light is coincident with the size of the cassette.

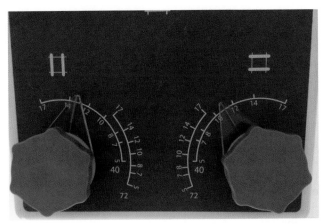

FIG. 9.19 Collimator size indicator. The outside partial ring is for 180 cm (72 inches). The inside ring is for 100-cm (40-inch) measurements.

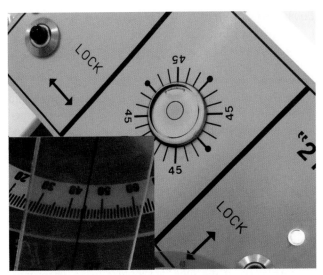

FIG. 9.20 This tube is angled to 45 degrees as evidenced on the protractor.

5. Repeat this for each size of cassette in the normal range of use in the facility.

Conclusion
- The indicators must be accurate for the size of the cassette.
- Correcting the indicators in the field by a service engineer can be difficult and expensive.
- Sometimes it is easier and less expensive to mark the correct measurements on the collimator in black marker for the size of cassette in the facility

Test 9. Angulation Indicator Is Correct
Objective
To ensure that the angulation indicator is accurate.

Equipment
- Carpenter's level
- Protractor with angles clearly marked

Procedure
1. Position the x-ray tube over the center of the table.
2. Ensure that the central ray is perpendicular to the tabletop (see Test 6).
3. Position the tube so that the angle indicator on the x-ray tube is at 45 degrees (Fig. 9.20).
4. Position the protractor so that the angle indicated is 45 degrees. Note that the collimator angle and the protractor angle are coincident.
5. Repeat this procedure for 60 degrees and 90 degrees.

Conclusion
- The angle indicator must be completely accurate.
- Some x-ray tubes do not have angle indicators. In this case if some views require an angled tube, it is necessary to keep the protractor in the x-ray room.

Test 10. Tube, Table, and Tube Stand Stability
Objective
To ensure that the x-ray table, the x-ray tube, and the tube stand do not move during an exposure (Fig. 9.21).

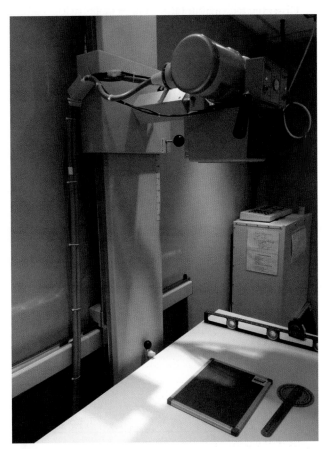

FIG. 9.21 X-ray tube and tube stand stability. The x-ray tube stand is moved to the end of the table and stopped. It must be mounted correctly so that it does not sway or move when the operator's hand is lifted from the handles. Standing at the end of the table, the operator should also note whether the tube is slightly angled front to back from the operator moving the tube while pulling downward on the handles.

Equipment

- X-ray tube, table, and tube stand
- Carpenter's level

Procedure

Note: Some x-ray tubes are mounted directly to the wall and do not move along the table. Some tube stands are mounted to the ceiling or the floor. Some x-ray tables are not mounted to the floor.

1. Position the tube stand at the center of the table.
2. Turn on the collimator light, and ensure that it is positioned exactly over the center of the table. If the table is not bolted to the floor, mark on the floor where the table legs must be before each exposure. It is vital that the table does not move at all, particularly if a grid is to be used.
3. Move the tube steadily and quickly along the table and then let go of the tube. It should remain where your hand left it and not move farther or swing from side to side.
4. Stand at the end of the x-ray table (either end is fine), and move slightly toward the tube-stand side of the table.
5. Observe whether the tube stand is vertical or is angled slightly toward the table.
6. Observe whether the collimator base is slightly angled across the table (from table front to table back).

Conclusion

- The tube stand must be stable and must not move once it is placed in position. The x-ray table must be bolted to the floor directly in line with the center of the central ray.
- The tube stand must not lean in toward the table.
- The tube hanger must be parallel to the floor and must not allow the tube to "sag" so that the bottom of the collimator is not absolutely parallel with the table front and back and side to side.
- The table and the bottom of the collimator must be parallel to one another both vertically and horizontally.

Radiobiology and Radiation Protection for the Patient and the Worker

This section discusses quality control as it relates to Chapter 3, Radiobiology and Radiation Protection for the Patient and the Worker.

The leaded products that are purchased for the x-ray room will deteriorate over time. Lead-impregnated rubber will

harden and crack. Leaded protective garments should be tested annually and logged on a chart (Fig. 9.22). Each apron, thyroid collar, and pair of gloves should be identified and dated when they are purchased and marked with an indelible marker.

Leaded Aprons

Leaded aprons are not intended to absorb primary radiation and therefore do not require high technical factors to penetrate the lead. Aprons should be stored on a hanger or specially made rack. They should not be folded or permanently bent over a wire hanger.

Equipment

- X-ray unit set at 60 kV and 6 mAs or whatever setting gives a density 1 + base + fog on the image through the leaded apron.
- Two 35- by 43-cm (14- by 17-inch) cassettes or a digital detector
- Numeric markers – these can be cut out of an old apron or a leaded mask and are used to identify each apron; coins of different denominations can also be used as long as a guide is kept matching the apron to the size of the coin

Procedure

- Place a 35- by 43-cm (14- by 17-inch) cassette crosswise on the tabletop. Place a leaded apron on the cassette so that the bottom of the apron is aligned with the lower edge of the cassette (Fig. 9.23A).
- Select an exposure on the x-ray unit that is 60 kV, 100 mA, and $\frac{1}{15}$ sec (6 mAs).
- Open the collimator to include the entire detector.
- Expose and process the film.
- The density on the film should be 1 + base + fog.
- Repeat the exposures, exchanging the cassette with each exposure and moving it up toward the neck with each repositioning until the entire apron has been tested.
- Remember to mark each section with the same identifier so that there is a referenced image for each section.

Takeaway Tips

Leaded products are not designed to be penetrated by primary radiation. They are designed for protection against secondary radiation. Therefore a high technical factors are not required to penetrate them with direct radiation. If the film image is

Date	Apron #1	Apron #2	T. Collar #1	T. Collar #2	Leaded Gloves / Masks Visual Inspection

FIG. 9.22 Leaded products integrity test.

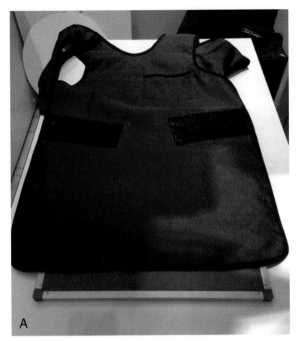
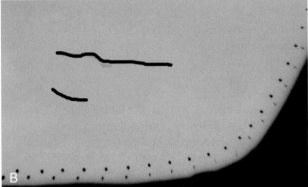

FIG. 9.23 A, Lead apron testing. The apron is spread over the cassette, which is placed horizontally on the tabletop. Two images are generated: one for the bottom of the apron and one for the top of the apron. **B,** Leaded apron radiograph showing the even stitch lines on the edge of the apron and two simulated apron cracks to demonstrate the difference between the stitch line and actual cracks (no one would agree to having their apron slashed even for the textbook!).

too dark, any cracks will not appear. If the film is too light, the cracks will still appear as dark gray lines. Do not be alarmed regarding the stitching on the sides of the apron. This will show up as a line of black dots. Any cracks or holes will show up as black lines or black holes. Areas of lighter density demonstrate overlaps or stretching of the lead sheets within the apron.

Thyroid Protectors
Procedure
These can be tested using the same technique as with the leaded aprons. They can be logged on the same chart. If the thyroid protector is attached to the apron, it should still be labeled individually.

Gloves/Leaded Rubber Masks/Blockers
Procedure
Because gloves are double-sided, it is impossible to test them individually using radiation, as one side will mask the other. Gloves must be pliable and easily folded when used. Old leather gloves and mitts can become stiff and unbendable. They should be replaced with new pliable mitts/gloves. The old gloves may be repurposed as leaded masks for absorbing scattered radiation. They should be labeled as masks with indelible marker.

Gloves should be examined manually by inserting a hand into the glove and palpating to identify any cracks or splits in the leaded rubber. Leaded masks should be examined regularly and should be stored lying flat.

Imaging on Film

This section discusses quality control as it relates to Chapter 4, Imaging on Film.

The image gallery in Chapter 4 demonstrates many different problems associated with film-based imaging. These problems are usually identified by their effect on the image after processing. The following are a few additional tests that may be necessary.

Testing Film/Screen Resolution

In radiography, recorded detail is measured and expressed as resolution. Resolution is the ability of the viewer to distinguish separate line pairs. A line pair is described as one black line and one white line in an image. Line pairs are expressed as lp/mm. The test tool that is used is a resolution test pattern (see Fig. 4.30).

Very-high-resolution images are 30 to 35 lp/mm (for extremity and mammography images in medical imaging). Standard full-speed x-ray film with appropriate 400-speed screens is typically 8 to 9 lp/mm. Advertised line pairs in digital imaging are typically 4 to 5 lp/mm.

The question of resolution is important throughout all areas of imaging. It is what defines a system—the system in this case being the cassette, intensifying screens, film, and all the other factors that are included in the process. Resolution becomes even more important when digital imaging is considered. The comparison between digital imaging and film/screen imaging is always, primarily, about resolution.

X-ray film alone has virtually infinite resolution. When a veterinarian looks at an image and attempts to diagnose a hairline fracture, he or she is looking at the combination of the technical factors used to produce the image: the cassette front, the film, the intensifying screens, any tabletop artifacts, the grid, processing artifacts, the patient's anatomy, and, finally, the illuminator. Each of these factors can degrade the image and yield a far-less-than-perfect result.

Equipment
- Resolution test tool
- Cassette with film
- X-ray unit

Procedure
1. Place the resolution test tool on one side of the cassette with a leaded blocker on the other side.
2. Set the x-ray unit factors to 55 kV and 3 mAs or whatever factors are required to expose the film to a density of 1 + base + fog outside of the resolution test tool.
3. Now move the leaded strip across to the unexposed side of the cassette.
4. Turn the resolution test tool 90 degrees and place it on the cassette.
5. Expose this side of the cassette and process the film.
6. Use the guide on the resolution test tool to determine the resolution of the film/screen system by counting the line pairs until they appear to run together and cannot be differentiated.

X-Ray Cassettes
Uniform Speed of Intensifying Screens
Objective
To identify the uniformity of the intensifying screens in your facility. (First ensure that the generator is correctly calibrated and has good reproducibility.)

Equipment
- Every film cassette in use in the facility
- Leaded numbers to identify each cassette (Cassettes may also be identified permanently by writing small numbers on the screen with a fine, black felt-tip marker. The same number should then be marked on the outside of the cassette.)
- X-ray generator that has been tested for reproducibility (See tests for reproducibility, p. 138). Each exposure must be the same as the one before and the one after.

Procedure
1. Place the cassettes on a table outside the x-ray room ready to test in ascending order of size.
2. Bring in one cassette at a time and remove it from the room once it has been exposed. (This will eliminatethe possibility of scattered radiation affecting the cassette.)
3. Place one cassette containing film on the tabletop and center it beneath the central ray.
4. Open the collimators to the size of the cassette. Set the generator to 50 kV, 100 mA, $\frac{1}{30}$ sec (3.3 mAs). (This is a typical technique for a 400-speed system. If your system speed is different, then adjust the mAs according to the chart in Table 4.1.)
5. Process your film and record the density. (If you do not have a densitometer, record the value that is different from or similar to the reference image (see Fig. 9.1).
6. Adjust the technique if necessary until the image is density 1 + base + fog.
7. Using the same technique, expose the film in all of the cassettes. (If you had to adjust the technique, then retest the original cassette.)
8. Check the speed of the intensifying screens, and compare the images using the same illuminator with the room lights turned off.
9. Slower screens produce a lighter image; faster screens produce a darker image. Ideally, all images should be the same density. Any screens that produce a vastly different density should be taken out of service and replaced so that every cassette in the hospital produces uniform densities.

The Blue/Green Question
Objective
To identify the color emission of a blue or green screen.

Frequently the cassettes in the x-ray room are replaced or added to by well-meaning veterinary clinics or local hospitals as they change systems and no longer require these particular cassettes. It is easy to identify the film that accompanies them, as blue-receiving film is green and green-receiving film is mauve or very light purple. Remove one sheet of film from the box, close the box tightly, and turn on the light. The type of film will be instantly recognizable.

The intensifying screens present a further challenge. It is not enough to assume that because the film that accompanied these cassettes is green-receiving film that the screens must be green-emitting screens. Many times the reason the cassettes are replaced with other systems, or even digital systems, is because the wrong color film is in the cassette and the hospital staff cannot produce a diagnostic image.

Before the "new" cassettes are put into use, always follow this procedure.

Equipment
- Cassettes to be tested, which were identified earlier
- X-ray generator

Procedure
1. Set the generator to 70 kV, 100 mA, and 0.25 ($\frac{1}{4}$) sec.
2. Turn off the lights in the room and ensure that it is completely dark.
3. Place an open cassette beneath the central ray.
4. Open the collimator to cover the open cassette.
5. Wait until the collimator light turns off (or turn it off if it is a manual switch).
6. Make an exposure and record the color of the light.

7. It is often useful with a mixed group of cassettes to write a large G for green or B for blue on the back of each cassette as it is tested.

Conclusion

Screens that are not the same emission as the ones already in use must be disposed of. If they are kept in the hospital because the cassettes may be used later, then they must be clearly labeled with the color of the screens.

Film/Screen Contact Testing

The intensifying screens must be held in the cassette in close overall proximity to the film. Any air gaps between the screen and the film will result in a fuzzy image (Fig. 9.24A–D). Early cassettes had metal bars that locked under the edges of the cassettes. These bars assisted with good film/screen contact, but many operators' fingers were pinched between the bars and the edges. This method was abandoned in favor of sliding bars that clipped closed (but also clipped open on the larger cassettes at inappropriate times).

Agfa cassettes (see Fig. 4.25) were made of a lightweight plastic that made the cassettes easier to carry, but the overall design detracted from good film/screen contact. An Agfa cassette is equipped with a magnetized rubber insert on the back and a metallic film beneath the screen on the front. The front screen is loosely held in place so that it can be drawn to the magnetized back (see Fig. 4.26). The engineering was critical and expensive. The magnet lost its holding strength over time and contributed to the loss of film/screen contact. These cassettes are clearly marked (they are bright orange and black) and should be checked with a screen contact test tool regularly or if a problem is suspected.

Most companies use foam rubber, which is glued to the back of the cassette, holds the screen evenly and permanently with the correct amount of pressure against the front screen, and maintains the film in good film/screen contact.

Equipment

- Screen contact test tool
- Cassettes to be tested containing film
- X-ray unit
- Leaded numbers or black markers to identify each cassette

Procedure

1. Place a cassette on the tabletop centered beneath the central ray.
2. Open the collimator light to cover the cassette.
3. Place the screen contact test tool on top of the cassette.
4. Set the technique at 55 kV 5 mAs. (This is a suggestion only and may have to be altered depending on the generator and film/screen combination.)
5. The density of the overall image should be 1 + base + fog (see Fig. 9.1).
6. Some technicians drill a small hole with a diameter of 0.635 cm ($\frac{1}{4}$ inch) in the center of the test tool. This enables a density reading to ensure that the technical factors are correct and that the screen speed is consistent with every cassette.
7. Once the correct density has been verified, test all the other cassettes in use within the facility.
8. Check the density in the center hole for every cassette to ensure that the screens in use are functioning correctly and have not lost speed.

Conclusion

Every film image should demonstrate a clear mesh pattern with no darkened areas. Dark areas within the pattern indicate areas of poor screen contact, which will degrade the image and make it fuzzy.

> ### ◆ APPLICATION INFORMATION
>
> All cassettes are vulnerable to problems and should be reviewed once per year. The films should be removed in the darkroom (or the cassette should be left unloaded after use). The cassette should be examined under room light to ensure that the foam rubber has maintained its integrity and that the hinges and latches are in good working order. The screens should then be cleaned with gauze dampened with distilled water to remove any dust or fingerprints. The cassettes should be stood open and upright on the tabletop for a minimum of 10 minutes until the screens are completely dry. A record should be kept to note any problems observed during the inspection.

Inspecting Cassettes for Stability and Integrity

Kodak cassettes (see Fig. 4.28) were rugged and sturdy, with rubber edges and hinges, which worked well when they were new. As they aged or were subjected to extreme temperatures, however, the rubber hardened and cracked on the hinge side and the cassette broke apart. Kodak also slightly bent the back of the cassette to improve film/screen contact. This worked well; however, it put extra strain on the hinge side, which also compromised the rubber. The screens can be removed from the broken cassette and placed into a new (or used) cassette.

Removing Screens From Broken Cassettes

If the latches break or the Kodak cassette rubber hinges break apart, the intensifying screens can be removed with caution and placed into a new cassette with no screens or a used cassette whose screens have deteriorated.

Equipment

- Double-sided tape
- Replacement cassette with old screens removed
- Sturdy table or floor space
- Distilled water
- 4 inch × 4 inch (10 × 10 cm) gauze pads

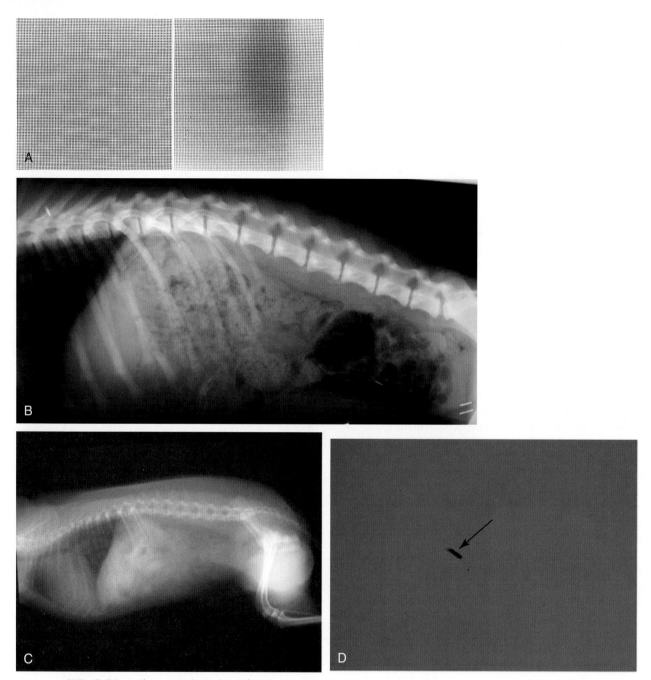

FIG. 9.24 A, This screen shows the perfect screen contact image. **B,** A problem with screen contact caused by the light being allowed to diffuse between the screen and the film. There is an area of "fuzziness" in the caudal thoracic and cephalic lumbar area of the spine. This corresponded with poor film screen contact when the cassette was tested. **C,** Poor screen contact across the entire image. The Kodak cassette had a split back, which the staff tried to correct using duct tape. The overall poor screen contact demonstrates that this method is not a solution. The screens must be changed into a new cassette. **D,** A small piece of dirt was discovered on the screen, causing a minus density artifact in the image. This artifact was in a different place each time. As the films were drawn out of the cassette, it would be moved around—but never out of—the image. (**A** from Fauber TL. *Radiographic Imaging and Exposure,* 4th ed. St. Louis; Mosby; 2013.)

Procedure

1. Place the cassette on a sturdy table, and peel a corner of the screen away from the back of the cassette.
2. Very carefully pull the screen back away from the corner, making sure that the screen does not crease or bend in any way. The emulsion of the screen can be "rolled" away, but it must not crease. This takes practice, and

it is best to practice on a used cassette where it doesn't matter if the screen is creased. Experience will teach you how much strength and pressure the screen will take before it creases. Kodak screens are difficult to remove because they are glued over the entire back surface. Other companies just use double-sided tape to attach the screens.

3. Make sure that the tabletop is clean and dust free.

4. If the foam starts to rip away, just pull the screen out carefully and place it face down on the tabletop.

5. Now peel away the foam from the screen. It will probably rip away in sections; this is fine as long as all of it comes away. This can be a messy job, as some of the older screens had a very thin rubber backing that deteriorated into a rubbery glue.

6. Once the screen is free of the backing, place double-sided tape on all four sides and place it in the cassette on the same side as it was in the original cassette. For example, if the screen you are working with was on the back of the cassette, then place this screen on the back.

7. The easiest method for replacing the screen is to place the front screen into the front of the cassette and then place the back screen on top of the front screen and close the cassette.

8. Now open the cassette and clean the screens with distilled water and gauze.

9. Stand your cleaned cassette upright on the tabletop to dry for at least 10 minutes before reloading it with film.

Takeaway Tips

This is a worthwhile exercise if you have Kodak screens. They are excellent screens and maintain their speed virtually indefinitely. Make sure that you do not crease the screen when you remove it from the cassette. If you need smaller screens and you have smaller cassettes, you can cut the screens with regular scissors.

Reinstating the Curve on Curved-Back Cassettes

DuPont and a few other cassette companies bent the back of the cassette slightly to enhance the film/screen contact (see Fig. 4.27A). Over time, the bend decreased as the cassette was opened and closed hundreds or even thousands of times.

Equipment

- Cassette to be adjusted
- Firm, stable tabletop

Procedure

Place the cassette over the edge of a table and carefully press gently but firmly and evenly on the back of the cassette (see Fig. 4.27B). The pressure does not have to bend the cassette very much, so gentle pressure and then a check to ensure that the back has been recurved is sufficient.

Takeaway Tips

These cassettes also have a very tiny "handle" that was added to assist the operator in opening the cassette (Fig. 9.25). This worked well if the cassette back popped up when the cassette was opened, but if the bend was eliminated and the cassette was opened without the back rising slightly, it became difficult to open the cassette once it was unlocked. Carefully rebending the cassette solves this problem.

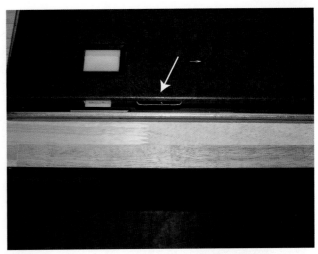

FIG. 9.25 These cassettes have a tiny handle that is useful for opening the cassette if the curved back is curved correctly.

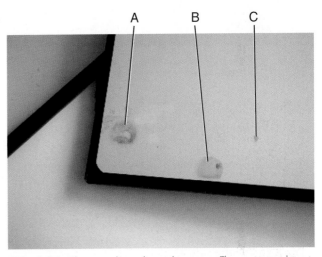

FIG. 9.26 Chemistry dripped onto this screen. The screen emulsion is porous and will absorb chemicals of any variety that are dripped onto it. It is important to remove the film and close the cassette when manually processing.

Miscellaneous Screen Artifacts

The emulsion of the intensifying screens can be compromised in various ways. A few of these problems are demonstrated in the following images. There is no particular test protocol to identify these problems because they are obvious once the cassette is opened in the light. The cause of the artifact that was clearly displayed on the image is now visible (Figs. 9.26 and 9.27; see Figs. 4.36 and 4.37).

Cassettes must be handled with care to ensure that the front remains undamaged and radiolucent. Any foreign material introduced into the cassette shell may show up superimposed on the image. Patient effluent, barium, or contrast material can leak between the front of the cassette and the back of the screen. If seepage occurs, the screen and backing must be removed and cleaned thoroughly.

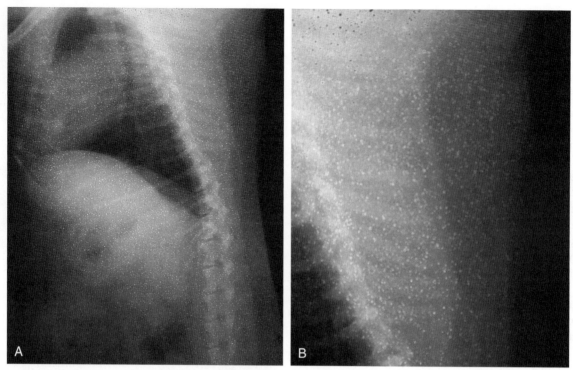

FIG. 9.27 A, A particular problem with DuPont Quanta 111 and later screens. In a humid environment, the screen emulsion absorbed moisture from the air and swelled into tiny raised points. These points broke up the lattice network of the image, causing small minus density artifacts. These artifacts started at the screen edge and migrated across the entire screen as the process continued. **B,** An enlarged view of a portion of part A. The screen is destroyed and must be replaced. There is no "fix" to this problem.

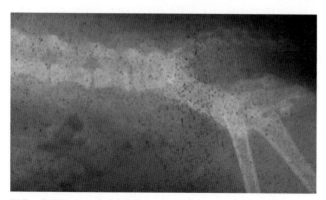

FIG. 9.28 An example of overuse of screen cleaner. Overuse of commercial screen cleaners build up residue on the screen, which eventually causes artifacts on the film as they case plus-density artifacts across the image. The artifacts are actually areas of the film that were affected by the components of the screen cleaner that caused the silver in the emulsion to coagulate.

Commercial Screen Cleaners

A number of commercial screen cleaners have been introduced over the years. There are also several home remedies for cleaning screens. A commercial screen cleaner can stain a screen if the particular brand does not match the brand of the screen. Screen cleaners can also leave a residue that builds up over the years send causes artifacts on the image (Fig. 9.28). If screen cleaners are mandatory for whatever reason, they should be used once per year followed by a distilled water rinse to remove the residue.

Home remedies such as alcohol and other cleaning agents should never be used on screens because they can dissolve the protective layer and damage the emulsion.

Cleaning Intensifying Screens
Equipment
- Cassettes to be cleaned that are open and have the film removed
- Distilled water
- 1 package 10 cm × 10 cm (4 inch × 4 inch) gauze pads

Procedure
This procedure is best carried out on the x-ray table, as it is a wide surface for cleaning the cassettes and standing them upright to dry after cleaning.
1. Open the cassette and remove the film in the darkroom.
2. Lay the open cassette on the x-ray table.
3. Dampen a 10 cm × 10 cm (4 inch × 4 inch) gauze wipe with distilled water. The gauze should be damp, not wet.
4. Wipe the screen lightly in one direction; then wipe again at a 90-degree angle. The screen should be very slightly damp with no visible water marks. Any surface dirt or dust is removed with this technique.
5. Stand the cassette upright on the table and leave it to dry for at least 15 minutes. The cassettes should be placed

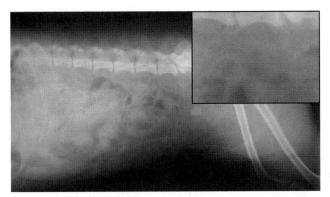

FIG. 9.29 Screen wear. The emulsion of the screen becomes worn over many years. The thinning emulsion is not as effective at converting x-rays to light. The lighter areas on the film replicate the wear areas on the screen. The insert demonstrates an enlarged part of the indistinct image.

upright so that dust in the room does not settle and adhere to the screens.

6. Check that the screen is dry and that it is adhering to the cassette front and back. If the screen is loose (as might be the case with Agfa cassettes and some generic brands), make sure there is no dirt or dust beneath the screen. (Use a flashlight if necessary.)

Takeaway Tips

Commercial screen cleaning agents are often specific to the manufacturer and can stain screens that are manufactured by other companies. Screen cleaners that are not matched to the manufacturer can discolor the screens, reducing their x-ray–to–light conversion (see Fig. 4.33). Screen cleaners often build up a residue, which eventually becomes visible on the images. Distilled water and lint-free gauze are the best combination to use to clean screens. It is very important that a screen is completely dry before reinserting the film. Film emulsion is manufactured to absorb moisture rapidly, and any remaining moisture on the screen would be absorbed into the film emulsion and would adhere to the screen, ruining the film as well as the screen. Stains and scratches that have penetrated the emulsion of the screen are not removed by the technique just described. If the emulsion from the screen is missing, there is no way to repair the screen.

Intensifying Screen Wear: Emulsion Loss

Older intensifying screens exhibit wear artifacts (Fig. 9.29). Over many years of use, the emulsion of the screens thins and then disappears completely as thousands of films are inserted into and removed from the cassette. There is no solution to this problem other than replacing the screen with one of similar speed.

Intensifying Screen Lag

In the late 1980s and early 1990s Agfa produced a screen using a unique phosphor. The images were excellent, but the screens retained a very small amount of phosphorescence. If

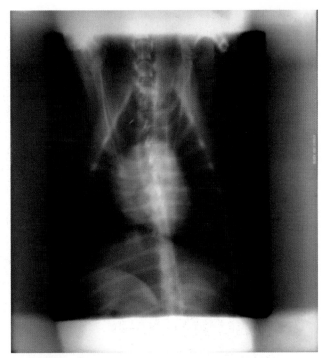

FIG. 9.30 Collimator splash. The image is overexposed. The boundaries of the collimator are clearly visible, yet the film has been exposed by secondary/scattered radiation beyond the collimator limits.

the cassette was used right away after being filled, there was no problem. However, if the film stayed in the cassette for any length of time beyond 5 minutes, the film became fogged and the next exposure was made on fogged film. Thousands of these cassettes and intensifying screens were taken out of distribution, but a number of them showed up in the veterinary market, given to the veterinarians as "free" cassettes.

Producing the Image

This section discusses quality control as it relates to Chapter 5, Producing the Image.

Testing for Extrafocal Radiation

This test is used to determine that the scatter/secondary radiation as seen in Fig. 9.30 is actually from the patient and not from extrafocal radiation, as is seen in Fig. 9.31.

Equipment

- Aluminum foil folded so that there are 8 to 10 layers in a strip about 4 inches wide and 15 inches long (10 cm × 40 cm)
- A market chicken about 5 pounds*
- X-ray unit

---

*This experiment can also be carried out in the veterinary hospital using live patients. It does not increase the dose to the patients, but rather solves a mystery as to why the extrafocal images are occurring.

Procedure

1. Wrap the aluminum strip around the x-ray tube hanger just at the attachment of the collimator to the bottom of the x-ray tube (Fig. 9.32).
2. Place the patient (or phantom) on the tabletop, and set the technical factors according to the technique chart.
3. Collimate to the edges of the patient's anatomy.
4. Process the film and view the image.

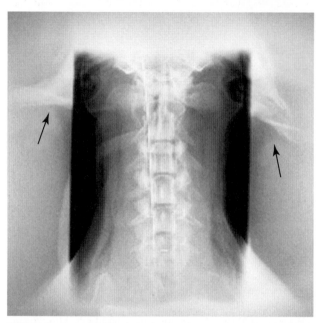

FIG. 9.31 An example of extrafocal radiation. This imprints the image of the dog's ears beyond the edges of the collimator.

Conclusion

If the images previous to this one demonstrated extrafocal radiation, the aluminum foil will absorb the soft radiation and the regions beyond the collimator will be clear. If the densities are caused by secondary/scattered radiation, it will remain the same, with or without the aluminum filter.

Optimizing the Image

This section discusses quality control as it relates to Chapter 6, Optimizing the Image.

Grids, Grid Lines, and Grid Artifacts

Grids are added to the x-ray unit after it is installed, and they should be checked annually as part of a routine quality control program. It is useful to know what grid is installed in your x-ray unit. If it is possible to remove the tabletop easily and safely, then do so and clean the grid with a glass cleaner. Look on the front of the grid to locate the label, which will tell you:

- The way the lines are running (the grid should be positioned so that the lines run vertically along the tabletop)
- The grid ratio
- The line pairs
- The number of lines per inch (or per cm)

A 10:1 ratio or 103 line pairs is ideal for use in a veterinary hospital using a film/screen combination. Any ratio lower than this will probably be visible on every image (Fig. 9.33). Any ratio higher than this will add to the dose, as it will require an increase in technique without a corresponding improvement in the image. Gridlines on the image detract from the resolution and imprint an image of the grid on every image taken with the cassette below the tabletop.

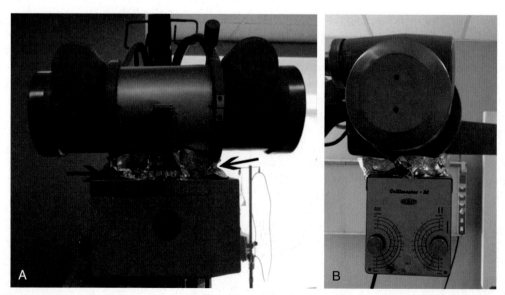

FIG. 9.32 A, Aluminum foil will reduce the effect of the extrafocal radiation if it is radiating from the front and sides above the collimator. The foil should be at least 8 to 10 layers thick and wedged tightly against the mounting brackets. **B,** The aluminum foil surrounds the collar of the x-ray tube. In this case the staff have rotated the collimator so that it is easy to turn on the light if it is necessary to hold the patient.

Grid Quality Test
Equipment
- Cassette with film
- X-ray unit containing a grid

Procedure
1. Place the cassette with film enclosed into the grid tray, and close the grid tray.

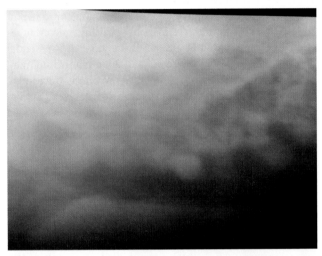

FIG. 9.33 This grid was an old metal door screen from about 50 years ago. A new veterinarian was puzzled by the artifacts that affected every image taken in the grid tray.

2. Do not put any object on the tabletop, and make sure the tabletop is clean.
3. Set the technical factors to 55 kV and 8 to 10 mAs (or whatever technique is necessary to expose the film to a density of 1 + base + fog).
4. Process the film and examine the resulting image closely.

Takeaway Tips
Any grid artifact will be immediately visible (Fig. 9.34). The image should be a gray film at density 1 + base + fog. Faint vertical lines may be visible, but they will be uniform, will be very faint, and will not affect the images.

Grid Artifact Images
These images are taken to demonstrate incorrect grid position. The grid artifact problems are easy to identify as shown in Figs. 9.34 to 9.36.

Illuminators: Characteristics and Test Tables
Once the film is processed and ready for viewing, the next piece of equipment in use will be the illuminator (Fig. 9.37). The illuminator is a vital link in the imaging chain. It is important to be aware that the illuminator provides light by ionizing the gas within the illuminator tubes. It does this by means of a ballast and an electric current. If the illuminator is mounted in the x-ray room and the room is also used as a darkroom, the gas will continue to ionize for up to 30 minutes

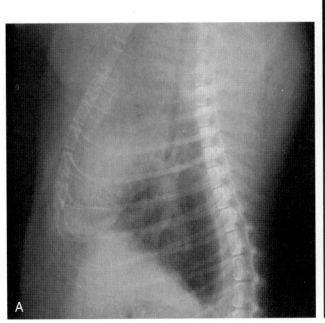
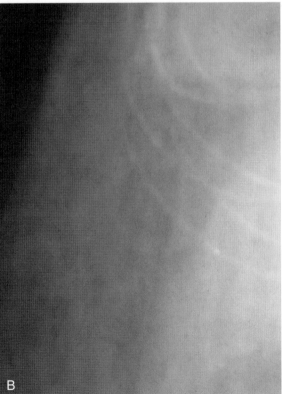

FIG. 9.34 A, Grid deterioration places an overall indistinct pattern of vertical lines on this image. **B,** Magnified view of part A. The vertical lines are more obvious. The film was positioned on the illuminator vertically to mask the lower portion of the illuminator, causing the artifact to become more visible.

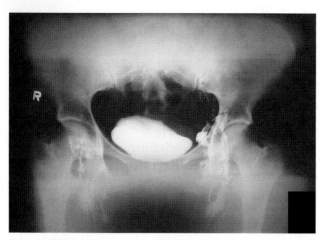

FIG. 9.35 This grid is placed in the holder upside down and horizontally. The grid lines should run vertically; that way if the tube is angled, there will be no grid cut-off.

after the illuminator is switched off. This situation will definitely fog any x-ray film within the room even though the light is not visible to the human eye. With older illuminators and fluorescent lights, the shape of the light is actually visible after the light is switched off. This is the reason why fluorescent lights should never be mounted in a darkroom.

The illuminators should be on the list of cleaning and maintenance protocols within the veterinary hospital. Each illuminator should be checked at least once per year or if any discrepancy is noticed between any of the light tubes in the facility (Fig. 9.38). Fluorescent tubes are sold in many different colors. The tubes for the veterinary hospital are standard tubes and can be purchased at any hardware store. It is essential that the light tubes are matched and are a blue-white light. They must not be any other color. X-ray film is tinted blue to reduce the glare of the illuminator when the veterinarian is viewing the images. The illuminator light tubes must be

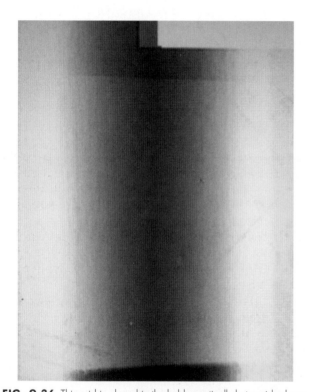

FIG. 9.36 This grid is placed in the holder vertically but upside down. Because it is a focused grid, the grid lines absorb the lateral radiation and only the center of the image shows the exposure.

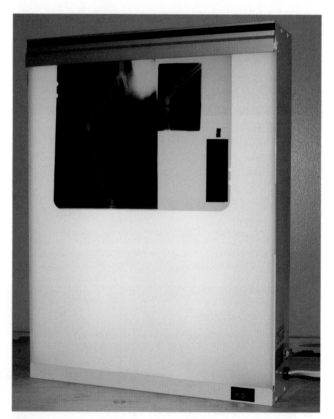

FIG. 9.37 The light from the illuminator with no mask is glaring to the eye of the viewer and decreases the brightness of the image so that small details are lost.

Illuminator Position	Color	Brightness	Both bulbs bright	Flicker?	Clean screen Y/N
X-ray room					
Examination room 1					
Examination room 2					

FIG. 9.38 Test table for illuminator condition.

blue-white to match the blue tone of the film base. The front of the illuminator is a specially treated glass that will diffuse the light from the light tubes. This glass is expensive and not readily available except from a radiography illuminator supply company. The back of the illuminator behind the light tubes must be a shiny white in order to reflect the light through the front of the illuminator.

An Illuminator Mask

A mask can be easily made from a 35 cm × 43 cm (14 inch × 17 inch) sheet of film (Fig. 9.39).

- Remove the film from the film box.
- Seal the box and then expose the film to the light.
- Process the film, and cut small or large holes in it to mask only the areas with no image.
- Keep the portion of the film that was cut away, and use it if a second hole is cut in the film to view a second image.
- The mask will eliminate light from around the image, causing small details to be seen more easily.

Processing the Image on Film

This section discusses quality control as it relates to Chapter 7, Processing the Image.

Protecting the unexposed film from any kind of exposure to heat, light, and chemicals is vitally important to the production of an optimized image. Containers for storing unexposed film are available, and they must be positioned in the darkroom with no possibility of light seeping in (Fig. 9.40).

Darkroom Integrity

Testing safelight integrity must always be completed using a film that has been exposed to radiation. The film is now 8 to 10 times more sensitive to any form of film fog or artifact.

Equipment
- Cassette with film
- Stopwatch preset to 2 minutes (to be turned on by pressing a switch)

Procedure
1. Position a cassette on the tabletop.
2. Collimate to the edges of the cassette.
3. Lightly expose the film using 50 kV and 2 mAs. When processed, the lightest section of the film should be considerably lighter than the density 1 + base + fog density.
4. Take the cassette to the darkroom and place it on the counter.
5. Turn the safelight off, secure the darkroom from any noticeable visible light, and open the cassette.
6. Remove the film from the cassette, and place three-quarters of the film beneath the cassette, leaving half exposed to any light leaks on the counter.
7. Press the stopwatch to start counting down from the 5-minute preset.

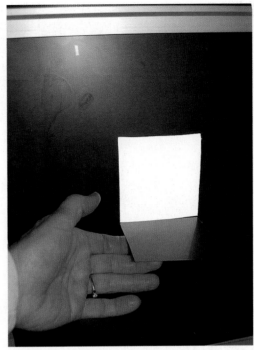

FIG. 9.39 A simple illuminator mask cut from a 35- by 43-cm (14- by 17-inch) film. A hole is cut in the mask and then taped onto the film. The "window" allows the light to illuminate the image but masks the brightness of the surrounding light.

8. While the stopwatch is counting down, slowly and carefully move around in the darkroom as your eyes acclimate to the dark (only after 5 minutes will you start to see light leaks). Look around to see if there is any visible light. Several places to look are:
   - Around the room where the walls join the ceiling
   - Around the placement of any exhaust fans
   - Around and through any electrical sockets near the countertop
   - Around all the edges of the door frame, especially below the door
9. Once the stopwatch counts down to zero, place the film on the feed tray and process the film.
10. Now look around and recheck all of the locations you checked the first time.
11. If there is a problem with the darkroom integrity, the half of the film that was exposed to the light will show a density that is not present on the half of the film that was beneath the cassette.

Safelight Testing

Testing safelight integrity must always be completed using a film that has been exposed to radiation (Fig. 9.41). The film is now 8 to 10 times more sensitive to any form of film fog or artifact.

Equipment
- Film in a cassette

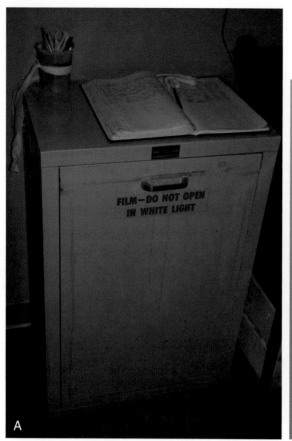
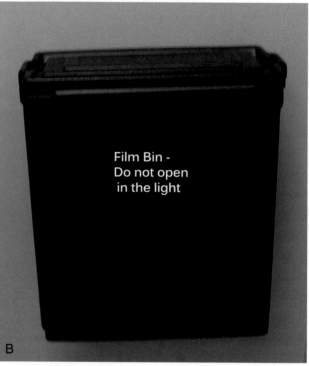

FIG. 9.40 A, An example of a standalone metal film bin. The metal bin is essential if the film is stored in the x-ray room. This one doubles as a counter. **B,** A plastic wall mount bin in the darkroom. This model holds two sizes of film.

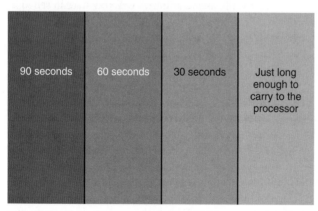

90 seconds	60 seconds	30 seconds	Just long enough to carry to the processor

FIG. 9.41 The safelight test film will quickly demonstrate that there is a problem with the positioning and brightness of the safelight.

Procedure

1. Expose a film in a cassette on the tabletop using 50 kV and 2.0 mAs or just enough radiation to cause a low density on the film. It does not have to be as high as density 1 + base + fog.
2. In the darkroom place the cassette on the counter.
3. Turn the safelight on, secure the darkroom, and open the cassette.

4. Remove the film from the cassette, and place three-quarters of the film beneath the cassette, leaving one-quarter exposed to the safelight. Count to 30 seconds.
5. Slide the next quarter of the film out from under the cassette, and count to 30 again. (Now half of the film has been exposed to the safelight.)
6. Repeat this once again so that three-quarters of the film has been exposed to the safelight.
7. Immediately remove the rest of the film from under the cassette, and process it.

The last quarter of the film was exposed to the safelight for just the length of time it took to take the film to the processor. If there is a problem with the safelight, the areas exposed will be darkened in proportion to the length of time that they were exposed to the light plus the amount of the original exposure. The total length of exposure time is 1.5 minutes (90 seconds).

Ideally the processed film will be completely clear with no fog on it. Fig. 9.41 shows the results of a safelight test where there was definitely a problem with the positioning or wattage of the safelight.

Processor Tests
Developing, Fixing, Washing, and Drying
Problems with artifacts in automatic processors can be a challenge to diagnose. Some problems, such as the ones in

the image gallery in Chapter 7, are easy to diagnose. Occasionally there is a problem that is more difficult or the veterinarian would like to evaluate two different films and the way they react to light from the intensifying screens.

As the film is placed on the entrance tray and is moved forward toward the entrance rollers, it is affected by the solutions in the developer, fixer, and wash. The dryer rollers can also cause artifacts, but this is rare.

Automatic Processors vs. X-Ray Equipment

The majority of processor problems occur in the developer. First, it must be determined that the problems occurred in the processor and are not a result of a problem with the x-ray equipment. A simple test for this follows.

Equipment

- Two cassettes loaded with film
- X-ray unit
- Processor at the correct temperature and ready to process film
- Leaded pencil

Procedure

1. Place the first cassette on the tabletop.
2. Set the technical factors at 50 kV and 5 mAs (or whatever factors are necessary to give a density of 1 + base + fog).
3. Press the exposure switch.
4. Remove the cassette from the x-ray room.
5. Place the second cassette on the table.
6. Use the same technical factors.
7. Expose the second film.
8. Take the cassettes to the darkroom and open them both.
9. With the leaded pencil mark the direction of travel of each film on the film itself.
10. Film #1 will be processed horizontally (long side in first).
11. Film #2 will be processed vertically (short side in first).
12. Process each film individually, one film after the other, through the center of the feed tray
13. Review Fig. 9.42.
14. If the artifact lines are horizontal on the one image and vertical on the next image that was rotated 90 degrees, then the artifact is caused by the x-ray unit and not the processor.
15. If the artifact lines stay in the same direction even if the film is rotated, then the artifact is caused by the processor.

Sensitometry/Densitometry

Sensitometry/densitometry is a method of tracking processing parameters. It has nothing to do with the x-ray equipment, as the x-ray equipment is not involved in this procedure. Sensitometry makes use of a device called a *sensitometer* (Fig. 9.43A). This unit has a stepped table on the bottom with a light beneath it. The table has 21 steps or small strips of graded densities that increase from base + fog level to the maximum blackness that the film will attain. It is manufactured so that when the light exposes a film, the middle step (Step 10) will

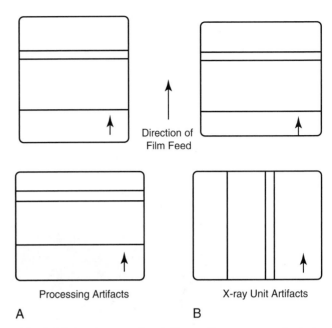

Direction of Film Feed

Processing Artifacts   X-ray Unit Artifacts

A   B

FIG. 9.42 A processor test film. **A,** The two films are processed individually at 90 degrees to one another. The artifacts do not rotate with the orientation of the film. This indicates that the artifact problem is in the x-ray equipment. **B,** The two different films are processed individually, and the artifacts change with the rotation of the film. This indicates the problem occurs within the processor.

be density 1 + base + fog (Fig. 9.43B). The top step will be base + fog only (D$_{min}$), and the bottom step will be the maximum density of the film (D$_{max}$).

The density will be read on a companion unit called a *densitometer* (Fig. 9.44). The densitometer contains a "platform" where the film is positioned for each of the 21 steps. These steps are then plotted on graph paper to produce a sensitometry curve (Fig. 9.45).

Every radiograph is made up of densities, from the clear areas on the film to the very black areas. It is the combination of these densities that demonstrates the anatomy/pathology of the patient (Fig. 9.46). Sensitometry is one easy method to sequentially arrange the densities on the radiographs to ensure that the processing parameters are stable day to day. A chart is filled in that measures two steps above density 1.0 (Step 12) and two steps below density 1.0 (Step 8) (Fig. 9.47). When the total of Step 12 minus Step 8 is filled in on the bottom line, the number should be virtually identical every day, only varying by 2 to 3 points.

If the processing varies from day to day as the chemistry in the processor becomes older and more contaminated, this would demonstrate that the replenishment is not working well and does not maintain fresh chemistry. The resulting films will become flat and lack contrast. This will show up quickly on the images, but the sensitometry strip will also confirm there is a problem even if no images are taken that day.

Another use of sensitometry is to compare the contrast and speed of two different films. If a sales rep convinces the

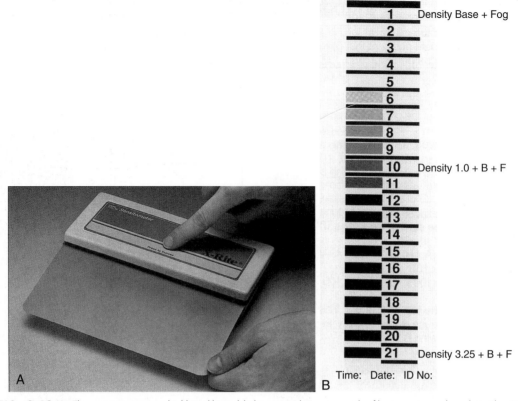

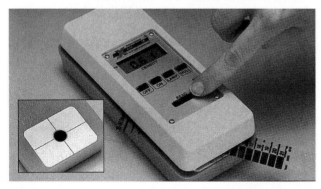

FIG. 9.43 **A,** The sensitometer is a highly calibrated light source that exposes the film to a stepped wedge. The 21 steps on the wedge are used to plot contrast and consistency of the processor. **B,** A sensitometry strip produced by the sensitometer and processed. The top step is base + fog only. The bottom step is the maximum density of the film. Step 10 is density 1 + base + fog.

FIG. 9.44 A companion densitometer. The inset shows the small area that the light shines through to read the film. The readout is a digital screen at the top of the unit.

veterinarian that his or her film is better than the present film in use in the hospital, the first thing that must be done is to determine the contrast and speed of the new film. Is it more black and white (higher contrast), and does it react faster to radiation (speed) than the present film? Both films should be tested in the darkroom before any exposures on patients. Speed will affect the technique chart, and contrast may enhance or degrade the image.

Fig. 9.48 demonstrates three films, and it is easy to read that the stepped wedge on the left is very low contrast

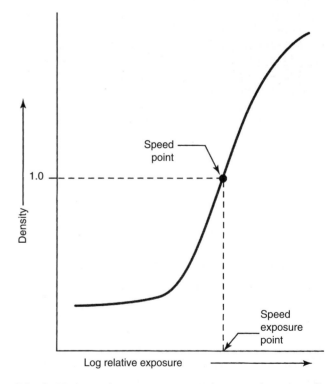

FIG. 9.45 A typical sensitometry curve. At the x-y axis there is virtually no density other than base + fog. As the steps increase, the density increases to step 21, which gives the maximum density.

and the film on the right is very high contrast. Fig. 9.49 demonstrates the curves plotted for two different films. The speed point should always be read at density 1 + base + fog. In these curves Film A is considerably faster (reacts to the radiation) than Film B. However, the contrast of both films is virtually identical. In this same figure the bottom row shows that in order to achieve density 1 + base + fog on Film A, you need to reduce your exposure from 2.0 to 1.5. This can be translated to a 25% speed advantage for Film A over Film B. Another film may be manufactured to show several different gray steps and never get to solid black.

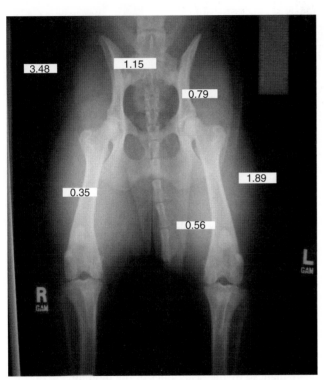

FIG. 9.46 It is possible to read all of the various densities in a radiograph using the densitometer. Sensitometry provides a way of arranging the densities in sequence from the lightest to the darkest density provided by that particular film.

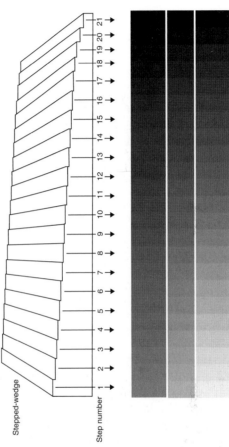

FIG. 9.48 Comparing three different sensitometry strips from three different films. The film to the left is very low contrast with many steps of gray. The middle film is a standard general radiography film with more contrast than film number 1. The film on the right is a specialty high-contrast film with few gray steps.

Month _____

Day	Mon	Tues	Wed	Thur	Fri	Mon	Tues	Wed	Thur	Fri	Mon	Tues	Wed	Thur	Fri	Mon	Tues	Wed	Thur	Fri
Date	3	4	5	6	7	10	11	12	13	14	17	18	19	20	21	24	25	26	27	28
Step 12																				
Step 8																				
Contrast																				

FIG. 9.47 Monthly chart plotting the sensitometry contrast levels every operational day.

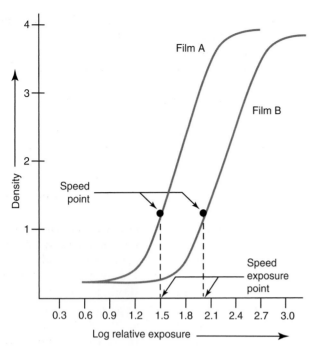

FIG. 9.49 Comparing two general radiography films from two different manufacturers. Film A reacts more quickly to the radiation than does Film B. The comparable densities are measured at density 1 + base + fog, which is known as the *speed point*. The bottom of the graph indicates the relative exposure levels.

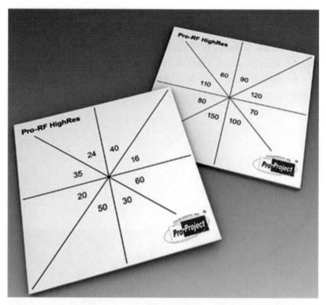

FIG. 9.50 Two test patterns for measuring fluoroscopy resolution on the monitor. Mesh (corresponding to the number on the front covers) is embedded between the two covers. The lower test tool measures a resolution of 16 to 60 mesh. The other measures a high-resolution screen from 60 to 150 mesh. These test tools can also be used to view edge distortion and lag.

Fluoroscopy

This section discusses quality control as it relates to Chapter 11, Fluoroscopy.

As veterinary hospitals become more sophisticated, fluoroscopy and real-time imaging become necessary. The equipment is more sophisticated, but a few simple tests can be easily carried out before any examinations. One is the fluoroscopy resolution test procedure.

Fluoroscopy/Image Intensifier Resolution

Objective

To identify the resolution of the fluoroscopy monitor and to log image lag or fade to identify if the image is severely distorted at the edges of the monitor screen.

Equipment

- Fluoroscopy unit with the monitor turned on
- Fluoroscopy resolution test tool (usually the lower-resolution test tool [16 to 60 mesh] is sufficient for most hospitals)

Procedure

1. Position the fluoroscopy unit over the tabletop so the image intensifier is as close to the table as possible.
2. Place the resolution test tool on the tabletop (Fig. 9.50). Position the central ray of the x-ray unit over the center of the resolution test tool.
3. All personnel in the room must wear leaded protection.

4. Stand close to the table and the resolution test tool so that a view of the image intensifier is unobstructed.
5. Depress the foot switch so the test tool appears on the monitor with the center of the test tool in the exact center of the monitor.
6. Identify the finest mesh that is visible on the monitor.
7. Release the foot switch and rotate the mesh 90 degrees. Depress the foot switch and verify your first reading.
8. Step 7 will identify if the mesh was correct or if it was enhanced by the raster lines of the monitor.
9. Record the finest mesh that was identified. This is a subjective test, so if you are wearing eyeglasses, ensure that they are clean and unmarked with fingerprints or dust.
10. Now move the image intensifier from side to side and watch the image. It should move and stop with no lag or "drag" of the image.
11. The mesh should now be located in the exact center of the monitor. If there is any distortion of the image at the edges of the monitor, it should be noted, as this may increase with the age of the monitor.

Takeaway Tips

As stated, this is a subjective test so the observer must make sure that his or her eyes are unobscured by fogged or marred eyeglasses. The minimum mesh should be 30 or higher. A mesh reading of 16 indicates that the unit should be recalibrated. This test should be repeated at least once every 6 months for every monitor in the facility. The distortion is a natural result of the curvature of the lens in the monitor. It can deteriorate as the monitor ages.

REVIEW QUESTIONS

1. Quality control and quality assurance are defined as follows:
   a. Quality control is concerned with performance of equipment; quality assurance is documentation of all factors.
   b. Quality control is concerned with performance of people; quality assurance is the assurance that people are working.
   c. Quality assurance is the performance of equipment; quality control is the documentation of assurance.
   d. Quality assurance is identification of the actions necessary to assure performance; quality control is the performance.

2. Correct line voltage is confirmed by reading the dial on the front of the generator. Which of the following statements is true?
   a. There is always a dial on the front of every generator.
   b. Modern generators do not have a dial; calibration is internal.
   c. There is no particular importance to reading the dial.
   d. Once the machine is turned on, every generator will recalibrate.

3. kV testing is carried out with a kilovolt meter. Which of the following statements is true?
   a. The typical allowance is ±8% of the station tested.
   b. Accurate kV is not important, as the unit will compensate.
   c. Testing of every mA station is unnecessary, as the unit is always consistent.
   d. The typical allowance is ±15% of the station tested.

4. Half-value layer is defined as:
   a. The amount of filtration that reduces the intensity of the x-ray beam by 50%
   b. The amount of aluminum that reduces the penetration of the beam by 50%
   c. The amount of filtration needed to calibrate the generator to 50%
   d. The amount of aluminum that reduces the output of the generator by 50%

5. mA linearity is described as follows:
   a. The mA stations are mathematically linked.
   b. The output of each station must be exactly the same or within 50% of each other.
   c. The output of each station must be linear; the output at 50 mA is 50% of the output at 100 mA.
   d. The output of a generator is dependent on its linearity; all the stations should be the same.

6. Collimator testing is essential to ensure that the area to be radiographed is exactly delineated. Which of the following statements is true?
   a. The minimum collimation is the same size as the smallest cassette.
   b. The indicated collimation must be in place and be accurate.
   c. The x-ray tube can be misaligned up to 5%.
   d. The alignment of the visual field and the x-ray field is coincident.

7. Testing leaded aprons involves:
   a. Placing the apron under the fluoroscope and scanning it
   b. Just testing the areas of concern on each apron
   c. Placing the apron on a cassette and radiographing it
   d. Setting a very high technique because it is made of lead

8. When an image consistently appears to be out of focus across the entire surface, one problem may be:
   a. The film/screen contact has been compromised
   b. The patients all move when this cassette is used
   c. The manufacturer built in a soft focus to this screen type
   d. The processing parameters are not functioning correctly

9. One cassette always appears to give lighter-than-normal images. Which of the following statements is true.
   a. The technician should mark this cassette and not use it.
   b. The technician should examine the screens to see if they are the same manufacturer and type.
   c. The veterinarian should throw out the screens and cassette and buy new ones.
   d. The staff should mark the cassette and always increase the technique when they have to use it.

10. One cassette always produces very gray films with little to poor contrast; a cause could be:
    a. The source-image distance is too great
    b. The screens emit blue light and the film is green receiving
    c. The screens emit green light and the film is blue receiving
    d. The processing chemistry is contaminated

11. One cassette always produces images with reasonable contrast but requires twice the radiation; a cause could be:
    a. The screens emit blue light and the film is green receiving
    b. The screens emit green light and the film is blue receiving
    c. The patient is very large with little contrast in its anatomy
    d. The source to patient distance is too great

12. The service person has just left, and the veterinarian brings you an image with an outline of the patient's ears on it. You diagnose this as:
    a. Scattered radiation and nothing can be done about it
    b. The service person left the collimator plates out of the collimator
    c. The problem is extrafocal radiation because the collar was left off the collimator
    d. The image is too dark and this is the result

13. The test for grid quality includes:
    a. The film in the grid tray and keys and syringes on top of the table for contrast
    b. The cassette on the tabletop and a very light exposure
    c. The cassette in the grid tray with nothing on the tabletop
    d. The film is exposed on the tabletop, and the grid lines should not be visible

14. The test for darkroom integrity includes:
    a. Turn out all the lights except the safelight, then look for light leaks
    b. Turn out the light and wait 5 minutes for your eyes to adapt before looking for light leaks
    c. Turn out the light and immediately look for light leaks, then process a film out of the film bin
    d. Expose a film, place it on the counter halfway beneath the cassette, turn all the lights off, and process after 5 minutes

15. The test for safelight integrity includes:
    a. Expose a film, place it on the counter three-quarters beneath the cassette, draw it out a quarter at a time, and then process
    b. Turn out the light except the safelight, look for housing cracks, and process a film from the bin
    c. Safelight is on; stand for 5 minutes, look for light leaks, and process a film
    d. Safelight is on; expose a film and process it, then look for cracks in the housing

16. Sensitometry is defined as:
    a. A method of testing processing parameters
    b. A method of testing the integrity of the x-ray equipment
    c. A testing device using a densitometer on exposed films
    d. A density measure for films exposed by the sensitometer

17. One type of artifact is the appearance of clear minus density "dots." Which of the following statements is true?
    a. The cause of this is unknown.
    b. The screen must be cleaned and dried before reuse.
    c. This is a rare occurrence with new screens.
    d. This is caused by minute areas of swollen emulsion.

18. Chemical spills and darkroom accidents:
    a. Damage screens and film and are preventable with good darkroom protocols
    b. Are easily wiped up with no further consequences
    c. Damage cassettes but are easily wiped off screens
    d. Cause fixer and developer to settle on film, prematurely developing it

19. Commercial screen cleaners:
    a. Are the best method for cleaning screens
    b. Should not be used without adequate ventilation
    c. Can build up layers and produce artifacts on the image
    d. Must be matched to the screens or they will not work

20. Heat and chemical fumes will fog the film and cause:
    a. The films in the box to stick together and be difficult to remove
    b. An increase in activity of the emulsion, which will produce a density on the film
    c. An image on the film that can be processed
    d. Artifacts that are identifiable on the film

21. One method of ensuring good resolution is to test each cassette:
    a. For good film/screen contact
    b. To ensure that they all have the same exposure response
    c. To ensure that they all require the same technical factors
    d. For its ability to mask artifacts and shadowing

Answers to Review Questions can be found on the Evolve website.

CHAPTER **10**
Ultrasonography

Robert F. Hylands, DVM

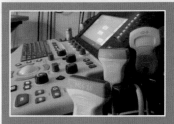

Ultrasound technology is becoming an invaluable diagnostic modality.

A mind that is stretched by a new experience can never go back to its old dimensions.
—Oliver Wendell Holmes, Jr., American author, 1841–1935

OUTLINE

LEARNING OBJECTIVES

When you have finished this chapter, you will be able to:

1. Understand the principles of real-time ultrasound imaging.
2. Recognize the artifacts and limitations of ultrasonography.
3. Identify the various transducer types and functions.
4. Describe the various image modes and discuss their applications.
5. Discuss clinical applications with regard to body systems.

APPLICATION

The application of the information in this chapter is relevant to the following areas:

1. Producing ultrasonographic images when alternative diagnostic imaging is required.

KEY TERMS

Key terms are defined in the Glossary on the Evolve website.

Acoustic impedance
B-mode
Brightness
Cine loop
Color flow Doppler

Continuous wave Doppler
Convex
Depth control
Gain control

M-mode
Microconvex
Phased array
Presets

Pulsed Doppler
Sector probe
Spatial resolution
Transducer

In the years since the first introduction of ultrasound to veterinary medicine, the use of this indispensable imaging tool has grown exponentially to include a vast number of applications. Ultrasound advances our diagnostic abilities in a safe and reasonably economical manner. In almost 30 years of rigorous studies focusing particularly on prenatally exposed children, ultrasound has been found to have no associated health risks. Studies in 1982 and 1987 by the Bioeffects Committee of the American Institute of Ultrasound in Medicine (AIUM) first demonstrated that there were no biological effects on the patient or instrument operators at intensities typical of diagnostic ultrasonography. In 1998 the World Health Organization stated that ultrasound imaging was both a safe and effective modality. This chapter will discuss basic principles in order to familiarize the technician with the goals of an ultrasound examination.

Throughout the chapter there are certain unfamiliar terms of which the reader should be aware. They are presented here so that the student may refer to them as they arise within the chapter.

Echogenicity: The appearance of the tissues on ultrasound, based on the ability of the tissues to reflect sound waves. This refers to the brightness of tissues that are being projected on a B-mode display.

Anechoic: A structure that is lacking in internal echoes or is echo free. Appears very dark to almost black on ultrasound.

Hyperechoic: The tissue of interest reflects back more intense sound waves and appears brighter than the tissues surrounding it. This is a subjective evaluation of adjoining structures.

Hypoechoic: The tissue of interest reflects fewer sound waves and with less intensity, making it appear darker than the tissues surrounding it. This is a subjective evaluation of adjoining structures.

Isoechoic: This a term used to describe two structures that have relatively similar echogenicity toward each other.

Attenuation: This is the loss of sound wave energy as it traverses the tissue or the medium due to absorption, reflection, or scattering.

Reverberation: The sound wave is repeatedly reflected between two highly reflective surfaces—for example, air and the ultrasound probe.

Near Field: The area of a structure of interest that is closest to the probe.

Far Field: The area of a structure of interest that is farthest from the probe.

Ultrasonography and Plain Radiology: A Comparison

One of the defining characteristics of ultrasound is the benefit of real-time imaging. During a scan, a continuous stream of live, digitized data is obtained. From this data, video recordings can be saved, which then can be transferred into a "cine loop." A cine loop is a continuous feed that allows the area of interest to be visualized over a prolonged period. In comparison, plain radiography catches the area of interest in a still frame during a split second of time when the exposure is taken.

The advantage of real-time imaging is seen when we use ultrasound for cardiac studies. We can watch the movement and function of the heart and internal structures over the course of a cardiac contraction. Newer matrix probes can even take this a step further by instantly projecting the acquired data in multiple planes. These planes are then reconstructed by computer and can allow visualization of the heart in a three-dimensional format. This is called *multiplanar reconstruction,* or MPR, and it allows the ultrasound equipment to project an image that is similar to that of more advanced technologies such as magnetic resonance imaging (MRI) and computed tomography (CT).

A second benefit to ultrasound is the ability to move the diagnostic probe in any direction that is required. In comparison, radiography usually requires standardized positioning and orientation. The ability to move the ultrasound probe over the area of interest gives us a much greater amount of information about the subject.

When we use high-quality ultrasound machines in this way, we are able to show fine anatomical detail through the use of multiple sensitive receptors in the ultrasound transducer (probe) (Fig. 10.1).

And finally, as mentioned in the introduction, the safety precautions required when using ionizing radiation (x-rays) are *not* required when an ultrasound is in use. There are no protective gowns and gloves, and multiple people may be in the room during the ultrasound study.

There are many other benefits to this modality, which we will explore as we continue through this chapter, including the ability to visualize detailed pathology through tissues and fluid, which could be difficult or impossible with conventional radiographic imaging.

The Ultrasound Machine

Principles

The basic principle of the ultrasound machine is the production of sound waves by an ultrasound probe (also known as the *transducer*) and the return of that reflected sound wave. Sound waves enter the tissues and are reflected back to the probe; the intensity and speed of the reflections are influenced by the tissue densities. The probe receives the reflected sound waves and then translates the information to the computer so that it can be read on the video screen by the operator.

The most important components of an ultrasound machine are the elements in the transducer. These elements are predominantly made of piezoelectric ceramics. These materials have unique properties that allow them to change shape in the presence of an electric current. When the ultrasound machine emits a desired frequency, strong but very short electrical pulses make the ceramics vibrate. This causes the crystals within the ceramics to emit a mechanical vibration at a preset frequency. The sound frequency emitted is usually

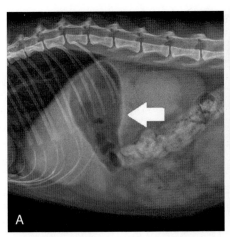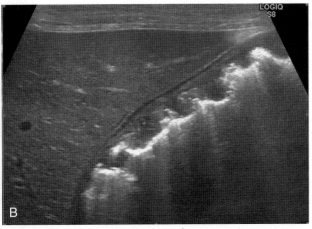

FIG. 10.1 A, The white arrow represents the outline of the stomach wall on a lateral radiograph of a canine abdomen. Very little information about the wall thickness or health can be extrapolated through this image. **B,** The photograph to the right is a high-resolution image of the stomach wall acquired in a near-field ultrasound examination. In the ultrasound study we can observe gastric motility and can visualize the detail of each anatomical layer of the stomach wall. (Images courtesy of R. F. Hylands.)

set anywhere between 2 and 18 megahertz (MHz), but can reach as high as 50 MHz in probes used for ophthalmic studies. The resulting sound wave pulses can then be directed, steered, or focused to the desired depth as set by the ultrasonographer. Each of the crystals is connected to an individual circuit known as an *element,* which allows them to be directed independently. This individual control allows the operator to steer and focus the image through timing delays.

When the sound waves are reflected back to the transducer from the various tissues, they again make contact with the transducer elements, distorting the shape of the individual ceramics and creating electrical energy that is now sent back to the machine to analyze. It is this electric current that is digitized to create a diagnostic image.

Practicality

Modern ultrasound machines come in a variety of formats, including larger cart models, laptop units, and even handheld portable devices. Each unique system offers different levels of image quality and software options. There are many considerations when selecting an ultrasound machine for use in a veterinary practice. For example, machines may vary based on their selection of available types and frequencies of their transducers, the computer processor speed, the quality of the viewing monitors, and many optional software applications. Some machines also vary by whether they will support either a cardiac or general imaging platform. Ideally, for small-animal veterinary practices, a machine with dual-function capability would be the most beneficial (both cardiac and general imaging).

Patient Preparation

Small animals are generally imaged in ventral recumbency on a padded trough, standing, or in lateral recumbency. In actuality, an animal can be examined in just about any position that achieves the desired imaging. Animals undergoing a cardiac study are often placed on a specialized cardiac table

that is customized so that the transducer may be directed through the small cut-out opening of the table top on the "down" side of the patient's chest.

Large animals are usually examined in a standing position.

It is important that the patient remain still in order to achieve an accurate ultrasound examination. Panting, struggling, and tensing up will all decrease the diagnostic capabilities of the sonographer by reducing image resolution and clarity. In these instances, a diagnostic study will require sedation.

Sound waves do not travel through air; therefore the probe must have direct contact with the skin surface. Ideally, fur is clipped away, and alcohol should be sprayed on the skin to remove superficial fats (Fig. 10.2). Next, an acoustic coupling gel is applied to the skin surface and to the surface of the probe to improve contact.

Grayscale

Ultrasonography visualizes a much wider range of tissue densities because the computer sees a larger "grayscale" than can be seen in plain radiographs (Fig. 10.3). Typically at least 256 shades of gray are incorporated into the display of an image obtained through ultrasound. This creates a much superior level of contrast compared with plain radiographs. For comparison, the human eye can only distinguish about 30 to 60 shades of gray (Fig. 10.4).

Modes in Ultrasound Imaging

In ultrasound imaging, the echo data collected can be formatted into specific images that represent different interpretations of the characteristics of the tissues being evaluated. The following list contains an abbreviated outline of the individual characteristics of each mode.

B Mode

In B mode, the "B" represents brightness. The intensity and speed of the returning echo are sent to the transducer,

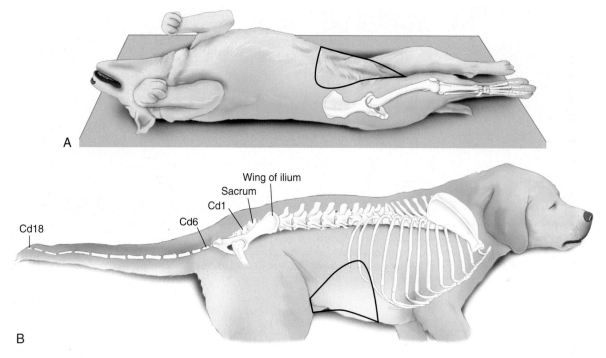

A

Wing of ilium

Sacrum

Cd1

Cd6

Cd18

B

FIG. 10.2 A, Generally when preparing a patient for an abdominal ultrasound, the abdomen should be shaved from the sternum to the distal border of the pubis. In deep-chested breeds the right ventral side of the thorax should also be included from the 11th to the 13th rib. This is to help visualize the gallbladder, common bile duct, and pylorus of the stomach. **B,** In preparing for cardiac studies a rectangle is shaved caudal to the axilla on both sides. To find this location, bend the elbow and find the spot where the point of the elbow touches the ribs.

interpreted, and then transformed into a digitized pixel within a two-dimensional image on screen. The pixel is either classified as hyperechoic (bright) or hypoechoic (dark) (Fig. 10.5).

The full spectrum of 256 shades of gray is used to create each pixel comprising an image. The spatial resolution (or distance) between pixels can be as low as 0.3 mm depending on the type of transducer and frequency used to perform the scan.

M Mode

"M" is interpreted as motion. In this mode, a cursor line is set over an area of interest as imaged in B mode. M mode simultaneously creates a B-mode image (light and dark) while displaying the motion of the tissues over a two-dimensional scale. This creates a continuous wave form and plots where each pixel intersects the cursor line.

M mode is particularly useful when evaluating the heart. Using this mode and plotting the movement of each light and dark pixel, we can determine the thickness and diameter of the ventricular wall through different stages of the cardiac cycle. We can measure cardiac dimensions and evaluate movement of the valvular leaflets within the ventricles (Fig. 10.6).

Doppler

This modality is used to image the flow of blood and other liquids while measuring their velocity. There are four different Doppler techniques.

Color Doppler

In color Doppler the information collected is presented as a color overlay above a B-mode image. This application was first introduced in the mid-1980s. There are different gradients of superimposed color, depending on the color map selected. In standard imaging, for instance, we track blood flow by using the color blue to show blood flow away from the transducer and the color red for blood flowing toward the transducer. This is best remembered through the acronym BART (blue away/red toward) (Fig. 10.7).

The addition of another type of more sensitive color mapping may add variances that detect abnormal turbulence within the normal laminar flow of blood.

Power Color Doppler

This is yet another form of color imaging that is highly sensitive to the flow of blood but does not identify its direction. It is used predominantly to detect lower velocities in tissues where the directional flow is less important than detecting the flow itself. An example of this would be in evaluating the vascularity (blood vessel pattern) of a neoplastic mass.

Pulse Wave Doppler

As the name implies, pulsed wave Doppler (PW) is produced by a transducer that alternates between sending and receiving sound signals. This allows the area being analyzed to be set to within a very small sample volume, or "gate." The sampling or listening area can be set anywhere along a cursor line that

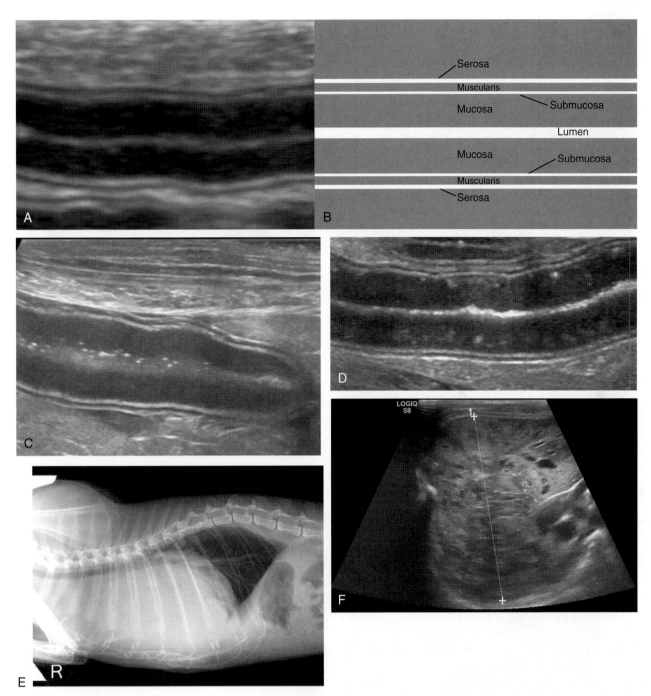

FIG. 10.3 A and B, Ultrasound image showing a segment of the canine jejunum and its structural components. Acoustic impedance gives contrast to the anatomical layering of the intestines, allowing them to be visualized on ultrasound as the sound wave traverses different tissue densities at variable velocities. These variables lead to different shades of gray representing each density. This can be useful in identifying different types of intestinal pathology, as each may be associated with changes in different individual layers. C and D, The second row of images illustrate a normal jejunum to the left and, on the right, hyperechoic densities within the mucosa. This pathology as seen on ultrasound represents dilated lacteals. E and F, Finally, the bottom set of images show a radiograph (below left) where there is a fluidlike radiopaque density filling the cranial aspect of the thoracic cavity *(white arrow)*. This radiograph cannot differentiate between the heart, fluid in the chest, and the outline of a mass. The ultrasound, (lower right) because of enhanced grayscale, clearly identifies the density as a large cystic mass. This was diagnosed as a thymoma. (A, C, D, E, F courtesy R. F. Hylands.)

transects the concurrent B-mode image. PW can read blood flow velocities in the 0.4 to 0.6 m/sec range, making it quite useful for small peripheral vessels. PW can detect blood flow velocities up to a maximum of 1.4 m/sec. At these velocities, the probe reaches what is called a *Nyquist point*. Above this point the transducer inaccurately displays as an inverse or flow reversal, making their true measurement impossible to quantify with any accuracy. At these velocities, continuous wave (CW) measurements should be taken instead of PW (Fig. 10.8).

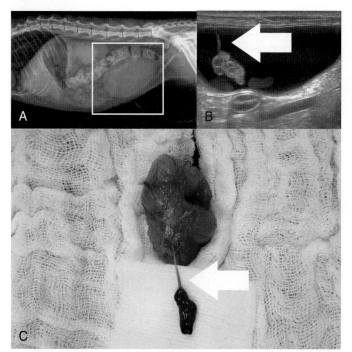

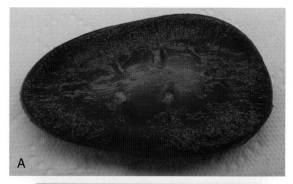

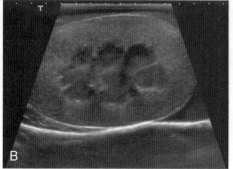

FIG. 10.4 A, The area outlined by the white box in the abdominal radiograph (top left) delineates the space that is usually occupied by the urinary bladder. Note that the tissue grayscale limitations in plain radiographs do not allow visualization of bladder contents other than fluid. **B,** Compare this to the significant difference in visualization of a urinary bladder polyp on ultrasound. This was previously undetected. Diagnosis of this polyp was only possible due to the increased contrast achieved through a wider dynamic range or grayscale. The fine detail is so sensitive that if you look closely, you can visualize a thin stalk **(C)** attached to the bladder wall *(white arrows)*. (Images courtesy R.F. Hylands.)

FIG. 10.5 B-mode image of a kidney illustrating the strong anatomical correlation between a transverse picture of a sectioned organ **(A)** and the accompanying ultrasound study **(B)**. (Images courtesy R.F. Hylands.)

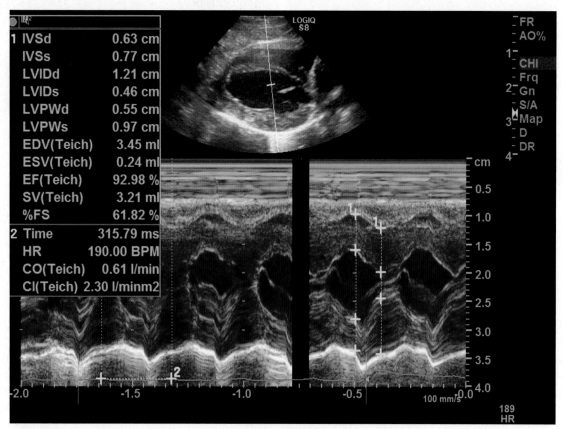

FIG. 10.6 M-mode study of the left ventricle of the heart. Note that it is a continuous graph representing motion of the myocardium along the thin transecting cursor line dissecting the heart. (Images courtesy R.F. Hylands.)

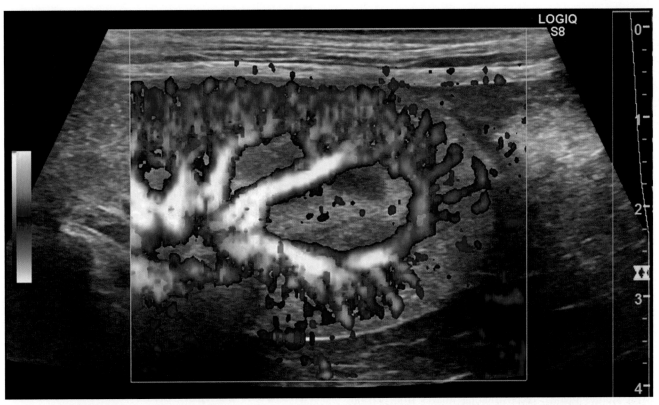

FIG. 10.7 A color flow image of a kidney demonstrating the blood flow within it. (Images courtesy R.F. Hylands.)

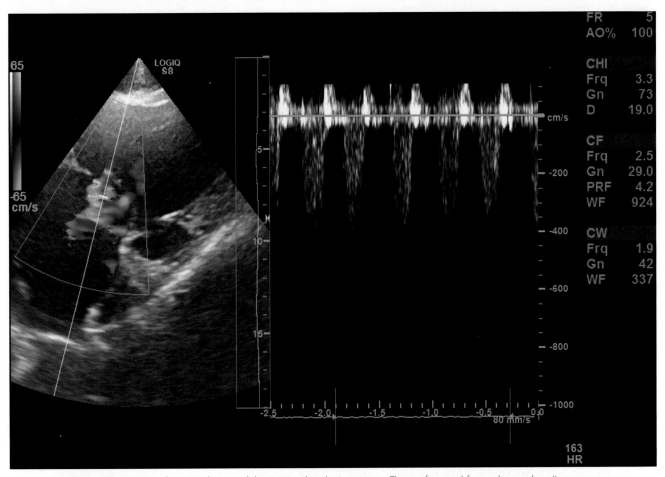

FIG. 10.8 Image depicting three modalities viewed at the same time. This is often used for cardiac studies. (Images courtesy R.F. Hylands.)

Continuous Wave Doppler

This type of Doppler imaging requires that the scanner have two different sets of crystals built within it that work together simultaneously. One set of crystals is continually sending out signals and the other set receives. This allows accurate measurements during studies of very-high-velocity blood flow found in many congenital heart conditions. It is, however, less accurate when it comes to selectively measuring flow at a certain depths, and it cannot be gated as with PW studies.

Harmonic Mode

The use of tissue harmonics helps decrease ultrasound artifacts (see the section on artifacts later) in very large or obese patients. In this mode either a single or multiple deep, penetrating frequencies are emitted into the body along with a harmonic overtone. The overall objective is to achieve deeper homogeneous penetration with fewer artifacts, as this mode utilizes software to filter the returning sound wave, which removes echoes that may interfere with a clearer image (considered "noise"). Other applications used to improve image quality include speckle reduction and compound imaging.

Multiplanar Reconstruction

MPR studies involve reconstructing images from various planes to allow simultaneous visualization on the monitor. Although MPR has been the norm in both CT and MRI studies for some time, it is a relatively new imaging format for the field of ultrasonography. Volume transducers are needed to acquire this image.

Three-Dimensional and Four-Dimensional Modes

Although currently of limited practicality in veterinary medicine, both stationary three-dimensional and time-lapsed four-dimensional reconstructions are available in human ultrasonography. This is currently used primarily for human fetal, obstetrical, and cardiac valve imaging. As newer applications arise, these technologies will likely migrate to veterinary use.

Postimaging Processing and Measurements

With the advent of digital technology, studies can be stored in their raw format for later review. This allows for a vast multitude of calculations to be made after a study is completed. The veterinary technician can be involved in reformatting the data to help complete the case study.

"Knobology"

Every ultrasound machine, regardless of manufacturer, shares a common set of instrument adjustments that can modify both the performance of the machine and its image quality. These adjustments are made either mechanically (manipulating knobs and boards) or by contact on a software-driven touch screen (Fig. 10.9).

Gain

The gain adjustment affects the brightness of the image. It affects what range of the grayscale is used to format the image for that particular study. Most machines will have a choice of preformatted grayscale and colored maps to start as the base image for the gain. These are chosen depending on the ultrasound study required. As an example, cardiac studies do not require the full grayscale range, but instead use a high-contrast image in order to better define the edges of the cardiac musculature. Abdominal studies, on the other hand, will benefit from a wide range of grayscale to better detect minor anatomical changes within an organ or tissue.

Depth

Every type and size of transducer has a set maximum and minimum depth at which it can send and receive sound waves. A common mistake when imaging an area of interest is to set the depth of the scan too deep. Although it may appear to give a better perspective of the tissue relative to the surrounding structures, it inevitably wastes valuable pixels that could give finer organ detail. As a rule of thumb, one should limit the depth of the scan so that the area of interest fills the full monitor screen for closer analysis.

Time Gain Compensation

This feature allows the operator to selectively adjust the gain at various depths. Echoes that return from deeper structures are more attenuated as they travel back through more tissues. This makes part of the far-field image appear to be darker. Time gain compensation (TGC) adjustments allow for one to compensate the gain to obtain a smooth grayscale image throughout the full depth of the scan view. This adjustment is often done through manipulating a series of sliding tabs that affect the level of brightness at various depths.

Presets

These are preinstalled settings programmed by the manufacturer. The settings included with the machine's software are meant to facilitate and maximize the performance of a transducer, depending on the type of study required. Selecting a preset for a cardiac study may affect such parameters as the

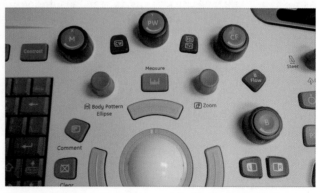

FIG. 10.9 Ultrasound machine panel displaying image control options. (Images courtesy R.F. Hylands.)

sensitivity and range of the Doppler reading for either adults or neonates. Presets will affect the dynamic range, gain settings, gray map selection, frequency of the transducer, number of focal zones, and scan depth. Some machines may also allow the operator to modify these presets or create and save their own, because personal preferences can vary.

Focal Zones

Adjustments to the focal zones will allow the ultrasound beam to converge more at a particular depth during the study. This will maximize the axial and lateral spatial resolution at the area of interest (see definitions). This focal setting works best if selected within the near-field imaging parameter of a transducer. A maximum of only two focal zones should be used at a time, even though some machines will allow the operator to select up to five.

Frequency Selection

Individual transducers generate sound waves with a set range of frequencies based on the properties of the piezoelectric ceramic crystals used within the ultrasound probe. The frequency selection "knob" allows the operator to change the frequency within the range allowed by that probe. This will affect the maximum penetration depth of the sound waves in the tissues. It is important to be aware that the depth of penetration is inversely related to the level of frequency used. The advantage of using higher frequencies is that they provide better optimization of the resolution of the area.

Optimization

Another option found on many newer machines is a single-step adjustment that automatically optimizes the settings in order to obtain the best image. Choosing this setting will affect the gain settings and the tissue harmonics in order to obtain the ideal image as the sound beam travels through a particular part of the body. Ultrasound manufacturers will have different names for this option, but the end result is relatively similar. It is meant to assist operators who have limited knowledge of individual settings and adjustments to quickly obtain the best possible image.

Transducers

As we have discussed earlier, the purpose of the ultrasound transducer (or probe) is to change electrical energy into mechanical energy (sound waves), which penetrate into the tissues, and then to receive the reflected sound waves, converting them back into electrical impulses, which are read by the computer. This is accomplished by piezoelectric crystal elements, which can change shape and vibrate in response to electrical or mechanical stimulation.

The greatest advancement in ultrasound imaging came in the early 1990s when there was an explosion in the development of high-speed digital electronics and the development of powerful computer platforms. With the advent of the digitization of the systems, many fine adjustments to the processing software could be implemented, resulting in a dramatic reduction in signal noise and artifacts. The numbers of elements on individual transducers can range from as low as 64 to over 500 elements per transducer head. At the same time improvements in the speed and quality of the receiving and processing can directly affect the image quality and resolution of the scan images for advanced studies.

Transducer Frequency

There is an inverse relationship between increasing the frequency output of a probe and the maximum depth that it can scan. This means that the higher the frequency of the transducer, the less it will penetrate. Second, there is a direct relationship between increasing the frequency of a transducer and the lateral spatial resolution (Fig. 10.10).

Lateral spatial resolution is the ability to distinguish between two objects or echoes that are adjacent to each other yet perpendicular to the sound wave. This is influenced by the sound beam's width. The lateral resolution is best when studied in the near field where the sound beam is narrowest.

Choosing a Transducer

A typical small-animal practice may require up to three or four different types of transducers, depending on the type of ultrasound studies that are being performed. For instance, a clinic that does both cardiac and abdominal scans will need more transducers than a clinic performing only general abdominal ultrasonography. In comparison, an equine practice devoted exclusively to lameness studies may require only a single high-frequency, linear transducer to perform most tendon studies.

Because the frequency or wavelength at which the ceramics are vibrating will affect the spatial resolution within an image, higher-frequency transducers will be required for detailed studies. Many higher-end ultrasound machines can reach frequencies of up to 22 MHz.

Transducers have single-frequency or multiple-frequency ranges on a single probe. In veterinary medicine, the wide range in both the sizes and weights of patients makes the use of single-frequency transducers difficult (Fig. 10.11).

Markers

Each ultrasound probe is tagged with a marker that may be in the form of an indentation, a raised surface, or an

Transducer Frequencies			
Increasing frequency			
• Decreases penetration capability			
• Increases fine detail. Provides better spatial resolution			
	Depth	Wavelengths	Max spatial resolution
3 MHz	20 cm	0.44 mm	0.76 mm
5 MHz	15 cm	0.31 mm	0.62 mm
7.5 MHz	10 cm	0.21 mm	0.42 mm
10 MHz	7 cm	0.15 mm	0.33 mm

FIG. 10.10 Comparison of transducer frequency with depth of penetration and spatial resolution. (Images courtesy R.F. Hylands.)

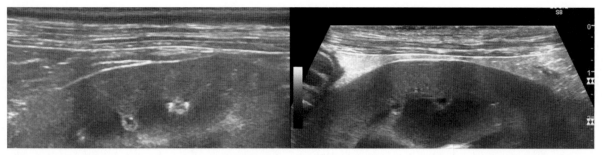

FIG. 10.11 Spatial resolution is improved when using a higher-frequency transducer in the near field. In the image of the kidney to the left, there is decreased detail noted over the transition point of the renal cortex to the medullary zone. Contrast this with the image to the right where minute changes in the echogenicity of the transitional zone can be noted with greater clarity. (Images courtesy R. F. Hylands.)

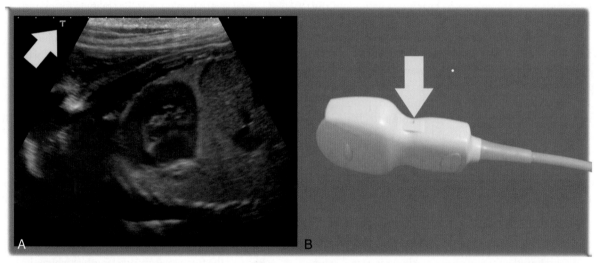

FIG. 10.12 A and B, Each transducer has an identifying mark that helps align the direction of the probe with that which is displayed on the monitor screen *(arrows)*. (Images courtesy R.F. Hylands.)

illuminated "in use" light. This marker will be associated with a similar identification tag on the upper-left corner of the ultrasound screen. Orienting the marker on the transducer toward the marker on the screen will assist in performing a standardized ultrasound (Fig. 10.12).

In keeping with standardized convention, in a sagittal scan plane, the cranial aspect of the patient's body should be displayed on the left side of the monitor, and when viewing transverse planes, the right side of the patient should be presented to the left of the screen as well. It is the marker icon that is represented on the screen, along with the reference point etched over the transducer, that assists the sonographer to properly orient and record the scan.

Transducer Types

A wide variety of different types of transducer probes are available to veterinarians (Fig. 10.13). The most commonly used in veterinary medicine are listed next. Other types of probes include those used within endoscopes, esophageal probes, and endocavity probes used for obstetrics. The size, frequency range, and conformation of the actual footprint shape (the part of the probe that makes contact with the patient) will vary between probes and between vendors as well.

Linear Transducer

The linear transducer design was one of the first probes to appear on the ultrasound scene. It has a flat contact surface, or footprint. The earlier designs would only scan in a limited rectangular view of tissues directly beneath the probe. This resulted in many artifacts, such as "side lobes," forming (see the Ultrasound Artifacts section later in this chapter). With the advent of digital technology and the ability to focus the sound beam, the linear probe now has the added option of trapezoid imaging. This keeps the high resolution of the linear probe and gives some of the broader advantages of the curvilinear probe. Software changes also have resulted in a dramatic reduction of artifacts, and the faster processing time has improved the linear probe's capability. Recently because of these adaptive changes, linear probes have reemerged in popularity as an ideal diagnostic tool for fine-detail imaging (see Fig. 10.13A).

Convex Transducer

The convex transducer (see Fig. 10.13B) is also known as a *sector or curvilinear probe* and was first introduced in the late 1970s and early 1980s. At the time, they exceeded the popularity of the linear probe because of their curvilinear shape,

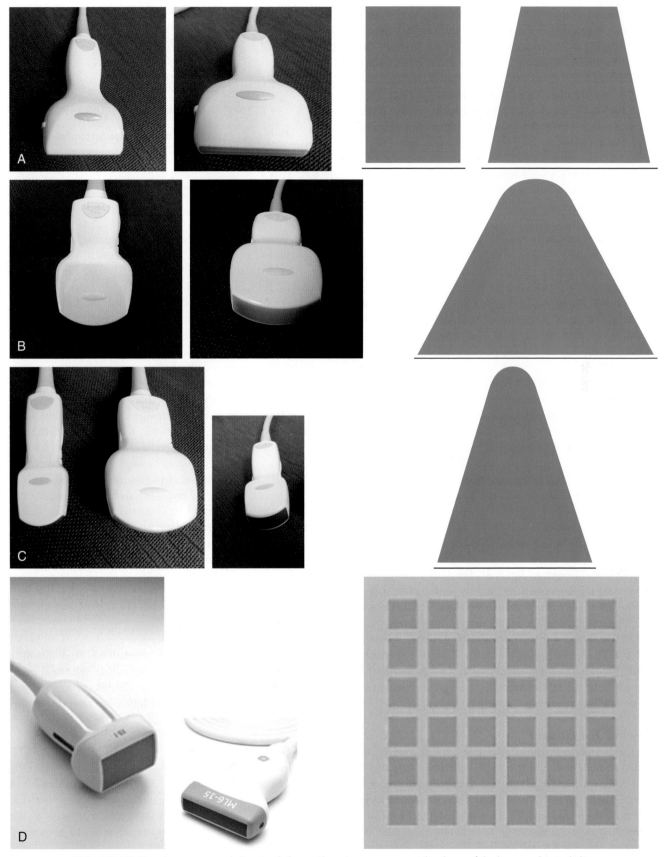

FIG. 10.13 Transducer types and directional shape. These images represent the shape of the linear probe, including their footprint. **A,** The linear pattern can produce either a rectangular box or a trapezoid shape. They are high-resolution superficial transducers. **B,** The images represent a typical curvilinear or convex probe. Note the curvature to the scan head itself. This results in a wider scan view. **C,** Microconvex transducer (left) versus convex transducer (right). These images illustrate the difference in the size of each of the footprints of the probes. **D,** The arrangement of extra rows of elements within the matrix volume transducer allows for either scanning in multiple directions at the same time or higher-resolution scanning. (Images courtesy R.F. Hylands.)

which offered a wider field of view at the sacrifice of spatial resolution (especially in human obstetrical studies). In some cases the wide footprint was excessive for small-animal use. As the trapezoid imaging of the linear probe has improved and increased the detail available in the scans, the convex and the linear probes have become almost equally popular. Many ultrasonographers will use the convex probe for a general scan and then switch to the linear probes for higher-resolution inspections.

Microconvex Transducer

Although similar to convex probes because of the curvilinear shape, the microconvex transducer has a much smaller footprint size (see Fig. 10.13C). This difference makes them more practical for smaller animal patients. This is especially true for intercostal studies where the distance between the ribs limits the probe's view and contact with the patient. The disadvantage of this size change is the reduced number of elements and the spread of the wide-angle view, which ends up sacrificing some degree of image quality. Microconvex probes are particularly useful in smaller canines, felines, and exotic patients.

Phased Array Sector Transducer

Phased array transducers contain piezoelectric elements that are stimulated in complex timing sequences and controlled by circuitry to provide focus and sound beam steering at different depths simultaneously. In these types of transducers, the crystals are electronically steered through firing time delays. They are most often used in cardiac studies, as they have the unique ability to offer a CW mode.

Matrix Transducer

The matrix transducer (see Fig. 10.13D) is the newest class of transducers and at the time of writing is only offered by a select number of vendors. This type of probe will likely replace many of the other probes as technology continues to improve and the size of the transducer becomes slightly more manageable. The probe offers the ability to scan in different planes at the same time due to the high density of elements installed within it. The two-dimensional matrix allows the operator to create three-dimensional images of an area in question, for example, heart valves. Unfortunately due to costs, it has limited use in veterinary medicine at the present time.

Volume Transducer

The use of volume transducers is quite limited in veterinary medicine, mainly due to their high individual cost and the need to use optimum machines with their extended processing power. These probes are necessary for four-dimensional reconstructions, and five-dimensional models are now being released. It is just a matter of time before they will be in common use within the veterinary profession.

Transducer Care and Cleaning Guides

Each ultrasound transducer can be worth thousands of dollars when new ($3000 to $16,000). When handling probes, care

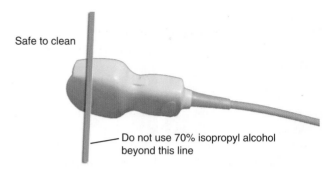

FIG. 10.14 Ultrasound transducer probe. (Images courtesy R.F. Hylands.)

must be taken to avoid dropping or jarring them, as the piezoelectric crystals can become damaged.

After each use, the technician should wipe off any remaining acoustic gel found on the probe with either a dry or water-moistened *soft* cloth. Contaminated fluids on the transducer may be gently cleansed with a 10% bleach solution, a glutaraldehyde-based disinfectant, or 70% isopropyl alcohol. Check with your manufacturer's service manual, as not all companies recommend this. Follow required cleaning practices carefully to avoid warranty disruption.

Alcohol should *never* be used beyond 2 cm from the tip of the transducer, as it can damage the housing joint seals. Never use alcohol on the transducer cables (Fig. 10.14).

For probes that are used in endocavity procedures a spray of mild disinfectant solution may be used. Although the rubber of the transducer's footprint can be immersed in fluids for very short periods, it is still not recommended. The connectors and distal cables should never be immersed. At no point should a transducer be autoclaved or gas sterilized with ethylene oxide. Care should be taken also to avoid contact with gels that contain lotions, mineral oil, or lanolin.

Applications for Ultrasound

Bovine and Ruminants

In these species an ultrasound examination is predominantly used for reproductive work, such as follicle detection, pregnancy examination, reproductive difficulties, and so on. Ultrasound-guided biopsies and follow-up monitoring also employ ultrasound.

Equine

Two distinct imaging services exist in the equine world: sports medicine and reproduction. Ultrasound is invaluable in identifying both tendon and ligamentous strain and injuries. It is also particularly useful for monitoring progress as the horse improves and returns to normal with the prescribed therapeutics.

Fertility is also an important consideration in equine medicine, and the use of ultrasound is the standard of care when following up on the early stages of gestation and fetal development.

Porcine

The main use for ultrasonography here is for the measurement of backfat levels found within animals destined for meat production.

Small Animals

The list of possible applications seems to be almost endless for small-animal studies because the size of the patient is ideal for the types of frequency ranges available to the practitioner. The scope of studies is only limited by the imagination of the ultrasonographer.

Abdominal studies include all of the gastrointestinal (GI) system, from the esophagus as it transverses the diaphragm, to the distal end of the colon, including the rectum, which is imaged through the perineal area. Abdominal ultrasound studies also include the imaging of the liver, gallbladder, and biliary tree. The pancreas, spleen, kidneys, adrenals, and regional lymph nodes are routinely imaged and evaluated. As an example, abdominal lymph nodes can be assessed for their level of inflammation and reactivity. The urinary bladder and excretory system (up to the bony interference from the pelvic rim) is also part of any examination, as are all of the components of both sexes' reproductive organs. The more distal structures can also be reached with more superficial scanning methods. The only major limiting factor is the obstruction from either bony structures or gas-filled organs.

Thoracic studies usually include full cardiac examinations with M-mode interpretations and Doppler vascular velocity assessments. In emergency medicine, ultrasonography is the diagnostic modality of choice when assessing trauma and suspected abdominal bleeding.

Ultrasound Artifacts

Ultrasound waves do not travel through air or bone. Because of this, there are situations where a reflected sound wave may occur that interferes with the diagnostic scan. One of the most common examples is the reflection of sound waves when the beam comes into contact with air. The resultant artifact reflection is called *reverberation*. A number of common ultrasonographic artifacts are presented next.

Comet Tail

The comet tail artifact (Fig. 10.15) appears as a series of closely interspaced and intense reverberations or reflections that appear to look like the tail of a comet. They can occur when there is reflection of the sound wave off small reflector targets, such as air pockets in the GI tract or metallic objects, a foreign body, or the tip of a biopsy needle. Fig. 10.15 shows typical illustrations of a comet tail artifact as noted in three different gastric images.

Edge Shadowing Artifact

Edge shadowing is a form of refraction, or redirection of the sound wave, as it passes through a fluid–tissue interface. It is associated with curved fluid-filled structures such as the gallbladder, urinary bladder, cysts, and even sometimes the kidneys. The phenomenon occurs in the far field of the object (away from the entrance of the beam). It appears like a hypoechoic linear shadow that diverges from the surface of the curved structure.

Edge shadowing can occur when the incident angle of the sound beam hits the leading edge of a circular object (the near edge). The objects in question must be composed of different attenuation material, such as a liquid and solid side by side, as in a cystic structure. The images in Fig. 10.16 show such an artifact (arrows) off the surface of the gallbladder.

Acoustic Enhancement

Acoustic enhancement occurs when the sound beam travels through a weakly attenuating structure such as a bladder filled with fluid. The sound beams traveling through tissues *around* the bladder will be slowed or attenuated, whereas the sound beams passing *through* the liquid will not have lost as much energy or intensity. When the sound beams hit the tissue at the far side of the bladder, the reflection will appear brighter (hyperechoic) compared with the surrounding tissues on the same plane. The resulting artifact appears as a distal

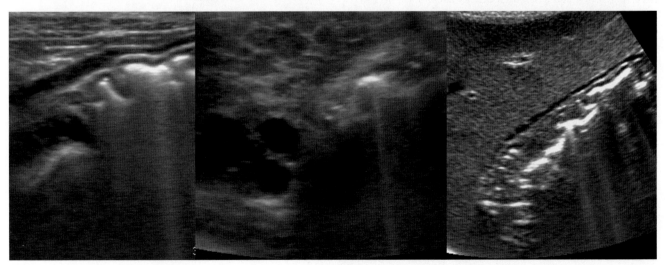

FIG. 10.15 Comet tail artifacts in three different gastric images. (Images courtesy R. F. Hylands.)

enhancement (brighter on the far side of the structure) on the B mode.

This predictable artifact is quite useful in differentiating certain hypoechoic masses from cystic or fluid-filled structures. The images in Fig. 10.17 show the increase in echogenicity in the area outlined between the two white lines. This is consistent with acoustic enhancement.

Mirror Image Artifact

The strong reflective surface between the diaphragm and the air-filled lungs is a common place to observe a distinct mirror image of tissues in the abdomen (Fig. 10.18). The sound beams reflected back from this interface are misinterpreted by the ultrasound machine, which then places a second image of the liver, for example, on the opposite side of the diaphragm. This artifact is important to recognize because an inexperienced ultrasonographer may interpret the artifact as a diaphragmatic hernia, a thoracic mass, or even lung pathology.

Reverberation

Reverberation is due to repeated back-and-forth reflection of echoes trapped between two strong reflectors. The resulting effect appears like a bright veil, similar to northern lights in the sky (Fig. 10.19). It is principally seen in a superficially positioned, gas-filled loop of bowel within the stomach. The bright echo display makes it difficult to see anything distal to the artifact. The result is that one cannot properly visualize the image of the opposing wall of the digestive tract.

Acoustic Shadowing

Acoustic shadowing is the simplest of all of the artifacts to understand (Fig. 10.20). When the sound beam contacts a

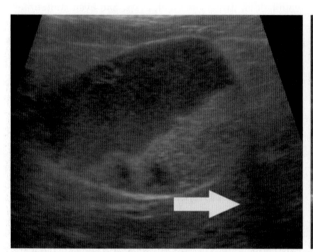
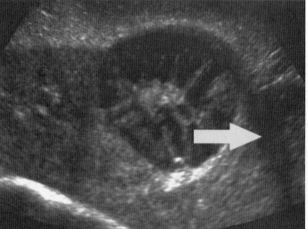

FIG. 10.16 Edge shadowing artifact off the surface of the gallbladder. (Images courtesy R. F. Hylands.)

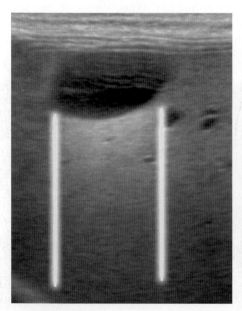
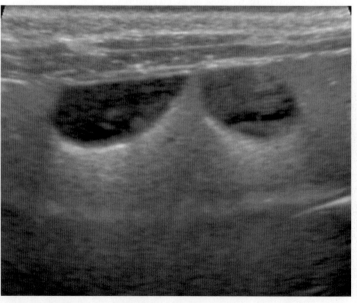

FIG. 10.17 Acoustic enhancement is apparent compared with tissues around the gallbladder. The indicator lines on the image to the left outline the area of relative increase in echogenicity just below the gallbladder. (Images courtesy R. F. Hylands.)

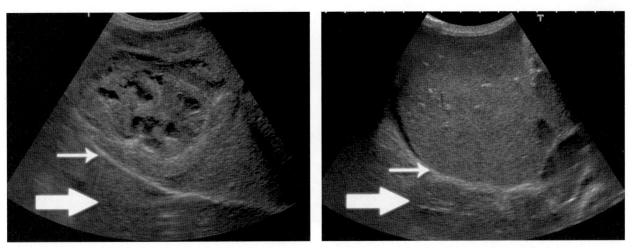

FIG. 10.18 Mirror image of the liver *(large arrow)* is seen on the opposite side of the diaphragm *(small arrow)* from its normal place in the abdomen. (Images courtesy R. F. Hylands.)

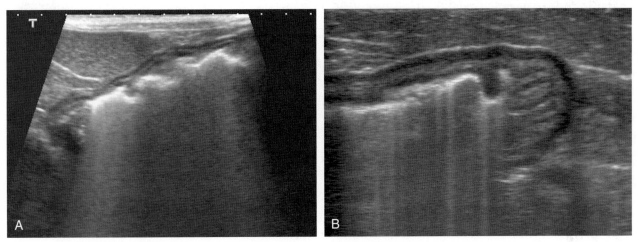

FIG. 10.19 Reverberation due to repeated reflection of sound waves off gas in the gastrointestinal tract. (Images courtesy R. F. Hylands.)

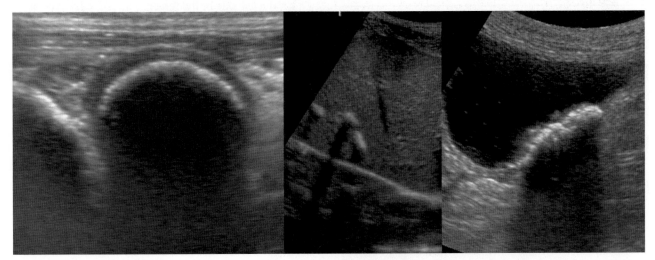

FIG. 10.20 Acoustic shadowing as seen distal to a foreign body in the jejunum (left), stones in the biliary tree of the liver (middle), and an aggregation of urinary bladder stones in the bladder (right). Note the dark shadowing below each dense structure. (Images courtesy R. F. Hylands.)

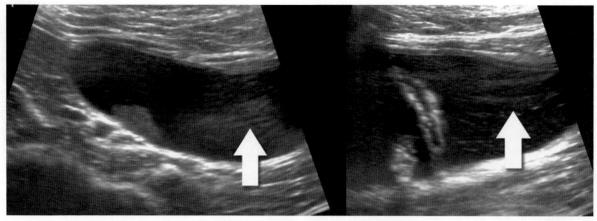

FIG. 10.21 Side lobe artifacts are secondary emissions usually seen when imaging anechoic structures such as urinary structures or the gallbladder. (Images courtesy R. F. Hylands.)

highly attenuating surface such as a urolith (bladder stone) or bone, most of the sound beam is either reflected away or absorbed. This creates a lack of echo information distal to the dense object. The absence of data is displayed as a dark streak or shadow below the object where the ultrasound beam has not penetrated. The shadow is lined up parallel to the direction of the emission of the sound beam from the transducer.

Side Lobe Artifacts

When a transducer is emitting sound beams, the majority of them are directed in a primary direction, but secondary lateral minor emissions are simultaneously created. These become more pronounced as a transducer is set at its upper threshold. These side lobe echoes can be displayed on the monitor even if they did not originate from the principle or main sound beam (Fig. 10.21). This artifact can be reduced by changing the position of the focal zone or by reducing the frequency of the transducer.

REVIEW QUESTIONS

1. In the following ultrasound image, what are the three artifacts highlighted by the letters A, B, and C?

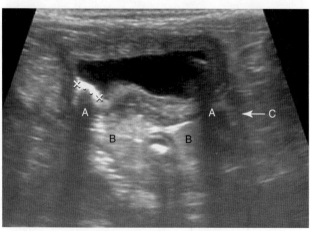

(Image courtesy of R. F. Hylands.)

a. Shadowing (A), acoustic enhancement (B), edge shadowing (C)
b. Shadowing (A), reverberation (B), comet tail (C)
c. Comet tail (A), reverberation (B), edge shadowing (C)
d. Shadowing (A), acoustic enhancement (B), comet tail (C)

2. One purpose of the gain control setting is:
a. To adjust the color intensity
b. To select for continuous Doppler
c. To control the brightness level of an image
d. To set the frequency of a probe

3. The piezoelectric materials within a probe can:
a. Convert electrical energy into mechanical energy
b. Convert mechanical energy into electrical energy
c. Convert electrical energy into mechanical energy and vice versa
d. All of the above

4. When recording an abdominal ultrasound, on which side of the monitor should the cranial quadrant be displayed on a sagittal view?
a. The far field of the image screen
b. The near field of the image screen
c. The left side of the screen
d. The right side of the screen

5. When performing a cardiac examination, what would be the ideal transducer to choose?
a. A convex probe
b. A linear transducer
c. A phased sector array probe
d. A sector transducer

Answers to Review Questions can be found on the Evolve website.

CHAPTER 11
Fluoroscopy

Lois C. Brown, RTR (Can/USA), ACR, MSc., P.Phys

Television is a medium because anything well done is rare.
Television is the triumph of machine over people.
—Fred Allen, American comedian, 1894–1956

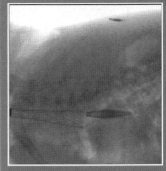

Fluoroscopy is real-time imaging.

OUTLINE

LEARNING OBJECTIVES

When you have finished this chapter, you will be able to:

1. Discuss the equipment necessary for fluoroscopy
2. Describe the functions of the fluoroscopic unit.
3. Explain the difference between radiographic and fluoroscopic images.
4. List the applications for fluoroscopy in veterinary medicine.

APPLICATIONS

The application of the information in this chapter is relevant to the following areas:

1. Fluoroscopic real-time scanning and imaging in small and large animals.

KEY TERMS

Key terms are defined in the Glossary on the Evolve website.

Fluoroscopy	Input phosphor	Photocathode	Pulsed radiation exposure
Image intensifier	Output phosphor	Photoemission	

Fluoroscopy is an emerging field in veterinary medicine, and because of its real-time imaging it is an invaluable tool in veterinary surgery and in interventional imaging. The insertions of catheters and lines and manipulation of structures can all be done using fluoroscopy. In large-animal orthopedic surgery, fluoroscopy is vital for the positioning of plates, pins, and screws. Static images can be captured from the output phosphor and recorded for later viewing or for the prearchives and postarchives.

Very shortly after the discovery of x-rays, scientists wanted to see moving images. Thomas Edison is credited with inventing the fluoroscope in the United States in 1896. Because Roentgen had patented the discovery of x-rays only in November of the previous year, Edison worked quickly to patent his new device before the end of the year. However, Edison's design did not intensify the image and so it was useless as a diagnostic tool. It wasn't until 1953 that a commercial image intensifier was produced by Westinghouse. It then became a useful diagnostic imaging system. The refinements over the years have enhanced the image considerably but have not changed the basic design dramatically (Fig. 11.1).

The primary function of fluoroscopy is to provide dynamic real-time imaging of anatomical structures. Static images are useful, but the imaging of certain activities within the body is enhanced if the veterinarian is able to view the activities as they happen. This is also true of fluoroscopically guided orthopedic surgery. Obtaining static images and processing them as the surgery progresses is time consuming, whereas anatomy may be imaged quickly in real time with fluoroscopy. Today the fluoroscope is connected to a radiographic camera, and a corresponding static image can be obtained without interrupting the dynamic examination.

Fluoroscopic Equipment

The fluoroscopic generator is virtually identical to a radiography unit. Many veterinary radiography units that are purchased from human hospitals have a fluoroscopy panel on the right side of the control panel.

The kilovoltage (kV), milliamperage (mA), and time values are the same as on a radiography unit. The difference is an added panel that allows the operator to select the "fluoro" mode, which switches the unit to a low mA (2-5) and a high kilovoltage (100-120) (Fig. 11.2). The time is not independently selected because the image is created in real time, and thus time is controlled by the operator as he or she watches the screen and obtains the imaging sequence necessary for diagnosis.

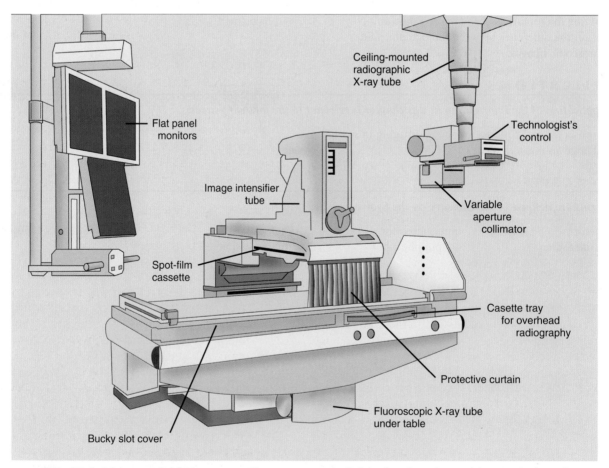

Flat panel monitors

Ceiling-mounted radiographic X-ray tube

Technologist's control

Image intensifier tube

Variable aperture collimator

Spot-film cassette

Casette tray for overhead radiography

Protective curtain

Fluoroscopic X-ray tube under table

Bucky slot cover

FIG. 11.1 A large, installed fluoroscopic unit. The two monitors usually hang from the ceiling, and the control is located in a shielded booth within the room. The operator will stand beside the table. Handlers will also stand beside the table assisting the patient and/or the veterinarian. All personnel in the room will wear protective aprons and accessories. (From Bushong SC. *Radiologic Science for Technologists*, 10th ed. St Louis: Elsevier; 2013.)

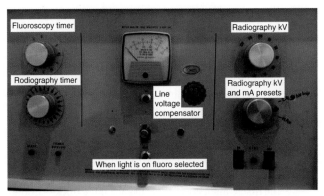

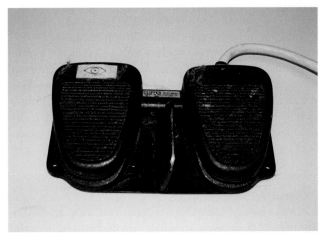

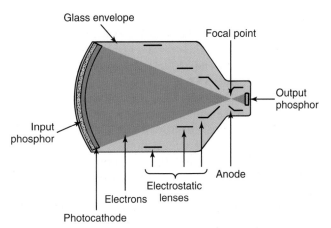

FIG. 11.2 An older-generation radiography/fluoroscopy unit. The switch to alternate between radiography and fluoroscopy is on the side of the generator.

FIG. 11.3 The foot switch (exposure switch) has two options. One side is a single-exposure switch, and the pedal on the right is used for continuous exposure (fluoroscopy).

A foot switch (Fig. 11.3) operates as the exposure switch, and x-rays are generated continuously if the switch is depressed. A timer on the unit alerts the operator at a preset time limit (1, 2, or 5 minutes). The image intensifier monitor looks very much like a television monitor and is the display for the dynamic images.

Fluoroscopic Doses to the Patient

It is important to remember that the milliampere-seconds (mAs) is a function of mA × time. If the mA value is 3 and the operator extends the exposure time to 1 minute, the resulting mAs to the patient is 3 × 60 sec, or 180 mAs. Patients can receive radiation burns from a fluoroscopy unit if it is too close to the skin and remains in exposure mode for too long.

There are no specific dose limits in veterinary medicine, but the operator should always be aware of the "as low as reasonably achievable" (ALARA) principle discussed in Chapter 3 and try to keep the dose as low as possible.

One way to reduce the dose to the patient considerably is to use the pulse function on the machine. With pulsed radiation, the radiation is turned on and off for very brief periods of time. The image that is visible to the eye is not affected,

FIG. 11.4 The image intensifier converts the remnant radiation from the patient into a bright visible image on the output phosphor. It is then converted into a digital image to be viewed on the monitor or stored in a picture archiving system for later review and diagnosis. (Redrawn from Bushong SC. *Radiologic Science for Technologists*, 10th ed. St Louis: Elsevier; 2013.)

but the radiation dose is reduced considerably. The radiation is pulsed, but the image on the screen is held for the brief period of time that there is no radiation. The pulse function can reduce the dose by one-half. Each manufacturer builds this function into the unit, so there is no specific time for each pulse. If the pulses are every one tenth of a second, for example, the image is not affected and the patient dose is reduced considerably.

The Image Intensifier

The image detector on a fluoroscopy unit is an image intensifier (Fig. 11.4). As with x-ray tubes, the image intensifier contains a cathode and an anode but with quite a different design. This electronic device receives the remnant radiation exiting from the patient and converts it into a visible light image of high intensity. Modern image intensifiers consist of 11 components, each of which is uniquely important:

1. **The glass envelope.** This is the vacuum housing for the unit and must be specifically designed to withstand the outside air pressure without collapsing. An ion pump device maintains the vacuum and removes any ions produced when the intensifier is operating.
2. **The input screen.** This is the vacuum window of the intensifier. It receives the x-rays emitted from the patient. It consists of the support layer, the input phosphor, and the photocathode.
3. **The support layer.** This serves as a backing for the input phosphor and the photocathode. It is usually a thin piece of aluminum purposely shaped to help focus the electrons toward the other end of the intensifier. It is very important that the electrons are not distorted as they are intensified and projected onto the output screen. If they are distorted, then the resulting image will be distorted.
4. **The input phosphor.** The concave surface of the input phosphor is usually coated with cesium iodide. Cesium

iodide crystals grow in long columns that function as pipes directing the remnant radiation toward the photocathode. This system is highly efficient, typically converting a single 60-kiloelectron volt (KeV) photon to more than 3000 light photons.

5. **The photocathode.** As light exits the input phosphor, it strikes the photocathode, which absorbs light and emits electrons. These two units are situated very close together to prevent the light from spreading.

6. **The photoelectrons.** These electrons are released by the photocathode in direct proportion to the amount of light that was absorbed. The conversion efficiency of the photocathode is between 10% and 20%. For every 60-KeV x-ray photon that is absorbed by the input phosphor, the photocathode releases about 400 photoelectrons.

7. **The electrostatic focusing lens.** These lenses line the sides of the image intensifier and direct the electrons to the positively charged anode. These lenses are highly positively charged and draw the electrons with considerable force toward the anode, which has a positive charge of about 25,000 to 30,000 volts of electricity.

8. **The focal point.** The electrons are drawn rapidly toward the anode. As they travel they cross each other at a spot known as the *focal point* (Fig. 11.5). This point enables the operator to control the magnification or minification of the image.

9. **The anode and the output screen.** The positively charged anode is immediately in front of the output screen. Once again, this prevents any image spread. The output screen displays the image and is read by

the monitor and by any other storage devices attached to the unit.

The anode merely attracts the electrons, which pass through a hole in the center of the anode. This does not interrupt the flow of electrons or distort the image as it arrives at the output phosphor.

10. **Output phosphor.** As the photoelectrons strike the output phosphor, they are converted back into light photons. Each photoelectron that strikes the output phosphor is converted into 1000 light photons.

11. **Output window.** This is the final viewing point on the image intensifier and is usually quite thick—around 14 mm. The sides of the window are coated with a black pigment to absorb any stray light reflected in the window.

There can be modifications to these basic components depending on the manufacturer. In addition, upgrades are available to eliminate artifacts associated with a moving image.

Originally units were supplied with a cassette holder, and individual exposures were possible. Today, with the advent of digital imaging, there is no longer a need for these holders. Now if a single exposure is required, it can be retrieved from the bank of dynamic images and stored in a separate folder. This improvement reduces the radiation exposure for the patient because individual static images are unnecessary.

C-Arm Configuration of the Fluoroscopy Unit

The original fluoroscopy units were mounted on a radiographic table and were exceptionally large and unwieldy. They required a motor drive just to move the unit over the table to examine the patient from head to toe. In the 1960s a portable configuration was developed and is still used today. With this two-part unit, the x-ray tube and image intensifier are mounted in a "C" configuration, and the monitors and recording devices are located in a separate cabinet (Fig. 11.6).

The C-arm is the most common veterinary fluoroscopy unit. Many units in veterinary hospitals are purchased from human hospitals, and because their use is limited to surgical procedures in human hospitals, they are usually in excellent condition (if somewhat cosmetically compromised). They are mounted on wheels and are portable, although a little awkward to move about. Such a unit can be stored in a separate room and brought into the radiography room or surgery when required. The components are fairly rugged and withstand the bumps and shocks of uneven flooring and elevator loading and unloading.

In recent years fluoroscopic units have been manufactured specifically for veterinary hospitals. They are virtually identical to human medical units and are operated in exactly the same manner.

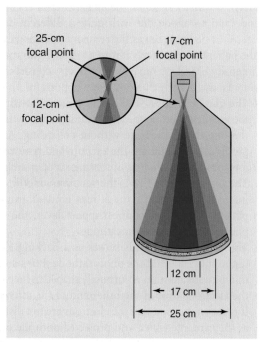

FIG. 11.5 The focal point of the electrons is in front of the photoanode and can be moved slightly to allow magnification of the image. (From Bushong SC. *Radiologic Science for Technologists,* 10th ed. St Louis: Elsevier; 2013.)

The Fluoroscopy Table

One factor that is often overlooked is the table on which the patient will lie for the fluoroscopic procedure. The tabletop

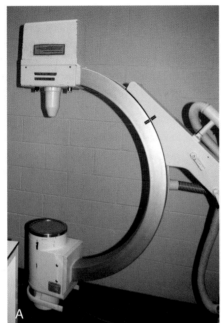
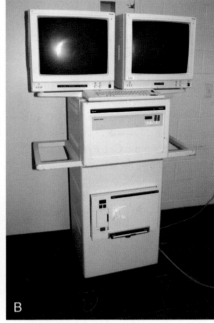

FIG. 11.6 **A,** The typical configuration of a veterinary fluoroscopy unit. In this case the image intensifier is positioned below the x-ray tube. The flexibility of the unit means that the arm can be rotated so that the tube is above the intensifier or positioned for a lateral view. **B,** The two monitors are mounted on a cabinet with the recording units below. The monitor on the left shows the image in real time. The monitor on the right provides a static last image held for comparison.

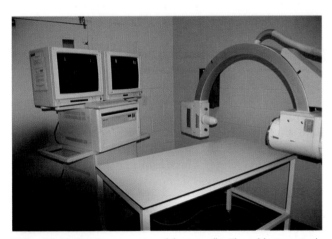

FIG. 11.7 The C-arm positioned horizontally. The table is a sturdy construction with the support rails situated so that the x-ray tube can move beneath it unobstructed. This x-ray tube is a stationary anode tube.

must be free of obstruction above and below and must be radiolucent. The radiation will travel through the patient and the tabletop, and the configuration must be accessible so that either the x-ray tube or the image intensifier can be placed beneath the table (Fig. 11.7).

An important consideration is the radiation absorption of the tabletop. A steel stretcher would act as a radiation filter, absorbing a considerable amount of radiation, and filtration would "flatten" the image, destroying contrast. With a wooden tabletop, the rings and lines of the wood grain are imprinted on the image, obscuring detail and reducing resolution. The best table is custom-made of 1-inch (2.54-cm) squared tubular steel, and the tabletop should be a composite material that is completely radiolucent. The pattern for building such a table

may be extrapolated from the images in the text or from the diagram provided on the Evolve website.

The tabletop may be ordered through an imaging supplier, and the table frame can be constructed by any welding shop. The outside dimensions are 56 in × 26 in (142 cm × 66 cm). The bracing of the legs can be at a 45-degree angle to each leg, or it can be in the form of rails, as shown in Fig. 11.7. The length of the image intensifier should be considered when the rails are mounted because it must be convenient to move the C-arm during surgery from the vertical position to the horizontal position. The table in Fig. 11.7 was manufactured so that the x-ray tube fits below it and the image intensifier is positioned above the patient. A surgical drape was custom made to completely encase the image intensifier. (The radiation penetrates the cloth drape.)

Radiation Dose and Service Considerations

On a standard medical unit, the x-ray tube is a high-end rotating anode tube. It must have a high heat capacity to withstand the long exposure times common in fluoroscopy. One method used to reduce the radiation dose to the patient is to pulse the exposures so that the radiation switches on and off at a predetermined rate. The image on the monitor is not affected because it is preprogrammed to react to a continuous stream and to ignore the pulses.

The x-ray tubes on a C-arm have a stationary anode, and particular care should be taken to limit the exposure times so that the tube does not overheat. Each unit is supplied with an anode cooling chart manual and x-ray tube specifications.

If a used unit is purchased from a medical hospital, all equipment manuals and service manuals must be supplied. These will give a history of any problems, as well as a wiring diagram for any future service. Each C-arm, like any automobile, is upgraded and changed year to year, with major changes occurring at regular intervals depending on the manufacturer. The wiring diagrams from 1 year ago are not necessarily relevant the following year, even if they are produced by the same manufacturer.

If no information is available from the C-arm manufacturer, it may sometimes be obtained from the Internet.

The Monitor Tower

Two monitors are mounted on a cart and are usually positioned at about eye level (5 feet, 5 inches [165 cm]) (see Fig. 11.6B). Older models of C-arms had only one monitor; however, the double monitor serves a useful purpose. One monitor presents the static image, and the second monitor shows the real-time dynamic image. During a surgical procedure, a prosthetic device or a catheter may not be in quite the right position. The surgeon may then hold the image on the left monitor, move the device under real-time imaging, and compare the two images.

A computer keyboard and picture archiving and communications system (PACS) are mounted beneath the monitors (Fig. 11.8). These are linked to the hospital radiology information system (RIS). The patient's information may be keyed in at the monitors or may be available through the RIS. The system may also allow measurements to be calculated or positioning angles to be determined on the monitor.

The Procedure

The animal is placed on the table and wheeled into position between the x-ray tube and the image intensifier. The configuration is movable around the patient, so the tube can move from the dorsoventral or ventrodorsal position to the lateral configuration easily without repositioning the patient.

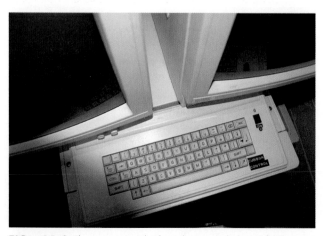

FIG. 11.8 The computer keyboard mounted beneath the two monitors.

In the surgery the unit is positioned after the animal is on the surgery table and has been draped appropriately. If the C-arm is to be moved during surgery, the unit must be thoroughly wiped down with antiseptic wipes. It can be cleaned with the same solutions used on all other operating room equipment.

Dark Adaptation

The images on the fluoroscopic screen are not in color and may be dim in comparison with the routine images read on the illuminator. The veterinarian must allow his or her eyes to become accustomed to the dim light of the room (known as *dark adaptation*) before starting the procedure.

The human eye is not very sensitive to dim light. The rods and cones within the eye must adapt to changes in illumination. The rods are sensitive to low light levels, whereas cones are most efficient at 100 lux and greater. (Lux, a unit of illuminance, is the comparative measure of light read by a light meter.) Cones have a greater ability to perceive fine detail, and so the eye must be allowed to undergo dark adaptation to see the image on the image intensifier most efficiently. Full dark adaptation for the average human eye takes about 15 minutes. The easiest method of dark adaptation is the use of dark sunglasses.

Archiving the Images

Once the image is configured at the output phosphor, it may be viewed in several different modes.

Just as an image detector in radiography displays an image, fluoroscopic images can be digitized and sent to various recording units. Typically, the dynamic image is stored on a hard drive attached to the unit. Because the image is actually a series of still images, just like those in a movie camera, individual "spot films" may be extracted from the "movie." If a particular pathology is demonstrated, the images may be started, fast-forwarded, reversed, and then stopped and captured. If the pathology is of sufficient interest, the images may be posted to a website and discussed by many veterinarians from anywhere in the world.

Individual images may also be printed on a laser printer, such as the one illustrated in Chapter 8.

Applications in Veterinary Medicine

Real-time imaging is useful as a surgical tool in equine radiography for a review of the equine extremities. The real-time imaging does not have the resolution of the film/screen or digital imaging, so it is used mainly for fracture reductions and as a screening tool for placement of catheters, stents, and endotracheal tubes.

Contrast media studies commonly use fluoroscopy to image the function of the gastrointestinal system, as well as narrowing or blockage of blood vessels in angiography studies. The form and function of the blood vessels can be studied with the use of a contrast medium that is injected into the veins and then concentrated and excreted by the kidneys.

Miniaturizing the C-Arm

The miniature C-arm was developed in the early 1980s. This unit was originally intended to be used in the emergency department of human hospitals to image the reduction of fractures and dislocations. It is light and very portable, and even though the image is of comparatively low resolution, it is very useful for the purpose for which it was developed (Figs. 11.9 and 11.10).

Shortly after it was introduced, the miniature C-arm became a valuable tool in scanning equine legs and the joints of the extremities. It is not very powerful, but it images the equine leg very well and can demonstrate an area of trauma or pathology that should be examined further by radiography, computed tomography, or magnetic resonance imaging.

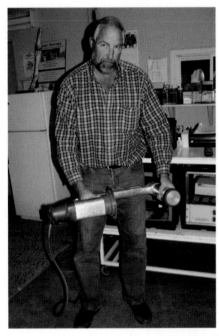

FIG. 11.9 Dan McMaster, DVM, holds the XiTec Mini C-Arm (XiTec LLC, Connecticut, USA) to demonstrate its small size and portability. The x-ray tube port is beside his left thumb, and the image intensifier is in front of his right hand. The monitor cart is behind him.

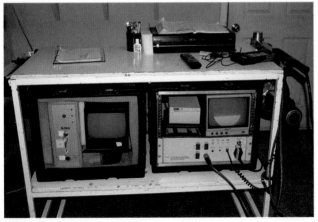

FIG. 11.10 The monitor cart for two miniature C-arms. This hospital uses one unit and stores the other for backup. The video recorder is mounted on top of the cart. A small thermal printer is mounted beside the monitor on the right.

Summary

When Edison first used a zinc cadmium sulfide screen to examine a patient, he placed the screen directly over the patient and then looked down at the images, which he viewed as very pale, yellow-green shadows. The image intensifier, which was developed in the 1950s and enhanced in the 1960s, is still a valuable diagnostic tool today and still uses Edison's zinc cadmium sulfide recipe. This chapter has reviewed the evolution of real-time imaging from the original plates to the sophisticated image intensifiers now used with digital imaging. It also explored the possibilities of the mini C-arm and its application in the equine hospital.

REVIEW QUESTIONS

1. The fluoroscope is an adaptation of a radiography unit used to:
   a. Check the function of the brain
   b. Provide dynamic real-time imaging
   c. Scope the internal structures of the gastrointestinal system
   d. View the radiographic images after they are processed
2. The value of fluoroscopy during surgery:
   a. Saves money by providing real-time imaging
   b. Saves time by providing on-the-spot images
   c. Provides a functional view of the internal organs
   d. Is useful because the patient is awake
3. Because the image on the fluoroscopy unit is produced as a series of individual images:
   a. Static images cannot be taken from it
   b. Static images may be extracted without disrupting the flow of the examination
   c. All of the images show movement, and static images are useless
   d. The images removed from the program do not have contrast
4. The technical factors for fluoroscopy are:
   a. High kV and low mAs
   b. Low kV and low mA
   c. A function of the time; the kV does not matter
   d. High kV and a low mA; time is not preset
5. The mAs on a fluoroscopy examination could be as high as:
   a. 50
   b. 75
   c. 150
   d. 180

6. The exposure time is controlled by the operator:
   a. Using a timer
   b. Using a hand switch
   c. Presetting the exposure time on the unit
   d. Depressing a foot switch; there is no preset limit
7. High doses of radiation are possible during fluoroscopy if:
   a. The x-ray tube is off and the patient is not wearing a lead shield
   b. The patient is protected and the tube is too close
   c. The operator does not pay attention to the timer
   d. The image intensifier is not turned on
8. Patient positioning during the examination:
   a. Is difficult because the patient must be rotated
   b. Takes place at the start of the procedure
   c. Is difficult if the patient is large and uncooperative
   d. Is complicated because the tube arm rotates around the patient
9. The image on the intensifier screens:
   a. Is immediately visible and clear to the human eye
   b. Is dull and flat in a grainy black and white
   c. Is enhanced when the human eye is correctly dark adapted
   d. Is clear when the image intensifier is warmed up correctly
10. The fluoroscopic system functions the same way as:
    a. A film/screen combination in radiography
    b. A detector in digital imaging
    c. The x-ray tube and detector in radiography
    d. A light bulb and an x-ray tube
11. The image intensifier consists of:
    a. A photocathode and a photoanode
    b. A light beam and an output phosphor
    c. The input phosphor and an output phosphor
    d. Input and output phosphors, which are the same

12. The process of converting x-rays to light is called:
    a. Phototransmission
    b. Phototropic
    c. Photoemission
    d. Thermionic emission
13. A method to ensure that the electrons accelerate to the output phosphor:
    a. Uses negative photons to guide them to the phosphor
    b. Uses positive electrons and a negative charge
    c. Uses a potential difference across the intensifier
    d. Uses a magnetic field within the tube
14. Each photoelectron that arrives at the output phosphor:
    a. Is intensified 50 to 75 times
    b. Produces 50 to 75 times as many light photons
    c. Produces more x-ray photons to radiate the patient
    d. Is absorbed by the input phosphor
15. The end result of the image on the fluoroscopy unit may be:
    a. Retained within the unit and reviewed on the image intensifier
    b. Converted into a WAV file and stored in a jukebox
    c. Stored on a hard drive and reviewed for diagnosis
    d. Stored on a hard drive and saved as a JPEG image
16. Applications for fluoroscopy are:
    a. Static extremity and pelvic images with contrast during surgery
    b. Contrast images of internal organs in real time converted from ultrasound
    c. Real-time images of archived radiographs converted from the films
    d. Real-time imaging of orthopedic surgery and function of the gastrointestinal system

Answers to Review Questions can be found on the Evolve website.

CHAPTER 12

Computerized Tomography

Lois C. Brown, RTR (Can/USA), ACR, MSc., P.Phys; and Stephanie Holowka, MRT(R), MRT(MR), MRSO(MRSC™)

Part of the inhumanity of the computer is that, once it is competently programmed and working smoothly, it is completely honest.

—Isaac Asimov, Science fiction writer and biochemistry professor, 1920–1992

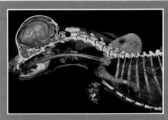

Sagittal cut plane. Volume-rendered CT scan of a dog showing placement of the endotracheal tube. (Courtesy of Animage Imaging.)

OUTLINE

LEARNING OBJECTIVES

When you have finished this chapter, you will be able to:

1. Understand the basic principles of tomography.
2. Discuss the basics of computerized tomography.
3. Understand the apparatus of the CT scanner.
4. Correlate tomography with computerized tomography.
5. Have a basic understanding of the application of computed tomography as a diagnostic tool.
6. Describe the concept of three-dimensional reconstruction.

APPLICATIONS

The application of the information in this chapter is relevant to the following areas:

1. The use of computerized tomography in veterinary medicine.

KEY TERMS

Key terms are defined in the Glossary on the Evolve website.

Algorithm
Analog
Archive
Attenuation coefficient

Computerized tomography
CT number
Detector

Digital
Gantry
Hounsfield unit

Image data
Pitch
Raw data

In the very early days of radiography, researchers were frustrated by the lack of resolution on the images they produced (Fig. 12.1A). In the early 1900s, several researchers worked independently in different countries with a common goal: to separate the superimposed shadows that necessarily result when complex structures of differing density are exposed to radiation and the exposure is recorded on a two-dimensional image receptor. How could the unwanted shadows be eliminated and the structures of interest left clear and unobstructed?

The first tomography unit was established in June 1921 when Andre Bocage filed a patent for an "apparatus for radiography on a moving plate." All refinements to this original patent have left Bocage's original concept untouched.

Tomography, from the Greek word *tomos,* meaning "cut" or "section," has been defined as a special technique to show, in detail, images of structures lying in a predetermined plane of tissue while blurring or eliminating detail in images or structures in other planes. A further clarification describes the original two-dimensional radiographic image as layers of images piled on top of one another. Pathology or contrast-enhanced anatomy in one layer may be obscured by dense anatomy in an area lying on top of or below the region of interest. However, if the layers of tissue can be separated and the areas above and below the region of interest are

blurred sufficiently, the anatomy in the plane of interest stands out in sharp focus against the blurred background (Fig. 12.1B).

The best way to demonstrate this concept is by visualizing the playground seesaw. A child sits on either end of a board that is placed on a midway support (Fig. 12.2). The distance of the arc the children travel as they ride on the ends of the board is determined by the length of the board and by the angle at the central support. If the children sit still, there is no travel and thus no angle. As the children start to travel through the arc, the angle at the ends of the board becomes larger and larger, whereas the midpoint becomes narrower and narrower. This narrow fulcrum is called the *region of interest (ROI)* (Fig. 12.3).

Principle of Rotation About a Fixed Point

The Focal Plane

The focal plane is the section, or layer, at which minimal blurring occurs (Fig. 12.4). The ROI is a fixed point in the anatomy of the patient. The structures above and below that point must be blurred out in order for the ROI to stand out in focus. If the x-ray tube and image receptor stay perfectly still, all of the structures will be in focus and the layers of

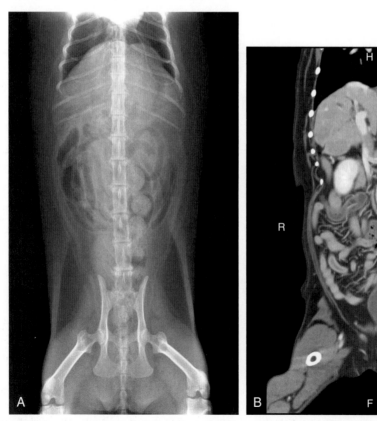

FIG. 12.1 A radiograph of an abdomen **(A)** next to a coronal reconstruction of an abdominal CT scan **(B)**. The benefit of the scan slice demonstrating each organ as the series is constructed is very obvious.

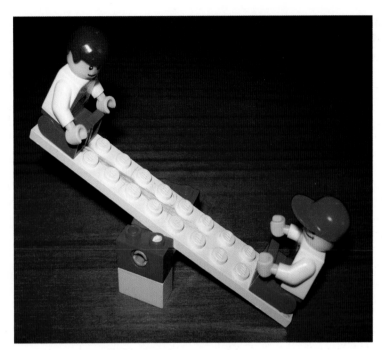

FIG. 12.2 The concept of the seesaw.

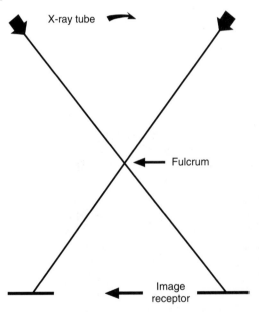

FIG. 12.3 Rotation about a fixed point.

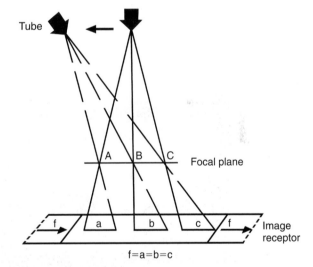

FIG. 12.4 Blurring of points outside the focal plane. The objects at levels A and C are projected onto different areas of the image receptor and are therefore blurred. The objects at level B are projected onto exactly the same place on the receptor and are in sharp focus.

anatomy will be superimposed. However, if the x-ray tube moves through an arc and the image receptor follows that arc exactly, then the structures at the fixed point will remain in focus and the structures above and below that point will be blurred (see Fig. 12.4).

In Fig. 12.5 the objects at levels A and C are projected onto different areas of the image receptor and are therefore seen as blur. The objects at level B are projected onto exactly the same place on the receptor and are in sharp focus.

Fulcrum

The fulcrum is the central support in the playground seesaw. It is also described as the central point about which a lever rotates. In tomography, the x-ray tube sits at one end of the seesaw, and the image receptor sits at the other end. The length of the lever does not change, but the point about which the lever rotates—the pivot point (fulcrum)—can be moved up and down. This then changes the level at which the anatomy is blurred.

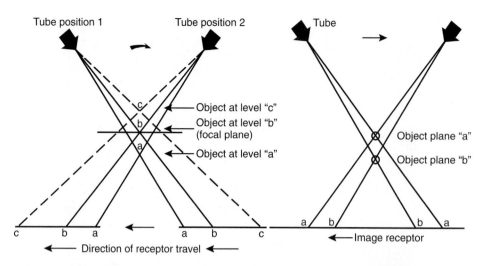

FIG. 12.5 As the x-ray tube moves coincident with the image receptor, the anatomy on the focal plane is projected onto the same place on the receptor. All other anatomy is blurred. This figure illustrates the fact that during the exposure and consequent tube and receptor movement, there is a "plane" or slice of tissue in focus, and not merely a point within the object.

◆ APPLICATION INFORMATION

Hold a yardstick (meter stick) vertically in one hand. Grasp it at a midway point, say, 18 inches (45 cm). Your hand has now become a fulcrum about which either end of the stick may be rotated evenly. Now move your hand down to the 9-inch (23-cm) mark. The length of the stick has not changed, but the fulcrum has moved significantly and the area of interest is now at the 9-inch (23-cm) mark.

Blur

Blur is the distortion or blurring of the anatomy above and below the ROI.

Computerized Tomography

The introduction of computers in the mid-1970s transformed standard tomography. The images could now be received and displayed on a computer, and the wealth of information far surpassed routine imaging on film. Invented in 1971 by Sir Godfrey Hounsfield, computerized tomography (CT), also known as *CT scanning* or *CAT (computerized axial tomography) scanning,* was the first imaging modality that enabled surgeons to noninvasively see the brain. CT took the standard analog images on film from conventional tomography and used computers to transform them into digital images. CT technology has evolved significantly over its 40-year history, but the basic working principles have remained the same.

When we image structures on a radiograph, we produce a two-dimensional image (length and width of the structure)—a matrix of pixels or picture elements. (A *matrix* is a series of boxes or individual shades of information.) A computerized tomographic image is a three-dimensional image—a matrix of voxels—that includes the third dimension, depth. If a wide matrix is imaged, the result is said to be pixilated (Fig. 12.6A). If the boxes of information are very small, the image becomes clearer (Fig. 12.6B).

CT uses an x-ray machine that acquires images that look like slices in a loaf of bread. As with conventional tomography, the CT machine uses a moving x-ray tube to create the series of images, but it also requires the use of detectors and a computer.

Translation to the Computer

An x-ray tube emitting a fan-shaped beam of x-rays rotates 360 degrees around a gantry (or opening in the center of the machine) and the patient within it (Fig. 12.7A). Mounted directly across from the x-ray tube is a series of x-ray detectors that rotate at the same speed around the patient. The x-rays pass through the patient, and the attenuated beam is collected by detectors. The detectors convert the photons to an electrical signal that is fed into an analog-to-digital converter. The digital signal, or raw data (also known as *scan data*), is sent to a computer that reconstructs the images and presents them in the operator's chosen format. As a CT scanner is acquiring images, the table moves forward in increments set by the operator, enabling several images/slices to be taken at various levels for a complete examination. The computer reassembles the images and displays them on a monitor so that as the operator reviews the images, each "slice" is displayed in perfect focus independent of its neighbor (Fig. 12.7B).

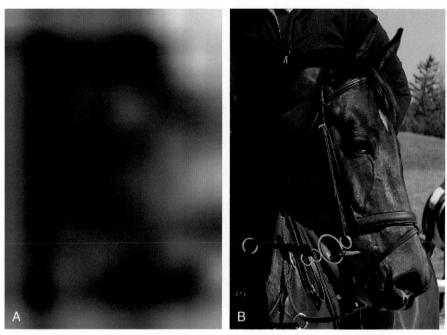

FIG. 12.6 A, The image is pixilated and the subject is unrecognizable (37 × 123 pixels/inch). **B,** The matrix is enhanced, the pixels are smaller, and the resolution is superior (750 × 1029 pixels/inch).

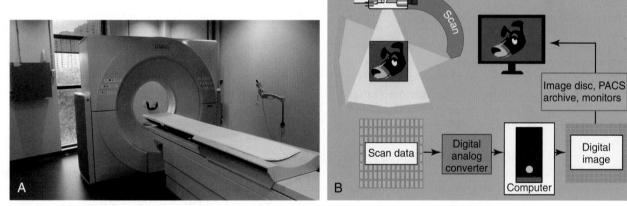

FIG. 12.7 A, A CT scanner in a veterinary clinic. To the right of the scanner is a power injector, which is used for injecting contrast media as the scanner images the patient. **B,** The basic workings of a CT scanner. The x-ray tube rotates around the patient, and the data are sent to the computer. The resultant images look much like slices in a loaf of bread.

◆ APPLICATION INFORMATION

As the x-ray beam passes through the patient, parts of it are absorbed by the tissues. The amounts that are absorbed by the various tissues are related to how many photons each type of tissue absorbs, or the *attenuation coefficient* of the tissue. In this text, the math is not important; the important part is that bone attenuates more x-rays than tissue, and fat and air attenuate about the same amount. Thus our image is made up of a series of densities reflecting the tissue types that were imaged.

The Hounsfield Genius

Normal x-ray practice is to take at least two views (90 degrees to each other) so as to display the anatomy free of superimposing structures. In CT, multiple views or projections are created by the rotation of the x-ray tube and detectors. The detectors are photodetectors that convert the x-ray photons into light and then into electric currents. Historically, the detectors were vacuum tubes containing xenon gas; however, modern-day CT scanners use solid-state detectors. The data or electric currents created by the detectors are fed into an analog-to-digital converter and then sent to the computer for reconstruction. The primary method of reconstructing CT images is a process called *filtered back-projection.* Back-projection is a method of calculating an unknown value from multiples of known values. The multiple views performed by a CT scanner create a large number of calculations, so a computer is required to do it in a timely manner. Take a look at the simplified picture of the process in this example of a back-projection calculation:

by calculation   x = 1

6	3	7	4
5	2	3	5
5	X	4	5
4	3	7	6

By calculation $x = 1$

In this simple depiction, one can calculate the value of x by subtracting it from all of the known values—both crosswise and diagonally. The calculated values appear in gray. The computer does a similar process in CT, but on the order of thousands of calculations. A mathematical filter or calculation is applied to the pixel calculations to cancel out any blurring artifact in the final image.

The numbers depicted in the example for back-projection can also be used to demonstrate another aspect of the CT image. When images are reconstructed for CT, they are constructed and displayed as a matrix. A matrix is made up of several pixels, or picture elements—the dots in a picture. The resolution of the image is tied to how many pixels are displayed in a given field of view. In the previous example, the resulting image would have a matrix of 2. The size of a pixel depends on its relationship to the field of view that is displayed.

An image's resolution can be calculated in mm² as follows:

$$\text{Resolution (in millimeters)} = \text{Field of view (in millimeters)} \times \text{Matrix}$$

In most modern-day CT scanners, the standard matrix used is 512×512.

Another factor in the setup of a CT scan image is the slice thickness (or, in the case of our seesaw, the fulcrum width). The operator chooses the slice thickness according to the anatomy to be displayed. Each image in CT is a three-dimensional slice of the subject because the image has length, width, and height (or thickness). Because images in CT are created as slices, the pixels making up the image are actually voxels, or volume elements, and the density displayed is averaged into each pixel of each slice. When one looks at a single CT slice, the image has height and width, but one does not look at the picture from the top or bottom. Rather, the thickness of the image is whatever the collimation has been set at the time the slice is acquired. The concept of slice thickness is discussed in more detail later in this chapter.

Each voxel in a CT image is also calculated into a density measurement called a *Hounsfield unit (HU)* or *CT number.* The value is calculated by this equation:

$$\text{Hounsfield unit} = K \frac{\mu p - \mu w}{\mu w}$$

where K is the constant (usually 1000), μp is the attenuation coefficient of the pixel, and μw is the attenuation coefficient of water. (An attenuation coefficient describes the ability of the pixel to absorb radiation. Bone absorbs more radiation, and fat and water absorb less radiation.)

This equation is significant to the CT scan for the following reasons:

1. It converts densities from tiny values of attenuation coefficients to usable units.
2. Every pixel can be interpreted as a particular density that can be used in diagnosis or postprocessing.
3. The Hounsfield unit sets up a direct relationship with creating and displaying the images.

Table 12.1 gives the conversions for various attenuation coefficients versus HUs. As shown in Table 12.1, the variances between the attenuation coefficients are very tiny (on the order of 10^{-3}), whereas the HU shows demonstrable and consistent differences for each of the tissue densities. This is also key for the visibility of various tissues in the body. On a normal x-ray, bone appears white because it is very dense, and soft tissues appear as shades of gray. It is difficult to see individual soft tissue organs on x-ray because their abilities to absorb x-rays are very similar; in addition, organs are superimposed on top of one another (Fig. 12.8A and B). However, as shown in Fig. 12.8C, a CT scan is able to show various soft tissue organs in cross-sections and in HUs.

Image Display

HUs also affect how images are displayed in terms of brightness and contrast. For CT images, the *window* of an image is the number of shades of gray making up the image (contrast). The *level* is the midpoint of the range of grays within a specific anatomical scanned area (density).

A brain, for example, may be windowed at 80 HU and leveled at 38 HU. This means that white and black make up

TABLE 12.1	Conversions for Attenuation Coefficients (AC) vs. Hounsfield Units (HU)	
SUBSTANCE	**AC**	**HU (at 120 kV)**
Air	0.0004	−1000
Fat	0.185	−50 to −150
Water	0.206	0
Blood	0.208	+80
White matter	0.213	34
Gray matter	0.212	38

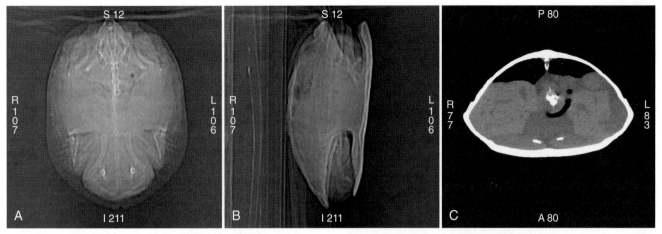

FIG. 12.8 A and B, Two x-ray images generated on a CT scanner showing how the turtle is not well demonstrated on simple x-rays. This is a classic issue for structures such as the brain and skull in other animals. C, The CT scanner allows the internal organs to be seen through the shell. Spleen, lungs, liver, and trachea are all visible on the CT scan.

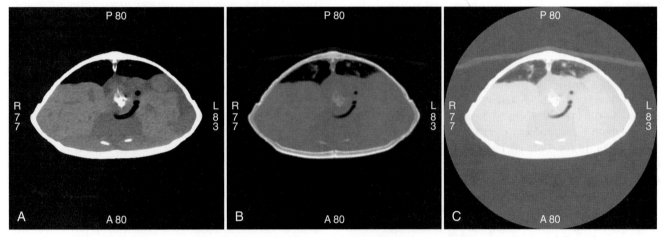

FIG. 12.9 Same image of the turtle but with different window levels. A, The internal organs are best on abdominal windows (W350, L40). B, The bone is best on a bone window (W2500, L250). C, The lungs are shown on a lung window (W 2000, L−700).

the image, as well as 78 shades of gray in between. So how does one come to this number? If 38 is the midpoint, it is half of the number for contrast. So 80 is divided by 2 (or a half), which is 40. To calculate the number of shades of gray visible, you add and subtract 40 from the level of 38: 38 − 40 = −2 and 38 + 40 = 78. This means that all of the shades of gray are visible from HUs −2 to 78. Bone, which is denser, simply appears as white because its HU is out of the visible range. Air and fat appear as black because, again, their HUs are less than what is visible as a gray level.

Let us try this calculation again. As stated before, bone is visible on a brain window only as white, so a different window/level (or contrast/brightness) is used to demonstrate bones. A typical window width is 2000, and a typical window level is 250. Half of 2000 is 1000. Now you add and subtract 1000 from 250 to get the visible range of grays. Because 250 is the midpoint, −750 to 1250 will be visible as shades of gray. Anything below −750 HU will be seen as black, and anything above 1250 will appear as white. This is a considerably wider window level. It is good for showing bone, but the brain is

not as visible because there are very few HUs or shades of gray between white matter and gray matter (Fig. 12.9A-C).

HUs also can be measured with a cursor to help the veterinarian determine the nature of a lesion. For example, when a veterinarian sees a lesion in the lungs, if a cursor reading is −50 HU, then the lesion may be fat. If it is 160 HU, then it is calcium. Blood reads at about 80 HU. Some scanners even have a feature that allows the operator to apply a set cursor that will read all of the HUs for each voxel.

The CT Data

The operator uses two types of data on CT scanners. The scan data (raw data) collected from the detectors are used to create the images. These data sets tend to be very large, and so storage is usually temporarily on the CT scanner itself. The operator will use the raw data to re-create images as needed, even after the patient is no longer on the table. Once the raw data are removed from the scanner (most scanners perform the removal automatically after a period), new images can no longer be produced. The image data are either photographed onto films or networked to a picture archival and communications system (PACS). Modern CT scanners are capable of producing hundreds, if not thousands, of images.

Just as in digital radiography, all images are stored, or archived, in a huge data bank. These banks may be local or they may be anywhere on earth.

For a CT scan operator, there are many ways that a scan or the images from it can be viewed. Some of the considerations that show the thinking behind the various methods are discussed in the following sections.

Field of View

In CT scanning, there are two types of field of view (the area seen in the image). The *scan field of view* (SFOV) is the number of detectors covered by the x-ray beam. This is important because if the patient's body part is outside the field of view (or chosen range of detectors), it cannot be reconstructed.

The *display field of view* (DFOV) is a key element in the resolution of CT images. DFOV will be either equal to or smaller than the SFOV. By decreasing the DFOV, one can increase the ability of the images to resolve structures. Although a maximum SFOV may be set by the manufacturer, the DFOV is a key factor that an operator chooses for his or her CT images (Fig. 12.10). Even after an animal has been removed from the CT scanner, a technologist can reconstruct the images using the scan or raw data to create images that have a desired DFOV.

Technical Factors Used in CT Scanning and Radiation Dose

As with x-ray units, CT scanners use kilovoltage (kV) and milliamperes per second (mAs) as scanning factors. Typically the kV tends to be much higher than in standard radiography—from 80 to 140 kV. The mAs value also tends to be much higher, ranging from 10 to 400 mAs. The *scan time* depends on the method of scanning (spiral or conventional) and usually means the time it takes the x-ray tube to rotate 360 degrees

around the patient for an exposure. By increasing the mAs, an operator can affect which structures are visualized.

Of course, increasing kV or mAs also increases the overall radiation dose emitted by the CT scanner. One unfortunate aspect of CT scanning is that the higher the technical factors, the prettier the images. CT has much more tolerance for high technical factors than does general radiography. In any imaging, there is a great desire to restrict dosage as much as possible and always adhere to the ALARA (as low as reasonably achievable) principle.

Slice Thickness

Slice thickness is a technical variable determined by the operator of the CT scanner and is a key factor in image resolution. Slice thickness is altered by prepatient and predetector collimators. The original CT scanners acquired images in slices 10-mm thick. If a lesion was less than 2 to 5 millimeters thick, it could be missed by the averaging of the 10-mm slice of anatomy. Modern-day CT scanners with multislice technology are able to acquire image slices thinner than a millimeter (Fig. 12.11).

Algorithms/Kernels

An algorithm is a mathematical calculation and is applied to each of the pixels creating the CT image to enhance certain structures. Some manufacturers give algorithms (or kernels) an actual number, whereas other manufacturers give these calculations a name. A soft or low-pass algorithm shifts the pixels to enhance structures that have very few increments of CT numbers (e.g., the brain). A high-pass or bone algorithm alters the images to enhance structures that have sharp edges. The use of an algorithm can be understood when comparing a soft tissue view to a bone view. Even with the proper window/level, a soft algorithm produces a blurry bone image, and a bone algorithm on a brain image produces a very grainy, noisy image. In CT scanning, as long as there are raw data (or scan data), a user can postprocess the images multiple times to show various structures.

Table Movement and Pitch

A key working part in CT scanning is the movement of the table during the procedure. Three types of table motion can

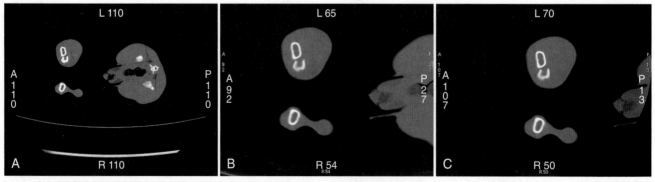

FIG. 12.10 A rabbit with a tibial fracture. **A,** This image was taken with a 22.0-cm display field of view. **B,** This image was acquired by magnifying the original scan. **C,** This image has the best resolution because the scan data were reconstructed into a 12.0 display field of view.

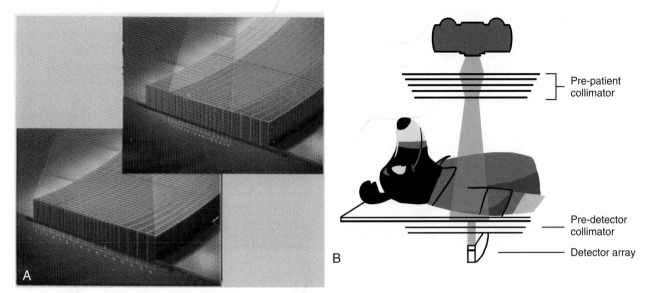

FIG. 12.11 These images show how slice thicknesses are determined on the CT scanner. **A,** On a multislice scanner, ranges of detectors acquire multiple images in a collimation. **B,** The operator selects a slice thickness or detector range. The scanner's prepatient and predetector scanners maintain that slice thickness for the images.

be chosen. When setting up the scans, a scout view (scanogram) may be taken. This looks much like a radiograph and allows the operator to choose the regions included in a scan. For the picture to be taken, the tube and the detectors remain in one location while the table passes through a chosen distance. For the actual CT scanning, the images are acquired in a conventional method or helical/spiral. The operator of the CT scanner has the ability to choose which type of scanning is best for a given image or pathology.

Conventional scanning refers to table motion as done by the original CT scanners. The scanner takes a slice (image) at one location. The table then moves a chosen distance, and another slice is taken. A whole stack of slices can be created in this manner. On older machines, the x-ray tube was connected by wires and cables to its generator and transformers in a separate box outside the gantry. The tube was therefore limited to moving in one rotation and then back. This motion also took time in CT scanners. Typically, the delay between slices on later-model conventional CT scanners was approximately 3.5 seconds.

In the late 1980s, a new phenomenon became available in CT scanning called *spiral* or *helical CT scanning*. The design of the scanner was changed to allow a slip ring and brushes (Fig. 12.12) to bring power to the CT gantry and x-ray tube. In turn, the same slip ring/brush assembly gave information back to the CT computers. This arrangement allowed the x-ray tube and detectors to rotate continuously, thus saving a delay between scans. In order for helical scanning to work, the CT scanners had to compensate for the motion of the scanner by using another calculation called an *interpolation algorithm*. Interpolation is the calculation of an unknown value based on two known values on either side. The scanner is thus able to calculate the slice in a straight plane rather than how it would appear (like a corkscrew). CT scanner manufacturers have used either a

180-degree or a 90-degree interpolation algorithm to correct helical images.

To lessen the CT dose, the helical scanner allows the technologist to choose a table motion greater than the slice thickness. Pitch is defined as the ratio between table movement (in millimeters) and CT slice thickness. How does this look in calculation?

$$\text{Pitch} = \frac{\text{Table movement (in mm)}}{\text{Slice thickness (in mm)}}$$

For example, if a table moves 5 mm for a 5-mm slice, then the pitch calculated is 1. If the CT operator chooses a pitch of 1.5 on a 5-mm slice, then the table will move 7.5 mm while scanning 5-mm-thick images.

The plus in using pitch is that it drops the radiation dose for the patient while keeping the image resolution. On single-slice CT scanners, the pitch can be increased up to 1.8 with no visible effect on image resolution. Scanner design has changed further with the advent of multiple-slice CT scanners. Now the table pitch must also take into account the numbers and width of the detectors chosen.

Prescribing a Scan and Protocols

The protocols or scan technical factors used in CT scanning are just as varied as the region or body area being scanned. All CT scanners allow operators to program protocols (labeled for body part or type of scan) and store them in the computer. Technologists can then enter the name (or select the name from a list created by the radiology information system) and then select the desired protocol, such as for a CT scan of the head. The technologist then completes a scanogram view or scout view (CT version of a radiograph) and from those images prescribes the actual CT scan.

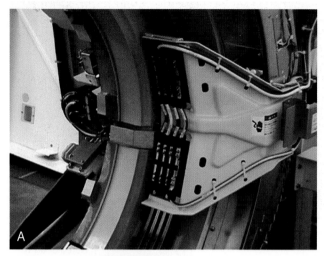

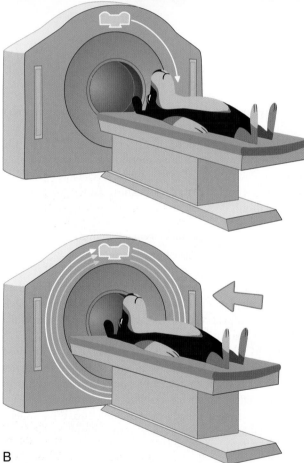

FIG. 12.12 A, Photograph of slip ring and brushes. The brushes are mounted onto the slip ring. **B,** As the x-ray tube and gantry rotate around, the slip rings transfer electrical signals and receive data.

The CT scanner always allows the technologist to make any desired change to a protocol setup as needed. On some protocols, an intravenous (IV) contrast agent may be required. IV contrast agents are iodine based and enhance veins, arteries, and some entire organs. Angiography can also be performed on CT; by rapidly injecting a contrast agent, an operator can show the arteries and veins in any given part of the body.

Abdominal scans typically need a contrast agent so that the organs can be better seen. Contrast agents may also be used to demonstrate infection in extremities. In cases in which a spinal pathology is suspected, a veterinarian may inject a contrast agent into the spinal canal (via a lumbar puncture) to show any disturbances of the spinal cord. This procedure is called a *myelogram*. (Only special contrast agents are used in the spinal canal; see Chapter 23). Fluoroscopy, radiographs, and CT scans may all be part of the imaging of a spinal cord.

Multislice CT Scanners

Within the past 15 years, CT scanning has seen a further evolution in the design of the detectors. Most scanners available now have multiple detectors. Instead of a single detector array, the fan beam originating from the x-ray tube is now wider to radiate a larger array of detectors. Modern multislice scanners can have up to 256 detectors in the width of their array. Because of this new technology, larger sections can be obtained in one scan while the images are reconstructed into submillimeter thicknesses. This has allowed most CT scan data sets to be collected as volume scans that can be reconstructed into three-dimensional pictures afterwards.

Indications and Postprocessing for CT Scanning

CT scanning used to be the primary modality for imaging the head and spine, but magnetic resonance imaging has now supplanted it. However, CT scanning remains an excellent diagnostic tool for assessing trauma and for body imaging. It is also good at demonstrating the skeleton.

Because of the evolution of the technology, CT scans are performed so that the images can be reconstructed in multiple ways. A single conventional exposure through a multislice scanner can create 32 images of 0.625-mm thickness. Whether the images are collected by a conventional scan or a spiral scan, they function as a volume if they have the same field of view, center, matrix, and algorithm. This means several slices can easily be stacked together and reconstructed into any two-dimensional plane or three-dimensional image.

In volume imaging, there are multiple ways to construct the objects. The simplest reconstruction is to angle the volume of images and reconstruct them into a two-dimensional view in a direction differing from the original scans. The operator can alter the slice thickness on the 2-dimensional reconstruction and the window/level so that he or she can better demonstrate the affected anatomy. A spine is always reconstructed through the sagittal or longitudinal plane. Typically, several images are constructed along each plane (Fig. 12.13).

Three-dimensional images can simply be created by a process called *shaded-surface display,* whereby a three-dimensional object is created by limiting the number of HUs seen. For bone, 160 HU and higher is selected. For a skin surface, the range might include −200 HU and higher. These objects can be modified by well-designed software. Another

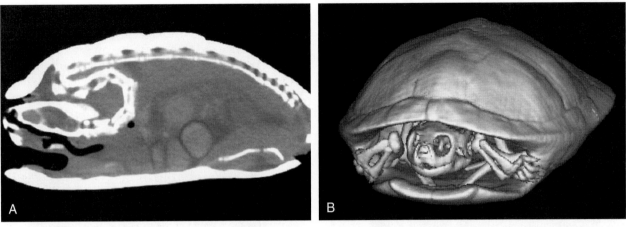

FIG. 12.13 A, Sagittal reconstruction of Waddle's spine from axial CT scans. **B,** A three-dimensional picture that is a shaded-surface display image demonstrating voxel values of 160 HUs and higher. Such three-dimensional images can be virtually angled and cut into to show various perspectives on anatomy.

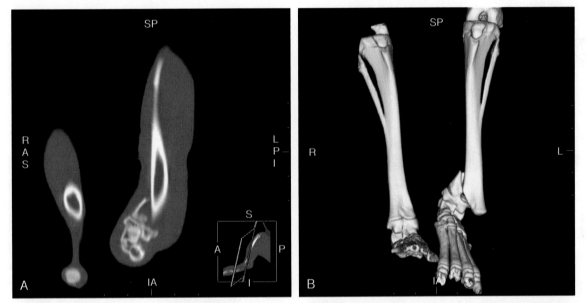

FIG. 12.14 Tools such as three-dimensional imaging greatly help in the understanding of pathology. Although the rabbit's fracture is visible in the two-dimensional coronal reconstruction or reformatted image **(A)**, the severity is much more apparent on the volume-rendered three-dimensional reconstruction **(B)**.

type of three-dimensional imaging is called *volume rendering* (Fig. 12.14). This process takes the entire range of HUs and includes them in the picture. The operator can then select the range of voxels that are opaque and those that are transparent.

soft tissue and bone structures. Images can be reconstructed in many formats, including two-dimensional reformat, three-dimensional imaging, and volume rendering. All of these formats can aid the veterinarian in the assessment and diagnosis of patients.

Summary

Computed tomography is a modality that uses x-radiation to create images in cross-section. It has the ability to demonstrate

Image Gallery

The CT scan images and reconstructions in Figs. 12.15 to 12.21 demonstrate various pathologies.

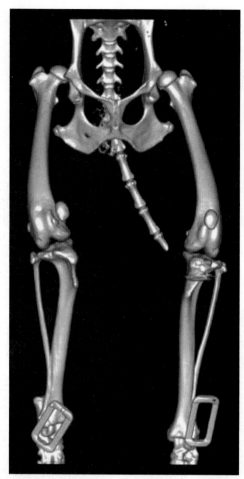

FIG. 12.15 Volume rendering of a CT scan taken of a patient's lower limbs. The right hip is completely displaced from the hip joint. The left hip is slightly dislocated.

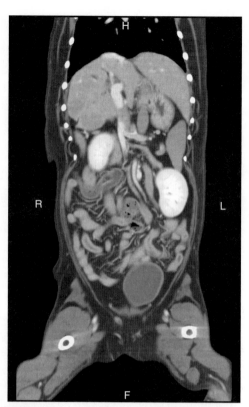

FIG. 12.16 Coronal reformat of arterial phase of CT scan of the abdomen. Liver, kidneys, spleen, stomach, and bladder are seen.

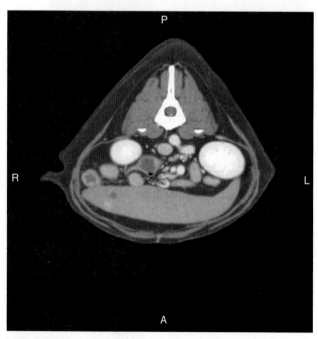

FIG. 12.17 Axial image of a contrast-enhanced abdominal CT scan. Two lesions are seen in the pancreas toward the patient's right side. One lesion is hypodense, and the other lesion is enhanced with intravenous contrast.

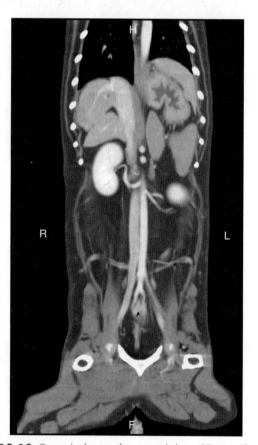

FIG. 12.18 Coronal reformat of an arterial-phase CT scan. The aorta and renal arteries are well demonstrated. Because of multislice technology and spiral scanning, various phases of intravenous contrast enhancement can be taken (arterial, capillary, and venous).

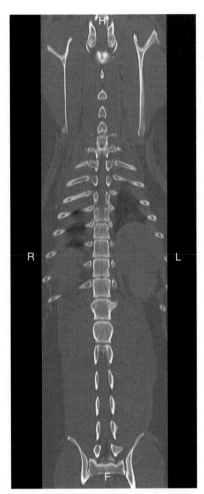

FIG. 12.19 Coronal reformat of bone algorithm images demonstrating the spine. This scan could have been reconstructed from neck, chest, and abdominal CT scans using the raw or scan data retrospectively. One can perform a single CT scan of a patient and then (without further radiation) reconstruct more images to enhance the demonstration of patient anatomy. This aspect of CT is very helpful in both cancer and trauma imaging of patients.

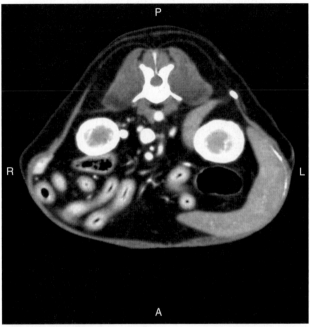

FIG. 12.20 Early phase of intravenous enhancement on this axial plane image. The phase of contrast is seen in the parenchyma of the kidneys and the splotchy appearance of the pancreas. The vertebrae is seen at the top of the image.

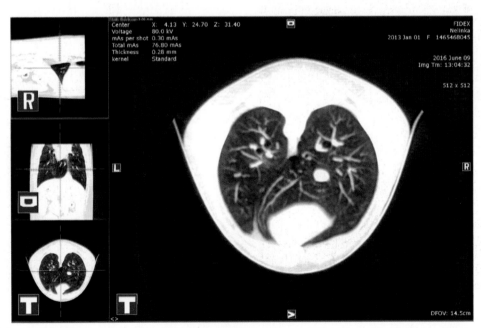

FIG. 12.21 Reformats of the lungs. The axial image shows a large nodule or tumor in the left lung parenchyma.

REVIEW QUESTIONS

1. A Hounsfield unit:
   a. Is a measurement of density on a CT scan
   b. Compares the density value of a pixel with that of water
   c. Is also called a CT number
   d. All of the above

2. If the scanning slice thickness is 5 mm and the table pitch is 2.0, the resulting table movement per rotation is:
   a. 5 mm
   b. 7.5 mm
   c. 10 mm
   d. 15 mm

3. Which method is the most common way to reconstruct CT scan images?
   a. Fourier transformation
   b. Filtered back-projection
   c. Back-projection
   d. Filtered optical transfer

4. What determines the slice thickness on the CT scanner?
   a. The prepatient collimators
   b. The predetector collimators
   c. The technician's choice
   d. All of the above

5. A technician has just finished scanning a patient. Which is the best way to magnify the images to show pathology?
   a. Magnify the picture using the scanner software.
   b. Use the raw data to magnify the picture.
   c. Decrease the field of view using the raw or scan data and reconstruct the images.
   d. Increase the field of view using the raw or scan data and reconstruct the images.

6. What does a slip ring assembly do in a CT scan?
   a. It allows the x-ray tube and detectors to rotate continuously.
   b. It allows for helical or spiral scanning.
   c. It makes the table move quickly.
   d. a and b
   e. b and c

7. Raw data or scan data:
   a. Are used to create more images
   b. Are archived regularly
   c. Are kept on the scanner for only a short duration
   d. Do not occupy much disk space on the scanner
   e. a and c

8. A CT scan of a patient's skull shows a fracture on the soft tissue images. The scan has been done on a multislice scanner. Which is the best way to show the skull fracture?
   a. Change the window/level to bone windows.
   b. Using the raw data, change the algorithm to bone or high-pass.
   c. Rescan the patient using thinner pictures.
   d. Reconstruct thinner pictures with a bone algorithm.

9. When may a veterinarian want contrast "on" for a CT scan?
   a. To show an infection
   b. To show a tumor
   c. To show the organs in the abdomen
   d. To show a fracture
   e. a, b, and c
   f. All of the above

10. What is the typical matrix used to show most CT scan images?
    a. 512
    b. 388
    c. 128
    d. 256

Answers to Review Questions can be found on the Evolve website.

CHAPTER 13
Magnetic Resonance Imaging

Stephanie Holowka, MRT(R), MRT(MR), MRSO(MRSC™)

The world is your mirror and your mind is a magnet. What you perceive in this world is largely a reflection of your own attitudes and beliefs.
—Michael LeBeuf, American author and management professor, University of New Orleans

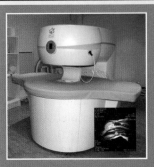

Magnetic resonance imaging is superior in demonstrating the brain, spinal cord, and soft tissue structures.

OUTLINE

LEARNING OBJECTIVES

When you have finished this chapter, you will be able to:

1. Discuss the equipment necessary for magnetic resonance imaging.
2. Understand the principles of magnetic resonance imaging.
3. Know the MRI machine.
4. Describe how MRI is used in diagnosis.
5. List the safety issues in MRI.

APPLICATIONS

The application of the information in this chapter is relevant to the following area:

1. Imaging using magnetism and resonance to determine pathology.

KEY TERMS

Key terms are defined in the Glossary on the Evolve website.

Atom
Echo time
Faraday cage/Faraday shield

Magnet
Magnetic field
Radio frequency

Repetition time
Resonance

Signal intensity
Specific absorption rate

Magnetic resonance imaging (MRI) came into existence in the early 1980s. Its creation was based on the principles of magnetic spectroscopy—the use of a magnetic field and radio frequencies to determine the chemical makeup of a substance. The chemical makeup of a substance can be determined by which radio frequencies are emitted by that substance and which are received in response from the substance.

MRI has become increasingly common in human medicine and is now found in specialized veterinary centers as well (Fig. 13.1). Because it shows the concentration of free-floating hydrogen molecules in tissue, it has much better subject contrast than a computed tomography (CT) scan and conventional radiography. MRI is superior in demonstrating the brain, the spinal cord (Fig. 13.2), and soft tissue structures such as the ligaments and cartilage in joints. MRI is also a desired modality in that it does not use any ionizing radiation in creating the images. This chapter gives an overview for understanding this fascinating and complex new technology.

Safety Notice

Magnets such as those used in MRI scanners are very dangerous machines, especially for untrained personnel (Fig. 13.3). Anyone walking into an MRI room must be screened for unsafe implants and any loose metal. The highest danger to staff and patients is the projectile effect—the launching of a metallic object into the magnet by magnetic force. A person cannot predict how an object will project into a magnet. People have been severely injured and even killed by such accidents. Only magnetically safe objects and safe people should be allowed to enter an MRI room. Only special stretchers, MRI-safe monitors, MRI-safe oxygen tanks, and so on can be used in an MRI room. Every MRI site must have policies and procedures in place to ensure the safety of patients and staff.

Principles

To understand the workings of MRI, one has to start at the atomic level. All atoms have protons, neutrons, and electrons. The protons and neutrons are found in the center, or core (nucleus), of the atom, and the electrons spin around on the outside. Every atom also spins and wobbles in space as well (Fig. 13.4). This wobble (much like how a top wobbles) is called *precession*.

Atoms join together to create molecules. All atoms and molecules (as in anything electrical) exhibit the ability to show magnetic polarity, or fields. When placed in a magnetic

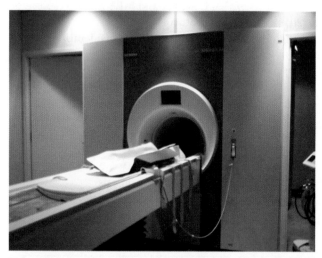

FIG. 13.1 An MRI machine in a veterinary clinic. This is a high-field (1.5-T) superconductor magnet. The machine was being prepared for a spine scan on a dog. It has the spine coil in place.

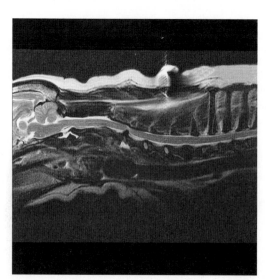

FIG. 13.2 A sagittal T2-weighted magnetic resonance image of a dog's spine. The scan shows that an intervertebral disc is bulging into the spinal canal and against the spinal cord. The compressed cord is brighter in that region, showing that it is swollen, or has edema.

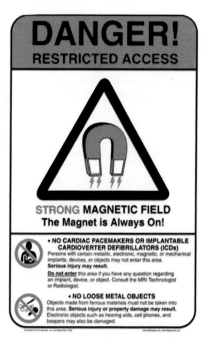

FIG. 13.3 An MRI warning sign. (Courtesy Magmedix, Inc., Ritchberg, Massachusetts.)

field, they will respond according to their own polarity (they align north and south).

How Does MRI Work?

In a most basic description, one puts an animal onto the table, which then enters the core of the magnet. All of the subject's molecules align on the basis of polarity and become magnetized (Fig. 13.5). In performing a scan, a technologist applies a radio frequency tuned to the precessing frequency of hydrogen atoms (Fig. 13.6A). The hydrogen atoms in the subject respond by resonating (or responding) into a higher energy state. They

also change the angle of their magnetization and wobble together. The radio frequency is removed, and the molecules return to their normal energy state (Fig. 13.6B). In doing so, they give off a radio frequency that the MRI scanner calculates into an image. The actual method is quite a bit more complicated, but this is the basic concept of MRI.

Magnets and Magnetism

A magnet is any object that exhibits a magnetic field or force. Magnetic force can be created in an object in several ways. It can occur naturally in some substances, such as iron and malachite. It can be induced into an object; some metallic objects become magnetized if exposed to a strong magnetic field and, as a result, act as magnets. A magnet can be created by electricity. When an electric current is applied through a series of copper windings, an electromagnet can be created. Magnetic force also exhibits polarity, in that there are two poles, north and south, like positive and negative in electricity.

In magnetism, opposite poles attract each other and pull two magnets together. Like poles repel and push two magnets away from each other.

The imperial unit of measurement for magnetism is the gauss (G). For example, the earth has a magnetic field of 1 gauss. The most common measurement of magnetism is the

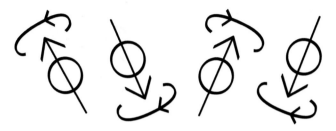

FIG. 13.4 Atoms in their normal random positions, spinning and wobbling. Arrows represent the positions of their magnetic polarities.

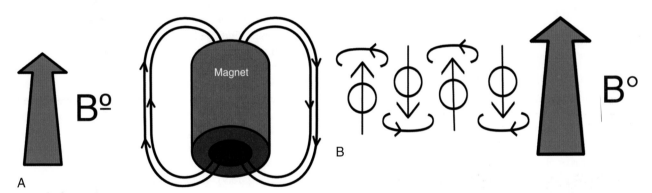

FIG. 13.5 A, A magnet and its magnetic field. The total magnetic force is represented by B0. **B,** What happens to atoms within a strong magnetic field. The atoms randomly align to their polarity, and B0 represents the total magnetization of the atoms.

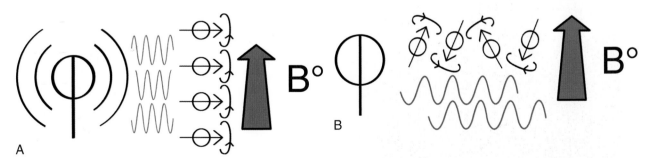

FIG. 13.6 A, What happens in magnetic resonance imaging. A radio antenna emits radio waves in a resonant frequency that causes certain atoms to go into a higher energy state. The hydrogen atoms respond to this frequency by aligning their magnetism *(black arrows)* to 90 degrees from their original orientation *(blue arrow)* within the magnet. They also wobble or precess together. **B,** When the radio waves are turned off, the atoms return to their original magnetization state and their energy state returns to equilibrium. The atoms give off radio waves, which are detected by the radio antenna.

metric equivalent, the tesla (T): 10,000 G = 1.0 T. The earth's magnetic field is 10^{-4} T. Tesla is the unit that people use in describing a medical magnet's field strength.

In medical MRI, three types of magnets can be in use. There are permanent magnets. These consist of two slabs of magnetic material facing each other (Fig. 13.7), and they tend to be lower field strengths—less than 0.3 T. There are electromagnets, or resistive magnets, created by an electrical charge applied through copper wire wrapped around a center. These also tend to be lower field magnets—less than 0.6 T. The most common medical magnets are called *superconducting magnets*. They are massive electromagnets made of windings that are superconductive in very low temperatures. Liquid helium (the coldest substance available on earth, with a temperature very close to absolute zero [−273° C/−459° F]) is used to keep the magnet active.

◆ APPLICATION INFORMATION

For the use of a superconducting magnet, great consideration is made in terms of the construction of the room surrounding the magnet. Special ventilation ducts must be created for quenching the magnet, a process whereby the liquid helium vents out rapidly and shuts off the magnet by increasing the resistance across the windings. Liquid helium has an expansion ratio of 1 to 700 liters. There are at least 1000 liters of liquid helium in a superconductor magnet, so the total expanded volume would rapidly exceed the size of any MRI room. It is these magnets (1.0 T or more field strength) that are never turned off. The very strong magnetic field is always on, even when the machine is not taking pictures.

Aside from the magnet, many other parts work together to make an MRI unit work correctly (Fig. 13.8).

Magnetic Shims or Shim Coils

Shims are pieces or plates of metal used to correct the magnetic field within the magnet. For an MRI unit to work properly,

the main magnetic field of the bore must be entirely homogenous. (All of the hydrogen atoms must synchronize exactly the same.) Any alterations of the main magnetic field could result in distorted images.

Gradients

Gradients are coils or assemblies within the magnetic bore that enable the machine to create images in any plane. An incremented current is applied across the gradient in an orientation chosen by the technologist, thus slightly varying the magnetic field in that direction. When the radio frequency is applied to the body, the variances in the frequency are calculated back to determine the "x-y-z" dimensions in space of each of the voxels of the image. The method used to reconstruct images from the gradients is called *two-dimensional Fourier transformation*. It is the design of the gradients that allows MRI to create images in any plane—axial (or transverse), coronal, or sagittal.

Radio Antenna

The radio antenna used in the MRI machine is quite strong, so strong that it could be used for a radio station. The antenna sends and receives radio waves to and from the patient. Radio waves are part of the electromagnetic spectrum, as are light, microwaves, and x-rays (see Chapter 1, Fig. 1.6). They are a form of energy but are not radioactive. Because the radio waves are important to the creation of images, MRI rooms have to be shielded with a Faraday cage against any external radio signals. Outside radio waves can cause artifacts on the magnetic resonance images.

Surface Coils

MRI machines are able to produce patient images from the main magnet (or body coil) itself; however, the radio signals received from smaller body parts have very poor resolution. Surface coils are devices that receive (and sometimes send) radio wave signals from a body part that is covered or contained by them (Fig. 13.9). There are specialized coils for many body

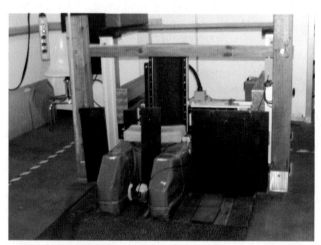

FIG. 13.7 A resistive magnet MRI unit used to image horse legs. The magnet covers only a specific field of view. A white spherical phantom (in between the two blue magnets) is covered by a surface coil.

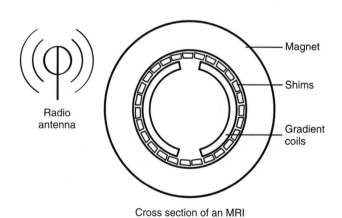

Cross section of an MRI

FIG. 13.8 A basic overview of the components needed to make up a basic MRI machine. A superconducting magnet would have a vacuum and helium chambers outside the actual magnet assembly but within the casing of the machine.

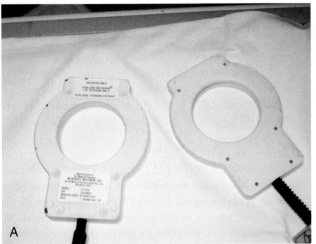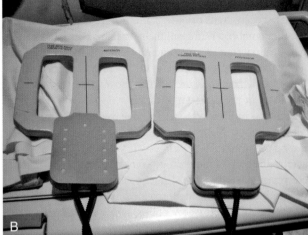

FIG. 13.9 Surface coils are used to get better images of smaller structures in MRI. **A,** 3-inch coils. **B,** Cardiac coils. These coils demonstrate well any body part that can be contained within their dimensions.

parts, including the brain, spine, shoulders, head and neck, and hocks. These coils are made or adapted to each vendor's scanner and are not usually interchangeable because of the plug-in design for the coil, which is specific to each scanner. Typically, the smaller the coil, the better the image.

Use of surface coils depends on what needs to be seen. On a small dog brain scan, for example, one could use a chimney (human knee) coil because it may show a smaller field of view better than a human-sized head coil. Most superconductor magnets are designed for adult humans, and so other sites, including veterinary, may have to make their own adjustments as to which coils are used. They may also have to create their own specialized coils. Coils and MRI technology are constantly advancing. Now many coils have multiple channels and settings to decrease the time of the scan and to increase the signal obtained from the body part. One rule to keep in mind with MRI is that any coil within the active scanner must be plugged in. Coils that are on the table but unplugged during a scan can be damaged or could burn a patient.

Computers

MRI scanners require computers to perform the reconstructions of the radio signals into images. The computers also enable the technologist to photograph, network, and manipulate magnetic resonance images once formed. Unlike CT, no raw data can be kept or stored with MRI. The images are acquired in their chosen field of view (like CT), matrix, slice thickness, and other factors. One cannot go back after a 5-minute MRI scan and change the resolution of the images as one can in CT.

Physics and Technique

As stated earlier, an MRI scanner uses radio waves to manipulate hydrogen atoms in and out of an excited energy state.

The actual application of this technique is quite a bit more complicated, and whole books are written on the physics and progress of this technology.

The frequency used by MRI to produce images is based on a calculation called the *Larmor equation.* All atoms have the ability to respond to radio waves in a magnetic field. This ability is called the *gyromagnetic ratio.* The frequency applied in MRI is calculated by the following equation:

$$Wo = Y\ B^0$$

where:

Wo is the radio frequency

B^0 is the magnetic field (typically in field strength of tesla)

Y is the gyromagnetic ratio

Medical MRI focuses on hydrogen, which also has the highest gyromagnetic ratio. The ratio for hydrogen is 42.56 MHz · T^{-1} or MHz/T. In a typical medical MRI, the field strength is 1.5 T. Using the previous equation yields the typical frequency for medical MRI, as follows:

$$42.56\ \text{MHz/T} \times 1.5\ \text{T} = 63.8\ \text{MHz}$$

When this frequency is applied by the radio antenna in a medical 1.5-T MRI scanner, the hydrogen atoms respond (or resonate) into a higher energy level and change the direction of their magnetization in the scanner. When the radio frequency is stopped, the atoms return to their equilibrium or prior state within the magnet. Because the atoms were excited into a higher energy state, they give off energy as they return in the form of radio waves that are detected by the radio antenna. The actual change of magnetic direction of the atoms on the return gives off two types of signals. The first is called *T1 decay,* which is the direct magnetic movement of the center of the atom from its tipped position (90 degrees or whatever has been chosen) to its original state. The second is called *T2 decay,* the signal received from the spinning of the atom back into its original state. Tissues and molecules in the body have different responses with regard to T1 and T2 decay; this difference is what allows the MRI to show various tissues so well with all of the different settings.

The actual radio waves in these decayed signals are very small. During an MRI scan, the scanner applies the radio frequency in multiple pulses, which continue to "tip" the magnetic direction of the hydrogen molecules again and again. These repeated radio waves dramatically increase the radio signals received. One factor in an MRI technique is the time between the radio frequency pulses, which is referred to as *TR* or *repetition time.* A lower repetition time—699 milliseconds (ms) or less—shows the T1 decay response of the tissues. A higher repetition time—1500 ms or greater—shows the T2 decay response and changes the contrast of the images.

Another factor used in MRI is the echo time, or TE (in ms). This is the time between responses showing the maximum signal. As for TR, shorter TE times demonstrate the T1 response of tissues. Longer echo times show the T2 responses of tissues. MRI, like CT, shows images in slices. For an MRI, several slices are acquired in a single scan or sequence.

Signal Intensity and the Weighting of Images: T1 vs. T2

In MRI, the various shades of gray seen in an image are referred to as *signal intensities,* not densities. If a part of the image is shown as bright or closer to white, it is described as having a *high signal intensity.* The reverse is true for anatomy seen in darker shades of gray; they are called *low signal intensity.* When looking at images from an MRI, people also refer to the T1 or T2 appearance of the tissues as *weighting.*

The most typical comparison are tissues that have opposite weightings—water and fat.

In a true T1-weighted image (TR < 699 ms, TE < 30 ms), cerebrospinal fluid (CSF) looks black (low signal intensity) (Fig. 13.10A). Fat (and skin) look bright or white (high signal intensity). A true T2-weighted image (TR > 2000 ms, TE > 80 ms) shows CSF as bright white and skin as black (Fig. 13.10B).

Signal-to-Noise Ratio

Many factors beyond TR and TE can be altered in MRI. Many can affect the quality, the resolution, and the amount of time it takes to obtain images. Technologists must take all these factors into account when entering a protocol for an MRI sequence. The goal in acquiring MRI images is to have a high signal-to-noise ratio. The higher the amount of signal, the better the pictures. Table 13.1 lists the effects of altering

TABLE 13.1	Effects of Altering Technical Factors in MRI		
TECHNICAL FACTOR ALTERATION	**INCREASE OR DECREASE**	**EFFECT ON SIGNAL-TO-NOISE RATIO**	**EFFECT ON IMAGE RESOLUTION**
Field of view	Decrease	Decrease	Increase
Pixel size	Decrease	Decrease	Increase
Bandwidth	Increase	Increase	Decrease
Number of excitations or acquisitions	Increase	Increase	Increase
Slice thickness	Increase	Increase	Decrease
Image matrix size	Increase	Decrease	Increase

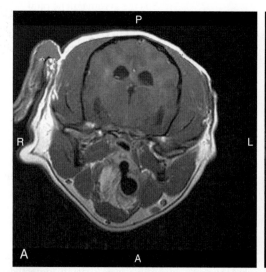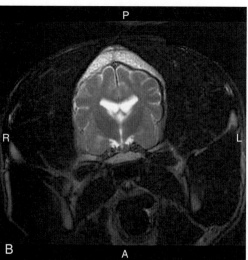

FIG. 13.10 Coronal plane images on magnetic resonance images of a dog's brain. **A,** A T1-weighted image. The cerebrospinal fluid in the ventricles is shown as black, and the skin and body fat are shown as white. **B,** A T2-weighted image. The T2 weighting can be identified from the longer TR and TE times listed, as well as from the facts that the fat either is not visible or is black and the ventricles are bright with high signal intensity.

individual technical factors in MRI in a classic spin-echo image (see later discussion of sequences).

In radiography, a technologist balances radiation dose and resolution or image noise. In MRI, the trade-off is between time and image resolution. A technologist may, for example, want thinner slices, which will drop the signal, and therefore may have to increase the number of excitations, which doubles the time of a sequence.

Specialty Sequences

In MRI, specialty sequences can be used to image various parts of the body. It is possible to image blood vessels by MRI without the use of a contrast agent. A couple of sequences are able to capture the phases of moving blood, for example. These specialty sequences are called *magnetic resonance angiography* or *magnetic resonance venography,* and they can show the anatomy of blood vessels. These volumetric sequences enable the anatomy to be reconstructed in three-dimensional images, which are typically called *maximum intensity projections* (Fig. 13.11). Also, the naming of sequences varies from vendor to vendor. Charts are now available that translate these names from machine to machine. For example, "turbo spin-echo sequence" on one scanner is the same as "fast spin-echo" on another. A three-dimensional T1-weighted volume acquisition scan can be called "MPRAGE" by one vendor, "3D SPGR" by another, and an "FFE, or fast field-echo," by a third. MRI technologists must constantly learn and upgrade their knowledge about the physics and techniques of their scanning.

Another aspect of MRI is the ability to suppress the fat signal. This is desired in places where the fat may alter the ability to see pathology, such as the orbits and in soft tissue structures. The expression for this is *fat saturation,* for which various MRI methods can be used.

Contrast and MRI

MRI does require the use of a contrast agent to highlight infection, tumors, or vascular disease. The contrast agent used in MRI is called *gadolinium* (Fig. 13.12); various chemical formulas include this molecule. Gadolinium is a paramagnetic—meaning that it has partially magnetic qualities. It alters the T1 properties of tissues so that they enhance, or light up, in the picture. After contrast is injected into the patient, only T1-weighted sequences (with or without fat saturation) will show the enhancement of tissues. Because gadolinium is removed by the kidneys, it is very important that a subject's kidney function is assessed before the MRI. In veterinary practice, because the patients are under general anesthesia when scanned, blood work assessing kidney function is always

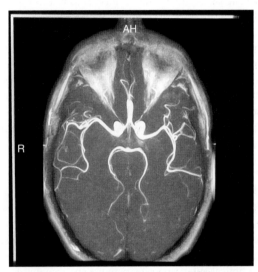

FIG. 13.11 A noncontrast magnetic resonance angiogram performed on a human patient. The vessels are visible as a function of the blood flow within them. It is reconstructed as a maximum intensity project (MIP) and viewed from inferior to superior view.

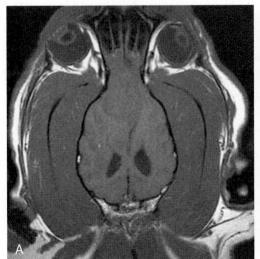
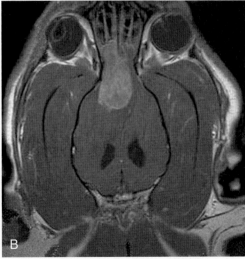

FIG. 13.12 The change in how a tumor is seen when gadolinium contrast is administered. **A,** The T1-weighted image without contrast. **B,** The T1-weighted image with contrast. Usually tissues enhance because the contrast decreases the T1 contrast of the pathology.

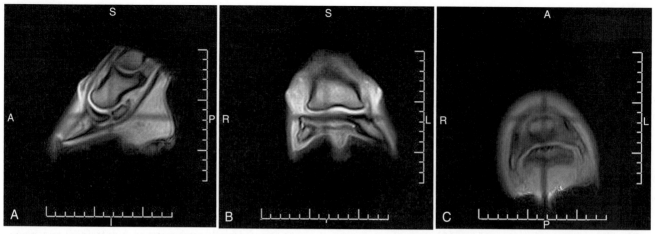

FIG. 13.13 Quick images in coronal **(A)**, sagittal **(B)**, and axial **(C)** planes showing the position of the horse's leg within the scanner.

performed with the preanaesthetic blood work. In humans, necrotizing systemic fasciitis, a very rare and irreversible complication, has occurred when gadolinium was given to patients with renal failure. In this condition, the skin and connective tissues permanently stiffen and retract, causing the patient to lose kidney function. For this reason, gadolinium is administered only to patients who have normal renal function.

Protocols

From this chapter, you have learned that there are many ways to scan a patient using MRI. Various surface coils and sequences can be used.

In a typical veterinary site, patients are accepted for MRI scans only when referred by specialists. The patient is prepared and evaluated before the MRI examination. These scans are not short in duration, with each sequence typically lasting around 5 minutes or so and an entire scan of body parts taking 20 minutes or longer. For this reason, patients are always anesthetized or sedated. The technologist or veterinarian chooses the most appropriately sized surface coils for the region to be covered. An MRI scan always starts with a low-quality, quick image called a *localizer*. The localizer allows the technologist to see the anatomy on MRI and to plan subsequent images. Most MRI sites have specific protocols for each body part, using multiple sequences in at least two planes (Fig. 13.13).

MRI has a great advantage over other modalities. It has excellent subject contrast, in that the soft tissues are better seen than even with CT. The images are also acquired in any plane or angle that the technologist may desire (see Figs. 13.13 to 13.16).

Further Safety Considerations

As described previously, MRI uses a high-field-strength magnet to produce images, so the safety of patients and staff is of

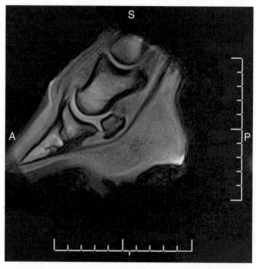

FIG. 13.14 A sagittal T1-weighted image of the horse's left forefoot. Several images in a plane were acquired in multiple settings.

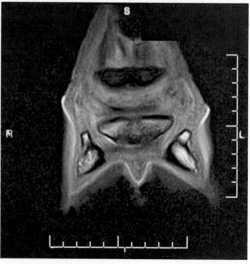

FIG. 13.15 Coronal T1-weighted image through a horse's forefoot.

utmost importance. As mentioned, the most dangerous aspect of MRI is the projectile effect, whereby an object launches into a magnet. Injuries and deaths have occurred from such accidents. MRI applies radio frequencies to the entire body of the patient. Implanted devices, such as pacemakers and certain aneurysm clips, cannot go near the magnetic field, which might cause them to move within the body. Another risk of implanted metal is heating, with possible burning of the patient. All implants must be screened for MRI safety with use of the written checklist or form given to anyone planning to enter the MRI room. Owners of animals must complete a form ascertaining that the animal has not had surgery involving metal clips and has not been shot with pellet guns, etc.

Another safety concern in MRI is the ability of the patient's body to dissipate heat from the interaction of the magnet and radio frequencies. Specific absorption rate (SAR) is a calculation made on the basis of the mass of the patient. Every written scan sequence in MRI lists the potential SAR value for the patient. This is much more significant in higher-field-strength magnets (>3 T) than with the weaker ones. MRI machines are also acoustically very noisy. Many MRI scans produce noise in excess of 60 to 90 decibels (dB). Ear shielding (ear plugs or head phones) is necessary for patients and anyone staying in the MRI room during a scan.

The static MRI field is not considered a risk for pregnant personnel. However, a pregnant woman should not remain in the room while a scanner is in use.

Further policies should be made within MRI departments in planning for emergencies. For situations such as fire, magnet quench, flood, and cardiac arrest, normal screening procedures cannot apply because it is impossible to rapidly screen everyone and every object entering the room to deal with an emergency.

Summary

Magnetic resonance imaging uses a very strong magnet and radio waves to create images. It has superior subject contrast because it demonstrates the molecular makeup of tissues. It is the best modality to image the brain, spinal cord, and other soft tissue structures such as joints. MRI should be performed only by trained individuals. For further reading, consult the Bibliography at the end of this chapter.

Image Gallery

Figs. 13.17 to 13.26 demonstrate use of the invaluable tool of magnetic resonance imaging. **Please note:** These reports are given according to the entire scan, not just the images presented here. Some of the components would be viewed on adjacent scans within the procedure.

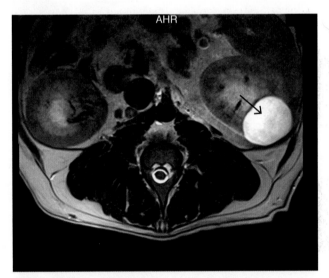

FIG. 13.17 Incidental finding, right kidney cyst *(arrow)*. A 2.8-cm multilobulated cyst is present in the craniolateral aspect of the left kidney, without evidence of other renal anomaly. (Patient was being examined due to ataxic hind end.)

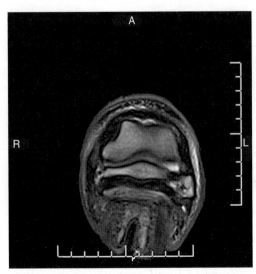

FIG. 13.16 Axial T2-weighted image taken through the horse's forefoot. These images were acquired with the MRI unit shown in Fig. 13.7.

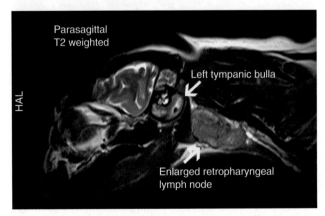

FIG. 13.18 Skull and cervical spine. An aggressive soft tissue process that invades the left tympanic bulla and caudoventral portion of the left occipital bone, with regional fat alteration and severe ipsilateral retropharyngeal lymphadenopathy.

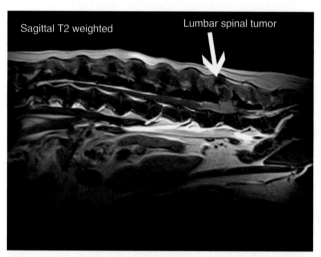

FIG. 13.19 T2-weighted lumbar spinal tumor. Lobulated soft tissue mass infiltrating L6 and compressing the nerves of the cauda equina, with characteristics consistent with an aggressive neoplastic process.

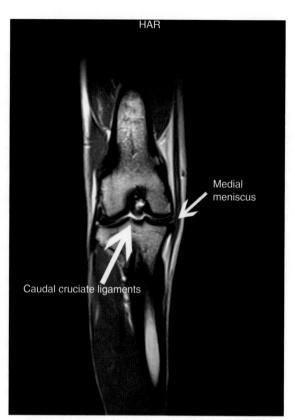

FIG. 13.20 Right stifle. Minimal synovial fluid in both stifles, but without evidence of effusion. All soft tissue components, including the cranial and caudal cruciate ligaments, collateral ligaments, and menisci, appear intact.

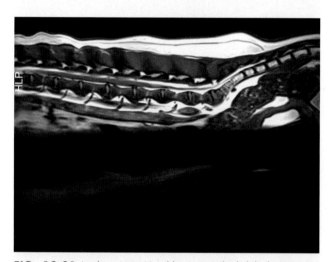

FIG. 13.21 Lumbar spine. Variable intervertebral disk degeneration throughout the spine in association with variable spondylosis deformans and endplate sclerosis.

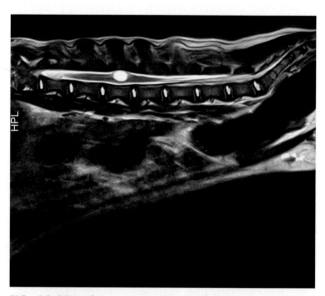

FIG. 13.22 Lumbar spine cyst at L3. Cystlike lesion in the middorsal portion of the spinal cord at L3 that may communicate with the central canal and that is likely congenital in origin. (The dog is 4 months old.)

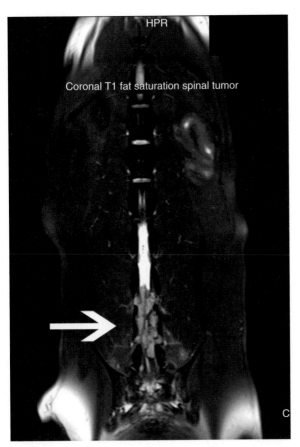

FIG. 13.23 Coronal view, spinal tumor. Coronal view T1 fat saturation demonstrating a tumor at the caudal level of the lumbar spine.

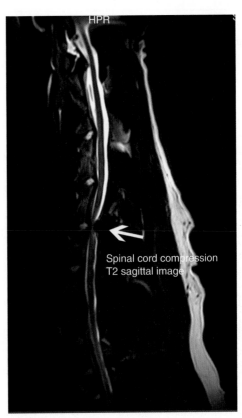

FIG. 13.24 T2 spinal cord compression, sagittal view, T2 weighted demonstrating cord compression.

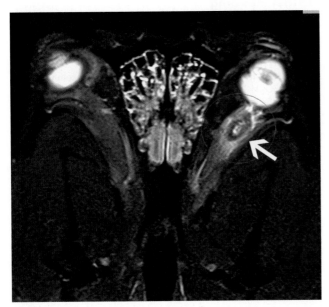

FIG. 13.25 Coronal right posterior orbit, porcupine quill. Left retroorbital soft tissue swelling with signs consistent with a migrating porcupine quill, with mild to moderate local pyogranulomatous infection.

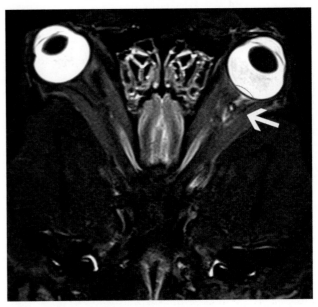

FIG. 13.26 Second view, coronal right posterior orbit. Same patient as in Fig. 13.25, but different level.

REVIEW QUESTIONS

1. What part of the MRI machine is considered the most dangerous to anyone walking into the room?
   a. The radio antenna
   b. The magnet
   c. The shim coils
   d. The surface coils

2. What must be done for every person or patient entering into an MRI room?
   a. A screening form must be filled out to check for implants or operations.
   b. All loose metallic objects need to be removed.
   c. Pregnant workers cannot enter.
   d. a and b

3. What purpose are the magnetic shims in an MRI?
   a. They are used to create the images.
   b. They are used to make the field within the magnet homogenous.
   c. They are used to produce the images.
   d. They are used to create the radio waves.

4. What is a T1-weighted magnetic resonance image?
   a. An MR image on which fat appears black
   b. An image on which CSF appears white
   c. An image for which TR is 2000
   d. An image on which fat appears white

5. What method of reconstruction is used for magnetic resonance images?
   a. Filtered back-projection
   b. Back-projection
   c. Two-dimensional Fourier transformation
   d. Three-dimensional Fourier transformation

6. What happens to atoms when they are placed in a magnet?
   a. They start to spin or precess.
   b. They move randomly.
   c. They reposition themselves with regard to their magnetic polarity.
   d. They shift to the north pole of the magnet.

7. A superconductor magnet is filled with which substance?
   a. Hydrogen
   b. Helium
   c. Carbon
   d. Liquid helium

8. Which part of an MRI scanner obtains better images of smaller body parts?
   a. Gradient coils
   b. Shims
   c. Body coil
   d. Surface coils

9. Why is the word *resonance* used in the term MRI?
   a. It uses radio waves and they are musical.
   b. It is the manner in which the atom's magnetic fields respond to a radio frequency.
   c. Resonance comes from the term used in spectroscopy.
   d. The atoms resonate to all of the radio waves.

10. For which atoms are MRI radio frequencies tuned to in order to create images?
    a. Hydrogen
    b. Carbon
    c. Oxygen
    d. Helium

11. What does "high signal intensity" mean in a magnetic resonance image?
    a. A high concentration of helium atoms is responding to the radio waves.
    b. More signal has been received from a tissue in an image with a given weighting.
    c. In a T2 image, the fat will show this.
    f. This refers to the dark part of an image.

Answers to Review Questions can be found on the Evolve website.

Further Reading

Hesselink JR: Basic principles of MR imaging. http://spinwarp.ucsd.edu/NeuroWeb/Text/br-100.htm.

MRI Glossary. FONAR Corporation; 2003. http://www.fonar.com/glossary.htm.

MRI-Technology Information Portal. http://www.mr-tip.com/serv1.php.

Shellock FG: MRI safety.com. http://mrisafety.com.

Westbrook C, Roth CK, Talbot J. *MRI in Practice*. 4th ed. Hoboken, NJ: Wiley-Blackwell; 2011.

CHAPTER 14

Nuclear Medicine and Introduction to Positron Emission Tomography

Lois C. Brown, RTR (Can/USA), ACR, MSc., P.Phys; Darryl Bonder, DVM; and Stephanie Holowka, MRT(R), MRT(MR), MRSO(MRSC™)

To raise new questions, new possibilities, to regard old problems from a new angle, requires creative imagination and marks real advance in science.
—Albert Einstein, German-born theoretical physicist, 1879–1955

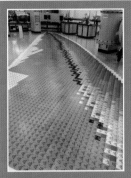

A unique linoleum incorporating a chart of the nuclides at a research laboratory at the University of Ottawa, Ontario, Canada. All known elements and their isotopes are listed on this tableau.

OUTLINE

LEARNING OBJECTIVES

When you have finished this chapter, you will be able to:

1. Understand the science of nuclear scintigraphy.
2. Know the etiology that indicates scintigraphy.
3. Define the term *isotope* and its use in nuclear scintigraphy.
4. Know the protocol for equine studies.
5. List the use of other isotopes for small animal studies.
6. Understand radiation protection in nuclear medicine.

APPLICATIONS

The application of the information in this chapter is relevant to the following area:

1. Diagnosis of skeletal trauma and pathology using an auxiliary diagnostic approach.

KEY TERMS

Key terms are defined in the Glossary on the Evolve website.

Annihilation
Attenuate
Attenuation profile
Cyclotron
Fludeoxyglucose

Half-life
Isotope
Millicuries
Nuclear scintigraphy
Osteoblastic activity

Photon
Positron
Positron emission tomography
Radioactive decay

Radioactive disintegration
Radioisotopes
Radionuclides
Scintigraphy

Nuclear Medicine

In the first section of this book, we spoke of the atom, the elements, and isotopes. A quick review is in order here because it is these isotopes that are used extensively in nuclear scintigraphy.

The Atom and Radioactivity

Each atom consists of three basic components: the electrons, which we manipulate in radiography; and protons and neutrons, which are contained in the nucleus. It is the neutrons that we will discuss now.

A stable atom such as helium, the second atom in the periodic table, has two protons, two neutrons, and two electrons. The protons determine the characteristic of the element. If the number of neutrons differs in a substance, it is an isotope of the element. Barium, a contrast medium with which we will are familiar, has seven naturally occurring isotopes.

> **? POINTS TO PONDER**
>
> Atoms that have the same atomic number but different atomic mass numbers are isotopes. Isotopes can occur naturally but also may be artificially produced in a laboratory.

Radioactivity describes atoms that are in an abnormally excited state characterized by an unstable nucleus. To reach stability, these atoms spontaneously emit particles and energy to transform themselves into other atoms. This process is called *radioactive disintegration* or *radioactive decay*. The method of determining the activity of a radioisotope involves establishing how long it takes for the isotope to decay to half of its original radioactivity. This is called its *half-life*. The atoms involved in this process are called *radionuclides*. An atom with any rearrangement of the nucleus is called a *nuclide;* therefore the atoms with nuclei that undergo radioactive decay are radionuclides.

In the 1940s and 1950s, a scientific branch of imaging was developed to examine radionuclides with respect to medical diagnosis. It was already known that infection produces heat, tumors attract cellular activity, and trauma causes an increase in blood supply around the wounded area. It was speculated that if a radioactive source was introduced within the patient either by swallowing or by injection, that source would gravitate to the area supplied by the most blood or with the highest cellular activity. The radiation emitted as the radionuclide decayed could then be imaged on a detection device that was connected to a camera. The substance ingested or injected must be nontoxic, other than the amount of radiation introduced, and it had to be capable of being excreted through the urine or via the bowels.

One other criterion that was very important to this study was the half-life of the radionuclide. The half-life is described as the length of time necessary to reduce the intensity of the radiation emitted by half. In medicine it is important that a radionuclide administered to a person or animal must decay within a relatively short period so that the patient is not a radiation hazard to itself or to people working in the area.

The Isotopes

Small Animals

The most common radionuclides used in veterinary medicine today are iodine-131 and technetium-99m. Iodine-131 is mainly used to treat hyperthyroidism in felines and is not normally used for imaging.

Although it has been around for more than 50 years, nuclear scintigraphy is still relatively unused in small animal veterinary medicine. The reason is because it uses radionuclides, which are both expensive and heavily regulated. In addition, the images derived from the studies are physiological in nature and therefore quite unfamiliar to most veterinarians. The heavy regulations and the high cost of the nuclides is also combined with the boarding and caring for animals while they are tested as the half-life of the nuclides disperse to a low enough level that they are not a risk to their owners and handlers. The other half of that equation then means that there are limited schools and courses for veterinarians to learn how to read the images produced by the cameras.

Large Animals

Technetium-99m is used for nuclear scintigraphy, particularly in equine studies. The quantity identifier for the radiation emitted by the isotopes is the curie (Ci), named after Marie and Pierre Curie, a husband-and-wife team who did very early research into radiation. The amount of radioisotope used for each examination is measured in millicuries (mCi).

The hospital or clinic that uses radioisotopes must be registered with the local atomic energy board. In Canada, it is the Canadian Nuclear Safety Commission (nuclearsafety. gc.ca). In the United States, it is the U.S. Nuclear Regulatory Commission (www.nrc.gov). Internationally, it is the International Atomic Energy Agency (www.iaea.org) that provides information regarding the regulations for various countries.

The Science of Nuclear Medicine

Nuclear scintigraphy is the science of diagnosis by means of radioisotopes. The patient is injected with or ingests a radionuclide, and the nuclear medicine camera detects the emission of the radioactivity from the patient.

Nuclear medicine is a very effective way to localize pathology or the results of trauma because the radioisotope is carried to the area with the most active blood supply. Certain isotopes are more readily attracted to certain types of tissue. Technetium-99m is attracted to bone. Iodine-131 is attracted to the thyroid gland.

Indications for Imaging With Nuclear Medicine

A subtle, severe, or multifocal lameness in horses may be very difficult to diagnose (Fig. 14.1). When radiography does not demonstrate the abnormality, a very effective option is a nuclear scan. Bone scans can also be used to monitor the healing process of fractures. In addition, they are significant tools in a prepurchase examination of a horse.

In the equine patient, some of the areas of concern are quite large and difficult to image via the traditional methods of imaging—computerized tomography (CT), magnetic resonance imaging (MRI), and radiography. Nuclear medicine scanning can rule out abnormalities in these areas or identify pathology or the evidence of trauma. The animal does not have to be anesthetized to undergo the study.

Procedure

The horse is injected with 160 to 180 mCi technetium-99m, which has an affinity for localization in bone. After a certain period, the horse is brought to the camera, which is very large and has a room of its own (Fig. 14.2). The horse's body is brought within the field of range of the camera, which detects the emission of radiation known as *gamma photon bursts* from the horse and records the activity on a computer. The camera is moved around by a gantry system.

An area of osteoblastic activity indicates accelerated metabolism within the bones, which will result in an indication of higher radiation emitted. It is termed a *hot spot.*

Phases of a Bone Scan

The vascular phase is not commonly used in horses unless a thrombosis is suspected. In this phase, the camera is positioned over the horse while the isotope is being injected. The course of the isotope can then be traced as it moves through the circulatory system. The radionuclide is spread fairly thin at this phase.

The soft tissue phase (Fig. 14.3) occurs approximately 5 to 10 minutes after injection. It detects the pooling of the nuclide and demonstrates tendons and ligaments in the equine lower limb.

The bone phase is the final phase as the nuclide is distributed throughout the bone (Fig. 14.4). This phase is usually performed 2 to 3 hours after the injection to ensure that the maximum amount of nuclide has gathered at the point of interest.

For the safety of the handlers regarding radiation exposure, the horse is then hospitalized for 48 hours in order for the isotope to decay. The half-life of technetium-99m is about 6

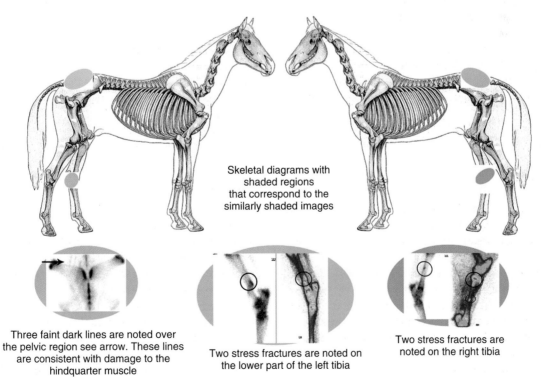

Skeletal diagrams with shaded regions that correspond to the similarly shaded images

Three faint dark lines are noted over the pelvic region see arrow. These lines are consistent with damage to the hindquarter muscle

Two stress fractures are noted on the lower part of the left tibia

Two stress fractures are noted on the right tibia

FIG. 14.1 A case of multifocal lameness. This young horse had a history of being "off" in the hind end. Nuclear medicine studies revealed four stress fractures (two right and two left hind) and muscle damage over the hindquarters (arrow).

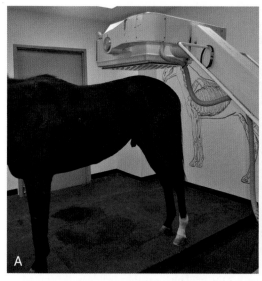
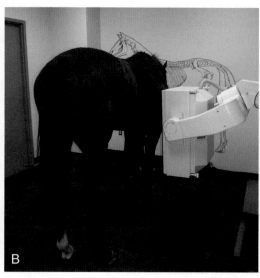
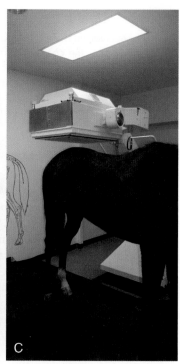

FIG. 14.2 A, B, and C, A horse stands quietly while the gantry is moved into various positions.

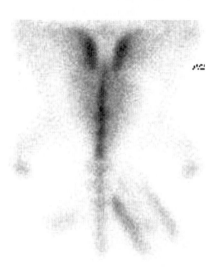

FIG. 14.3 Exertional rhabdomyolysis. An example of posttraumatic injury demonstrated in the soft tissue phase.

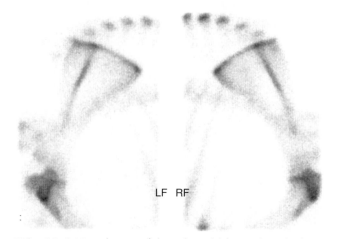

FIG. 14.4 Normal scans of the right and left scapulae. The bone phase of the scan reveals a normal set of scapulae in this case.

hours, and it must go through several half-lives before the animal can be safely handled and sent home.

The Images

Because the images are demonstrating function and not anatomy, they are plotted out on the computer as a series of dots. These dots indicate radioactive bursts emitted from the horse. The structure of the anatomy is visualized so that the area of interest is easily identified. Newer cameras count the radiation bursts and display the results in color. The color red (hot) indicates high activity, and blue (cool) indicates low activity (Fig. 14.5).

The following sections demonstrate normal and abnormal bone activity in horses and are identified as such.

Diagnosis

The veterinarian reading the scan compares the images from the left and right sides of the horse in order to make a diagnosis. Some areas of high activity are normal for certain breeds. Certain areas in young horses (the epiphyseal growth plates) should be highly active, and this is one reason why comparisons are essential. If one growth plate is not as active as the other, this finding could be a cause for concern (Figs. 14.6 and 14.7).

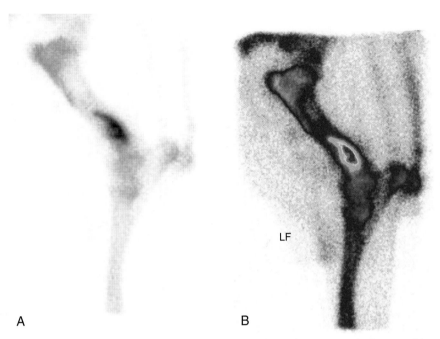

FIG. 14.5 A left humerus fracture **(A)** becomes more evident when color represents the location of the injury **(B)**.

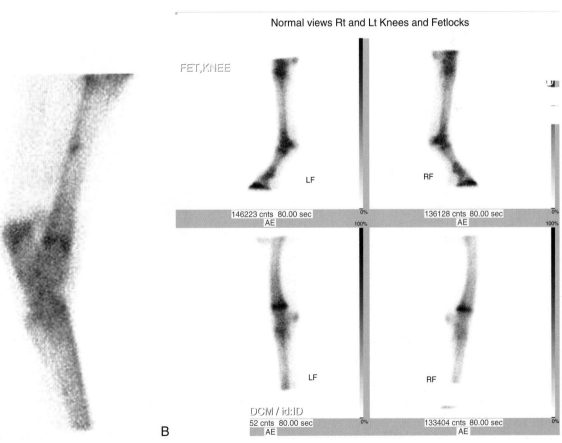

FIG. 14.6 A, Right tibial stress fracture. The heightened activity in this scan demonstrates a fracture, whereas absence of activity could signify tissue necrosis. **B,** Comparison views of right and left knees, fetlocks, and tibiae.

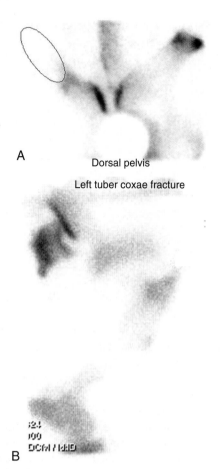

A

Dorsal pelvis

Left tuber coxae fracture

B

FIG. 14.7 A particularly serious fracture of the pelvis. This horse was discovered in the stall in the morning refusing to bear weight on the left hind leg. **A,** The oval area indicates the portion of the pelvis that is missing. **B,** The lateral view shows a tuber coxae fracture with displacement.

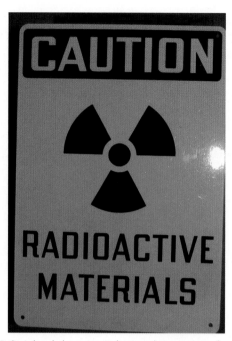

FIG. 14.8 A legal door sign indicating the presence of radioactive sources. In some countries the sign would read "Danger–RadioHazard Materials."

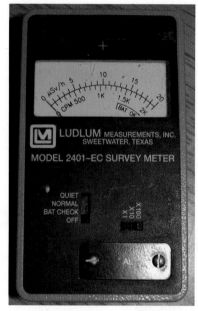

FIG. 14.9 A radiation dosimeter. The horse is kept at the facility until the dose count on this dosimeter is below 4 microsieverts/hour. Usually the count is less than 1 after 48 hours.

Radiation Protection

Nuclear medicine studies take place only in an approved site where radiation safety is ensured (Fig. 14.8). The patient is the radiation emitter, and the half-life of the radioisotope must be taken into consideration when patient care and length of stay are issues. The half-life of technetium-99m is 6 hours, which means that if you start with 160 mci at the time of injection, only 80 mci will be present 6 hours after the injection, and 40 mci would be present 12 hours after the injection. The typical equine protocol is to retain the horse at the hospital or clinic for a minimum of 24 hours or, more typically, for 48 hours.

When the radioisotope has been injected into the horse, its body and its waste products are radioactive. The waste products must be retained in a lead-lined container in a designated area for 48 hours. The staff handling the horses must wear laboratory coats, latex gloves, disposable boots, and dosimeters because of the risk of effluent contamination. The scan room and the camera should be scanned with a survey meter (Fig. 14.9) before each examination to ensure that there is no contamination between examinations. The room is scanned at the start of the examination with a Geiger counter to establish a baseline. Fluorescent lights and concrete may emit a certain amount of radiation, which will be included in the count of a sensitive gamma camera (Fig. 14.10).

Summary of Nuclear Medicine

From the very early days of searching for a method to evaluate areas of heightened activity within the anatomy of their patients, scientists can now not only search the form of the pathology but also evaluate the function. This ability is

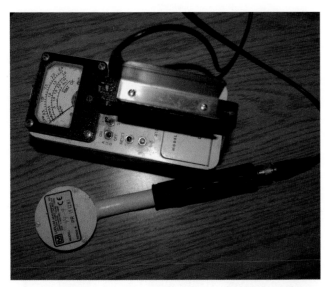

FIG. 14.10 A Geiger counter is set to measure in kilocounts/minute (Kc/min).

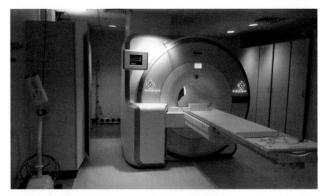

FIG. 14.11 MR/PET scanner built by Siemens Electric Company. The two gantries are positioned one behind the other so that there is no interruption in the flow of the examination.

particularly valuable in equine studies, in which often the structures are so large that routine radiographs do not demonstrate the extent of trauma and pathology.

We can now move to small-animal imaging in a nuclear medicine field using the positrons emitted by a nuclide and combining them with either CT or MRI.

Positron Emission Tomography— Hybrid Imaging PET/CT, PET/MR

Introduction to PET

Imaging is a rapidly advancing field staffed by the curious: If this works, what if I combine it with this? Such is the case with nuclear medicine. An imaging system that demonstrates function but not form needs to be paired with an imaging system (or systems) that demonstrate form but not function. Now you have the best of both worlds. So nuclear medicine in the form of positron emission tomography (PET) is now paired with MRI, and in another facility it is paired with CT.

We have presented this science in this text as an introduction to the future of imaging. These units are available today to the veterinary market and are at times shared with the medical market in the interests of costs and efficiency. It is beneficial to the veterinary community to understand superficially how these modalities function and how they can be of use to the patients. Fig. 14.11 is an illustration of a Siemens Electric Company PET/MR unit. This unit is used by human patients during the weekdays and by veterinary patients evenings and weekends.

Principles of PET

PET (or PET scan) is an imaging modality that is a form of nuclear medicine technology. PET has been available since the 1970s and has become a hybrid technology that is normally combined with either CT or MRI.

PET uses the injection of a radioisotope that emits gamma rays (Fig. 14.12). The PET unit consists of a series of scintillating sensors (like nuclear medicine cameras) arranged in a ring, and this allows for the images to be acquired and then reconstructed like slices in a loaf of bread.

The most common isotope used is fludeoxyglucose (FDG), and it is used both for the mapping of brain function and for the mapping of malignant tumors. It is the glucose in FDG that is metabolized in active brain tissue and cancerous tumors, appearing as "hot spots" or places of increased activity on a PET scan. FDG and other PET isotopes must be produced with a device called a *cyclotron*. The FDG isotope has a fairly short half-life of 110 minutes, which means that the place of its production must be located near the scanner. When an examination is scheduled, the isotope must be ordered and then delivered quickly.

Other isotopes can be used for PET studies, such as ammonia (for heart imaging). The reactions are the same as those in nuclear medicine; photons or beta decay with a predictable energy—511 keV. The positrons collide with electrons in the body, where they annihilate into two gamma photons that move 180 degrees from another.

The PET scanners are designed to both detect photons and calculate their origin (in space and time) within the body. In PET imaging, the scintillation chambers (like gamma cameras) are arranged in multiple rows on a ring, and the table moves following the imaging of each slice. As with nuclear medicine, the photons are a form of radiation similar to x-rays with regard to body tissues. They can be attenuated or absorbed differently by various body tissues, especially bone.

In the original design of a PET machine, a special scan is performed using germanium to predict the absorption of the gamma ray photons. The data collected are then used to calculate an absorption correction (attenuation profile), which would take into account various anatomical structures. A PET scan is then performed, and the computer of the scanner calculates the images using the attenuation profile it created on that specific patient. During both scans and in between,

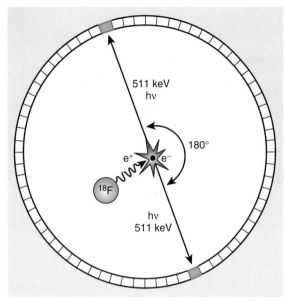

FIG. 14.12 The production of positrons from the nucleus. When positrons join with electrons, they break apart in a fixed pattern. This is called *annihilation*. They break apart into two photons that move 180 degrees away from each other. The PET unit is computed to detect where the particle originated and the timing of the annihilation. (From Hoppe R, Phillips T, Roach M. *Liebel and Phillips Textbook of Radiation Oncology*, 3rd ed. Philadelphia: Saunders; 2010.)

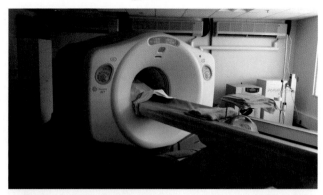

FIG. 14.13 CT/PET scanner by General Electric Company.

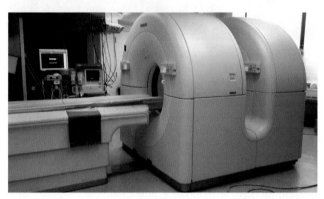

FIG. 14.14 CT/PET scanner by Philips. Here the two units are clearly visible.

the patient must remain very still. The attenuation profile allows the images to more accurately show the slice-by-slice metabolism of the FDG isotope.

The slice data collected from PET scanners tend to be high in spatial resolution, 5 to 10 mm thick—much more accurate than a similar nuclear medicine scan.

How Did PET Become a Hybrid Technology?

One of the disadvantages of PET is that it produces images that look similar to those of nuclear medicine. Brain images show the uptake of the positron isotope (specifically glucose), but show very little recognizable anatomy. Combining PET with CT accomplishes two aspects of the scans: 1) the x-ray radiation used in the CT scan has similar penetrating abilities to that of the produced photons; therefore it can be used to create the attenuation profile; and 2) CT scans provide more anatomical information for the body part being imaged. The CT scans or PET/CT scans can also be fused together to correlate functional data with anatomical data (form and function in one image).

Several designs of CT/PET scanners have been created, but all machines feature a CT scanner, which can be used on its own, and a PET scanner, which is used in combination with the CT. For some vendors, the gantry is in one piece and appears like a CT scanner with a longer tunnel (Fig. 14.13), and in another one the two units are separated and can be moved apart (Fig. 14.14). The gantries on CT/PET

machines are not able to be angled, unlike a regular CT scanner. Still, the CT scanner does function much like a clinical multislice CT scanner and so clinics and hospitals are able to use the machine for regular CT work in between PET studies.

PET/CT Studies

A PET/CT study starts with the injection of the isotope about 45 minutes before moving the patient onto the scanner. Because the FDG isotope may be taken up by active muscles, animals may be anesthetized so that they keep still. This ensures no false uptake occurs. The first part of the study is performed on the CT scan. The patient is positioned in a dorsoventral or ventrodorsal position. Intravenous contrast for the CT scan (for cancer detection) may be given. The anatomical images are now acquired. The computer is able to extract the density information from the CT detectors to create the attenuation profile for the PET study. The CT scan part takes less than a minute. Depending on the anatomy being imaged, the PET study can take from 20 to 40 minutes. The PET study can be seen both in its original state and then corrected by the attenuation profile. Ultimately they can be fused against the CT scan images and show both comparable anatomical and functional data.

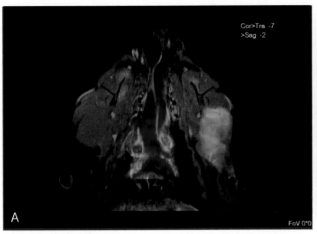
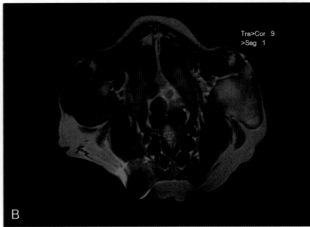

FIG. 14.15 A and B, Patient views from an MRI/PET scanner showing the degree of pathology in the left side of the skull.

PET/MR Studies

MRI is the best modality to show soft tissues. Now, hybrid machines are able to provide both MRI and PET scans in the same examination (Fig. 14.15).

The MRI/PET machine looks much like a regular MRI except that the tunnel or gantry is longer. The PET part is behind the MRI. The MRI will work much like a regular MRI scanner. Specialized surface coils have been created to work in MRI but not attenuate the gamma radiation used in PET. The patient is imaged with the MRI first. For the PET portion of the scan, some machines have to be told which body part is imaged on the MRI, and the attenuation profile is calculated from that site's images. The PET scan is acquired in a set volume of slices from body section to body section and then merged with the MRI. The veterinarians can look at both the high-resolution MRI anatomy and the PET images—either fused together or separately— to see where the glucose is being metabolized. The main advantage of this type of hybrid imaging is that a lump of tissue may be seen as cancerous or as active disease.

Summary

The images here show that technology moves forward each year to more and more interesting imaging solutions. The veterinary community is moving rapidly with it. CT/PET and MR/PET are two new modalities that we can safely offer clients with a view to capturing an obscure diagnosis.

REVIEW QUESTIONS

1. The science of nuclear medicine uses:
   a. Isobars, which are emitted from technetium
   b. Isotopes, which are not radioactive
   c. Radiation to activate technetium
   d. Radioisotopes to image structures

2. The camera in nuclear medicine is used to:
   a. Help the technician obtain good pictures
   b. Detect any background radiation
   c. Detect the emissions of the isotope technetium
   d. Promote the use of the isotope

3. The isotope that is most highly attracted to bone is:
   a. Iodine-131
   b. Technetium-99m
   c. Technetium-131
   d. Uranium-133

4. During the procedure, the equine patient:
   a. Is heavily sedated and usually does not react to the substance
   b. Is moved into several positions around the camera
   c. Stands and waits until a burst of radioactive activity is complete
   d. Stands quietly while its body emits radioactive signals

5. The camera used in nuclear medicine:
   a. Is actually a gamma detector that collects bursts of activity
   b. Records the patient's internal movements as the isotope detects a signal
   c. Records the radioisotope as it collects in the area of interest
   d. Senses the radioactivity and reacts to it with light bursts

6. Once the horse has been injected with the isotope:
   a. It is then radioactive and needs special handling
   b. It is then radioactive but no protection is necessary
   c. The radioisotope emits just enough for the camera to detect
   d. The radioisotope is not very strong so it does not emit anything

7. The diagnosis from the images is made on the basis of:
   a. All the information from the chart and the monitor
   b. The camera images and the half-life of the isotope
   c. The collection of radioactive bursts by the camera
   d. The high-resolution images from the camera

8. After the examination, the patient must:
   a. Be isolated for at least 24 hours in order to allow the radioisotope to decay
   b. Be isolated for an hour and then sent home with special instructions
   c. Not be handled or fed until the radioisotope's half-life decays and it is safe to go home
   d. Not be ridden for at least 24 hours, until a diagnosis is made
9. Positron emission technology uses radioisotopes that must be created with a machine called a:
   a. Reactor
   b. Cyclotron
   c. Camera
   d. Scintillator

10. The process by which photons are created by positrons colliding with electrons is called:
    a. Decay
    b. Bremsstrahlung
    c. Annihilation
    d. Fusion
11. What calculation is used to compensate for the differences in absorption of gamma photons by various tissues?
    a. Attenuation profile
    b. Attenuation coefficient
    c. Absorption coefficient
    d. Interpolation

Answers to Review Questions can be found on the Evolve website.

PART TWO

Radiographic Positioning and Related Anatomy

In the positioning chapters the following will be stressed:

Describe the proper radiographic positioning techniques for all anatomic areas of small, large, and exotic animals so that for each position you are able to demonstrate:

- The normal views and protocol
- Where you measure
- Where you center the beam
- The collimation and the peripheral boundaries
- How you ensure that the patient is properly positioned
- Important concerns, idiosyncrasies, and anatomy

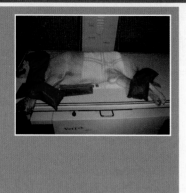

CHAPTER 15
Overview of Positioning

Marg Brown, RVT, BEd Ad Ed

*In the end we will conserve only what we love; we will love only what we understand;
and we will understand only what we have been taught.*

—Baba Dioum, Senegalese poet and environmentalist, b. 1937

OUTLINE

LEARNING OBJECTIVES

When you have finished this chapter, you will be able to:

1. Understand the proper anatomical positioning terminology used in veterinary radiography.
2. Indicate the common rules for radiographic projections that are used when identifying and radiographing animals.
3. Apply the various principles of nonmanual restraint and animal handling so that the patient does not need to be manually restrained when being radiographed.
4. Demonstrate radiation and patient safety procedures that should always be followed when any radiograph is taken.
5. Describe patient preparation that should be completed before radiographic exposure.
6. Describe the advantages and disadvantages of the various positioning aids available.
7. Understand the required views.
8. List positioning guidelines to ensure production of high-quality diagnostic images.
9. Explain how the three important principles of radiation safety are used to protect the radiographer.
10. Describe when and how cassette masks should be used in film/cassette imaging.
11. Understand the importance of collimation, particularly with the digital image.
12. Describe important issues for labeling and identifying an image.
13. Correctly display radiographs on a monitor or illuminator.
14. Determine whether a radiograph is diagnostic using a checklist.

KEY TERMS

Key terms are defined in the Glossary on the Evolve website.

Caudal (Cd)	Dorsopalmar (DPa)	Palmar (Pa)	Sagittal plane
Caudocranial (CdCr)	Dorsoplantar (DPl)	Palmarodorsal (PaD)	Skyline
Cranial (Cr)	Dose creep	Plantar (Pl)	Transverse plane
Craniocaudal (CrCd)	Lateral (L)	Plantarodorsal (PlD)	Ventral (V)
Distal (Di)	Lateromedial (LaM)	Proximal (Pr)	
Dorsal (D)	Medial (M)	Recumbent	
Dorsal plane	Oblique (O)	Rostral (R)	

TECHNICAL NOTE: To preserve space, the radiographs presented in this chapter do not show collimation. For safety, you should always collimate so that the beam is limited to within the image receptor edges. In film radiography, you should see a clear border of collimation (frame) on every radiograph. In some jurisdictions, evidence of collimation is required by law.

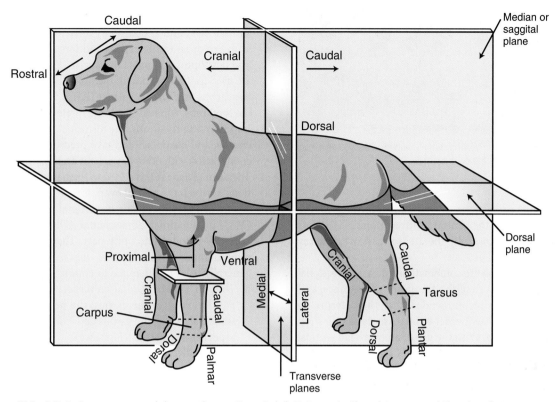

FIG. 15.1 Correct anatomical directional terms. (From Colville T, Bassert J. *Clinical Anatomy and Physiology for Veterinary Technicians*, 3rd ed. St Louis: Elsevier; 2016.)

art Two of this text educates the radiographer on how to properly position animals, with a focus on nonmanual restraint. In no other diagnostic imaging field is the patient held by the radiographer. Often patients in veterinary medicine are held while exposures are made, thereby needlessly exposing personnel to harmful radiation. With simple tools and common sense, most exposures can be completed without exposing the radiographer to direct or secondary radiation.

If proper positioning is to occur with nonmanual restraint, the patient should be immobilized by chemical restraint (sedation or general anesthesia) and/or positional devices. Please refer to a good anesthetic text for possible chemical agents. Overt manual restraint should be minimized. Even if chemical restraint is contraindicated, common behavior, restraint, and positioning principles can be applied to minimize radiographer exposure. The welfare of both the patient and the radiographer should be kept in mind during the production of accurate diagnostic radiographs.

If manual restraint is necessary, the radiographer must take all available precautions to minimize being exposed to ionizing radiation. All personnel in the radiographic suite during exposure must be shielded properly with the appropriate leaded apparel. (See Chapter 3 for proper manual restraint and shielding guidelines.) As is also stressed in the chapter on safety, judicious adherence to distance, protection, and exposure time will help minimize radiation exposure to the restrainer. A familiarity with the normal anatomy of the species and the proper terminology is essential. A basic

BOX 15.1	Positional Terminology
Dorsal (D)	Caudal (Cd)
Ventral (V)	Rostral (R)
Lateral (L)	Palmar (Pa, P)
Medial (M)	Plantar (Pl, P)
Left (L/Le)	Oblique (O)
Right (R/Rt)	Distal (Di)
Cranial (Cr)	Proximal (Pr)

understanding of what is normal assists in producing diagnostic radiographs for accurate interpretation and diagnosis by the veterinarian.

Positional Terminology

It is important to understand the correct terminology. Most associations still use the *Nomina Anatomica Veterinaria* as the point of reference. The American College of Veterinary Radiology (ACVR) terms are also shown in Fig. 15.1. The basic terms used are listed in Box 15.1.

Rules of Positioning

There are a few rules to keep in mind based on ACVR (see Fig. 15.1):

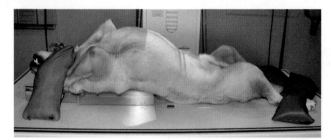

FIG. 15.2 Patient lying in ventrodorsal recumbency. The beam enters the abdomen and exits out the back or spine.

1. Radiographic projections are named according to the direction in which the central beam anatomically enters the body part, followed by the area of exit of the x-ray beam.
2. Many projections require combinations of basic directional terms to accurately describe the point of entrance and point of exit. It is recommended that these terms be combined in a consistent order to increase standardization of the nomenclature. With the use of an overhead vertical beam, the position in which a patient lying on its:
   a. Back (dorsal recumbency), is called *ventrodorsal (VD)*. The beam goes in the ventral (V) portion—the abdomen—and exits out the dorsal (D) aspect, or the patient's spine (Fig. 15.2).
   b. Abdomen (ventral recumbency), is called *dorsoventral (DV)*. The beam goes in the *dorsal (D)* portion—the spine—and exits out the *ventral (V)* aspect, or the abdomen.

> **TECHNICIAN NOTES**
>
> According to etymological rules, when two terms are combined, the combining vowel (generally "o") is used to connect them.

3. For lateral recumbency, the image is labeled according to the side the patient is lying on. Conventionally, for ease of description, only the area of exit is included.
   a. Thus in a right lateral image, the patient is lying on its right side. The right limb in this case would be the side against the image receptor, and it is called a *right lateral* (area of exit).
   b. Technically a right lateral radiograph is properly referred to as a *Le-RtL*, although this term is not commonly used.
4. The terms *right* and *left* should precede any other terms (e.g., right lateral).
5. The terms *medial (M)* and *lateral (L)* should be subservient (follow) when used in combination with other terms (e.g., dorsomedial).
6. On the head, neck, trunk, and tail, the terms *rostral (R)*, *cranial, (Cr)*, and *caudal (Cd)* should take precedence (go first) when used in combination with other terms (e.g., caudoventral).

Limb Terminology

1. Cranial (Cr) and caudal (Cd) refer to the portion of the limb proximal to the carpus and tarsus.
2. The descriptors dorsal (D), palmar (Pa), and plantar (Pl) are used for that portion of the limb distal to and including the carpus and tarsus. Palmar (Pa) is used in reference to the forelimbs, whereas plantar (Pl) refers to the hind limbs.
3. In describing the limbs, the terms *dorsal, palmar, plantar, cranial,* and *caudal* should take precedence when used in combination with other terms—for example, dorsoproximal.
4. The term *oblique (O)* is added to the names of those projections in which the central ray passes obliquely (not parallel) to one of the three major directional axes—mediolateral (ML), dorsopalmar/dorsoplantar (DP), or craniocaudal (CrCd)—through the body part. They are named in the same manner as the standard views. The term *oblique* is generally used in reference to equine limbs.
   a. Thus in a dorsomedial-palmarolateral oblique (DM-PaLO) image of the carpus, the beam enters the dorsomedial side of the carpus and exits the palmarolateral aspect of the carpus (Fig. 15.3).
   b. Technically, if this view was made by positioning the x-ray tube 60 degrees medially from the dorsal side, the designation would be D60°M-PaLO. Oblique terminology is discussed further in Chapter 24.
5. In those views requiring a combination of directional terms, a hyphen should be inserted to separate the point of entry and point of exit.
   a. For example, dorsoproximal-palmarodistal (DPr-PaDi) of the front digit of a horse means that the beam comes from the front of the foot and exits at the back of the foot (distal to and including the carpus). The plate is placed at the back of or under the foot, depending on the anatomy.
6. The tangential and skyline views require no special designation because the point of entry to point of exit method describes these views concisely.
   a. For example, palmaroproximal-palmarodistal (PaPr-PaDi) in reference to an equine forelimb navicular region means that the beam is aiming strictly at the palmaro- (back) aspect of the foot starting at the top (proximo-) and ending toward the sole of the hoof (disto-). Further terminology will be discussed in Chapter 24.

Patient Positioning

The Patient

The comfort and welfare of the patient should be considered at all times. Patience is vital, especially with animals that cannot be sedated, are critically ill, are compromised in any way, or are in pain. Make sure that any required supplies or monitoring equipment are close at hand. Constantly assess and monitor the patient.

Animals are often put in positions with which they are not familiar, but if they feel secure, patients will generally tolerate abnormal positions. To minimize anxiety, animals

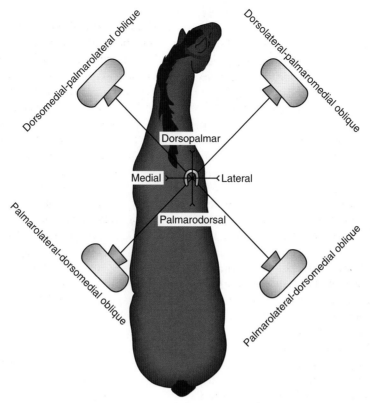

FIG. 15.3 Correct anatomical directional terms for oblique views.

should be handled in a slow, quiet manner in a darkened room:

- Animals often respond to a calm, soft voice and gentle stroking.
- Quick, loud movements and severe restraint usually result in a frightened, tense, and even aggressive patient.
- Permit the patient time to settle, either with or without sedation.

Do not underestimate the value of a muzzle. Muzzles often distract the patient, as well as being a "technician saver." Cats especially do not respond to overrestraint, but are often uncooperative. The combination of patience with mild sedation and strategically placed positioning aids generally produces highly diagnostic radiographs.

The rotor noise (spinning of the rotating anode) of the x-ray tube often startles animals. When working with patients exhibiting signs of anxiety, consider starting and releasing the rotor switch just before taking the radiograph so the patient becomes accustomed to the noise. However, be careful not to cause rotor damage.

To prevent retakes, make sure that proper exposure factors are used and that the patient is correctly positioned. Use a collimator, limiting the field of view to cover only the area of interest plus the peripheral borders (Fig. 15.4). You should see evidence of a border of collimation (frame) on each image, ensuring that the field of view is still included. Thus it is essential to include the full anatomy of the area of interest and know the peripheral borders that should be included for each position (e.g., the thorax should include the shoulder

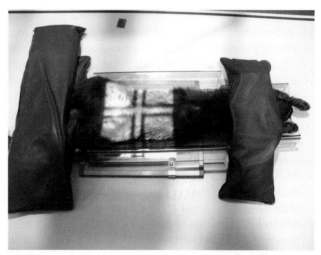

FIG. 15.4 Limit the image receptor to include the area that is being radiographed and its peripheral borders to prevent unnecessary radiation and excess secondary radiation.

joint and diaphragm). Peripheral borders will be stressed for each position in the relevant chapters. Proper collimation not only further protects the patient and positioner from secondary radiation but also increases the radiographic contrast of the image.

Always wear protective equipment if you must hold the patient or be in the room when an exposure is made. For film/screen systems, use a fast combination to lessen the milliamperage and exposure time needed. In digital radiography, minimize dose creep, or the tendency to increase your kV and mAs.

There is also the temptation to obtain more rather than fewer radiographs because digital images are easy to delete. An increased number of radiographs means increased exposure to the patient and personnel, so do limit the number taken by being correct the first time. It is essential to collimate the beam as much as possible to minimize secondary radiation.

Carefully plan and complete as much technical preparation for the exposure as possible before positioning the patient on the table to minimize the length of time the patient is being restrained. This includes measuring the patient, setting the exposure technique on the machine console, positioning the cassette, making the label (if needed), collimating the beam, gathering positional aids, and donning any protective gear. Proper preparation may mean being able to temporarily step away from the beam and secondary radiation even without chemical restraint. Aim for excellent diagnostic images the first time.

 TECHNICIAN NOTES

Always measure the animal in the position it is to be radiographed.

Patient Preparation

The patient should be clean and free of any debris. If the hair coat of the patient is wet or full of debris, confusing artifacts can appear on the radiograph. Collars, harnesses, and leashes of any sort, especially those made of metal, should be removed (Fig. 15.5). Remove bandages, splints, and casts before radiography unless there is a definite medical reason for leaving them in place. Pedal radiography of the horse may require removing the shoe and cleaning the frog of the foot to minimize any artifacts that may obscure an area of interest.

For radiography of the small animal abdomen, the gastrointestinal tract must be free of ingesta and fecal material. A cathartic such as an enema or a laxative may be indicated to remove the obstructive material. A more detailed discussion of patient preparation for abdominal studies is provided in Chapter 23.

TECHNICIAN NOTES

Always remember the safety rules of time, distance, and shielding when working with x-rays. What you don't see can cause you future damage and impair your health. Protect yourself.

Positioning Aids for Human Safety

To assist in the positioning of the patient, devices such as sandbags, foam blocks and wedges, wood blocks, and a radiolucent trough can be used (Fig. 15.6). Tape is essential;

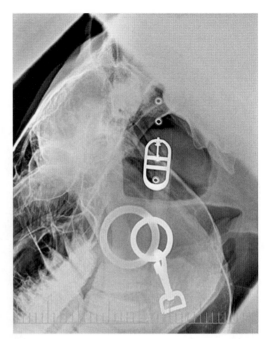

FIG. 15.5 It is important to remove any object that could interfere with the image. The harness was not removed from this horse's head before exposure.

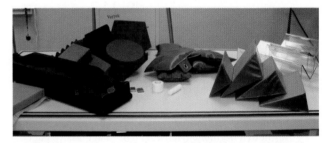

FIG. 15.6 Positioning devices available for nonmanual restraint.

gauze, rope, bungee cords, and compression bands are also useful positioning aids. Any reusable aids should be waterproof, washable, and stain resistant, as well as easy to store.

Positioning devices are commercially available. Prepared sandbags are generally prefilled with clean silica sand, permanently sealed, and often made of vinyl or nylon with plastic linings. Other material, such as bean bags, which are filled with polyester beads, can also be used; however, they do not offer the same support as sand does. Sand and bean bags are radiopaque, so should not be in the field of interest.

Commercial foam, available in various shapes and sizes, is generally covered in washable heavy vinyl covers (Fig.15.7A). Triangular and rectangular foam blocks are the most common. Foam tends to produce an air density shadow and, if not properly covered, absorbs and retains liquids that may be radiopaque when dry. The cover on foam blocks may also leave density shadows on the processed radiograph.

U- and V-shaped troughs are essential to maintain a patient in dorsal recumbency. Generally they are clear plastic or vinyl covered. The plastic/acrylic troughs are radiolucent,

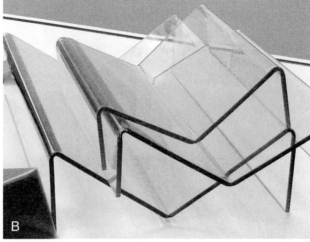

FIG. 15.7 **A,** Positioning devices should be covered for easy cleaning and sanitation. **B,** Acrylic positioning devices.

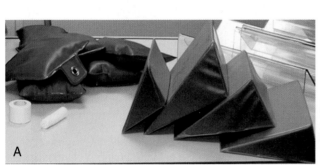

FIG. 15.8 Soft Velcro strapping can be attached to the table for easy patient positioning of any body part. (Image courtesy and permission of Ashley Jenner, RVT, Toronto, Ontario).

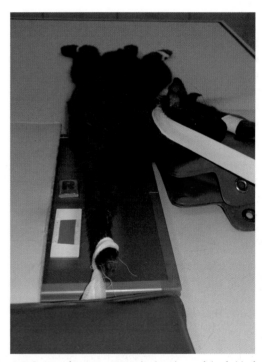

lightweight, and easy to clean (Fig. 15.7B). U-shaped troughs offer good head support. Those with acrylic rods can be used to maintain the shape of the skull. When using troughs for abdominal or thoracic radiographs, ensure that the entire field of view is either on or off the trough; otherwise, the radiograph may display distortion, artifacts, or asymmetry. Positioning troughs used for areas such as the pelvis should be fully outside the collimated area for the same reasons.

Tape, gauze, and compression bands are extremely effective. These must be functional to be satisfactory. Rope and gauze, using a half-hitch knot or variation (placing the end through the loop and then around the object), can be tied to the table if the patient is heavily sedated or anesthetized, or held by a person who can then back away from both the primary beam and secondary radiation. Velcro on the underside of the table allows soft Velcro straps to stick and is effective for many views (Fig. 15.8).

Adhesive tape can be used to extend and hold limbs, rotate limbs, secure the patellae and femurs for a hip dysplasia view, widen the space between the toes, temporarily secure a head out of the field of view, and so on (Fig. 15.9). A wooden spoon can be used to keep a cat's head out of the field of view so the radiographer is farther away from the primary beam.

Compression bands and hook-and-loop tape (Velcro) can be applied. Clothes pegs/clothes pins for cats, commercially available cat scruffers (Fig. 15.10), or nylon towel clamps

FIG. 15.9 Use of tape to secure the head out of the field of view.

applied to the dorsal neck region (a feline behavior principle that the queen uses with her kittens) is a valuable tool for feline patients and is almost as effective as sedation, especially if the positioning is quick and the patient is not in pain. Place the sandbag over the device. Wrapping a cat in a towel ("cat burrito") can be effective if you need to pull out the limbs for imaging or even for abdominal and thoracic views. Sandbagging the towel keeps cats in position. Wrapping does allow many angry cats to become compliant.

Your own devices can be made at a fraction of the cost of the commercially available positioning devices. Sandbags can easily be sewn and filled with sand. Empty sealable bags that

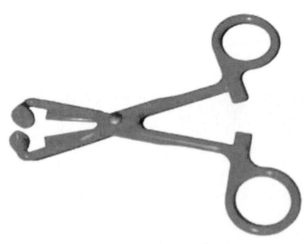

FIG. 15.10 Commercially available cat scruffer. Clipnosis binder clips also induce pressure on the neck, just behind the ear, to help calm a cat. Keep in mind that the American Animal Hospital Association (AAHA) and American Association of Feline Practitioners (AAFP) have made statements that scruffing cats does not allow a sense of control, often increasing fear and fear aggression.

can be filled with sand are also available. If you are making your own out of canvas (jean legs work well) or thick vinyl, make sure to use very narrow stitching so the sand does not leak out. Fabric sand bags are not easily disinfected, so before each use, wrap them in disposable plastic. Most fabric stores sell foam that can be cut into desired shapes with a scalpel blade or electric knife. Covering the bags and wedges is essential for disinfection between patients and for keeping the devices dry to minimize radiographic artifacts. With these devices, and sedation if necessary, minimal manual restraint can be used.

Any nonmanual restraint used must always focus on the safety and comfort of the patient. The devices should be quickly applied and released and should never compromise the patient. Positioning aids should give the patient the illusion that it is being held. Strategically placed sandbags or compression devices over the neck and limbs, judicious use of tape, a dimly lit room, calm deliberate movements, and a gloved hand placed over the head and held until the rotor is depressed may keep patients, especially dogs in lateral recumbency, calm long enough for the restrainer to step back at least 6 feet.

The moment the rotor is depressed, slip your hand out of the glove, leaving it over the animal's head so the patient assumes that you are still there. Keep talking to the patient as you quietly step back. Move forward as soon as the radiograph has been taken. Another person should be depressing the exposure buttons on the console; if you are using the foot pedal, step back as far as possible. Increasing your distance from the beam drastically reduces your exposure.

If there is no alternative but to restrain a patient, it is imperative to look away from the field of view and lean back as far as possible while taking the radiograph. At no point should any part of your body be in the field of view. Protective equipment protects you from secondary radiation, not from the primary beam.

Acrylic tubes, stockinette material, pillowcases, paper bags, and plastic containers can also be strategically used for the positioning of exotic animals. Please see Chapter 25 for more detail on this subject.

Equine radiographers are less likely to practice nonmanual restraint because of perceived physical safety for both the handler and the horse. However, every effort should be made to practice the three essential components of radiation safety (time, distance, and shielding). See Chapter 24 for further information on equine positioning.

> ### ✎ TECHNICIAN NOTES
>
> Have everything ready before taking the exposure. This includes measuring the animal, turning on the machine, setting the main voltage calibration if required, having proper source image distance, using a grid or not, and collimating and setting the exposures. Have the cassettes or plates ready. Positioning devices should be close at hand, but any objects or distractions should be removed.
>
> The patient should be clean, have no artifacts in the area of interest, and be chemically restrained if possible.

Required Views and Positioning Guidelines

The following guidelines assist in producing high-quality images:

- Two views of each anatomical area taken at right angles to each other are the minimum recommended exposures. You are trying to visualize a three-dimensional body on a two-dimensional image, so details will be missed if two perpendicular views are not taken (Fig. 15.11). There may be exceptions if the patient is debilitated or in trauma, or if positions other than the lateral will cause undue stress to the animal. A horizontal beam radiograph should then be considered so that you still have two perpendicular views (Fig. 15.12).
- Position the area of interest closest to the image receptor to reduce distortion and magnification of the area under examination (Fig. 15.13).
- When radiographing a limb, especially in immature or older patients, consider imaging the opposite corresponding limb to allow the pathological structure of one limb to be compared with the normal anatomy of the other.
- When the tabletop technique is used, an image receptor can be divided to image more than one view, limiting the number of films utilized (Fig. 15.14).
  - Place a lead sheet over half of the cassette (cassette mask) to prevent exposure while the other side is being radiographed.
  - The image receptor should still be collimated to the image only so that secondary radiation will not cause unnecessary fogging of the image.
  - Lead sheets, which can be purchased from most x-ray supply companies, are usually supplied in preselected sizes; or larger sheets can be purchased and cut to the desired size.

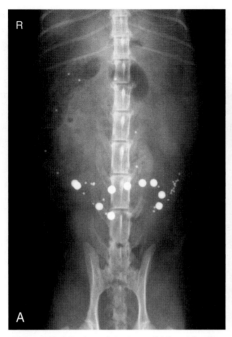

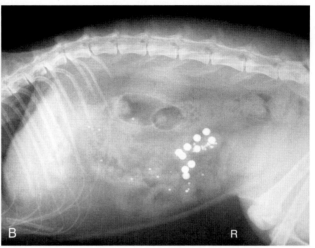

FIG. 15.11 A and **B,** It would be difficult to determine exactly where the barium-impregnated polyurethane spheres (BIPS) are positioned without the two perpendicular views. Note the proper placement for viewing of VD and lateral radiographs.

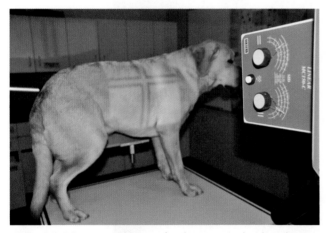

FIG. 15.12 Horizontal beam of a dog in a standing lateral view.

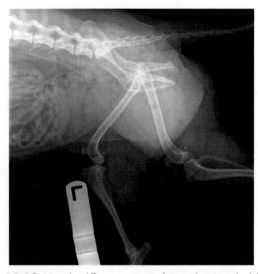

FIG. 15.13 Note the difference in magnification between the left limb, which is closer to the plate, and the opposite right limb, which is raised from the image receptor. Also note that the bone edges are not as defined on the right limb.

- The lead should be at least 2 mm thick. If a lead sheet is unavailable, a lead glove can be placed over the area to be shielded.
- When using the tabletop technique, place a nonslip pad, such as a rubber shelf liner, under the cassette to keep it from slipping (Fig. 15.15).
- When two separate views will be positioned on a radiograph, both views should be facing the same direction. For limbs, this would mean that the toes are facing the same side of the cassette; for the skull, the nose is in the same direction on each view.
- In general, the central ray should be centered directly over the area of interest.
  - If there is a known lesion, however, it is important to center the beam directly over this area, especially

to visualize fracture healing in limbs or spinal lesions.
- If the central ray is not directly over the area of interest, distortion and misdiagnosis may occur.
- The measurement for any anatomical region is generally taken over the thickest part.
  - This practice ensures that all regions of the area of interest will be penetrated with sufficient exposure factors.

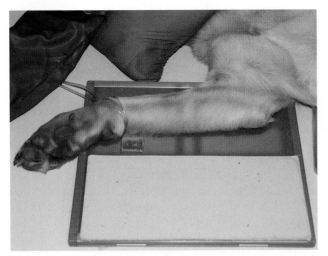

FIG. 15.14 Divided image receptor view of a dog extremity. Through the use of a lead shield, both views can be exposed on one plate. The receptor is not divided when a grid is used.

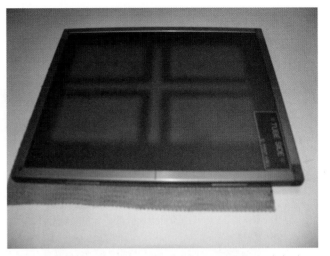

FIG. 15.15 Placing a grip pad under the image receptor helps keep the cassette from sliding when using the tabletop technique. Note also how the beam is collimated inside the cassette.

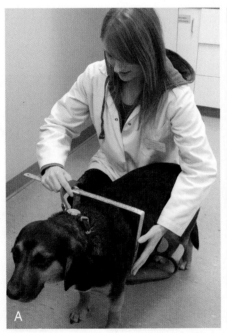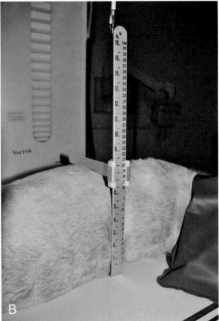

FIG. 15.16 A, Measuring with a caliper in this position may lead to extra tissue thickness. **B,** Calipers are properly used when the patient is measured lying in the radiographic view to be projected. This patient measures 17 cm.

- A caliper is used to measure the anatomical area of interest so that proper exposures can be made. This is an inexpensive device that measures part thickness in centimeter increments (Fig. 15.16).
- The patient should be measured in the same position used for the radiograph; if the animal is measured while standing, for example, the tissue thickness measurement will be greater than when the animal is recumbent, especially for soft tissue studies (see Fig. 15.16A-B).
  - If there is a large difference in tissue thickness between the cranial and caudal borders, which is not uncommon

  in the abdomen and thorax of a deep-chested dog, two separate exposures may need to be taken.
  - A compromise is best made if there is only a small difference in tissue density.
- Use an image receptor that is large enough to cover the body area being radiographed. Specific anatomy must be included for each anatomical area.
  - For example, all radiographs of long bones (humerus and femur) should include the shaft of the bone, as well as the joints both distal (Di) and proximal (Pr) to the bone.

- For joint radiography, the central ray must be centered over the joint space, and the beam should include a portion of the long bones distal and proximal to the joint.
  - Proper centering and inclusion is further expanded in Chapters 18 and 19.
- Have the thickest part of the area of interest toward the cathode side so that the most penetrating x-rays can assist in proper exposure (Fig. 15.17; see Chapter 2).

Image Identification

Identification (ID) of the radiographs is important both for legal purposes and for knowledge that the radiographs belong to the patient in which you are interested. Please see Chapter 7 for further details. Be sure that each radiograph contains the following information: owner and patient ID, date of examination, name and location of the facility, veterinarian, and other state or provincial requirements. Additional helpful information includes age, breed, and sex of the patient that should be written in the radiography log.

Positioning markers (right, left, front, hind) should be used so that the radiographs may be correctly interpreted. This is especially true for equine radiographs of areas distal to the carpus and tarsus or symmetrical anatomical areas such as a skull. Conventionally, markers are placed laterally (as opposed to medially) for DP, CrCd, or CdCr and oblique limb radiographs.

Place the markers cranially for lateral radiographs. In DV or VD views, place the appropriate L or R marker on the correct side of the patient. When a lateral projection of the body is taken, the marker should indicate the side that is directly on the table or cassette. Thus an R would indicate a patient lying in right lateral recumbency. The marker or label would generally be placed cranially and ventrally (Fig. 15.18).

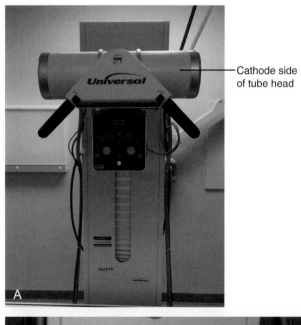

Cathode side of tube head

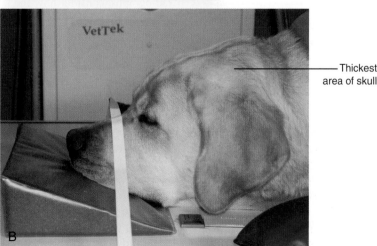

Thickest area of skull

FIG. 15.17 A, The thickest part of the area of interest should be toward the cathode, which is usually to the right side of the tube head. **B,** Positioning for radiograph.

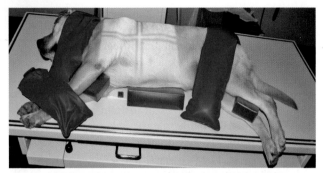

FIG. 15.18 The patient is in right lateral recumbency, lying on the right side. Note that the marker is placed cranially and ventrally.

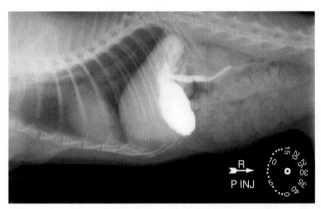

FIG. 15.19 The time clock indicates that the radiograph was taken 7 minutes after administration of barium. The feline patient is lying on its right side.

When a special procedure is performed, such as a gastrointestinal contrast study that is part of a series, time elapsed or order taken is also important. In film radiography this designation can be made on the lead tape label. Specialized time clocks can be used in which it is easy to adjust the time lapse (Fig. 15.19). Gravity markers that indicate a patient is standing are also available, although not frequently used.

✎ TECHNICIAN NOTES

Quickly go through a mental checklist such as this one before pushing the exposure button:
- Are the settings correct?
- Is the plate/cassette/machine/grid in position?
- Is the thickest part toward the cathode, if applicable?
- Are the markers and ID (if using) in the proper location and away from relevant anatomy?
- Do you have the correct body part and view?
- Is the patient properly centered? Are the peripheral borders correct?
- Is the x-ray beam correctly collimated?
- Is the patient properly prepared, positioned, and restrained so that the body part is parallel to the image receptor and so that the central ray is perpendicular to both?
- Is the patient in the correct phase of respiration if applicable?

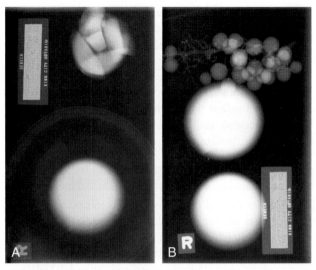

FIG. 15.20 Mystery radiographs. What do you think the different objects are in this figure?

Viewing Radiographs

To assist in understanding normal radiographic anatomy, you should always view radiographs on the illuminator or monitor in the following manner (see Fig. 15.11):

Lateral radiographs: The cranial part of the animal is to your left.

Dorsoventral/ventrodorsal radiographs: The cranial part of the animal points up, and the animal's left side is on your right (as if you are going to shake its paw).

Lateromedial/mediolateral or oblique radiographs of the limbs: The proximal part of the limb points up, and the cranial or dorsal aspect of the limb is to your left.

DP/PD/CrCd/CdCr radiographs: The proximal end of the extremity is at the top of the illuminator or monitor.

For proper illumination specifications and concerns, see Chapter 7. Consistency is important. When labeling film radiographs, consider how the labels and markers are positioned so that they can easily be read when the radiographs are viewed in the proper positions.

Fig. 15.20 is a mystery radiograph. Review it and answer the question presented with it.

Radiographic Checklist

Before submitting the radiographs to the veterinarian, you should ask yourself the following questions to ensure that you have optimal diagnostic and legal radiographs:
- Is the image label present and legible?
- Are positional lead markers present?
- Do you have good exposure with appropriate contrast and density?
- Is your image properly centered?
- Is the body part properly positioned, with no rotation?

- Are the appropriate borders included, and is there evidence of collimation?
- Is there no evidence of a human exposure, such as a glove?
- Is the film properly processed (if applicable)?
- Have artifacts been kept to a minimum to prevent interference with the image?

If the answer is no to any of these questions, consider the next two:

- Is the image diagnostic?
- Does the image need to be repeated?

✳ KEY POINTS

1. The radiographic projection is described according to where the beam first enters and then exits the area of interest.
2. Label the side that the animal is lying on for lateral radiographs.
3. For pectoral limbs, use the term *dorsopalmar (DPa)/ palmarodorsal (PaD)* to designate the area distal to and including the carpus. For pelvic limbs, dorsoplantar (DPl)/plantarodorsal (PlD) is used to designate the area distal to and including the tarsus. Craniocaudal (CrCd)/caudocranial (CdCr) is used for areas proximal to the carpus and tarsus.
4. The area of interest should be closest to the image receptor.
5. Keep human safety in mind at all times, utilizing the three important safety principles of time, distance, and shielding.
6. Careful planning and preparation help minimize retakes.
7. Use chemical restraint if possible and nonmanual restraint.
8. Knowledge of the proper positioning technique along with creativity leads to inventive and effective use of positioning aids and nonmanual restraint.
9. Generally utilize slow and deliberate movements in a dimly lit room to keep the patient calm.
10. When identifying limbs, place the markers laterally for DP, CrCd, or CdCr views and cranially for lateral views.
11. When looking at radiographs on the viewer, position for a VD/DV so that you are "shaking its paw" or looking at the ventral aspect. For a lateral view, have the animal's head to your left.

REVIEW QUESTIONS

1. A cat is lying on its abdomen with its limbs extended. The view of the tarsus in this position would be called:
   a. Palmarodorsal (PaD)
   b. Plantarodorsal (PlD)
   c. Craniocaudal (CrCd)
   d. Caudocranial (CdCr)

2. Sandbags are considered:
   a. Radiolucent and can be in the field of view
   b. Radiolucent and should not be in the field of view
   c. Radiopaque and can be in the field of view
   d. Radiopaque and should not be in the field of view

3. It is important to collimate the beam as much as possible so that there is less:
   a. Contrast and density on the image
   b. Secondary exposure to the patient and restrainer
   c. Chance of magnification or distortion
   d. Likelihood that the patient will move

4. An image of the radius/ulna of a dachshund has been collimated to include the humerus and metacarpus. This is:
   a. Correct, as the joints above and below the area of interest have been included
   b. Incorrect, as not enough of the limb has been included
   c. Incorrect, as it should be collimated to include from the elbow to the carpus
   d. Incorrect, as only the radius and ulna should be included

5. You are going to divide an image receptor for a feline skull. You should:
   a. Have the nose in each view pointing in the same direction
   b. Do so when utilizing a grid
   c. Use a lead sheet to cover the side being radiographed
   d. Place the marker at the caudal aspect of the skull in each case

6. You are radiographing a right craniocaudal humerus of a standard poodle. The "R" marker is best placed:
   a. Under the humerus
   b. At the toes on the right side
   c. Along the medial side of the humerus
   d. Along the lateral side of the humerus

7. You can be farther from the beam when the image is exposed if you:
   a. Wear appropriate apparel and hold your patient
   b. Use the shortest exposure time possible
   c. Utilize positioning aids whenever possible
   d. Measure at the thickest part

8. You are to radiograph the full abdomen of a sedated Doberman. The thickest part measures 20 cm. You are best to radiograph the:
   a. Cranial aspect and then remeasure and radiograph the caudal aspect
   b. Full abdomen on one large image receptor using the cranial measurement
   c. Average of both the cranial and caudal measurements of the abdomen
   d. Thickest part only and not include the caudal abdomen

9. When placing an image of an extremity on the illuminator for the veterinarian to read, you should position it so that the digits are pointing:
   a. Upward
   b. Downward
   c. To the left
   d. To the right

10. The veterinarian required a follow-up radiograph of the abdomen of a patient. The technique chart was correctly followed, but your image was darker than the one taken by your colleague a month ago. This could be because:
    a. Your patient has gained weight
    b. You measured at the thickest part while the patient was on the table
    c. You collimated more than your colleague did
    d. You measured while the patient was standing

11. The veterinarian requests a right lateral of the thorax of a Pomeranian. The patient will be tranquilized and:
    a. Lying on its right side
    b. Lying on its left side
    c. Standing so that its right side is against the plate
    d. The beam will enter the patient from the right side

12. The collimation for this Pomeranian patient in Question 11 will extend to the:
    a. Thorax and abdomen because both will fit on the image
    b. Heart and lungs, as this is the area that the veterinarian is interested in
    c. Third rib cranially and the 12th rib caudally, as this is the area of interest
    d. Diaphragm and shoulder joint, as the full thorax should be included

13. You are to radiograph a lateral abdomen of a well-behaved golden retriever. To keep your patient in position so you can move away from the beam, you should place:
    a. Sandbags over the chest and abdomen
    b. Sandbags over the head/neck, pelvis, and limbs
    c. Foam pads over the head/neck, pelvis, and limbs
    d. A scruffer over the neck region behind the ears

14. A dorsolateral-palmaromedial oblique (D60°L-PaMO) of an equine right carpus means that the beam is entering the right limb at 60 degrees from the:
    a. Front and lateral side of the limb
    b. Front and medial side of the limb
    c. Back and lateral side of the limb
    d. Back and medial side of the limb

15. The (D60°L-PaMO) of an equine right carpus in Question 14 means that the image receptor is against the:
    a. Dorsal and medial side of the limb
    b. Dorsal and lateral side of the limb
    c. Palmar and medial side of the limb
    d. Palmar and lateral side of the limb

Answers to Review Questions can be found on the Evolve website.

Bibliography

American College of Veterinary Radiology (ACVR). *Radiology 2—Equine*. ACVR; 2009.

Aspinall V, Cappello M. *Introduction to Veterinary Anatomy*. London: Butterman-Heineman; 2009.

Colville T, Bassert J. *Clinical Anatomy and Physiology for Veterinary technicians*. 3rd ed. St. Louis: Elsevier; 2016.

Done SH, Goody PC, Stickland NC, et al. *Color Atlas of Veterinary Anatomy, The Dog and Cat*. London: Mosby; 2009.

Dyce KM, Sack WO, Wensing CJG. *Textbook of Veterinary Anatomy*. 4th ed. St. Louis: Saunders; 2010.

Evans H, de Launta A. *Guide to the Dissection of the Dog*. 8th ed. St. Louis: Saunders; 2017.

Fauber TL. *Radiographic Imaging and Exposure*. St. Louis: Elsevier; 2017.

Han C, Hurd C. *Practical Diagnostic Imaging for the Veterinary Technician*. 3rd ed. St. Louis: Mosby; 2005.

Jenner A. Non-manual radiography: radiation and patient safety. *RVT Journal, Ontario Association of Veterinary Technicians*. Winter 2016, Volume 39, Issue 2.

Morgan JP, Doval J, Samii V. *Radiographic Techniques: The Dog*. Hannover: Schlutersche GmbH & Co; 1998.

Owens JM, Biery DN. *Radiographic Interpretation for the small Animal Clinician*. St. Louis: Ralston Purina; 1999.

Reid CF, Bathurst NW: Large animal radiography nomenclature, 1995, University of Pennsylvania School of Veterinary Medicine. http://cal.vet.upenn.edu/projects/larad/names/name.htm.

Romich J. *An Illustrated Guide to Veterinary Medical Terminology*. 4th ed. Stamford, CT: Cengage Learning; 2015.

Ryan G. *Radiographic Positioning of Small Animals*. Philadelphia: Lea & Febiger; 1981.

Sirois M. *Principles and Practice of Veterinary Technology*. 3rd ed. St. Louis: Elsevier; 2011.

Sirois M, Anthony E, Mauragis D. *Handbook of Radiographic Positioning for veterinary Technicians*. Clifton Park, NY: Delmar Cengage Learning; 2010.

Smallwood JE, Shively MJ, Rendano VT, et al. A standardized nomenclature for radiographic projections used in veterinary medicine. *Vet Rad*. 1985;26:2-9.

Thrall DE. *Textbook of Veterinary Diagnostic Radiology*. 6th ed. St. Louis: Elsevier; 2013.

Ticer J. *Radiographic Technique in Small Animal Practice*. Philadelphia: WB Saunders; 1984.

Tighe M, Brown M. *Mosby's Comprehensive Review for Veterinary Technicians*. 4th ed. St. Louis: Mosby; 2015.

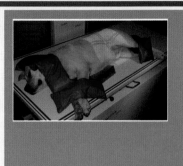

CHAPTER 16
Small Animal Abdomen

Marg Brown, RVT, BEd Ad Ed

By three methods we may learn wisdom: first, by reflection, which is noblest; second, by imitation, which is easiest; and third by experience, which is the bitterest.
—Confucius, Chinese philosopher, 551–479 BCE

OUTLINE

LEARNING OBJECTIVES

When you have finished this chapter, you will be able to:

1. Properly and safely position a dog or cat for the common abdominal views, with an emphasis on nonmanual restraint.
2. Correctly measure and center the patient to include the peripheral borders.
3. Ensure that the abdomen is parallel to the image receptor and the central ray is perpendicular to the field of view (FOV).

4. Be familiar with alternative positions for abdominal radiography as required.
5. Identify normal radiographic abdominal anatomy.

KEY TERMS

Key terms are defined in the Glossary on the Evolve website.

Brachecephalic
Cachexic
Chondrodystrophic
Coxofemoral joint

Decubitus
Field of view (FOV)
Focal radiograph
Horizontal beam

Intervertebral foramina
Positioning terminology
Sagittal
Spinous process

Transverse process
Vertebral bodies
Xiphoid

TECHNICAL NOTE: To preserve space, the radiographs presented in this chapter do not show collimation. For safety, always collimate so that the beam is limited to within the image receptor edges. In film radiography, you should see a clear border of collimation (frame) on every radiograph. In some jurisdictions, evidence of collimation is required by law.

Positioning for the abdomen is relatively straightforward, but visualization can be difficult due to the similarity in densities of multiple organs. The subtle differences in tissue densities of the abdomen offer significantly less natural contrast than are found in the thorax. Visualization of contrast depends on the gas and ingesta within the gastrointestinal (GI) tract and the fat in the peritoneal and retroperitoneal areas. Contrast media are often required to visualize differences.

Radiographic Concerns

- Appropriate kilovoltage (kV) and milliampere-seconds (mAs) should be used to differentiate the various shades of gray between organs and structures.
  - Because of low comparative contrast of the organs in the abdomen, use the appropriate kV to provide a longer scale of contrast (more shades of gray to differentiate the organs).
  - Use the highest mA and lowest kV that will produce the highest-quality film.
  - Higher mA means you can use fewer seconds for a shorter exposure and less chance of motion artifacts.
- The "enhanced contrast resolution of digital imaging" makes exposure factors less critical, but a technique chart needs to be adhered to.[1]
- Because of the differences in thickness between the chest and caudal abdomen, deep-chested dogs exhibit a marked difference in density between the cranial and caudal halves of the abdomen, which is especially evident in the ventrodorsal (VD) view. Two separate exposures measured at the thickest part of each site may be needed. If there is only a minimal difference in anatomical thickness, a compromise can be made.
- Using the same technique with digital radiography may be possible for the entire abdomen of such dogs.
- The two positions commonly viewed are the right or left lateral and ventrodorsal (Box 16.1). The right lateral is the most common, but it is important to be consistent so that abnormalities can quickly be visualized. Contrast studies and other situations may require additional views.

BOX 16.1	Protocol for Abdominal Radiography
Routine Views	**Ancillary Views**
• Right or left lateral	• Dorsoventral
• Ventrodorsal	• Lateral decubitus
	• Modified lateral/lateral oblique

- If a right lateral view is used, the animal is lying on its right side. Technically the correct terminology is *left-right lateral (Le-RtL)*, if one considers the "point of entrance of the beam to point of exit"; however, this term is not generally used in small animals.
- Take advantage of the anode heel effect (the thickest part toward the cathode) to help reduce density differences, especially in the VD or dorsoventral (DV) views.
- Use a 14 in. × 17 in. image receptor for large dogs. A very large dog will likely require two radiographs measured at the cranial and caudal abdomen, respectively.
- A grid should be used if the measurement exceeds 10 cm to prevent scatter that causes fogging, which further decreases the contrast.
- Expose the radiograph at the end of expiration, when a brief pause often occurs before inspiration. During expiration there is a maximum amount of space for the abdominal contents as the lungs contract and the diaphragm relaxes cranially.
- Routine abdominal studies generally do not require fasting or an enema. Chapter 23 outlines preparation for contrast studies or specific concerns.
- Nonmanual restraint should be utilized whenever possible to minimize radiation exposure to personnel. Use of a sedative or tranquilizer may be needed. Nonmanual restraint is illustrated in most of the following positions.
- Try to give the patient the illusion that it is being held by appropriate use of sandbags, tape, behavioral strategies, and other methods. For further suggestions, please see Chapter 15.

✎ **TECHNICIAN NOTES**

Measure the animal in the position in which it is to be imaged so that you are using the correct measurement to determine the settings from the technique chart.

✎ **TECHNICIAN NOTES**

Have everything ready before taking the exposure. This includes turning on the machine, setting the main voltage calibration if required, having proper source image distance, measuring the abdomen in the correct position, and setting the exposures. Have the image receptors ready. Positioning devices should be close at hand. Position your patient. To minimize scattered radiation, remove any objects or distractions not utilized.

The patient should be clean, should have no artifacts in the area of interest, and should be chemically restrained if possible.

Positions

Lateral—Routine

Positioning

Place in: Lateral recumbency.

Head: Keep in a natural position. Appropriately, place a sandbag over the neck, being careful not to restrict breathing.

Forelimbs: Pull cranially and sandbag. Place a small foam pad between the forelimbs to help eliminate rotation of the cranial abdomen.

Hind Limbs: Pull together slightly caudally and sandbag to prevent superimposition of the femoral muscles, which can mask portions of the urinary bladder and prostate. Place a foam pad of suitable thickness between the femurs to help eliminate rotation of the caudal abdomen and pelvis.

Sternum: Elevate with wedged sponges so the sternum is at the same plane as the thoracic vertebrae.

Comments and Tips

- Place any ID or markers at the ventral aspect of the abdomen.
- Ensure that the sternum and spine are on the same plane and are parallel to the image receptor; the central ray is perpendicular.
- The cranial border for routine abdominal views can also be determined by palpating the xiphoid process of the sternum. Place the cranial portion of the collimator light two finger widths cranial to the xiphoid process.

- The horizontal line of the collimator light should bisect the abdominal cavity into equal dorsal and ventral portions.
- Expose immediately at the end phase of expiration.
- Minimize skin folds to prevent overshadowing folds of tissue.
- Keep hind limbs perpendicular to the spine if organ crowding in the caudoventral abdomen is of concern.[1]
- Focal radiographs using gentle pressure with a compression paddle such as a wooden spoon or plastic paddle may effectively isolate organs such as the kidneys or move an underlying organ to improve the visualization of a suspected pathology in a VD position.[1] Remember to remeasure the patient and use this thickness to obtain the proper settings.
  - The decreased thickness allows for less scatter and a lower kVp and thus more contrast.
- There is better longitudinal separation of the kidneys[1] in a right lateral view, and the spleen is more consistently identified. Left lateral is preferable in vomiting patients, because gas is moved to the pyloric antrum.
  - This contrast between the gas and the structure may potentially highlight a foreign body that may not be as obvious on the right lateral.
- A left lateral view may also be required in contrast studies after the administration of contrast media.

MEASURE: Caudal aspect of 13th rib at the thickest area (unless interested in a specific region).

CENTRAL RAY:

Canine: Over caudal aspect of 13th rib at level of L2 to L3.
Feline: Two to three finger widths caudal to 13th rib.

BORDERS: Collimate cranially from about 1 inch cranial to the xiphoid of the sternum (include the full diaphragm and heart apex) and caudally to the greater trochanter to include the coxofemoral joints.

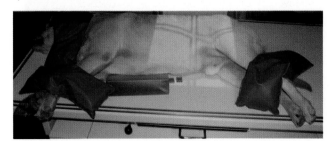

FIG. 16.1 Proper positioning for the lateral abdomen view of a canine.

> ### ✐ TECHNICIAN NOTES
>
> Remember to go through your mental checklist before pushing the exposure button. See Chapter 15. Always be conscious of radiation safety.

> ### ✐ TECHNICIAN NOTES
>
> To get maximum expiration:
> - If the patient is panting, cup or blow on the nose to momentarily stop breathing.
> - Apply light pressure on the abdomen to facilitate expiration.
>
> Breathe with the patient for a few breaths to determine the proper point of exposure. If a two-step rotor is available, have the exposure switch depressed (initial button of the two-step process) so that the moment breathing is paused, the exposure can be taken.

Continued

Lateral—Routine—cont'd

✎ TECHNICIAN NOTES

Ways to determine whether a normal animal is properly positioned[1-3]:

Lateral View
- Rib heads are superimposed.
- Intervertebral foramina are the same size.
- Transverse processes are superimposed at the origin from the vertebral bodies, appearing as Nike swooshes.[4]
- Coxofemoral joints and wings of the ilia are superimposed.

Ventrodorsal View
- Relevant spinous processes are aligned in the center of the vertebral bodies appearing tear-dropped in shape.
- Rib and abdominal symmetry.
- Wings of the ilium are symmetrical.
- Obturator foramina are symmetrical.

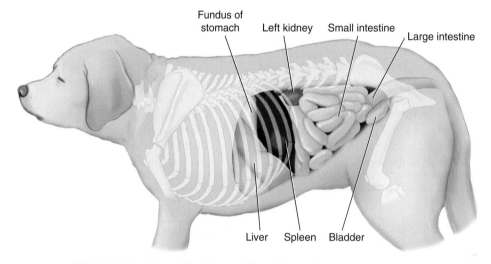

FIG. 16.2 Right lateral (Le-RtL) view of the abdomen showing major organs.

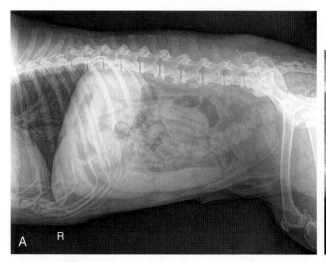
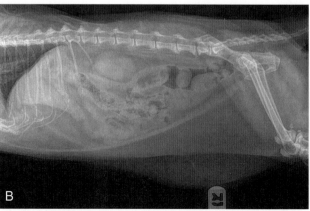

FIG. 16.3 A, Right lateral radiograph of the abdomen of a dog. **B,** Right lateral radiograph of the abdomen of a 17-year-old domestic shorthair. (**A** courtesy Vetel Diagnostics, San Luis Obispo, California, and Seth Wallack, DVM, DACVR, AAVR, Director and CEO of Veterinary Imaging Centre of San Diego; **B** courtesy Rosedale Animal Hospital.)

Ventrodorsal—Routine

Positioning

Place in: Dorsal recumbency. If a trough is needed to prevent rotation, place the device under the thoracic region, not the area being radiographed, so that distortion and artifacts are minimized.

Head: Keep the muzzle forward and straight so it is as parallel to the table as possible. Carefully position a sandbag over the head and neck, taking care not to restrict breathing.

Forelimbs: Extend forward with sandbags, positioning a sandbag over the limb just proximal to the elbows if possible. An alternative is either to tie each limb separately or to place a sandbag over each limb at the carpus and pull cranially.

Hind Limbs: Keep in a natural frog-leg position, and place a sandbag over each limb.

MEASURE: Caudal aspect of the 13th rib at level of umbilicus (about L2–L3). The area of the liver is generally the widest part. If interested in another area, measure that location.

CENTRAL RAY:

Canine: Center on midline over caudal aspect of 13th rib at level of umbilicus (L3).

Feline: Two to three finger widths caudal to 13th rib.

BORDERS: T9 vertebrae (about 1 inch cranial to the xiphoid of the sternum—full diaphragm) cranially to the greater trochanter caudally to include the coxofemoral joints (pubic symphysis).

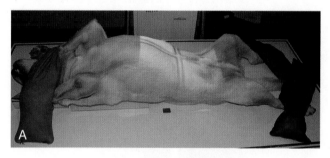

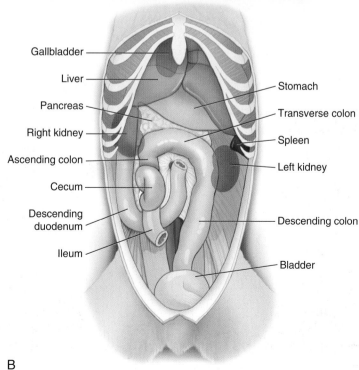

Gallbladder

Liver

Pancreas

Right kidney

Ascending colon

Cecum

Descending duodenum

Ileum

Stomach

Transverse colon

Spleen

Left kidney

Descending colon

Bladder

B

FIG. 16.4 A, Proper positioning for the ventrodorsal abdomen view. B, Ventral anatomy of the abdomen.

Continued

Ventrodorsal—Routine—cont'd

Comments and Tips

- Place any ID or markers adjacent to the corresponding side of the abdomen.
- Ensure that the body is evenly positioned so that the two sides of the rib cage appear equidistant.
- Ideally a straight line should be imagined connecting the point of the nose with the caudal midline. It may be difficult in brachycephalic or chondrodystrophic breeds to position the muzzle almost parallel with the table. Keep the head and neck of these breeds straight in front of the body with no rotation.
- Ensure that the sternum and spine are superimposed and are parallel to the image receptor; the central ray is perpendicular.

- Expose immediately at the end phase of expiration (this ensures that the diaphragm is positioned cranially and is not compressing the abdominal contents).

> 🖉 **TECHNICIAN NOTES**
>
> If radiographs of both the abdomen and thorax are required, complete both lateral views before imaging the VD views. The positioning is the same for the lateral views of the two areas; only the central ray and borders change.

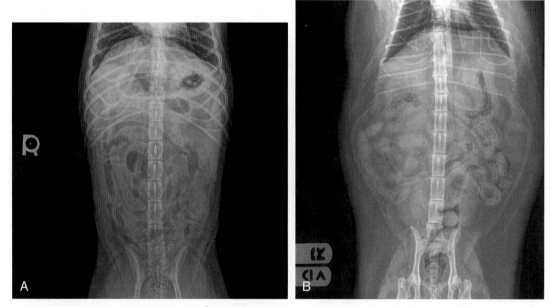

FIG. 16.5 A, Ventrodorsal radiograph of the abdomen of a canine. **B,** Ventrodorsal radiograph of the abdomen of a 17-year-old feline.

Further Views

In case of injury, for gastric contrast studies, or concern with fluid or free air, other views can be taken.

Dorsoventral—Ancillary

The DV view can be used in lieu of the VD view if the animal is compromised in the VD position or if an alternative view is needed for regular or contrast studies.

Positioning

Place in: Ventral recumbency.

Head: Keep straight and forward, carefully placing a sandbag over the neck and head, taking care not to restrict breathing.

Forelimbs: Extend slightly forward in a fairly natural position. Place sandbags over each elbow.

Hind Limbs: Keep in a natural position. Place a sandbag over each limb near the stifle.

Comments and Tips

- Place any identification or markers adjacent to the correct side of the abdomen.
- Ensure that the body is evenly positioned so that the two sides of the rib cage appear equidistant.
- Ideally a straight line should be imagined connecting the point of the nose with the caudal midline.
- Ensure that the sternum and spine are superimposed and that the image receptor and central ray are perpendicular to both.
- Expose immediately at the end phase of expiration.

MEASURE, CENTRAL RAY, BORDERS: Same as for the VD view.

> ✎ **TECHNICIAN NOTES**
>
> Collimate; ensure that labels/markers are included and that a clear frame is visible for every image.

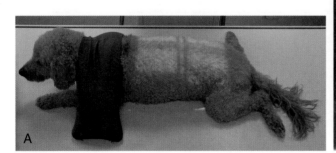
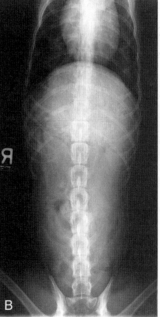

FIG. 16.6 A, Dorsoventral positioning. **B,** Dorsoventral radiograph of the abdomen of a canine. (**A** courtesy Jocelyn Affleck and Katerina White, Seneca College, Toronto; **B** courtesy Joshua Schlote, BS, LVT, Northeast Community College, Norfolk, Nebraska.)

Lateral Decubitus (Ventrodorsal View With Horizontal Beam)—Ancillary

The lateral decubitus should be considered if fluid or free gas is suspected, in order to evaluate gas-capped fluid levels that may be found in an abscess or in a bowel loop, or if the animal will be harmed if placed in an alternative position. Small amounts of fluid may not be identified radiographically.

Positioning

Place in: Right lateral recumbency on a thick foam pad or equivalent (to allow the dependent portion of the abdomen to be in the field of view).

Head: Keep in a natural position and place a sandbag over the neck, taking care not to restrict breathing.

Forelimbs: Pull cranially and sandbag. Place a small foam pad between the front limbs to help eliminate rotation of the cranial abdomen.

Hind Limbs: Pull slightly caudally to prevent superimposition of the femoral muscles that can mask portions of the bladder and prostate area. Place a sandbag over the limbs. Placing a foam pad of suitable thickness between the femurs helps eliminate rotation of the caudal abdomen and pelvis.

Sternum: Elevate the ventral abdomen with wedged sponges so the sternum is at the same plane as the thoracic vertebrae.

Comments and Tips

- The position is described according to the side on which the patient is lying (i.e., right decubitus if the patient is in right lateral recumbency).
- Place the image receptor vertically behind the patient.
- The horizontal beam will be directed ventrodorsally, entering the sternum and exiting the vertebrae.
- Expose immediately at the end phase of expiration.
- Ensure that the sternum and spine are on the same plane and parallel to the image receptor; the central ray is perpendicular.
- If free gas is suspected, wait at least 5 minutes once the patient is in position before imaging to allow dorsal collection of the gas.[5]

MEASURE, CENTRAL RAY, BORDERS: Proceed as for the ventrodorsal view.

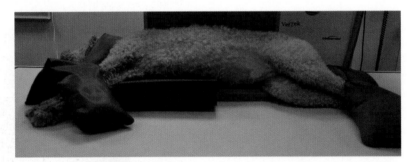

FIG. 16.7 Positioning of a dog for lateral decubitus—ventrodorsal view with a horizontal beam. (Courtesy Jocelyn Affleck and Katerina White, Seneca College, Toronto.)

Modified Lateral and Lateral Oblique—Ancillary

If evaluation of the entire length of the urinary tract is of concern in a male, the hind limbs may mask the ischial arch and os penis in a true lateral position. This is of concern especially if urinary calculi are suspected.[1-3,5] Two alternatives could be considered: the modified lateral and lateral oblique.

Modified Lateral—Ancillary
Positioning
Place in: Right lateral recumbency.

Head: Keep in a natural position, and restrain appropriately with a sandbag over the neck. Be careful not to restrict breathing.

Forelimbs: Pull cranially and sandbag. Place a small foam pad between the forelimbs to help eliminate rotation of the cranial abdomen.

Hind Limbs: Pull both limbs as cranially as possible without causing rotation of the body off the table. An appropriately sized foam pad placed between the femurs may help eliminate rotation of the pelvis. Place sandbags over the limbs.

Sternum: Elevate the ventral abdomen with wedged sponges so the sternum is at the same plane as the vertebrae. Have the central ray be perpendicular to both.

Comments and Tips
- Ensure that the pelvic limbs are not superimposed over the caudal aspect of the os penis.
- Expose immediately at the end phase of expiration.

BOTH POSITIONS

Measure: Over the ischium.

Central Ray: Over the cranial wing of the ilium unless the rectum is of interest; in that case have the central beam over the pelvis.

Borders: For a bladder, prostate, or caudal contrast study, include L4 and the caudal aspect of the rectum.

> ### ✐ TECHNICIAN NOTES
> For safety and to minimize scatter, remember to collimate only to the required borders. Include the markers in the image.

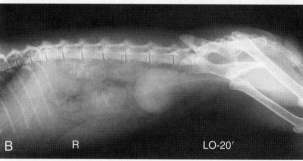

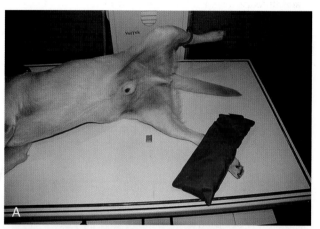

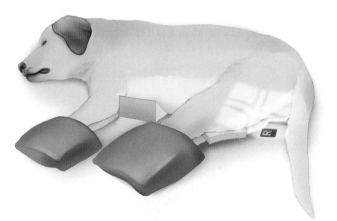

FIG. 16.8 Positioning for a modified lateral view of a male dog for contrast studies. The hind limbs are pulled cranially as far as possible for evaluation of the membranous and penile urethra.

FIG. 16.9 **A,** Positioning for lateral oblique view of the canine abdomen. Ensure that the pelvic limbs are not superimposed over the caudal aspect of the os penis. **B,** Lateral oblique radiograph of the abdomen of a feline patient during an excretory urography using iodine.

Continued

Modified Lateral and Lateral Oblique—Ancillary—cont'd

Lateral Oblique—Ancillary
Positioning
Place in: Right lateral recumbency.
Head: Keep in a natural position and support appropriately with a sandbag over the neck.
Forelimbs: Pull cranially and sandbag.
Hind Limbs: Pull the dependent limb caudally and place a sandbag over the femur to keep in position. Raise the contralateral limb and pull dorsally out of the field of view. To help keep the limb out of the field of view, tie a bungee cord, Velcro, or gauze around the tarsus and metatarsus and secure to the table, tube stand, or sandbag.

Comments and Tips
- Ensure that the pelvic limbs are not superimposed over the caudal aspect of the os penis.
- Expose immediately at the end phase of expiration.
- For male dogs, this view may be needed for specialized studies, as the penis may be superimposed over the bladder in the VD view.
- Oblique views can also be achieved by placing the patient in the VD or DV positions and rotating the body 15 to 30 degrees. This moves the esophagus, stomach, colon, and urinary bladder away from the vertebrae to allow better visualization.
- The criteria for proper symmetry will not apply to the oblique views.

Anatomical Abdominal Radiographic Concerns

Fig. 16.10 shows the various positions of a Sheltie during expiration, which is when the abdomen exposure should be completed. Figs. 16.11 to 16.16 show further anatomical features. Table 16.1 indicates how the radiographic anatomy changes as the patient's position changes.

✎ TECHNICIAN NOTES

Strategically used positioning aids give the patient the illusion it is being held. A sandbag over the neck and limbs and/or the use of tape or alternatives is essential if the patient is not appropriately sedated. Avoid holding the patient and step away from the primary beam. Reducing your x-ray exposure depends on your diligence.

A brief overview of normal radiographic anatomy is presented in Appendix C on the Evolve website so that the imager understands the implications of failure to properly position the patient: radiographic changes may be seen that are not attributable to disease processes or other findings. Also, the term *"normal"* may not be straightforward, because every organ or structure has particular normal findings, based on the shape, size, location, position, margins, number, and opacity, as well as being affected by superimposition of other tissues.

Variations in images depend on factors such as age and body condition, which can affect the interpretation of the peritoneum and retroperitoneal space.

Fat in the abdomen serves as a contrasting opacity to help identify the structures. Thus you see various body images much better in a fat cat than in an emaciated one because of the various types of fat present.

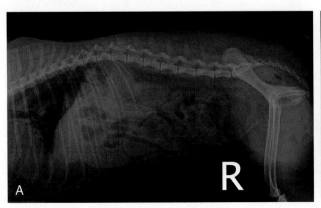
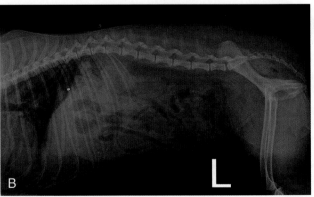

FIG. 16.10 Radiographs showing the various positions of a Sheltie during expiration. **A,** Right lateral. **B,** Left lateral.

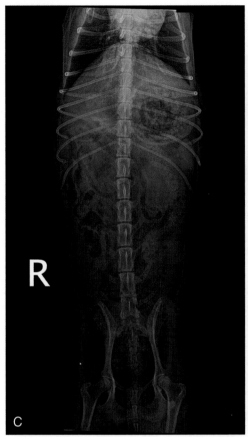

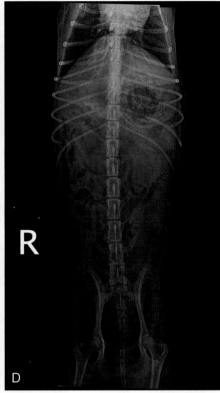

FIG. 16.10, cont'd C, Ventrodorsal. D, Dorsoventral.

Fat types include subcutaneous fat, retroperitoneal fat, and fat within the falciform ligament ventral to the liver. If there is no body fat, such as in immature or cachexic patients, it will be hard to distinguish the peritoneal or retroperitoneal organs.

Retroperitoneal and peritoneal fluid and gas also change the extent to which kidneys and other organs are obscured. Keep in mind that not all normal structures that are present anatomically are visible radiographically. However, abnormalities such as enlargements and increased opacities may cause such organs to become visible and may cause variations in positions of other organs.

See Appendix B on the Evolve website for specific organ overview (see also Fig. 16.11).

Fig. 16.17 is a mystery radiograph. Review it and answer the question presented with it.

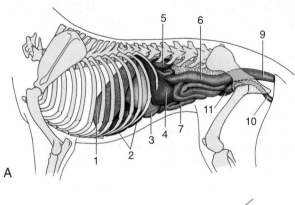

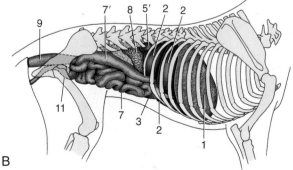

FIG. 16.11 Visceral projections on the left **(A)** and right **(B)** canine abdominal walls. *1,* Diaphragm; *2,* liver; *3,* stomach; *4,* spleen; *5* and *5',* left and right kidneys, respectively; *6,* descending colon; *7,* small intestine; *7',* descending duodenum; *8,* pancreas; *9,* rectum; *10,* female urogenital tract; *11,* bladder. (From Singh B. *Dyce, Sack and Wensing's Textbook of Veterinary Anatomy,* 5th ed. St Louis: Elsevier; 2018.)

Note

For information on alternative modes of imaging, please see Chapters 10 to 14.

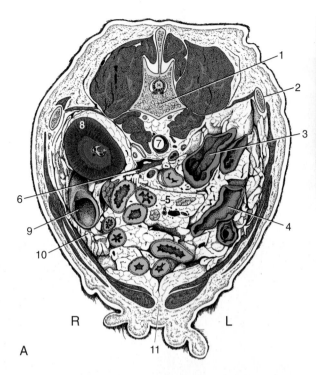

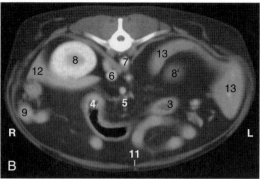

FIG. 16.12 **A,** Transverse section of the patient abdomen at the level of the first lumbar vertebra to show location. **B,** Corresponding computerized tomography (CT) scan slightly more caudal than the section shown in A; the patient was lying on its back during the CT procedure. *1,* First lumbar vertebra; *2,* last rib; *3,* descending colon; *4,* transverse colon; *5,* lymph nodes and blood vessels in mesentery, with the jejunum ventral to them; *6,* caudal vena cava; *7,* aorta, between crura of diaphragm; *8,* right kidney; *8′,* cranial pole of left kidney; *9,* descending duodenum and pancreas; *10,* greater omentum; *11,* linea alba; *12,* liver; *13,* spleen. (From Singh B. *Dyce, Sack and Wensing's Textbook of Veterinary Anatomy,* 5th ed. St Louis: Elsevier; 2018.)

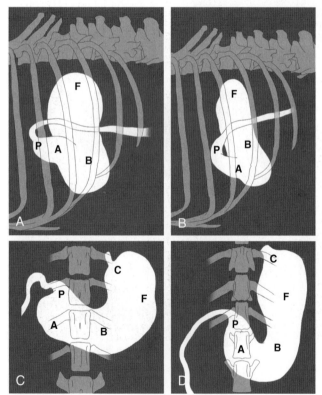

FIG. 16.13 Diagrams of normal canine or feline stomach in lateral and ventrodorsal projections. **A,** Canine stomach in lateral recumbency. **B,** Feline stomach in lateral recumbency. The gastric axis is parallel with the ribs. **C,** Canine stomach in dorsal (ventral) recumbency. The gastric axis is perpendicular to the spine, and the stomach is slightly U-shaped. **D,** Feline stomach in dorsal recumbency. The pylorus is located at the midline, and the stomach has more of an acute angle, appearing J-shaped. The major areas of the stomach are *F,* fundus; *B,* body; *A,* pyloric antrum; *P,* pyloric canal; *C,* cardia.

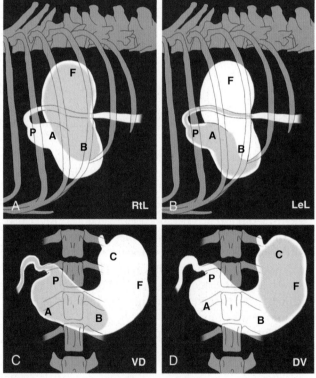

FIG. 16.14 Effects of positional changes as shown in the canine stomach, keeping in mind that air rises. **A,** Right lateral (RtL); gas is in the fundus (F) and dorsal body of the stomach (B). **B,** Left lateral (LeL); gas is in the main to distal body, pyloric antrum (A) and canal (P), and duodenum. **C,** Ventrodorsal (VD); gas is in the pyloric antrum, body near the midline, and descending duodenum. **D,** Dorsoventral (DV); gas is in the fundus and cardia (C).

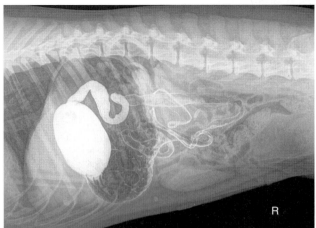

FIG. 16.15 Right lateral radiograph showing the air in the fundus and body of the stomach and barium in the pyloric region and the duodenum. Further contrast studies can be found in Chapter 23. (Courtesy Rosedale Animal Hospital.)

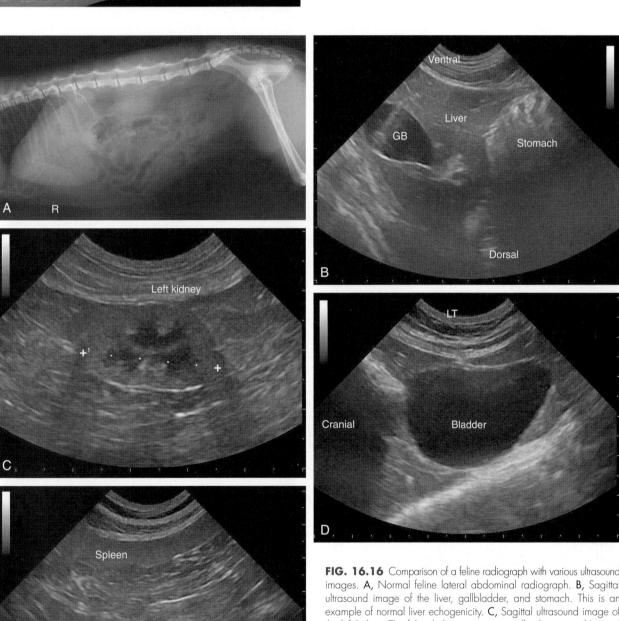

FIG. 16.16 Comparison of a feline radiograph with various ultrasound images. **A,** Normal feline lateral abdominal radiograph. **B,** Sagittal ultrasound image of the liver, gallbladder, and stomach. This is an example of normal liver echogenicity. **C,** Sagittal ultrasound image of the left kidney. This feline kidney measures smaller than normal (normal is >3 cm in length) but does have a smooth margin. **D,** Sagittal ultrasound image of the urinary bladder. This is an example of a normal urinary bladder. **E,** Sagittal ultrasound image of the spleen. This is an example of a normal feline spleen. **Note:** Although only one view is being shown here, all studies should be obtained with a minimum of two orthogonal views. (**A** courtesy Joshua M. Schlote, BS, LVT, Northeast Community College, Norfolk, Nebraska; **B** to **E** courtesy Vetel Diagnostics, San Luis Obispo, California.)

TABLE 16.1	Radiographic Anatomy With Positional Changes Using a Vertical Beam*
RADIOGRAPHIC ANATOMY	**POSITIONAL CHANGE(S)**[1–5]

Right Lateral View (See Figs. 16.2, 16.3, 16.10A, 16.14A, 16.15, 16.16)

Fundus and body of the stomach	Gas filled and in the dorsal and cranial aspects of the abdomen; fundus caudal to the left crus of the diaphragm
Pyloric antrum	Contains fluid and ingesta; soft tissue opacity ventrally, just caudal to the liver
Axis of stomach	Appears vertical
Liver	Appears larger than in left lateral; appears smaller in expiration
Spleen	Distal extremity more noticeable in dogs (caudal and slightly ventral to pylorus or liver), but may not be seen as separate structure due to overlap of the liver
Left kidney (upper)	Appears more bean shaped, is slightly magnified; caudal to right kidney
Crura of diaphragm	Appear parallel

Left Lateral View (See Figs. 16.10B, 16.14B)

Fundus	Fluid filled and difficult to identify unless filled with contrast medium
Duodenum, pyloric antrum, and canal (± body)	Gas filled
Axis of stomach	Appears vertical
Liver	Appears smaller than in right lateral
Entire shadow of spleen	May be hidden under small intestines
Right kidney (upper)	Appears larger, is more bean shaped; cranial to left kidney
Crura of diaphragm	Sometimes appear to cross

Ventrodorsal View (See Figs. 16.4B, 16.5, 16.10C, 16.12, 16.14C)

Body near midline, pyloric antrum/ descending duodenum (±)	Gas filled
Cardia, fundus	Partially fluid filled and may be difficult to see
Axis of stomach	Appears horizontal
Ascending colon and cecum	On patient's right
Descending colon	On patient's left
Colon	Question mark shape
Spleen	Left craniodorsal abdomen, under liver. The proximal extremity appears as a small triangle caudolateral to fundus of stomach, medial to the body wall, and craniolateral to left kidney
Right kidney	Cranial to left kidney

Dorsoventral View (See Figs. 16.10D, 16.12, 16.14D)

Fundus and cardia	Gas filled and caudal to the left diaphragmatic crus
Ventral part of the body and the pyloric antrum	Difficult to see; filled with fluid
Axis of stomach	Appears horizontal
Ascending colon and cecum	On patient's right
Descending colon	On patient's left
Colon	Question mark shape
Spleen	On left, under liver; appears as small triangle caudal to fundus of stomach
Right kidney	Cranial to left kidney

*Due to a variety of other factors the appearance may not always be as described in the table.

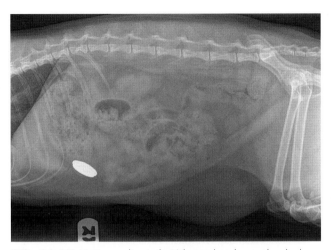

FIG. 16.17 Mystery radiograph. What is the abnormal radiodense material, and where do you think it is located? (Courtesy Rosedale Animal Hospital.)

✳ KEY POINTS

1. The lack of natural contrast inherent in the abdomen necessitates particular attention to appropriate exposure factors for proper diagnosis.
2. As with other body areas, correct positioning and technique are required for proper interpretation. This includes where to measure and center, what to include, and how to ensure that the positioning shows proper symmetry.
3. Routine positions for the abdomen are the right lateral (generally) and VD.
4. Proper positioning is essential to minimize misdiagnosis. Knowledge of normal radiography assists in ensuring that perfect radiographs are presented.
5. Not all abdominal organs are visible radiographically, so other modalities such as ultrasound, magnetic resonance imaging, and computerized tomography may be required to view the abdomen, as well as to further augment diagnosis of visible radiographic structures.

REVIEW QUESTIONS

1. The normal radiographic views of the abdomen are generally the:
   a. Left lateral and ventrodorsal
   b. Left lateral and dorsoventral
   c. Right lateral and dorsoventral
   d. Right lateral and ventrodorsal
2. Abdominal radiographs are best taken at:
   a. Maximum inspiration
   b. Maximum expiration
   c. Midinspiration
   d. Midexpiration
3. For positioning of a deep-chested dog, the head of the dog should be toward the:
   a. Cathode
   b. Anode

4. How should the hind limbs be positioned for a regular right lateral abdomen view?
   a. The right limb should be slightly forward and the left limb as far back as possible.
   b. The left limb should be slightly forward and the right limb as far back as possible.
   c. Both limbs should be pulled cranially and superimposed.
   d. Both limbs should be pulled slightly caudally and superimposed.
5. To ensure that there is symmetry in your final ventrodorsal radiograph of the abdomen:
   a. The rib heads, transverse processes, and coxofemoral joints should be superimposed
   b. The intervertebral foramina should be the same size
   c. The sternum and spine are superimposed
   d. The transverse processes are superimposed and appear as Nike swooshes
6. When measuring and centering for a ventrodorsal canine abdomen, you should:
   a. Measure and center over the caudal aspect of the 13th rib
   b. Measure and center at the level of T13
   c. Measure at T13 but center over the caudal aspect of the 13th rib
   d. Center at T13 but measure over the caudal aspect of the 13th rib
7. You have collimated for this VD radiograph 1 inch cranial to the xiphoid of the sternum and have included the coxofemoral joints. This is:
   a. Correct because the VD should include these peripheral borders
   b. Incorrect because the cranial border does not need to include the diaphragm
   c. Incorrect because the image does not need to extend caudally to the hip joint
   d. Incorrect because the image only needs to be from the edge of the liver to the bladder
8. You are ready to take the image and are breathing with your patient so that you will properly depress the exposure button during this VD canine abdomen at:
   a. Mid-expiration
   b. Peak inspiration
   c. The beginning of inspiration
   d. The end of expiration
9. The veterinarian had asked you to apply gentle pressure in this VD abdomen with a wooden paddle to isolate what she suspects might be a tumor. You do so and find the radiograph is darker with less contrast than your original one without any applied pressure. This is because you used:
   a. A grid for this image and not the first one
   b. Less kVp than your first image
   c. The same setting for both images
   d. A thicker measurement than the first image

10. The veterinarian asks you to image a beagle in which he suspects peritonitis. You do have an adjustable tube head unit. In order to properly evaluate whether there is fluid in the abdomen, you should place your patient in:
    a. VD position and utilize a vertical beam
    b. Dorsal recumbency and utilize a horizontal beam
    c. Ventral recumbency and utilize a horizontal beam
    d. Right lateral recumbency and utilize a horizontal beam

11. The veterinarian wants you to take a modified lateral of a golden retriever. The hind limbs should be:
    a. Pulled as cranially as possible to cause rotation of the body off the table
    b. Positioned perpendicular to the spine to prevent crowding in the caudoventral abdomen
    c. Pulled as cranially as possible without causing rotation of the body off the table
    d. Caudally with the upper limb raised and out of the field of view

12. The settings for your 12-cm abdomen of a bulldog that will not be sedated are 60 kV and 10 mAs. You are best to use:
    a. 400 mA and $\frac{1}{40}$ of a second
    b. 300 mA and $\frac{1}{30}$ of a second
    c. 200 mA and $\frac{1}{20}$ of a second
    d. 100 mA and $\frac{1}{10}$ of a second

13. In a right lateral view as opposed to a left lateral abdomen:
    a. There is greater longitudinal separation of the kidneys
    b. The fundus and body of the stomach are closer to the film
    c. The liver appears slightly smaller
    d. The axis of the stomach is more vertical

14. The veterinarian asks you to complete a ventrodorsal view with a horizontal beam. If the patient is lying on its right side, this view is properly termed:
    a. Right lateral
    b. Right decubitus
    c. Left decubitus
    d. Ventrodorsal

15. The veterinarian asks you to complete a series of abdominal radiographs. You inadvertently left the markers off. The image in front of you shows the duodenum, pyloric antrum, and distal body of the stomach filled with gas and the axis of the stomach appearing vertical. This view is likely a:
    a. Ventrodorsal
    b. Left lateral
    c. Right lateral
    d. Dorsoventral

References

1. Thrall DE. *Textbook of Veterinary Diagnostic Radiology.* 6th ed. St. Louis: Elsevier; 2013 [Chapters 35-45].
2. Muhlbauer MC, Kneller SK. *Radiography of the Dog and Cat: Guide to Making and Interpreting Radiographs.* Oxford: Wiley-Blackwell; 2013 [Chapter 6].
3. Holloway A. *BSAVA Manual of Canine and Feline Radiography and Radiology: A Foundation Manual.* Suffolk: BSAVA.; 2013 [Chapter 6].
4. Morgan JP, Doval J, Samii V. *Radiographic Techniques: The Dog.* Hannover: Schlutersche GmbH & Co.; 1998.
5. Owens JM, Biery DN. *Radiographic Interpretation for the Small Animal Clinician.* St. Louis: Ralston Purina; 1999.

Bibliography

Aspinall V, Cappello M. *Introduction to Veterinary Anatomy.* 3rd ed. London: Butterman-Heineman; 2015.

Ayers S. *Small Animal Radiographic Techniques and Positioning.* Oxford: Wiley-Blackwell; 2013.

Colville T, Bassert J. *Clinical Anatomy and Physiology for Veterinary Technicians.* 3rd ed. St. Louis: Mosby; 2016.

Done SH, Goody PC, Stickland NC, et al. *Color Atlas of Veterinary Anatomy, the Dog and Cat.* London: Mosby; 2009.

Dyce KM, Sack WO, Wensing CJG. *Textbook of Veterinary Anatomy.* 4th ed. St. Louis: Saunders; 2010.

Evans H, de Launta A. *Guide to the Dissection of the Dog.* 8th ed. St. Louis: Saunders; 2017.

Han C, Hurd C. *Practical Diagnostic Imaging for the Veterinary Technician.* 3rd ed. St. Louis: Mosby; 2005.

Romich J. *An Illustrated Guide to Veterinary Medical Terminology.* 4th ed. Stamford, CT: Cengage Learning; 2015.

Ryan G. *Radiographic Positioning of Small Animals.* Philadelphia: Lea & Febiger; 1981.

Sirois M. *Principles and Practice of Veterinary Technology.* 3rd ed. St. Louis: Mosby; 2011.

Sirois M, Anthony E, Mauragis D. *Handbook of Radiographic Positioning for Veterinary Technicians.* Clifton Park, NY: Delmar Cengage Learning; 2010.

Smallwood JE, Shively MJ, Rendano VT, et al. A standardized nomenclature for radiographic projections used in veterinary medicine. *Vet Rad.* 1985;26:2-9.

Ticer J. *Radiographic Technique in Small Animal Practice.* Philadelphia: WB Saunders; 1984.

Tighe M, Brown M. *Mosby's Comprehensive Review for Veterinary Technicians.* 4th ed. St. Louis: Elsevier; 2015.

Answers to Review Questions can be found on the Evolve website.

CHAPTER 17

Small Animal Thorax

Marg Brown, RVT, BEd Ad Ed

A good head and a good heart are always a formidable combination.
—Nelson Mandela, South African antiapartheid activist and president, 1918–2013

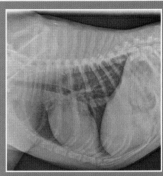

(Courtesy Jenn White, Mississauga Oakville Veterinary Emergency Hospital and Referral Group, Oakville, Ontario.)

OUTLINE

LEARNING OBJECTIVES

When you have finished this chapter, you will be able to:

1. Properly and safely position a dog or cat for the common thoracic views with an emphasis on nonmanual restraint.
2. Correctly measure and center the patient to include the peripheral borders.
3. Ensure that the thorax is parallel to the image receptor and the central ray is perpendicular to the field of view (FOV).
4. Be familiar with views that may need to be completed as an alternative.
5. Identify normal thoracic radiographic anatomy.

KEY TERMS

Key terms are defined in the Glossary on the Evolve website.

Atelectasis
Dependent
Diaphragmatic crura
Heel effect

Hemithorax
Hilar region
Horizontal beam

Mediastinum
Object-film distance (OFD)
Opaque/radiopaque

Orthogonal
Parenchyma
Positional terminology

TECHNICAL NOTE: To preserve space, the radiographs presented in this chapter do not show collimation. For safety, always collimate so that the beam is limited to within the image receptor edges. In film radiography, you should see a clear border of collimation (frame) on every radiograph. In some jurisdictions, evidence of collimation is the law.

Thoracic radiography is a common diagnostic procedure in small-animal practice, with specific indications including suspicion of heart disease, pneumonia, or neoplasia (primary or metastatic) and treatment or disease follow-up.

Radiographic and Positioning Concerns

- High-quality images require emphasis on accurate positioning and centering of the x-ray beam, with appropriate collimation. A symmetrical image is essential, as any displacement of the x-ray beam or rotation of the patient will cause marked changes in the imaging of the thoracic anatomy.

- There should be a minimum of two orthogonal views: either a lateral view or a ventrodorsal/dorsoventral (VD/DV) view; however, further views are often required for proper diagnosis. Diagnosis can be missed if enough views are not taken. Keep in mind that because of the increased opacity of the dependent lateral lung due to recumbency-associated atelectasis, the lateral view appears more opaque than the VD/DV views, so orthogonal views should always be used to rule out suspected lung disease simply caused by atelectasis.[1] Consider taking the DV/VD view first to minimize the length of time that the patient has been lying in lateral recumbency.

- If pneumonia is suspected, both lateral views (right and left) are recommended in addition to a VD view.[1-3] If cardiac disease is suspected, either a right or left lateral and DV views are often imaged. For a metastasis examination, both lateral views (right and left) and a VD or DV view are recommended.

- On rare occasions, a further view to consider is the DV or VD oblique view, made at 20 to 30 degrees from center. This angle moves the area of interest away from the spine or cardiac shadow and may help identify rib lesions or pulmonary lesions in the hilar region. Decubital views may also be required as needed to rule out disease process.

- The protocol and patient preparation are the same for both dogs and cats (Fig. 17.1). Make sure the patient has a clean, dry hair coat, and remove collars or leashes. A thick hair coat, especially the matted hair of cats, can cause prominent artifacts. Animals are best sedated or anesthetized to avoid manual restraint.

- Patients in respiratory distress and geriatric patients may require more sternal time, flow by oxygen, and breaks. Critically ill patients can decompensate at any time, so it is essential to have any supplies and emergency drugs specific to their needs easily accessible. Monitoring is critical for these patients.

- The thorax is best radiographed in film/screen systems using a long contrast scale with many shades of gray, which is obtained with higher kilovoltage (kV) and lower milliampere-seconds (mAs). Correct exposures are critical, as underexposure may lead to an incorrect diagnosis of interstitial opacification, and overexposure or images taken with oversaturated digital systems can hide subtle lung

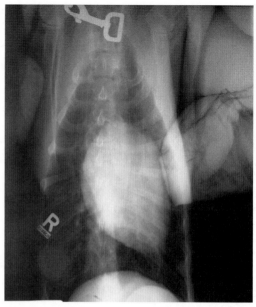

FIG. 17.1 Make sure the patient has a clean, dry hair coat, and remove collars or leashes. Artifacts on this radiograph include the marker, sandbags, and leash clip.

lesions or lead to a false diagnosis of pneumothorax. If a mediastinal mass or pleural fluid is suspected, increase the kVp exposure by 15% to 20%.

- Contrast and density in the digital system can be manipulated after the image is obtained, so exact exposures are not as critical digitally, although the closer to the correct technique, the better the image.

- Grids should be considered for measurements over 10 cm to minimize scattered radiation on the film that decreases contrast further.

- Once the mAs has been determined, use the highest mA and shortest time possible to minimize respiratory motion artifacts that can induce blurring.

- Exposure should be taken at peak inspiration by increasing aeration of the lung field so there is maximum contrast between the gas-filled lungs and soft tissue pulmonary structures. There is also greater separation of the cardiac silhouette and diaphragm at peak inspiration, especially in the lateral view. Panting is not uncommon. Holding the patient's mouth shut as the preexposure button is depressed and then releasing at the time of exposure may assist in having the dog take a deep breath so that the image is exposed at peak inspiration.

- Sedated and overweight animals often do not ventilate as fully as nonsedated animals, leading to possible misinterpretation of an alveolar pattern or interstitial pattern. If the patient is connected to the anesthetic machine, positive ventilation can be applied to synchronize inspiration with the exposure time.

- The full lung field needs to be included, from the cranial thoracic inlet to the most caudodorsal lung field. Keep in mind that the thorax is inside the rib cage so include the full rib cage. Generally a 14 × 17 plate will accommodate most large dogs, but if a dog is too large to allow full inclusion of the lung field on one image, each view may have to be divided into cranial and caudal sections.

- Because of the massive shoulder muscles, use the heel effect to advantage by having the thickest part toward the cathode, especially in medium and larger dogs. The cranial thoracic vertebrae are underexposed due to overlying shoulders.
- Diagnostic-quality thoracic radiographs are obtained by using short exposure times ($\frac{1}{60}$ second or less), making the exposure at peak inspiration, and using strict positioning, especially on the VD/DV projection.
- Keep in mind that any image is only an instantaneous picture of the thorax in a particular point in time.

Table 17.1 lists the protocol for thoracic radiography.

TABLE 17.1	Protocol for Thoracic Radiography
VIEW	**PROTOCOL**
Routine	Right and/or left lateral
	Dorsoventral and/or ventrodorsal
Ancillary	Lateral decubitus view
	Alternate lateral views with a horizontal beam:
	Standing lateral
	Lateral recumbent view
	Dorsoventral or ventrodorsal 20-30 degrees oblique
	Dorsoventral—thoracic inlet view
	Expiratory radiographs

TECHNICIAN NOTES

Always measure the animal in the position in which it is to be imaged to avoid incorrect settings.

TECHNICIAN NOTES

Strategically used positioning aids give the patient the illusion that it is being held. A sandbag over the neck and limbs and/or the use of tape is essential if the patient is not properly sedated. Have the room darker; use slow, methodical movements; keep speaking in a low, calm voice; and take advantage of the behavioral characteristics of the patient.

TECHNICIAN NOTES

With exceptions, generally consider the DV position to image the heart and the VD position to image the lungs.

TECHNICIAN NOTES

Collimate, ensuring that labels/markers are included and borders are visible for every image.

TECHNICIAN NOTES

Good-quality thoracic radiographs[1,3] have the following characteristics:
- Primary x-ray beam centered on the heart
- Include all the ribs between the sternum and spine
- No rotation
- No motion artifacts
- Exposed at peak inspiration
- Proper contrast and density to evaluate the heart and lungs adequately

The lateral view is properly positioned when:
- Rib heads are superimposed and ribs do not extend dorsal to the spine
- Dorsal spinal processes are faintly visible through scapulae
- Intervertebral foramina are the same size
- Transverse processes are superimposed at the origin from the vertebral bodies, appearing as Nike swooshes[1]
- Ribs over the heart are superimposed and faintly visible over the cardiac silhouette
- Costochondral junctions are at the same level

The DV/VD view is properly positioned when:
- Sternum and spine are superimposed
- Ribs and thorax are symmetrical so that the distance from the central spine is equidistant to both sides of the thoracic wall
- The intervertebral spaces are underexposed over the heart but visible cranial to the heart
- Vertebral bodies are visible over the cardiac silhouette
- Dorsal spinous processes do not extend beyond the lateral edges of the vertebral bodies

Positions

Lateral Thorax—Routine

> ✎ **TECHNICIAN NOTES**
>
> The thorax is inside the rib cage, so include the full rib cage on the image.

If only one lateral is required, personal preference dictates the view. Most right-handed imagers prefer that the patient be lying on its right side, producing a right lateral view. The left lateral view makes distinguishing between right and left cranial lobe pulmonary vessels easier (because there is no superimposition of other structures[3]), as well as more accurately determining relative vessel size.

When a patient is in lateral recumbency, the dependent lung is more perfused and less inflated than the nondependent lung. Atelectasis of the downward lung occurs in less than 5 minutes due to the effects of gravity,[3] the heart compressing the lung, less movement of the dependent rib cage due to the compression, and cranial movement of the dependent portion of the diaphragm.[1] Thus when a patient is in right lateral recumbency, lesions may be obscured in the lung on the right side. Aeration of the upper lobes enhances contrast, so if a lesion is suspected in the right lung, a left lateral should be taken, and vice versa. In addition, increased object-film distance (OFD) will magnify the lesion, which may further assist diagnosis.

Technically the correct terminology for the right lateral is *left-right lateral* if one considers "point of entrance to point of exit"; however, this term is not generally used (see Figs. 17.3A and 17.4A) in small animals. Instead only the side that the patient is lying on is included, so the patient would be lying on its right side for a right lateral.

Radiographs should be taken at maximum inspiration. If required, radiographs taken during expiration may aid in detection of small amounts of pleural fluid or pneumothorax, as well as in the diagnosis of tracheal or bronchial collapse (Figs. 17.2 through 17.8).[1]

Positioning

Place In: Right or left lateral recumbency.

Head: Keep in a natural position. Hold appropriately with a sandbag over the neck so as not to restrict breathing.

Forelimbs: Pull as far cranially as possible without rotating the thorax. Place a small foam pad between the forelimbs to help eliminate rotation of the thorax, and support with a sandbag.

Hind Limbs: Pull together caudally; place a small foam pad between the limbs if needed, and support with a sandbag.

Sternum: Elevate with wedged foam pads so it is at the same plane as the thoracic vertebrae to eliminate rotation.

MEASURE: Caudal border of the scapula over the thickest part of the thorax.

CENTRAL RAY: At the caudal border of the scapula, between the fifth and sixth ribs (where you feel the strongest heartbeat), approximately midway between the spine and sternum.

BORDERS: Spine, sternum, and palpate from the cranial point of the scapulohumeral articulation (thoracic inlet) to a few centimeters caudal past the last rib (the thorax is inside the rib cage, so include all the ribs).

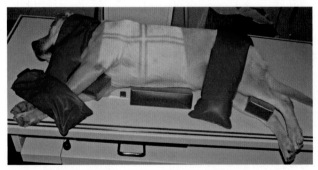

FIG. 17.2 Positioning for the lateral thorax view. Place positioning devices appropriately to eliminate rotation of the thorax. The marker should be placed cranially and ventrally. It can be placed under the foam pad. (Courtesy Seneca College of Applied Arts and Technology, King City, Ontario.)

Lateral Thorax—Routine—cont'd

Comments and Tips

- Place any identification (ID) or markers on the ventral aspect of the abdomen near the axilla.
- Ensure that the sternum is parallel to the table and at the same level as the vertebrae and that the beam is perpendicular to both. Rotation of the sternum may separate the mainstream bronchi mimicking left atrial enlargement or a heart mass.[3]
- The forelimbs need to be pulled as far cranially as possible without causing rotation to prevent any superimposition of the brachium muscles over the cranial lung field.
- Expose immediately at full inspiration.
- If your patient is critically ill or compromised, make sure to have any emergency supplies or equipment close at hand and constantly assess and monitor the patient.
- In addition to positioning devices, folds of skin, nipples, and fatty masses ventral to the sternum can cause artifacts (see Fig. 17.5).

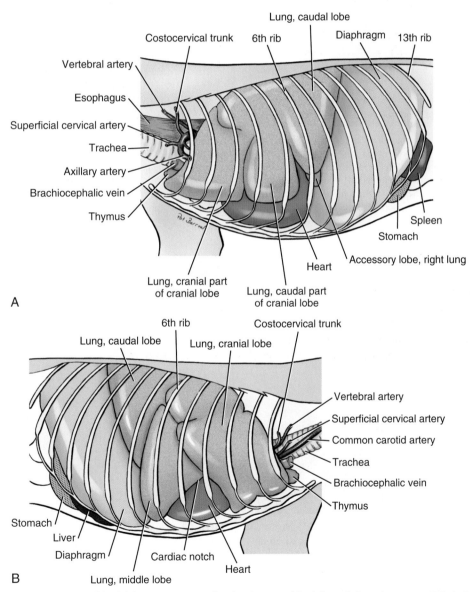

FIG. 17.3 A, Diagram of the left thoracic viscera within the rib cage of this left-to-right lateral projection (RtL). B, Diagram of the right thoracic viscera within the rib cage of this right-to-left lateral projection (LeL). (From Dyce KM, Sack WO, Wensing CJG. *Textbook of Veterinary Anatomy*, 4th ed. St. Louis: Saunders; 2010.)

Continued

Lateral Thorax—Routine—cont'd

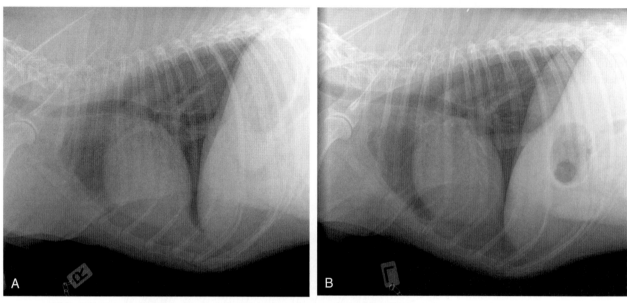

FIG. 17.4 A, Radiograph of the right lateral thorax in inspiration. The thorax is inside the rib cage. In a normal average dog, the heart measured at the base is about 2½ to 3½ times the width of an intercostal space, depending on the breed. In comparison with the left lateral view, the heart base appears more conical or oval on the right lateral view. **B,** Radiograph of the left lateral thorax in inspiration. Note that on the left lateral view, the apex of the cardiac silhouette is displaced from the sternum, making the overall cardiac shape appear more rounded than on the right lateral view. (Courtesy Jennifer White, Mississauga Oakville Veterinary Emergency Hospital and Referral Group, Oakville, Ontario.)

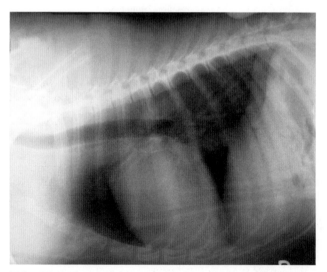

FIG. 17.5 The parallel horizontal lines over the ventral portion are folds of skin. Nipples, papillomas, or fatty masses can also cause artifacts.

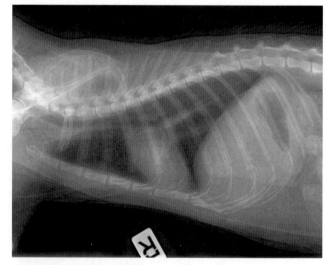

FIG. 17.6 Right lateral radiograph of the feline thorax. The apex is usually more pointed in a cat than in a dog. Normal width is two intercostal spaces. (Courtesy Jennifer White, Mississauga Oakville Veterinary Emergency Hospital and Referral Group, Oakville, Ontario.)

Lateral Thorax—Routine—cont'd

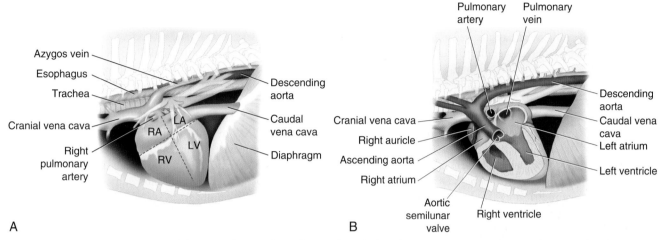

FIG. 17.7 Anatomy of the canine heart and vessels. **A,** Left-to-right lateral (RtL) projection. Note the vertical waist at the junction of the cranial vena cava and the right atrium and the horizontal waist at the atrioventricular groove at the junction of the left atrium and left ventricle, dividing the heart into the four chambers. *A,* atrium; *L,* left; *R,* right; *V,* ventricle. **B,** Right-to-left lateral projection (LeL).

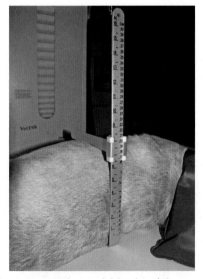

FIG. 17.8 Measure at the caudal border of the scapula over the thickest part. In a thick, muscled dog, the thickest part should be toward the cathode to take advantage of the heel effect.

> ### ✎ TECHNICIAN NOTES
>
> Inspiration is required to inflate the lungs and provide better contrast between the soft tissues of the thorax and air in the lungs.
>
> To obtain maximum inspiration from the patient:
> - Breathe with the patient, and depress the rotor of a two-step system at the point of either expiration or partial inspiration (depending on the patient's respiratory rate). Press the second stage at maximum inspiration.
> - If the patient has an endotracheal tube (ET), squeeze the anesthetic bag or use an Ambu bag (bag valve mask).
> - If the patient is not sedated and will tolerate it, administer a puff of air in its face either by blowing or using an Ambu bag, and then watch for maximum inspiration.

> ### ✎ TECHNICIAN NOTES
>
> Quickly go through your mental check list *before* pushing the exposure button; the checklist includes, but is not limited to, the following:
> - Settings correct
> - Image receptor/grid in position
> - Proper location of markers and ID (if using at this stage)
> - Correct body part and view
> - Properly measured and centered
> - Borders correct and collimated
> - Thickest part to the cathode
> - Patient properly prepared, positioned, and restrained so the thorax will be perpendicular to the central ray and parallel to the image receptor
> - Maximum inspiration

Ventrodorsal Thorax—Routine

The VD thorax view is suggested for images of the lung, ventral pulmonary fields, cranial and caudal mediastinum, accessory lung lobes, and caudal vena cava, as well as in cases of pleural effusion. Changes in the descending aorta and great vessels are more noticeable in the VD than in the DV, and the accessory lung lobe is better aerated to allow for more accurate assessment of the caudal mediastinal or for accessory lobe pathology. In severely ill animals, a VD view may cause compression of remaining functional lung fields. If your patient is critically ill or compromised, make sure to have any emergency supplies or equipment close at hand and constantly assess and monitor the patient. The VD is often easier to position more symmetrically than the DV, especially in cats.

Positioning

Place In: Dorsal recumbency in a radiolucent V-trough if needed.

Head: Pull gently forward. Carefully position a sandbag over the head and neck, being sure not to restrict breathing. Keep the head straight and nose parallel to the table.

Forelimbs: Extend cranially with the nose between them. Secure with sandbags. If a sandbag is positioned proximal to the elbows over the limbs, the head and neck can also be held in place. An alternative is to either tie each limb separately or to place a sandbag over each limb at the carpus.

Hind Limbs: Keep the hind limbs in a natural position and support with sandbags.

MEASURE: Over the caudal border of the scapula at the highest point of the sternum.

CENTRAL RAY: Midline over the superimposed spine and sternum at the caudal margin of the scapula or between the fifth and sixth ribs.

BORDERS: Cranial point of the scapulohumeral articulation (thoracic inlet) to a few centimeters caudal past the last rib (the thorax is inside the rib cage, so include all the ribs).

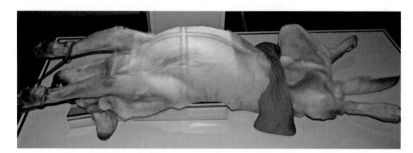

FIG. 17.9 Positioning of the ventrodorsal thorax is generally suggested for views of the lung. The forelimbs are pulled cranially. Make sure there is no rotation of the thorax. (Courtesy Joshua Schlote, BS, LVT, Northeast Community College.)

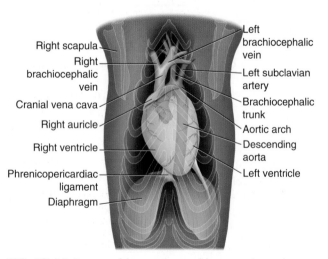

FIG. 17.10 Diagram of the ventral view of the canine thorax showing the heart (VD).

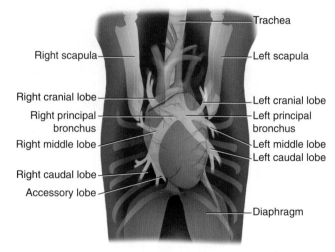

FIG. 17.11 Diagram of the ventral view of the canine bronchial tree in the ventrodorsal position.

Ventrodorsal Thorax—Routine—cont'd

Comments and Tips

- Place any ID or markers adjacent to the appropriate side of the thorax near the axilla.
- Positioning devices in the area of interest may affect the image.
- Evenly position the body so that the two sides of the rib cage appear equidistant.
- Ideally a straight line should be imagined connecting the point of the nose with the caudal midline.

- Ensure that the sternum and spine are superimposed; they should not be seen as separate structures; the central ray is perpendicular to both.
- Expose immediately at full inspiration.
- A nonroutine VD thoracic view can also be taken with the thoracic limbs pulled caudally. This is used to rotate the scapula and associated muscles away from the cranial thorax to aid in evaluation of the mediastinum, lungs, and pleura.[3]
- In large-breed dogs, a cranial and caudal image may be required.

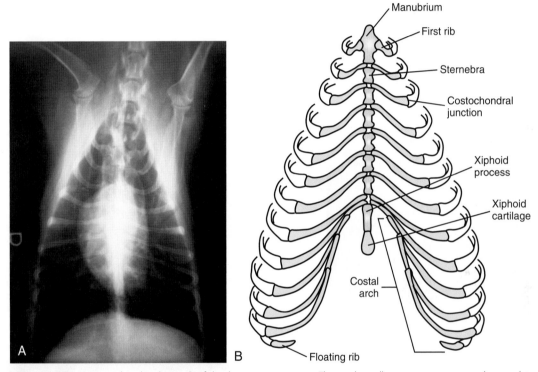

FIG. 17.12 A, Ventrodorsal radiograph of the thorax in inspiration. The cardiac silhouette appears more elongated in the VD than the DV because of increased object-film distance (OFD). **B,** Canine costal cartilages and sternum. Include the full rib cage in thoracic images.

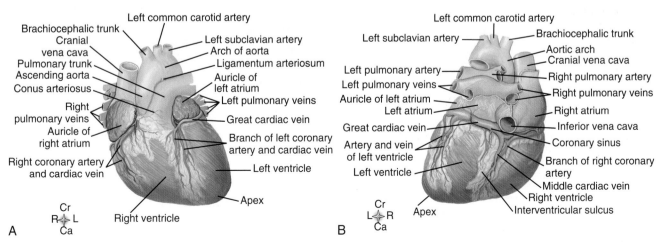

FIG. 17.13 Diagrams of the heart and great vessels. **A,** Ventral view. **B,** Dorsal view. (From Patton KT, Thibodeau GA: *Anatomy and Physiology,* 9th ed, St Louis: Saunders; 2016.)

Dorsoventral Thorax—Routine

The DV thorax view is generally considered the best position for the heart, which will lie in a more natural position. This offers a consistent cardiac silhouette, evaluation of the pulmonary lobar vessels, and better evaluation of the structures in the dorsal thorax, such as hilar lymph nodes, the caudal dorsal lungs, trachea, mainstem bronchi, and left atrium.[3] The DV view is also helpful for evaluating pneumothorax[4] and should be used for patients in respiratory distress (Figs. 17.14 and 17.15).

Positioning

Place In: Ventral recumbency in a radiolucent V-trough if needed.

Head: Gently pull forward, and carefully place a sandbag over the neck and head so it is not in the field of view. The chin can be supported on a pad to keep the cervical vertebrae at the same plane.

Forelimbs: Extend cranially. Slightly supinate the paws so that the elbows are together and the scapulae lie lateral to the lung field. Place sandbags over the limbs to maintain position.

Hind Limbs: Keep in a natural position, and sandbag.

MEASURE: Over the caudal border of the scapula or at the highest point.

CENTRAL RAY: Midline at the caudal margin of the scapula or between the fifth and sixth ribs.

BORDERS: Spine dorsally, sternum ventrally; palpate from the cranial point of the scapulohumeral articulation (thoracic inlet) to a few centimeters caudal past the last rib (the thorax is inside the rib cage, so include all the ribs).

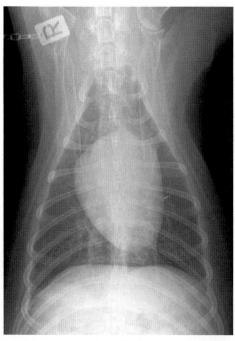

FIG. 17.14 Dorsoventral radiograph of the thorax in inspiration. Include from the shoulder joint to the first lumbar vertebra. The right side of the heart appears more rounded than in a VD position. The diaphragm is displaced cranially and generally only has one convex shape (the cupula) projecting into the thorax in the DV. This displacement tends to push the heart cranially and into the left hemithorax.[4] Air is noted in the fundus. (Courtesy Jennifer White, Mississauga Oakville Veterinary Emergency Hospital and Referral Group, Oakville, Ontario.)

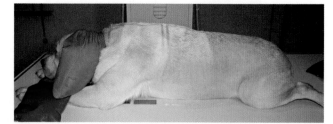

FIG. 17.15 Positioning for the dorsoventral thorax view. Because the heart lies in a more natural position, this view is generally preferred over the VD for the heart. Make sure there is no rotation.

Dorsoventral Thorax—Routine—cont'd

Comments and Tips

- Place any ID or markers near the axilla in the collimated area.
- Ensure that the body is evenly positioned so that the two sides of the rib cage appear equidistant.
- Keep the head straight. Ideally, a straight line should be imagined connecting the point of the nose with the caudal midline.
- Ensure that the sternum and spine are superimposed; the central ray is perpendicular to both.
- Expose immediately at full inspiration.
- If the limbs cannot be supinated, the forelimbs can be positioned with the elbows lateral to the thoracic inlet. This is easier, but the scapulae will be superimposed over the lung field.
- A slippery table may make a patient anxious, so consider using a radiolucent foam mat, towel, or sandbags surrounding the paws to help the patient feel more secure.
- If the patient is critically ill or compromised, make sure to have any emergency supplies or equipment close at hand and constantly assess and monitor the patient.
- There is a suggestion that the DV is not more accurate for evaluating heart disease as long as the difference in positioning is accounted for.[1]

> ✎ **TECHNICIAN NOTES**
>
> A common mistake is to center too far caudally. Center directly over the heart (palpate) and make sure to include cranially from the shoulder joint. Include the full rib cage.

Ancillary Views

Horizontal Beam Radiography—Ancillary

The x-ray tube is positioned so that the x-ray beam is horizontal across the table. The patient may be in lateral, ventral, or dorsal recumbency or may be standing. The horizontal beam is used to verify fluid or free air, or for a patient that would be compromised if placed in the VD or DV position. The horizontal beam can be helpful if fluid is to be removed from an area or to identify a mass. Sharp fluid lines will be noticed in horizontal beam radiographs only if there is a free fluid–free gas interchange.[1] If free air is suspected, keep the patient in position at least 5 minutes before exposure to allow dorsal collection of the air.[4]

General Comments and Tips for the Horizontal Views

- The side or position that the patient is lying on is referred to as *decubitus*, and the beam is parallel to the horizon.

- Place the image receptor vertically behind and close to the patient, using a positioner if needed. In some cases it is easier to drop the cassette slightly below the level of the table top.
- This view is not possible in digital units unless the plate is removable.
- Place the marker cranial to the axilla indicating the side closest to the image receptor within the collimated area.
- Expose at full inspiration.
- The correct source image distance must be used.

> ### ✎ TECHNICIAN NOTES
>
> The term *decubitus* means lying down, so in radiology a right lateral decubitus view means the patient is lying on its right side and the x-ray beam is parallel to the horizon. This is for an alternative VD or DV view depending on the beam direction.

Lateral Decubitus View (Ventrodorsal View With Horizontal Beam)—Ancillary

Positioning, Comments, and Tips

- Position as for lateral recumbency (Fig. 17.16) except that the patient should be on a thick foam pad or equivalent to allow the dependent portion of the thorax to be in the field of view.
- The position is described according to which side of the patient is closer to the table (i.e., right decubitus if it is lying on its right side).

- The horizontal beam will be directed in a VD direction, entering the sternum and exiting the vertebrae.
- Ensure that the sternum and spine are on the same plane.

MEASURE: Caudal border of the scapula over the thickest part of the thorax.
CENTRAL RAY: At the caudal border of the scapula, between the fifth and sixth ribs approximately midway between the superimposed spine and sternum.
BORDERS: Palpate from the cranial point of the scapulohumeral articulation (thoracic inlet) to a few centimeters caudal past the last rib (the thorax is inside the rib cage, so include all the ribs).

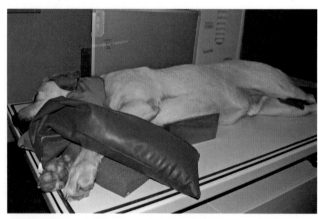

FIG. 17.16 Positioning for the lateral decubitus view (ventrodorsal view with horizontal beam). The beam enters as for a VD. The patient is best raised with a foam pad, or the cassette can be positioned lower than the table. (Courtesy Seneca College of Applied Arts and Technology, King City, Ontario.)

Dorsoventral or Ventrodorsal Decubitus View (Horizontal Beam Lateral Radiograph)—Ancillary

Positioning, Comments, and Tips

- Use gravitational markers such as a Mitchell marker.
- **Dorsoventral Decubitus View:** Position as for a DV view with the patient in ventral recumbency on a thick foam pad or equivalent. Use a radiolucent V-trough if needed.
- **Ventrodorsal Decubitus View:** Position as for a VD view with the patient in dorsal recumbency on a thick foam pad or equivalent. Use a radiolucent V-trough if needed.

- The beam will be directed horizontally through the patient laterally.
- Ensure that the body is evenly positioned so that the sternum and vertebrae are superimposed; the image receptor and central ray are perpendicular to both.
- Ideally a straight line should be imagined connecting the point of the nose with the caudal midline.

Standing Lateral View (With a Horizontal Beam)—Ancillary

Positioning, Comments, and Tips

- Have the patient in a natural standing position. There will be superimposition of the shoulder musculature over the cranial lung field. See Fig. 17.17.
- The beam will be directed horizontally through the patient laterally.

- The position is described as a standing right or left lateral, with the marker placed cranial to the axilla within the collimated area indicating the side against the image receptor.
- Use gravitational markers such as a Mitchell marker.

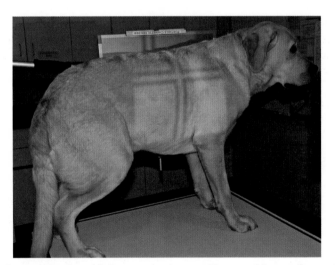

FIG. 17.17 Positioning for a standing lateral (LeL) view with a horizontal beam and the use of a portable cassette holder.

Ventrodorsal Oblique View—Ancillary

The position is designed to see lesions of the thoracic wall and pleura that may be obscured because of overlying tissue or the tangential or perpendicular angle of the beam.[3]

Positioning, Comments, and Tips

- Measure and position as for VD.
- Then rotate the sternum away from the side of interest. The x-ray beam is centered on the lesion.
- Utilize peripheral borders as needed.

Dorsoventral Thoracic Inlet View—Ancillary

The purpose of this view is to see the thoracic inlet without superimposition of the shoulder musculature. This position can be used for contrast studies of the esophagus to note the cross-sectional appearance of trachea[4] and is sometimes referred to as *the skyline or craniodorsal-caudoventral view.*[3]

Positioning

Place In: Ventral recumbency in a radiolucent V-trough if needed.

Forelimbs: Extend cranially in a natural position, and place a sandbag over the limbs.

Hind Limbs: Keep in a natural flexed position.

Head: Hyperextend the head so that the nose is pointing up and caudal; secure with tape to keep in position.

Comments and Tips

- Place any ID or markers in the collimated area.
- Ensure the body is evenly positioned so that both sides of the rib cage appear equidistant.
- Ensure that the sternum and spine are superimposed.
- Expose at expiration.
- The imaging technique should be decreased because of decreased tissue density.

MEASURE: Place the calipers between the ventral thoracic inlet and sternum just caudal to the limbs.

CENTRAL RAY: Over the thoracic inlet at a 45-degree craniocaudal angle. The beam will be directed ventrally to the neck.

BORDERS: Cranial point of the scapulohumeral articulation (thoracic inlet) to the caudal border of the scapula.

Further Information

Patient Positioning Changes and Anatomy Concerns

Variation in patient position, as well as the phase of respiration, does alter the radiographic appearance (Figs. 17.18 through 17.20). These changes are more prominent in medium and larger dogs and less so in cats and small dogs. Being familiar with these changes will assist you in providing diagnostic images.

Effect of Positional Changes and Phase of Respiration on Thoracic Radiographs

See Table 17.2.

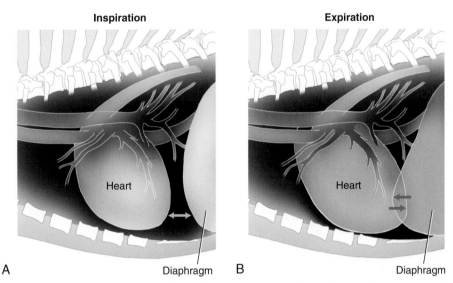

FIG. 17.18 A, During inspiration in a lateral view, the heart appears smaller and the vessels appear more elongated. There is increased distance from the apex of the heart to the diaphragm and less sternal contact. The intrathoracic portion of the trachea widens, and the lungs appear more inflated and less radiopaque. **B,** During expiration, the heart appears larger and the lung lobes smaller and more radiopaque. There is increased sternal contact of the right side of the heart and superimposition of the apex over the diaphragm with dorsal elevation of the trachea.

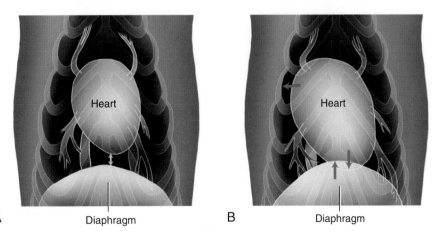

FIG. 17.19 A, During inspiration in either the ventrodorsal (VD) or dorsoventral (DV) view, the heart appears smaller and the vessels appear more elongated. There is increased distance from the apex to the diaphragm. **B,** During expiration in either the VD or DV view, the heart appears larger. There is increased sternal contact on the right side. The diaphragm is superimposed on the caudal cardiac border. The lungs appear more radiopaque.

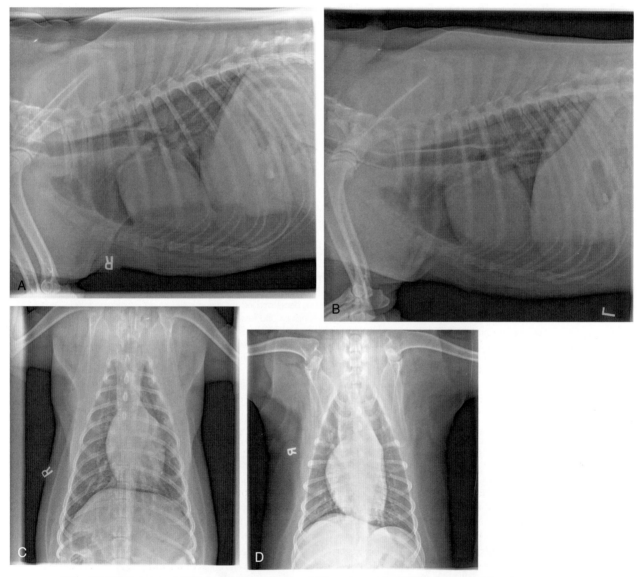

FIG. 17.20 Right lateral (**A**), left lateral (**B**), dorsoventral (**C**), and ventrodorsal (**D**) radiographs taken during expiration. Note that the heart is slightly rounder in the lateral views in expiration. There is more contact with the diaphragm in all views and greater radiopacity of the lungs in these thoracic views than in corresponding views in inspiration. (Courtesy Jennifer White, Mississauga Oakville Veterinary Emergency Hospital and Referral Group, Oakville, Ontario.)

TABLE 17.2	Effect of Positional Changes and Phase of Respiration on Thoracic Radiographs[1-4]
RIGHT LATERAL THORAX	**LEFT LATERAL THORAX**

(See Figs. 17.3A, 17.4A, 17.5, 17.6, 17.7, 17.20A, 17.25)
- Heart is more "conical" or oval—the cardiophrenic ligament prevents the heart from moving to dependent portion of pleural cavity.
- Right lateral recumbency causes more superimposition of the right and left pairs of cranial lobe vessels.
- Diaphragmatic crura are parallel to each other—the dependent right crus will be more cranial.
- The caudal vena cava will merge with cranial right crus, so it is only visible between the cardiac silhouette and diaphragm.
- More difficult to assess the size of pulmonary arteries and veins because there is overlap between the right and left cranial lobe pulmonary vessels.
- There may be air in the fundus of the stomach behind the left diaphragmatic crus.

(See Fig. 17.3B, 17.4B, 17.10, 17.20B)
- The apex of the cardiac silhouette is displaced from the sternum, making the overall cardiac shape appear more rounded.
- The dependent left crus of the diaphragm is more cranial.
- The right and left crura diverge from each other ventrally to dorsally (appear to cross).
- Easier to determine vessel size and to distinguish between right and left cranial lobe pulmonary vessels.
- Caudal vena cava silhouettes with right crus, usually caudal to the left crus.
- The right cranial lobar artery and vein are best seen because the contralateral right lung is better inflated.
- The fundic portion of the stomach is caudal to the left crus.

Inspiration for Both Laterals (See Figs. 17.4, 17.6, 17.18A)
- Heart appears smaller.
- Vessels appear more elongated.
- There is increased distance from the apex of the heart to the diaphragm.
- Less sternal cardiac contact because the lungs extend to the sternum.
- The lungs appear larger and more inflated.
- Intrathoracic portion of trachea widens, and the cervical portion of the trachea narrows.
- The dependent diaphragm is displaced cranially.
- In extreme inspiration, the diaphragm is more vertical on the image, and the shape moves from convex to straight.
- Caudal vena cava is horizontal or parallel with the spine.

Expiration for Both Laterals (See Figs. 17.18B, 17.20AB)
- Heart appears larger, and lung lobes smaller and more radiopaque.
- Increased sternal contact of the right side of the heart.
- Superimposition of apex over the diaphragm.
- Dorsal elevation of trachea.
- Intrathoracic portion of the trachea narrows, and cervical portion widens.

DORSOVENTRAL (DV) THORAX	**VENTRODORSAL (VD) THORAX**

(See Figs. 17.14, 17.20C)
- Cardiac shape more round due to upright position.
- Cardiac silhouette often displaced to the left by the cranially displaced diaphragm (left side looks almost straight). The cranial and right borders are rounded—appearance of lopsided egg more noted.
- The cranially displaced diaphragm pushes the heart cranially and into the left hemothorax,[4] which is more evident in medium and large dogs than in cats or small dogs.
- There are clear left and right crura with medially located cupula so that the diaphragm appears as a single convex shape unless the x-ray beam is centered caudally, in which it may appear as three humps.[3] Especially noted in deep-chested patients.
- Accessory lung lobe region is less aerated due to cranial diaphragm placement.
- There is improved pulmonary inflation in the DV view and better visualization of the caudal lobar pulmonary vessels and bronchi— more magnified and perpendicular to the beam than in the VD view.
- Caudal lobar vessels are significantly magnified due to increased object to film distance.
- Superimposition of cardiac silhouettes, great vessels, trachea, and esophagus.[1]
- Vertebrae appear more magnified.

(See Figs. 17.10, 17.11, 17.12, 17.20D, 17.21B)
- The cardiac silhouette is more elongated (increased OFD), and the cardiac apex shifts to the left laterally and dorsally. In dogs with deep and narrow chests, the heart may appear more rounded than oval because of upright orientation.
- Minor changes in size and shape of the cardiac silhouette are not as accurate in VD because of magnification, especially in large breed dogs.
- Right and left diaphragmatic crura and the cupula project into the thorax appearing as three humps unless the x-ray beam is centered caudally, in which case the diaphragm will appear as a single convex shape.[3]
- Changes of descending aorta and great vessels are more noticeable.
- Accessory lung lobe region is better aerated and is elongated between the cardiac silhouette and diaphragm; less air is noted in the dorsocaudal lungs.
- Pulmonary arteries sometimes superimposed over the heart.
- Thymus in puppies appears as a triangular-shaped soft tissue opacity in cranial mediastinum.

Continued

TABLE 17.2	Effect of Positional Changes and Phase of Respiration on Thoracic Radiographs[1-4]—cont'd
DORSOVENTRAL (DV) THORAX	**VENTRODORSAL (VD) THORAX**

Inspiration for VD and DV (See Figs. 17.12, 17.19A)

- Heart appears smaller.
- Vessels appear more elongated.
- There is increased distance from the apex to the diaphragm.
- DV radiographs produced during deep inspiration show the apex of the heart nearer to the midline.

Expiration for VD/DV (See Figs. 17.19B, 17.20CD)

- Heart appears larger.
- Increased sternal contact on the right side.
- The diaphragm superimposes the caudal cardiac border.
- The lungs appear more radiopaque.

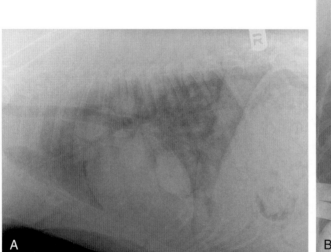
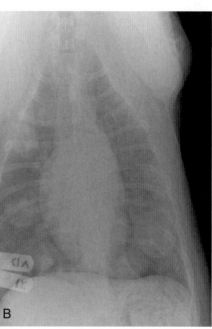

FIG. 17.21 Right lateral **(A)** and ventrodorsal **(B)** radiographs showing metastatic lungs. All views are suggested to see the extent of the metastases. (Courtesy Secord Animal Hospital.)

Normal Thoracic Radiographic Anatomy

The four basic anatomical regions of the thorax are generally considered to be the extrathoracic region, the pleural space, the pulmonary parenchyma, and the mediastinum. The mediastinum divides the thorax into right and left sides and is formed by the parietal pleura of the right and left hemithoraces and contains important structures, including the trachea, esophagus, heart, aorta and its major branches, thoracic duct, lymph nodes, and nerves (Figs. 17.22 and 17.23). Please see Table 17.2 for the effect of positional changes and phase of respiration on thoracic radiographs. Appendix C on the Evolve website outlines an overview of normal thoracic radiography and further radiographic concerns. Figs. 17.10, 17.11, 17.13, and 17.26 show further anatomy of the related areas. Fig. 17.24 indicates anatomy identification in the VD/DV position using the face clock analogy. Measurement of heart size is demonstrated in Fig 17.25.

Fig. 17.27 shows how the heart is visualized on a radiograph compared with two types of ultrasound images. See Chapter 10 for information on ultrasound.

Fig. 17.28 is a mystery radiograph. Review it and answer the question presented with it.

✳ KEY POINTS

1. Proper positioning and technique are essential for proper interpretation of thoracic images. This includes where to measure and center, what to include, and how to ensure that the positioning shows proper symmetry.
2. Lateral and DV thorax views are generally completed for evaluation of the heart, whereas lateral and VD views are suggested for visualization of lung parenchyma.
3. Additional and alternative views are often needed, depending on the suspected conditions.
4. Lung lesions are best identified on a lateral view of the nondependent position (lesions in the left lung will be more noticeable in right lateral recumbency).
5. Measurement is made over the caudal border of the scapula, the central ray is over the heart, and the full rib cage should be included.
6. The exposure is generally taken at maximum inspiration unless the thoracic inlet is being examined.
7. A long scale of contrast, obtained by higher kVp and lower mAs, is suggested for film-screen imaging;

underexposure or overexposure may lead to misdiagnosis.
8. A change in patient position, central ray, inaccurate positioning, or phase of respiration affects the radiographic appearance, so it is essential that the technician is aware of the changes that occur.
9. The four basic anatomical regions of the thorax are generally considered to be the extrathoracic region, the pleural space, the pulmonary parenchyma, and the mediastinum, including the heart and great vessels. Knowing the normal anatomy of these areas helps the technician take proper radiographs and, ultimately, enables the veterinarian to make the correct diagnosis.
10. Other modalities such as ultrasound, magnetic resonance imaging (MRI), or computerized tomography (CT) are more diagnostic and may be required to properly view the thoracic anatomy or augment diagnosis of radiographically visible structures.

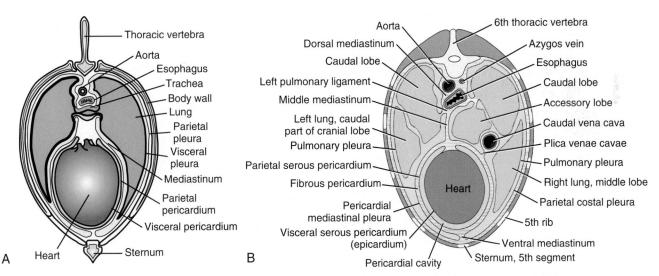

FIG. 17.22 **A,** Diagram of a cross-section of the thorax through the heart to visualize thoracic contents. **B,** Schematic transverse section of thorax through the heart, caudal view. (**A** from Colville T, Bassert J: *Clinical Anatomy and Physiology for Veterinary Technicians,* 3rd ed, St Louis: Elsevier; 2016.)

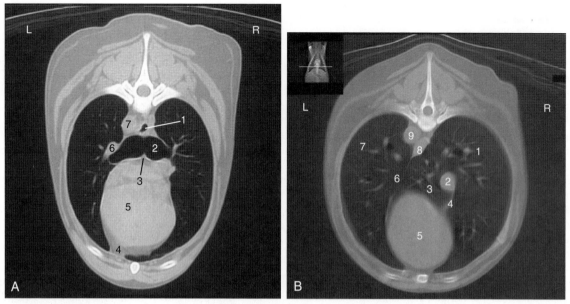

FIG. 17.23 A, Computerized tomography (CT) scan at midthorax. *1,* Esophagus; *2,* right principal bronchus; *3,* carina of trachea; *4,* ventral mediastinum–phrenicopericardial ligament; *5,* heart; *6,* left pulmonary artery; *7,* aorta. **B,** CT scan at caudal thorax. *1,* Right caudal lobe; *2,* caudal vena cava; *3,* accessory lobe; *4,* plica venae cavae; *5,* heart; *6,* caudal mediastinum; *7,* left caudal lobe; *8,* esophagus; *9,* aorta.

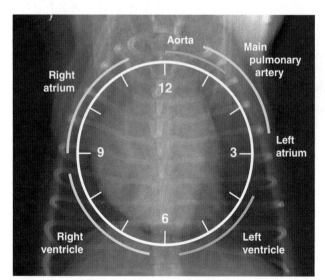

FIG. 17.24 The cardiac silhouette can be evaluated with a clock face analogy as noted in either the DV or VD position. In the cat, the left atrium forms the left heart border from 2 o'clock to 3 o'clock and the left ventricle from about 3 o'clock to 6 o'clock. In the dog the left atrium is not visible in this area and does not make up the heart border. The left ventricle forms the left heart border from 2 o'clock to 6 o'clock in the dog. The right atrium is at 9 to 11 o'clock. When evident, the main pulmonary artery is noted at 1 to 2 o'clock. The left pulmonary artery extends beyond the heart at about 4 o'clock, and the right pulmonary artery is found at about 8 o'clock.[1] The lateral radiograph would show the aorta at about 10 to 11 o'clock, the main pulmonary artery and right atrium at 9 to 10 o'clock, the right ventricle at 5 to 9 o'clock, and the left ventricle at 2 to 5 o'clock.

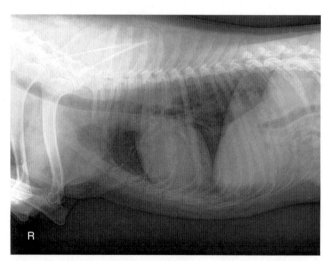

FIG. 17.25 Heart size can be measured with use of the vertebral heart scale, which measures the lengths of the long and short axes of the heart and scales them against the length of the vertebral bodies that lie dorsal to the heart, beginning with T4. In this image, the vertebral heart scale is 17.5.[4]

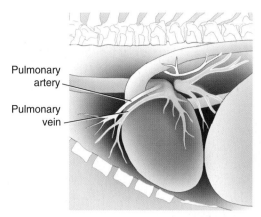

FIG. 17.26 In the lateral radiographic projection of the normal canine thorax, it is difficult to differentiate pulmonary arteries from the veins. The artery is always dorsal to the vein in the cranial lung lobes. In general the size of the pulmonary arteries should have the same size and shape as that of the corresponding pulmonary veins at the same level.[1]

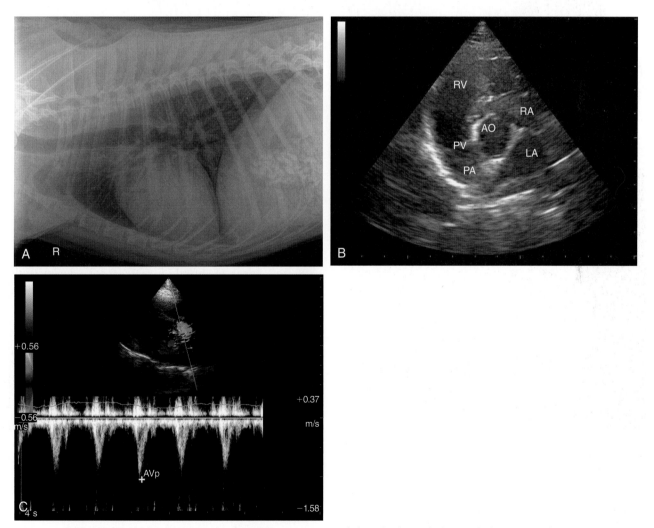

FIG. 17.27 The heart as imaged in three different ways. **A,** Right lateral radiograph showing the heart. **B,** An ultrasound scan shows the right-sided short axis of heart chambers and vessels. Greater diagnostic information is available. *AO,* aorta; *LA,* left atrium; *PA,* pulmonary artery; *PV,* pulmonary vein; *RA,* right atrium; *RV,* right ventricle. **C,** Pulsed wave Doppler ultrasonograph (see Chapter 10) evaluating blood flow across the aortic valve. There is normal velocity across the valve (approximately 1 m/sec) and a normal high resistance flow pattern. The flow of blood can be tracked: blue indicates blood flowing away from the transducer, and red shows blood flowing toward the transducer (remember BART: blue away/ red toward). Further color shows greater variances that detect abnormal blood flows.

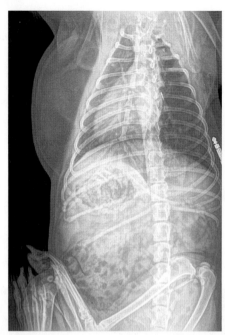

FIG. 17.28 Mystery radiograph. What position could this patient be in? How can the position be more diagnostic? (Courtesy Vetel Diagnostics, San Luis Obispo, California, and Seth Wallack, DVM, DACVR, AAVR, Director and CEO of Veterinary Imaging Centre of San Diego.)

REVIEW QUESTIONS

1. The veterinarian requests that you image a beagle for routine thoracic radiographs before surgery. For proper diagnosis your image should have a:
   a. Long scale of contrast, meaning higher kVp and lower mAs
   b. Long scale of contrast, meaning lower kVp and higher mAs
   c. Short scale of contrast, meaning higher kVp and lower mAs
   d. Short scale of contrast, meaning lower kVp and higher mAs

2. The veterinarian requires thoracic radiographs of a beagle, which should be measured at the thickest part, or the:
   a. Thoracic inlet
   b. Point of the heart
   c. Cranial border of the scapula
   d. Caudal border of the scapula

3. The peripheral borders for the beagle thoracic radiograph are the:
   a. Caudal border of the scapula to the first lumbar vertebral body
   b. Point of the heart to the first lumbar vertebral body
   c. Shoulder joint to just past the 13th rib
   d. First thoracic vertebra to the 13th thoracic vertebral body

4. You will expose the thoracic radiographs for the beagle:
   a. At maximum expiration
   b. At maximum inspiration
   c. Halfway between maximum inspiration and expiration
   d. At any point in the respiratory cycle

5. You check that you have taken proper inspiration images for this beagle. On the image, the heart in either lateral or DV taken during inspiration will appear:
   a. Smaller. The vessels are more elongated, and there is increased distance from the apex of the heart to the diaphragm.
   b. More conical or oval. The diaphragm is more caudal, and there is dorsal elevation of the trachea.
   c. Smaller. The vessels are more shortened, and there is decreased distance from the apex of the heart to the sternum.
   d. Larger. The vessels are larger, and there is greater sternal contact and a clear left and right crus with a medially located cupula.

6. To minimize rotation when positioning for the lateral for this beagle, you should:
   a. Not place any foam pads between the limbs or under the sternum
   b. Place thick foam pads between the limbs and under the sternum to rotate vertebrae
   c. Place foam pads only under the sternum because none are required between the limbs
   d. Place foam pads between the limbs if needed and to elevate the sternum

7. When positioning for the lateral view, you want to ensure that the front limbs are pulled as far:
   a. Cranially as possible without rotating the thorax
   b. Cranially as possible with slight rotation of the thorax
   c. Caudally as possible with a wedge between if needed
   d. Caudally as possible, causing the sternum and vertebrae to be on the same plane

8. You forgot to include a marker, but you know that you did provide the right lateral image of this beagle because on the image you note that:
   a. The diaphragm is not touching the heart
   b. The heart is more conical
   c. The heart is rounder
   d. Air is noted in the pyloric antrum

9. You are confident that you are presenting the veterinarian with well-positioned DV radiographs of this beagle because on the image you see:
   a. The sternum and spine are superimposed
   b. Intervertebral foramina are the same size
   c. Ribs over the heart are superimposed
   d. The "Nike swoosh" of the transverse processes

10. A routine VD is required on a feline patient. It is generally best to pull the front limbs:
    a. Caudally and have the nose pointing up equidistant between the front legs
    b. Caudally and have the nose parallel to the table equidistant between the front legs
    c. Cranially and have the nose pointing up equidistant between the front legs
    d. Cranially and have the nose parallel to the table equidistant between the front legs

11. The veterinarian suspects a lesion in the right lung of a poodle. She would like you to complete both laterals, but the most important one in this case is the:
    a. Right lateral
    b. Left lateral

12. The veterinarian would like you to complete a DV decubitus view on a springer spaniel, as fluid is suspected. This means that the patient should be in:
    a. DV position with a vertical beam
    b. Lateral recumbency with a horizontal beam
    c. Dorsal recumbency with a horizontal beam
    d. Ventral recumbency with a horizontal beam

13. In the DV decubitus view of the springer spaniel with fluid, the original exposure factors were 72 kV and 10 mAs. You are best to:
    a. Keep the same exposure factors
    b. Increase the kV to 80 and keep the mAs at 10
    c. Increase the kV to 80 and decrease the mAs to 5
    d. Increase the source image distance and keep the same factors

14. Pneumonia is suspected in a retriever. The recommended views are:
    a. Both laterals and a ventrodorsal
    b. Both laterals and a dorsoventral
    c. The right lateral and a ventrodorsal
    d. The right lateral and a dorsoventral

15. The mediastinum contains the:
    a. Heart solely
    b. Heart, trachea, esophagus, aorta and major branches, thoracic duct, lymph nodes, and nerves
    c. Trachea, esophagus, aorta and major branches, thoracic duct, lymph nodes, and nerves
    d. Stomach, liver, kidneys, diaphragm, gallbladder, intestines and bladder

Answers to Review Questions can be found on the Evolve website.

References

1. Thrall DE. *Textbook of Veterinary Diagnostic Radiology*. 6th ed. St. Louis: Saunders; 2013.
2. Ayers S. *Small animal radiographic techniques and positioning*. Oxford: Wiley-Blackwell; 2013.
3. Muhlbauer MC, Kneller SK. *Radiography of the Dog And Cat: Guide to Making and Interpreting Radiographs*. Ames, IA: Wiley Blackwell; 2013:[Chapter 5].
4. Morgan JP, Doval J, Samii V. *Radiographic Techniques: the dog*. Hannover: Schlutersche GmbH & Co; 1998.

Bibliography

Colville T, Bassert J. *Clinical Anatomy and Physiology for Veterinary Technicians*. 3rd ed. St. Louis: Mosby; 2016.

Done SH, Goody PC, Stickland NC, et al. *Color Atlas of Veterinary Anatomy, the Dog and Cat*. London: Mosby; 2009.

Dyce KM, Sack WO, Wensing CJG. *Textbook of Veterinary Anatomy*. 4th ed. St. Louis: Saunders; 2010.

Evans H, de Lahunta A. *Guide to the Dissection of the Dog*. 7th ed. St. Louis: Saunders; 2010.

Han C, Hurd C. *Practical Diagnostic Imaging for the Veterinary Technician*. 3rd ed. St. Louis: Mosby; 2005.

Jenner A. Non-manual radiography: radiation and patient safety. *RVT J Ont Assoc Vet Tech*. 2016;39(2).

Owens JM, Biery DN. *Radiographic Interpretation for the Small Animal Clinician*. St. Louis: Ralston Purina; 1999.

Romich J. *An Illustrated Guide to Veterinary Medical Terminology*. Clifton, NY: Delmar Cengage Learning; 2015.

Ryan G. *Radiographic Positioning of Small Animals*. Philadelphia: Lea & Febiger; 1981.

Sirois M, Anthony E, Mauragis D. *Handbook of Radiographic Positioning for Veterinary Technicians*. Clifton Park, NY: Delmar Cengage Learning; 2010.

Sirois M. *Principles and Practice of Veterinary Technology*. 3rd ed. St. Louis: Mosby; 2011.

Ticer J. *Radiographic Technique in Small Animal Practice*. Philadelphia: WB Saunders; 1984.

Tighe M, Brown M. *Mosby's Comprehensive Review for Veterinary Technicians*. 4th ed. St. Louis: Elsevier; 2015.

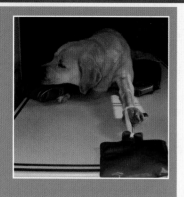

CHAPTER 18
Small Animal Forelimb

Marg Brown, RVT, BEd Ad Ed

How many legs does a dog have if you call the tail a leg?
Four. Calling a tail a leg doesn't make it a leg.
—Abraham Lincoln, U.S. president, 1809–1865

OUTLINE

LEARNING OBJECTIVES

When you have finished this chapter, you will be able to:

1. Properly and safely position a dog or cat for the various common positions of the forelimb with an emphasis on nonmanual restraint.
2. Correctly measure and center the patient to include the peripheral borders.
3. Ensure that the bone or joint is parallel to the image receptor and the central ray is perpendicular to the field of view (FOV) and receptor.

4. Identify views that may need to be completed as an alternative.
5. Identify the normal anatomy found on a radiograph.

KEY TERMS

Key terms are defined in the Glossary on the Evolve website.

Articular margin
Caudocranial/craniocaudal
Craniodistal-cranioproximal
Flexed

Hyperextended
Hyperflexed
Mediolateral

Oblique
Occult
Osteochondritis dissecans

Positional terminology
Skyline
Stressed view

TECHNICAL NOTE: To preserve space, the radiographs presented in this chapter do not show collimation. For safety, always collimate so that the beam is limited to within the image receptor edges. In film radiography, you should see a clear border of collimation (frame) on every radiograph. In some jurisdictions, evidence of collimation is required by law.

Diseases of the musculoskeletal system most often affect the dog's ability to move. Skeletal and joint disorders are the most common, but other problems in the musculoskeletal system can also indicate further issues.

Bone disorders can be developmental, infectious, nutritional, due to trauma or tumors, or be of unknown etiology. Bone diseases are generally present at birth or the result of nutritional deficiencies or injuries. Movable joints are vulnerable to joint diseases or disorders affecting their membranes, as well as related ligaments, cartilage, and bone. The emphasis in this and the next chapter will be the imaging of the appendicular skeleton (Fig. 18.1A) to detect fractures, pain, or lameness.

High-quality radiographs are essential so there is no misdiagnosis. Joint studies are generally completed non–weight bearing so it is often difficult to overtly evaluate joint space on the radiographs. Radiographic changes are often subtle because bone is a matrix of different tissues that continuously remodel through life as animals mature and respond to disease and trauma. Immature bones have an open physis between the epiphysis and the metaphysis seen as a translucent line that should not be confused with a fracture (Fig. 18.1B). There can be a large number of incidental findings and anatomical variants. Often it is not possible to determine the significance of lesions based on radiological appearance alone.

✎ TECHNICIAN NOTES

If you mentally place the patient in sternal recumbency for the distal portion of the limb and in dorsal recumbency for the proximal portion, the positional terms will make sense.

Radiographic and Patient Concerns

- There are many factors to consider in the production of high-quality radiographs.
  - Except for the shoulder and scapula in some dogs, most projections are completed tabletop. A grid is not generally used because the tissue thickness of the forelimb is less than 10 cm.
  - It is important to collimate the field as tightly as possible to reduce scatter radiation. Doing so also helps achieve higher contrast, which is particularly true in digital imaging (see Chapter 8).
  - Use a small focal spot to maximize spatial resolution.
  - Use low kV and high mAs technique to maximize radiographic contrast, and do not overexpose the image. One should clearly see the soft tissues and trabecular pattern of the bone.
  - Separate exposures may be required of the proximal and distal humerus of large dogs.
  - When a joint is to be imaged, always center on the joint; otherwise, there will be geometrical distortion due to the divergence of the x-ray beam.
  - Most digital systems have a software scaler for orthopedic measurements. If the unit does not, consider a scaler for digital radiographs, such as a coin or object of known size, for orthopedic templating.[1]
- Obtain orthogonal views in all cases to properly diagnose three-dimensional objects. Therefore in addition to a lateral (L) view, the patient is generally placed in dorsal recumbency to acquire a view of the proximal portion of the limb (shoulder, scapula, and humerus) or in sternal recumbency for the distal portion (elbow, radius and ulna, carpus, metacarpus, and digits) (Fig. 18.2).

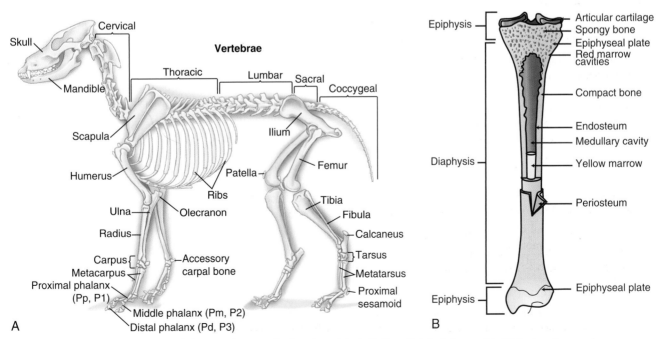

FIG. 18.1 A, Canine skeleton. B, Structure of a long bone (tibia). (B, From Colville T, Bassert JM: *Clinical anatomy and physiology for veterinary technicians,* ed 3, St Louis, Elsevier, 2016.)

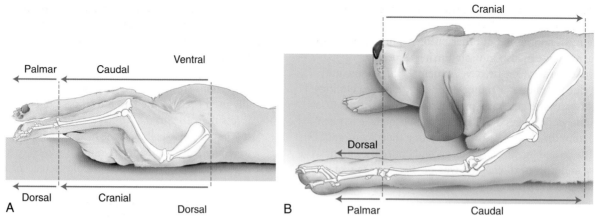

FIG. 18.2 A, Patient in dorsal recumbency for the contralateral image of the proximal limb: scapula, shoulder, and humerus. The humerus is referred to as the caudocranial (CdCr) view in this position. The thorax is termed ventrodorsal in this view. **B,** For positioning of the distal forelimbs (elbow, radius/ulna, carpus, metacarpus, and digits), the patient is generally in sternal recumbency. Note that the terminology changes at and including the carpus. Thus in this position the view of the elbow is craniocaudal (CrCd) and the carpus is dorsopalmar (DP or DPa).

TABLE 18.1	Protocol for Pectoral Limb Radiography	
ANATOMICAL LOCATION	**ROUTINE VIEWS**	**ANCILLARY VIEW(S)**
Scapula	Lateral, Caudocranial	
Shoulder	Lateral, Caudocranial	Extended or flexed lateral Skyline for the bicipital groove Craniocaudal
Humerus	Lateral, Caudocranial	Craniocaudal
Elbow	Lateral, Craniocaudal	Caudocranial (horizontal beam), hyperflexed lateral, obliques
Radius/ulna	Lateral, Craniocaudal	
Foot: carpus, metacarpus, and digits	Lateral, Dorsopalmar	Extended or flexed lateral, obliques

- Thus for the pectoral limb, along with the lateral view of each part, the common views are termed (Table 18.1):
  - Caudocranial (CdCr) for the shoulder, scapula, and humerus
  - Craniocaudal (CrCd) for the elbow, radius and ulna
  - Dorsopalmar (DP/DPa) for the carpus, metacarpus and digits. (Sometimes this is referred to as *anterior/posterior [AP]*; however, this is a human term and not correct for animals.)

- The lateral view is relatively straightforward to image, but the CrCd/CdCr views can be especially challenging in dogs because of the difficulty in keeping the bones parallel to the table to minimize geometrical distortion. In cats, it is generally easier to obtain symmetry with CrCd/CdCr views. Chemical restraint is highly suggestive for proper CrCd / CdCr views.
- Further ancillary views such as oblique positioning are generally not used in small animals but may be useful for the humerus, elbow, carpus, metacarpus, or digits. The purpose of obliques is generally intended to project different edges of a joint or region that may be overlooked unless projected tangentially where they are visible at the periphery.[2] Flexed views of the elbow and carpus may also be taken. Stress radiography of joints that involves application of traction, rotation, or a wedge to the joint is useful for sprains to show subluxation that might not be demonstrated on standard radiographic views.[2]
- If it is too painful for the patient to complete the perpendicular view to the lateral, use of a horizontal beam should be considered if available.
- Radiographs of the opposite limb are a valuable reference if there are any anatomical variant concerns, such as in physically immature patients. Many joint conditions are bilateral (e.g., osteochondritis dissecans, cranial cruciate disease, elbow dysplasia), so occult pathology might be missed if contralateral limbs are not imaged. A comparison with the opposite limb is often suggested in lameness of younger or older dogs. In this case a survey of both limbs from the shoulder joint to the elbow is recommended. Cats generally do not have developmental dysplasia of the bones and joints that leads to lameness; trauma is the most likely reason for imaging feline limbs.
- The field of view:
  - For long bones generally includes the proximal and distal joints.

- For joints includes one-third each of the long bones, proximal and distal to the joint.
- Along with ensuring that the required anatomy is included, it is also essential to achieve symmetry for proper diagnosis. There should be no rotation.
- The marker is placed at the dorsal or cranial aspect of the limb for lateral views and on the lateral aspect of the limb for the opposite views.

> **TECHNICIAN NOTE**
>
> For long bones, the field of view includes the joints proximal and distal. For joints, include one-third each of the bones proximal and distal.

- When tabletop views are indicated, both positions can be placed on the same image receptor if the size of the animal and body part allow, but center only on one limb at a time. If the film cassette is to be split into sections, point the toes of each view in the same direction. Collimate tightly and use a lead shield to cover the side not being imaged to prevent scatter radiation from decreasing the contrast. Splitting of the detector is not possible in digital imaging.
- Unless otherwise indicated, a vertical beam is used.
- Keep in mind that musculoskeletal radiographs are often performed on patients who may be in pain, so be conscious of positioning and consider the use of analgesics. Chemical restraint is required, as manipulation may be painful. If trauma is suspected, ensure that any concurrent issues such as thoracic pathology is addressed before radiography. Hair coat should be clean, dry, and free from dirt because debris may mimic foreign bodies.
- Emphasis in this book is placed on nonmanual restraint. Review the suggestions in Chapter 15 on techniques that can be used.
- For nonmanual restraint, it is essential to give the patient the illusion that it is being held with judicious use of sandbags, V-troughs, soft Velcro straps, compression bands, tape, etc. Use positioning devices in the field of view appropriately, because they may affect exposure or cause image artifacts. If splints and casts are not removed, compensate with increased exposure factors.
- See Box 18.1 for some terms relating to radiographic anatomy associated with bones.
- Other imaging modalities that are commonly available are ultrasonography, computerized tomography, and magnetic resonance imaging (MRI). MRI is particularly useful when evaluating tendons and ligaments around joints. Nuclear medicine or scintigraphy is used in equines and is expanded on in Chapter 14.

> **TECHNICIAN NOTES**
>
> For high-quality orthopedic radiographs:
> - Low kV and high mAs technique.
> - Tabletop technique except for proximal limbs of large dogs.
> - Small focal spot.
> - Measure the patient at the thickest part and in the position it is to be radiographed.
> - Minimize object-film distance (OFD).
> - Center on the area of interest.
> - Collimate and include only what is required.
> - Keep the bone parallel to the image receptor.
> - Keep central ray perpendicular to bone and image receptor.
> - No rotation.
> - Minimize superimposed structures.
> - Label correctly.
> - Obtain orthogonal views.
> - Radiograph the contralateral limb for comparison when required.

> **TECHNICIAN NOTES**
>
> Collimate and ensure that labels/markers are included and that borders are visible for every film image taken.

> **TECHNICIAN NOTES**
>
> For efficiency and ease of positioning, ensure that the body parts that are not in the beam are positioned and secured first. Then position the area of interest.

> **TECHNICIAN NOTES**
>
> Remember to always collimate as closely as possible.

> **TECHNICIAN NOTES**
>
> Remember to place the label or marker cranial to the bone or joint for the lateral view and on the lateral aspect of the limb for the opposite views.

Scapula

Lateral (Mediolateral) View of the Scapula—Routine

Positioning to View Body of Scapula

Place in: Lateral recumbency with the affected side down.

Head and Neck: Arch the head and neck dorsally so they are at 135 degrees to the thoracic spine, placing sandbags over the neck to keep it in position and taking care not to restrict breathing. Think of the head and limbs as being in a T-shaped position—the head and contralateral limb form the top of the T, and the affected limb its main stem (Fig. 18.3AB).

Hind Limbs: Leave in a natural position and support with sandbags if needed.

Forelimbs: To visualize the body of the scapula, pressure is forcibly applied to the affected limb to position the full scapula dorsal to the vertebral column. Pull the contralateral limb ventrally and caudally so the thorax will rotate slightly and further isolate the scapular body. Tie in place or use a sandbag. Grasp the affected limb below the elbow joint, keeping the joint extended so it cannot flex. Push the limb perpendicular to and dorsally toward the line of the neck and upper limb until the spinous processes can be seen bulging dorsal to the thoracic vertebral spinous processes. Use a heavy sandbag over the elbow to keep the limb in position. Manual restraint may be required.

Comments and Tips

- The goal is an unobstructed view, positioning the scapula dorsal to the vertebral column.
- Pulling the opposite limb slightly rotates the thorax, which further isolates the scapula dorsal to the body.
- If the upper limb is overextended dorsally, the upper shoulder musculature will be over the area of interest.

MEASURE: Dorsally at the cranial border of the scapula at about the site of the first vertebral body.

CENTRAL RAY: Center of the scapula.

BORDERS: Shoulder joint and caudal border of the scapula.

✎ **TECHNICIAN NOTES**

Remember to go through your mental checklist before pushing the exposure button. See Chapter 15.

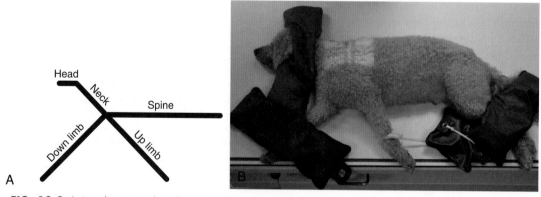

FIG. 18.3 A, Line drawing to show the correct alignment or T-position for lateral radiographs of the shoulder and scapula. B, Positioning for the scapula dorsal to the vertebral column. The affected limb is pushed up dorsally if the full scapula is to be above the thoracic spine.

Lateral (Mediolateral) View of the Scapula—Routine—cont'd

Superimposition of the Scapula Over the Cranial Thorax to View the Scapular Neck

- To view the scapular neck, if the patient is in pain or manipulation is not possible, the positioning is altered so that the affected limb is pulled cranially and ventrally; the upper limb is extended caudally.

- Force is not applied to push the limb dorsally.
- This places the body of the scapula over the radiolucent lung fields to allow visualization of the neck and body ventral to the thorax.

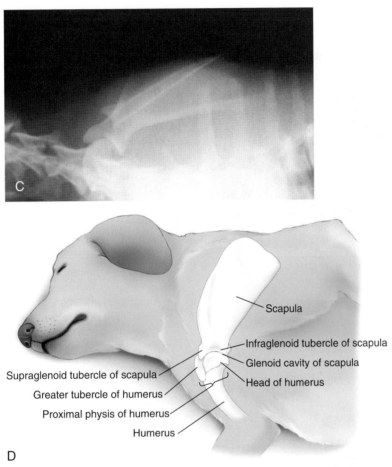

FIG. 18.3, cont'd C, Mediolateral radiograph of the scapula, dorsal to the vertebral column. The affected limb should be pushed up more dorsally if the full scapula is to be above the thoracic spine. **D,** Medial view of the right shoulder joint and scapula. (**A** redrawn from Muhlbauer MC, Kneller SK: *Radiography of the Dog and Cat: Guide to Making and Intepreting Radiographs.* Oxford: Wiley-Blackwell; 2013; **B** courtesy Seneca College of Applied Arts and Technology, King City, Ontario.)

Caudocranial View of the Scapula—Routine

Positioning

Place In: Dorsal recumbency in a trough or with the use of tape if needed.

Head and Neck: Push the head slightly laterally from the affected limb to avoid superimposition of the cervical spine over the joint. Place a sandbag over the neck if required, taking care not to restrict breathing.

Hind Limbs: Leave in a natural position and support with sandbags if needed.

Forelimbs: Tape and extend both limbs cranially, especially the affected limb. Use sandbags or tie the affected limb to the table so that the humerus is almost parallel to the table.

Comments and Tips

- Rotate the patient's sternum from the scapula about 10 to 12 degrees to avoid superimposition of the scapula and ribs and to have the spine of the scapula perpendicular to the table.

MEASURE: At the level of the scapulohumeral articulation (shoulder joint) so that the calipers are extended over the first thoracic vertebral body.

CENTRAL RAY: Center of the scapula.

BORDERS: Shoulder joint and caudal border of the scapula (about level of eighth rib).

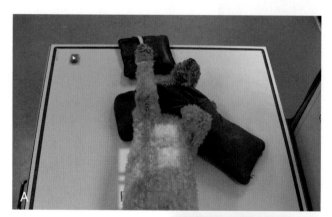

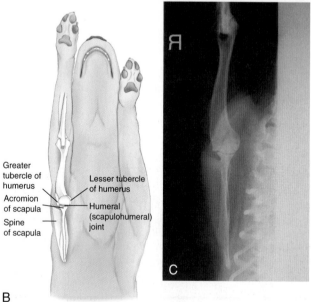

Greater tubercle of humerus

Lesser tubercle of humerus

Acromion of scapula

Humeral (scapulohumeral) joint

Spine of scapula

FIG. 18.4 A, Positioning of the caudocranial scapula. B, Caudal view of the right shoulder joint and scapula. C, Caudocranial radiograph of the scapula, humerus, and shoulder joint. (A courtesy Seneca College of Applied Arts and Technology, King City, Ontario.)

BOX 18.1	Terms Related to Radiographic Anatomy Associated With Bones[3]

- Condyle—rounded projection on the bone for articulation with another bone.
- Diaphysis—the shaft or body of the long bone.
- Epicondyle—a projection of bone on the lateral edge above its condyle.
- Epiphysis—the end of the long bone, with each long bone having a distal and proximal epiphysis.
- Epiphyseal plate or growth plate—plate of cartilage at the junction of the proximal and distal epiphysis with the diaphysis that ossifies as the animal matures.
- Foramen—opening or passage into or through a bone.
- Fossa—hollow or depressed area on a bone usually filled with muscles or tendons.
- Metaphysis—the wide portion of a long bone between the epiphysis and the narrow diaphysis that contains the growth plate.
- Trochlea—usually grooves in bone that allow tendons to act as pulleys.
- Tuberosity/trochanter/tubercle—protuberances on the bones, usually for muscle attachment.
- A long bone is described as having a head, shaft (body), and neck.

Shoulder Joint

Lateral (Mediolateral) View of the Shoulder—Routine

Positioning

Place in: Lateral recumbency with the affected limb down.

Head and Neck: Arch the head and neck dorsally so they are 135 degrees to the thoracic spine, placing sandbags over the neck, taking care not to restrict breathing.

Hind Limbs: Leave in a natural position and support with sandbags if needed.

Forelimbs: Pull the contralateral limb caudally in line with the neck and either secure with a sandbag or tie the limb. The affected limb should be extended perpendicular to the line of the neck downward and cranial, so the shoulder joint will be ventral to the sternum. Support with a sandbag.

Comments and Tips

- This is like the T position as described for the scapula, with the head and contralateral limb forming the top of the T, but the difference is that pressure is not applied to the affected limb.
- The extension of the head and neck places the shoulder joint ventral to the sternum and air-filled trachea, and puts the trachea dorsal to the scapulohumeral articulation, separating the joint surfaces.
- Palpate the shoulder joint by feeling along the humerus.
- The sternum will be slightly rotated from the thorax. Avoid overrotation of the thorax, which would place the shoulder joint in an oblique position and make evaluation of the articular surfaces of the shoulder joint difficult.[2]
- The shoulder joint should not be superimposed with the trachea.
- To visualize the articular margin of the humeral head, which aids in better determining whether there are osteochondrosis lesions, the affected limb can be slightly pronated and then slightly supinated (generally more effective)[4] to cause slight obliquity.
- Shoulder instability can be assessed by comparing two laterals: with and without pulling on the limb (applied traction).

MEASURE: At the level of the shoulder joint. Extend the caliper to the point of the unaffected shoulder, but be careful not to include that limb.

CENTRAL RAY: Palpate the proximal head of the humerus and the glenoid fossa of the scapula, and center at the scapulohumeral articulation[5] (shoulder joint).

BORDERS: Proximal third of the scapula through the proximal third of the humerus.

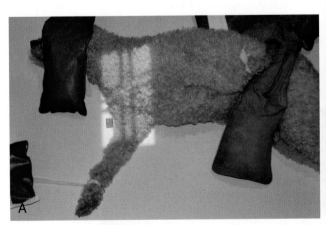

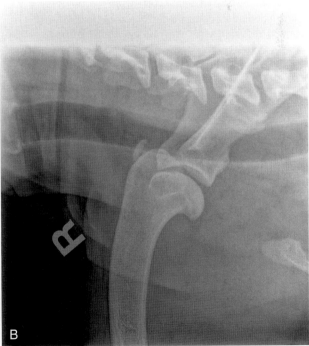

FIG. 18.5 A, Positioning of the lateral projection of the shoulder joint. The limb is fully extended to avoid superimposition, and the unaffected limb is pulled caudally in line with the neck. **B,** Mediolateral radiograph of the shoulder joint.

Caudocranial View of the Shoulder—Routine

Positioning

Place in: Dorsal recumbency in a trough or with the use of tape if needed. Foam pads can also be placed under the midthoracic and midabdominal regions.

Head and Neck: Push the head slightly laterally from the affected limb to avoid superimposition of the cervical spine over the joint.

Hind Limbs: Leave in a natural position and support with sandbags if needed.

Forelimbs: Extend both forelimbs cranially. Use sandbags or tie/tape the affected limb to the table so that the humerus is almost parallel to the table.

Comments and Tips

- The patient should be maintained in a true ventrodorsal position.

- The dog's or cat's body and ribs should fall slightly away from the scapula to avoid superimposition on the scapula and to have the spine of the scapula perpendicular to the table.
- Avoid overrotation of the humerus, which would produce an oblique shoulder joint.
- If the joints need to be compared, both can be included and the beam centered between the joints. However, if the patient is particularly broad chested, then each view should be completed separately.
- Craniocaudal radiographs (ancillary view), with the patient in dorsal recumbency and the limbs pulled caudally along the side of the thorax, can be taken to eliminate superimposition of the scapula over the cranial thorax.

MEASURE: At the level of the scapulohumeral articulation (shoulder joint). Extend the calipers over the caudal cervical vertebral bodies, but do not include the opposite limb.

CENTRAL RAY: Palpate the proximal head of the humerus and the acromion of the scapula at the center of the scapulohumeral articulation (shoulder joint).

BORDERS: Proximal third of the scapula through the proximal third of the humerus.

✎ TECHNICIAN NOTES

Use a modified abdomen technique chart for the scapula, shoulder, and humerus. The bone chart produces images that are too dark due to the increased tissue measurement, and the thorax settings produce images that are too light.

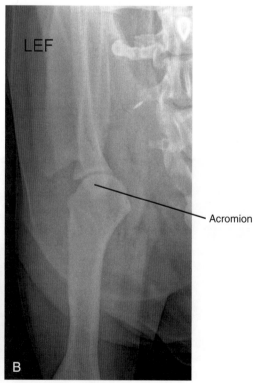

LEF

— Acromion

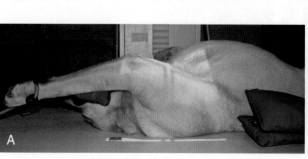

FIG. 18.6 A, Positioning of the caudocranial shoulder joint. **B,** Caudocranial radiograph of the shoulder joint.

Skyline (Cranioproximal-Craniodistal) View of the Shoulder for the Bicipital Groove—Ancillary

Positioning

To find calcified bodies in the bicep brachii or supraspinatus tendon,[2,4] the skyline view of the shoulder may be required with the patient in sternal recumbency.

Place In: Sternal recumbency

Head and Neck: Move the head and neck slightly away from the affected shoulder without any thorax rotation. Place the head and neck on foam pads and place sandbags over the neck to maintain the position, taking care not to restrict breathing.

Hind Limbs: Leave in a natural position and support with sandbags if needed.

Forelimbs: Keep the unaffected limb in a fairly natural position with a sandbag. Flex the elbow joint of the affected limb to project the shoulder joint over the proximal third of the radius and ulna. The film/screen cassette is placed in the crook of the elbow joint.

Comments and Tips

- Exposure factors should take the decreased source image distance (SID) into account.
- Most digital receptor (DR) panels are locked in place beneath the table, so this procedure is not feasible with digital units.

MEASURE AND CENTER: At the head of the humerus, palpating for the bicipital groove.

BORDERS: Proximal humerus with tight collimation.

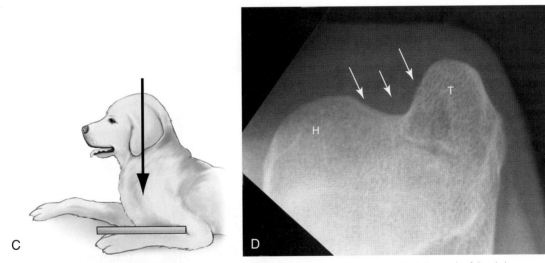

C

D

FIG. 18.6, cont'd C, Skyline positioning for the bicipital groove with film cassette. **D,** Radiograph of the skyline view (cranioproximal-craniodistal) of the shoulder/proximal humerus to project the bicipital groove *(white arrows) H,* Humeral head; *T,* greater tubercle). (**B** courtesy Jennifer White, Mississauga Oakville Veterinary Emergency Hospital and Referral Group, Oakville, Ontario; **D** from Thrall DE: *Textbook of Veterinary Diagnostic Radiology,* 6th ed. St Louis: Elsevier; 2013.)

Humerus

Lateral (Mediolateral) View of the Humerus—Routine

Positioning

Place In: Lateral recumbency with the affected limb down.

Head and Neck: Move the head and neck upward, placing sandbags over the neck to maintain the position and taking care not to restrict breathing.

Hind Limbs: Leave in a natural position and support with sandbags if needed.

Forelimbs: Extend the contralateral limb caudally and secure it to avoid superimposition. The affected limb should be extended downward and cranially. Secure with a sandbag or tie.

Comments and Tips

• Larger dogs may require two views if there is a significant difference in tissue density between the elbow and the shoulder. Measure each area separately.

MEASURE: Toward the proximal humerus at the level of the scapulohumeral articulation (shoulder joint).

CENTRAL RAY: Midshaft of the humerus.

BORDERS: Proximal to shoulder and distal to the elbow joints.

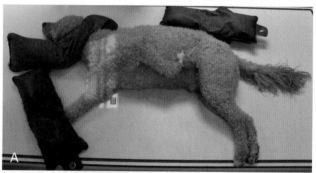

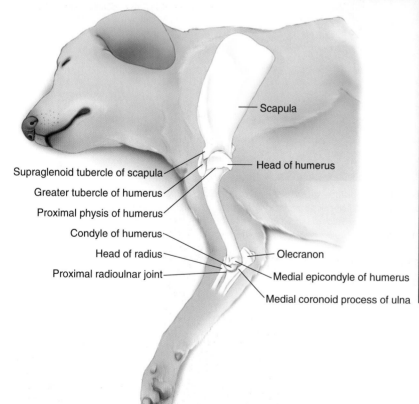

Scapula

Head of humerus

Supraglenoid tubercle of scapula

Greater tubercle of humerus

Proximal physis of humerus

Condyle of humerus

Head of radius

Proximal radioulnar joint

Olecranon

Medial epicondyle of humerus

Medial coronoid process of ulna

B

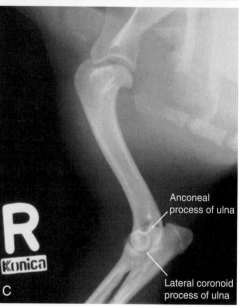

Anconeal process of ulna

Lateral coronoid process of ulna

FIG. 18.7 A, Positioning for the mediolateral (lateral) view of the humerus. **B,** Medial view of the right humerus. **C,** Mediolateral (lateral) radiograph of the humerus. (**A** courtesy Seneca College of Applied Arts and Technology, King City, Ontario.)

Caudocranial View of the Humerus—Routine

Positioning

Place In: Dorsal recumbency in a trough or with the use of tape if needed.

Head and Neck: Keep the head and neck fairly parallel to the humerus, and secure with a sandbag if needed, taking care not to restrict breathing.

Hind Limbs: Leave in a natural position so that the spine is perpendicular to the table. Support with sandbags if needed.

Forelimbs: Tape and extend both forelimbs cranially, especially the affected limb. Use sandbags or tie the affected limb to the table, keeping the humerus almost parallel to the table.

Comments and Tips

- There is some distortion as a result of increased OFD. Pull the limb as cranially and as close to the image receptor as possible.
- This positioning may not be tolerated by patients with fractures or severe degenerative joint disease. Consider using a horizontal beam if required in these situations.

Horizontal Beam of the Humerus—Ancillary

- The lateral decubitus view (caudocranial view with horizontal beam) may be useful if the patient is compromised in the dorsoventral position due to extensive trauma or other concerns.
- Center, measure, and include as for the caudocranial view.
- The patient is in opposite lateral recumbency with the extended affected side resting uppermost on a large sponge.
- The film-screen cassette is positioned against the cranial aspect of the affected forelimb.
- The tube head is directed horizontally from the caudal aspect of the limb and perpendicular to the humerus and image receptor.
- In cats, it may be difficult to place the cassette proximally enough to view the humeral head and the shoulder with a horizontal beam.

🖉 **TECHNICIAN NOTES**

Note that for the lateral and caudocranial views of the scapula, shoulder, and humerus, actual positioning procedures are similar, with slight variations.

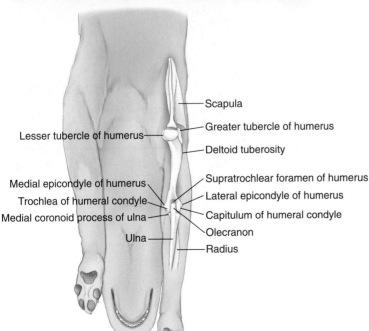

MEASURE: Midshaft toward the proximal aspect; across at the level of T1.

CENTRAL RAY: Midshaft of the humerus.

BORDERS: Proximal to the shoulder and distal to the elbow joints.

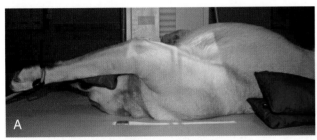

Scapula
Greater tubercle of humerus
Lesser tubercle of humerus
Deltoid tuberosity
Medial epicondyle of humerus
Supratrochlear foramen of humerus
Trochlea of humeral condyle
Lateral epicondyle of humerus
Medial coronoid process of ulna
Capitulum of humeral condyle
Ulna
Olecranon
Radius

B

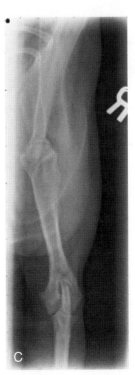

FIG. 18.8 A, Positioning for the caudocranial view of the humerus. **B,** Caudal view of right canine humerus. **C,** Caudocranial radiograph of the humerus. (B and C from Thrall DE. *Textbook of Veterinary Diagnostic Radiology,* 6th ed. St Louis: Elsevier; 2013.)

C

Craniocaudal View of the Humerus—Ancillary

Positioning

Place In: Dorsal recumbency in a trough or with the use of tape if needed.

Head and Neck: Keep the head and neck fairly straight, and secure with a sandbag if needed, taking care not to restrict breathing.

Hind Limbs: Leave in a natural position and support with sandbags if required.

Forelimbs: Extend the unaffected limb cranially and secure. The affected limb is flexed at the shoulder and pulled as far caudally as possible so that the humerus is parallel to the table. Tie to the table or carefully place a sandbag over the limb. The unaffected limb is left in a natural position.

Comments and Tips

- Use the craniocaudal view when adequate extension of postoperative patients cannot be achieved for the caudocranial view.
- The humerus is more nearly parallel to the table, but there is increased OFD.
- If the veterinarian suspects incomplete ossification of the humeral condyle, a CrCd is the best view, with a slight 15-degree craniomedal to caudolateral oblique.[2]
- Alternatively the patient can be placed in sternal recumbency with the limbs pulled forward. Extend the affected limb (Fig. 18.9B).

MEASURE: Midshaft of the humerus toward the proximal aspect.

CENTRAL RAY: Midshaft of the humerus.

BORDERS: Proximal to the shoulder and distal to the elbow joint.

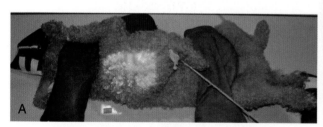
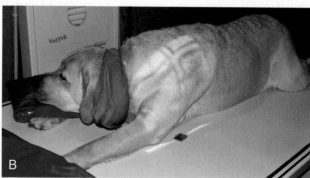

FIG. 18.9 A, Positioning for the craniocaudal view of the humerus in dorsal recumbency. B, Alternative positioning for the craniocaudal humerus view. (A courtesy Seneca College of Applied Arts and Technology, King City, Ontario.)

Elbow

Lateral (Mediolateral) View of the Elbow—Routine

The lateral view of the elbow joint can show a fragmented process.[6]

Positioning

Place In: Lateral recumbency with the affected limb down.

Head and Neck: Move dorsally, placing sandbags over the neck to keep in position, taking care not to restrict breathing.

Hind Limbs: Leave in a natural position and support with sandbags if needed.

Forelimbs: Extend the contralateral limb caudally and secure with ties or sandbag. Place the affected limb cranially and ventrally so that the degree of flexion is between 45 and 90 degrees, depending on veterinarian preference. Depending on the patient type, a small foam wedge can be placed under the metacarpus and/or the shoulder region.

Comments and Tips

- A small foam pad under the shoulder and distal region of the affected limb may help maintain lateral symmetry of the structures.
- Avoid rotation and superimposition of adjacent structures.
- A properly positioned elbow should show superimposition of the distal humeral condyles and a clear view of the olecranon.

MEASURE: Thickest part of the elbow at the distal humerus.

CENTRAL RAY: Palpate and center on the distal humeral condyles (elbow).

BORDERS: Distal third of the humerus to proximal third of the radius/ulna.

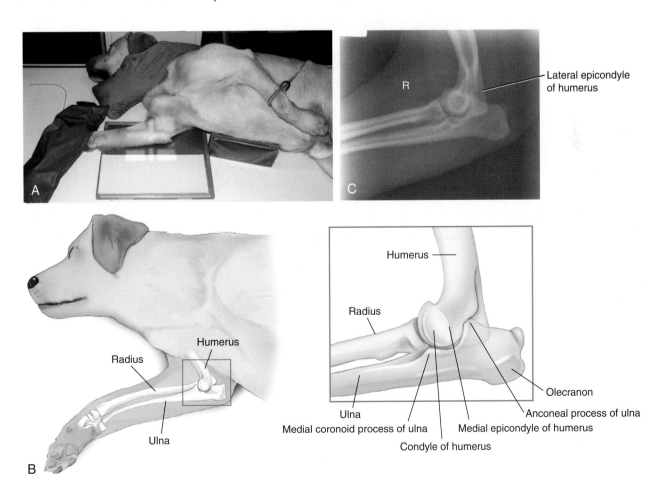

FIG. 18.10 A, Positioning for the mediolateral (lateral) view of the elbow joint. **B,** Medial view of the elbow joint. **C,** Mediolateral (lateral) radiograph of the elbow joint. (**B** and **C** courtesy Dana Greves and Jenn White, Mississauga Oakville Veterinary Emergency Hospital and Referral Group, Oakville, Ontario.)

Craniocaudal View of the Elbow—Routine

Positioning

Place In: Sternal recumbency.

Hind Limbs: Leave in a natural position to keep the spine straight and support with sandbags if needed. A V-trough may be used for stability of the caudal portion of the body.

Forelimbs: Extend both front legs forward. Pull the unaffected limb, placing a small foam pad under the elbow to prevent rolling and rotation. Extend the affected forelimb and secure it with a sandbag at the distal portion or tie to the table or to a sandbag.

Head and Neck: Pull away from the affected limb and the beam. Support the head at a natural height with foam pads. Tape can be placed around the head to keep it out of the field of view.

MEASURE: Thickest part of the elbow at the distal humerus.

CENTRAL RAY: Palpate and center on the humeral condyles at the level of articulation. Angle the beam distoproximally 10 to 20 degrees to visualize the joint surfaces if full extension is not possible.

BORDERS: Distal third of the humerus to proximal third of the radius/ulna.

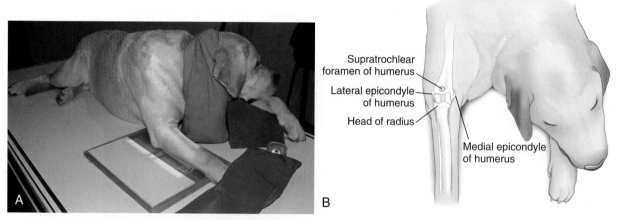

Supratrochlear foramen of humerus

Lateral epicondyle of humerus

Head of radius

Medial epicondyle of humerus

FIG. 18.11 A, Positioning for the craniocaudal projection of the elbow joint. Putting a sponge under the opposite elbow and head helps keep the olecranon in true CrCd position. B and C, Cranial views of the right elbow. D, Craniocaudal radiograph of the elbow joint.

Craniocaudal View of the Elbow—Routine—cont'd

Comments and Tips

- Symmetry is essential.
  - Move the patient's body slightly until palpation reveals the olecranon of the ulna to be in the center of the joint.
  - The olecranon should be positioned midway between the lateral and medial humeral epicondyles on the finished radiograph.
- The slight raising of the opposite limb helps place the olecranon between the humeral epicondyles.

- This keeps the radius and ulna parallel and the humerus at a slight angle to the tabletop.
- The paw of the affected limb is not flat on the table for a true craniocaudal elbow view.
- A craniocaudal view can also be completed with the patient in dorsal recumbency and the affected limb pulled caudally.
  - Keep the humerus parallel to the table.
  - To prevent superimposition of the ribs, abduct the affected limb slightly away from the thorax.

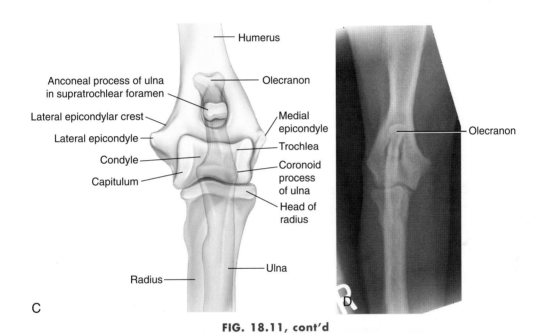

C

D

FIG. 18.11, cont'd

Hyperflexed (Mediolateral) View of the Elbow—Ancillary

- Hyperflexion allows evaluation of the ulnar anconeal process. This view is indicated when an ununited anconeal process (failure of the anconeal process to unite with the ulna, resulting in a fracture through the growth plate), a fragmented coronoid, or osteochondrosis is suspected.
- Elbow dysplasia is seen primarily in young dogs of large breeds and can cause varying degrees of weight-bearing lameness and arthritis.
- Extreme flexion of the medial to lateral view is required if radiographs are being sent to the Orthopedic Foundation of Animals for elbow dysplasia evaluation.[7]

Positioning

Place In: Lateral recumbency with the affected limb down.

Head and Neck: Move dorsally, placing sandbags over the neck to keep in position.

Hind Limbs: Leave in a natural position and support with sandbags if needed.

Forelimbs: Secure the unaffected limb caudally. Keep the carpus in a true lateral position as you move it toward the neck. Flex the affected elbow as much as possible by bending the limb dorsally and securing the paw under the head with a sandbag or tape. Tape is preferred. Place tape on the metacarpal region, flex the limb, and fasten the tape on the lateral aspect of the metacarpus. Affix the tape to the table under the cranial cervical region.

Comments and Tips

- A sponge under the shoulder may prevent the flexed elbow from moving medially.
- The limb should be flat on the table in a true lateral position with no rotation.
- If the tape was secured on the medial aspect, upward rotation would occur, causing the site of interest to be oblique.
- The elbow is positioned directly over the center of the digital plate. Tight collimation is essential.

MEASURE: At the distal humerus with the elbow in the flexed position.

CENTRAL RAY: Palpate and center on the humeral condyles.

BORDERS: Distal third of the humerus to proximal third of the radius/ulna.

> **✎ TECHNICIAN NOTES**
>
> Flexion assists in full examination of the joint.

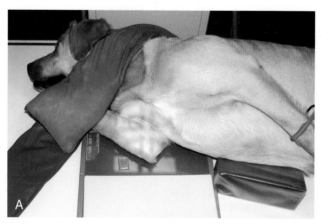

FIG. 18.12 A, Positioning for the mediolateral (lateral) flexed view of the elbow joint.

Hyperflexed (Mediolateral) View of the Elbow—Ancillary—cont'd

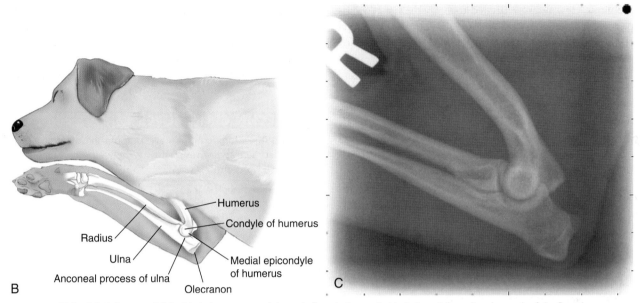

B, Medial projection of the right flexed elbow.

Humerus
Condyle of humerus
Radius
Medial epicondyle of humerus
Ulna
Anconeal process of ulna
Olecranon

B

C

FIG. 18.12, cont'd B, Medial projection of the right flexed elbow. C, Mediolateral (lateral) radiograph of the flexed elbow. (B and C courtesy Dana Greves and Jenn White, Mississauga Oakville Veterinary Emergency Hospital and Referral Group, Oakville, Ontario.)

Craniocaudal View With a Horizontal Beam of the Elbow—Ancillary

The CrCd elbow view (lateral decubitus) could also be taken with a horizontal beam if required:

- Measure, center, and include as for the craniocaudal view at the elbow joint.
- The patient would be in lateral recumbency with the extended affected side uppermost, resting on a large sponge, and with the head hyperextended away from the x-ray beam.
- The cassette is positioned against the caudal aspect of the upper forelimb.
- The tube head is directed horizontally from the cranial aspect of the limb and perpendicular to the elbow and the cassette. (See Fig. 18.16 as an example of using the CrCd view with a horizontal beam. The centering and borders would differ for the elbow.

Oblique View of the Elbow—Ancillary

An oblique view may be needed to properly visualize the supratrochlear foramen of the humerus and the anconeal and coronoid process of the ulna (Fig. 18.13).

- Measure, center, and include as for the craniocaudal view.
- Support the patient and limb with foam pads and sandbags.
- Pull and support the affected limb as cranial as possible and rotate the elbow joint:
  - Laterally about 30 degrees for the medial oblique and to see the medial coronoid process (craniolateral-caudomedial oblique) view
  - Medially (toward the patient) about 30 degrees for the lateral oblique (craniomedial-caudolateral oblique) view.
- Include only the structures making up the articulation.

Comments and Tips

- If the position is used to visualize increased joint space and see the medial coronoid process, extend the limb and angle the x-ray beam 20 degrees craniodistal to caudoproximal.[4]

✎ TECHNICIAN NOTES

For a true craniocaudal view, palpate the olecranon, making sure that it rests midway between the humeral epicondyles.

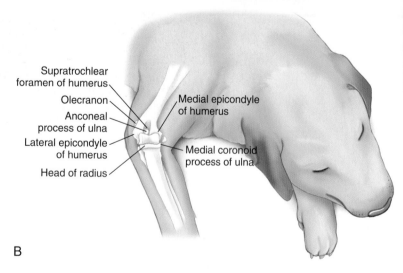

A

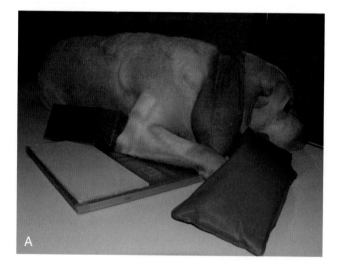

Supratrochlear foramen of humerus
Olecranon
Anconeal process of ulna
Lateral epicondyle of humerus
Head of radius
Medial epicondyle of humerus
Medial coronoid process of ulna

B

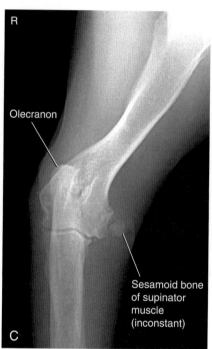

R

Olecranon

Sesamoid bone of supinator muscle (inconstant)

C

FIG. 18.13 A, Positioning for an oblique projection of the elbow joint. This is the craniolateral-caudomedial (medial) oblique position. Ideally the limb should be pulled more cranially. **B,** Medial oblique view of the right elbow joint. **C,** Craniolateral-caudomedial (medial) oblique radiograph of the right elbow. (**B** and **C** courtesy Dana Greves and Jenn White, Mississauga Oakville Veterinary Emergency Hospital and Referral Group, Oakville, Ontario.)

Radius/Ulna

Lateral (Mediolateral) View of the Radius/Ulna—Routine

Positioning

Positioning is the same as for the lateral extended elbow view:

Place In: Lateral recumbency with the affected limb down.

Head and Neck: Move the head and neck dorsally, placing sandbags over the neck to keep in position and taking care not to restrict breathing.

Hind Limbs: Leave in a natural position and support with sandbags if needed.

Forelimbs: Extend the contralateral limb caudodorsally and secure with a sandbag or tie. Place the affected limb parallel to the edges of the image receptor or table and support with a sandbag. Slightly flex the carpus to avoid supination of the limb. Depending on the patient anatomy, a small foam wedge can be placed under either the metacarpal region or the shoulder region to keep a true lateral view of the elbow.

Comments and Tips

- Placing foam under the humerus and cranial thorax may help keep proper alignment.
- Make sure the image receptor is large enough to include both the proximal row of carpal bones and the proximal olecranon.
- If the distal portion of the radius and ulna is the area of interest, measure at the midshaft of the bone to minimize overexposure.

MEASURE: Site of the distal humerus.

CENTRAL RAY: Midshaft of the radius and ulna.

BORDERS: Proximal to elbow joint and distal to carpal joint.

🖉 **TECHNICIAN NOTES**

Note the similarity in positioning procedures for the elbow, radius and ulna, and foot.

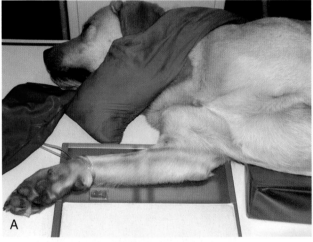

A

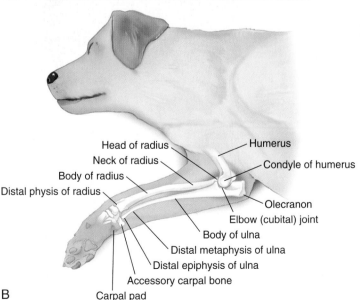

Head of radius
Neck of radius
Body of radius
Distal physis of radius
Humerus
Condyle of humerus
Olecranon
Elbow (cubital) joint
Body of ulna
Distal metaphysis of ulna
Distal epiphysis of ulna
Accessory carpal bone
Carpal pad

B

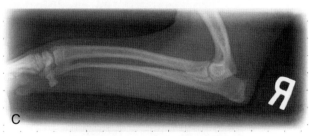

C

FIG. 18.14 A, Positioning for the mediolateral (lateral) projection of the radius and ulna. B, Medial view of the right radius and ulna. C, Mediolateral (lateral) radiograph of the radius and ulna. (B and C courtesy Dana Greves and Jenn White, Mississauga Oakville Veterinary Emergency Hospital and Referral Group, Oakville, Ontario.)

Craniocaudal View of the Radius/Ulna—Routine

Positioning

Positioning is the same as for the CrCd elbow view.

Place In: Sternal recumbency.

Head and Neck: Move away from the affected limb and beam. Support the head in a comfortable position with foam pads. Sandbags or tape can be placed around the head to keep it out of the field of view.

Hind Limbs: Leave in a natural position to keep the spine straight and support with sandbags if needed. A V-trough may be used for stability of the caudal half of the body.

Forelimbs: Place a small foam pad under the elbow of the unaffected limb to prevent rolling or rotation. Extend the affected forelimb and hold it with a sandbag or tie to the table or to a sandbag.

Comments and Tips

- Palpate to confirm that the olecranon is positioned midway between the humeral epicondyles for a true CrCd view of the radius/ulna.
- A thin foam pad placed between the point of the elbow and the image receptor may stabilize the elbow.
- Make sure that the image receptor is long enough to incorporate the carpus and elbow as well as the radius/ulna.
- If the distal portion of the radius and ulna is the area of interest, measure at the midshaft of the bone to minimize overexposure.
- A horizontal beam (lateral decubitus) can also be taken to show the CrCd view of the radius and ulna (Fig. 18.16).

MEASURE: Site of the distal humerus.

CENTRAL RAY: Midshaft of the radius and ulna.

BORDERS: Proximal to the elbow joint and distal to the carpal joint.

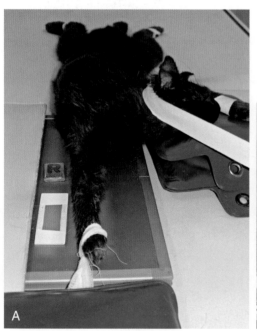
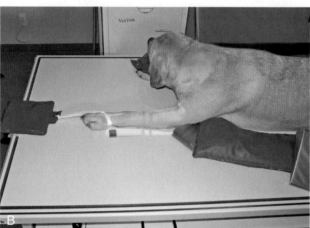

FIG. 18.15 A, Positioning for the craniocaudal view of the feline radius and ulna. Tape can be used to keep the head out of the field of view. **B,** Positioning for the craniocaudal view of the canine radius and ulna.

Craniocaudal View of the Radius/Ulna—Routine—cont'd

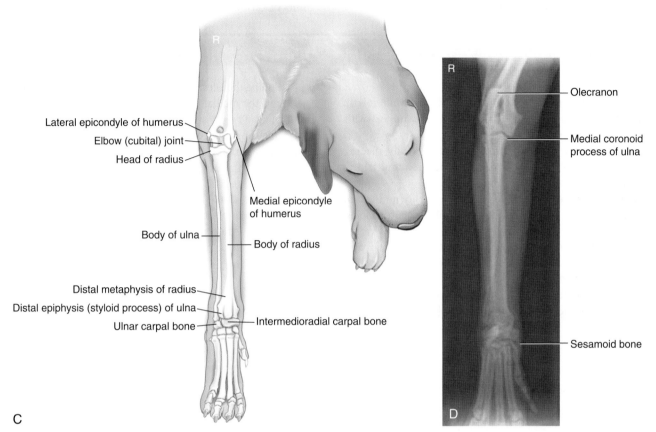

Lateral epicondyle of humerus
Elbow (cubital) joint
Head of radius
Medial epicondyle of humerus
Body of ulna
Body of radius
Distal metaphysis of radius
Distal epiphysis (styloid process) of ulna
Ulnar carpal bone
Intermedioradial carpal bone

Olecranon
Medial coronoid process of ulna
Sesamoid bone

C

D

FIG. 18.15, cont'd C, Cranial view of the right canine radius and ulna. D, Craniocaudal radiograph of the right canine radius and ulna.

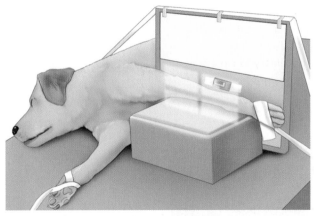

FIG. 18.16 Positioning for a craniocaudal view of the radius/ulna using a horizontal beam.

The Foot: Carpus, Metacarpus, and Digits

The carpus, metacarpus, and digits are typically radiographed in one view. If there is a particular area of interest, center and measure on this site. See Fig. 24.29C for anatomy of the carpal joints of various species.

Lateral (Mediolateral) View of the Foot—Routine

Positioning

Place In: Lateral recumbency with the affected limb down.

Hind Limbs: Leave in a natural position and support with sandbags if needed.

Head and Neck: Move the head and neck dorsally, placing sandbags over the neck to keep the position and taking care not to restrict breathing.

Forelimbs: Extend the contralateral limb caudally, and secure with a sandbag. Extend the affected limb cranially, placing sandbags on the proximal portion of the limb. Tie or support the distal metacarpus to the table or a sandbag.

Radiographing the Digits: Separate the digits to prevent superimposition. This is best completed by:

- Separately taping around the toenail of the lateral (fifth) phalanx and the medial (second) phalanx.

- Pulling the lateral phalanx slightly cranially and laterally and the medial phalanx slightly caudally and laterally.

Tape can also be put around the digit itself, or cotton or foam (manicuring pads) can be placed between the toes, although the latter method does not separate the phalanges as effectively.

Comments and Tips

- A wooden or plastic paddle supported with a sandbag can assist in positioning.
- The foot can be flexed by applying slight dorsal pressure to the digits.

MEASURE: At the site of interest:

Carpus: At the carpal joint.

Metacarpus or Phalanges: At the site of the phalangeal-metacarpal articulation.

CENTRAL RAY: Centered on the area of interest:

Carpus: Middle row of carpal bones.

Metacarpus or Phalanges: Center of the phalangeal-metacarpal articulation.

BORDERS:

Carpus: Distal third of the radius and ulna to proximal third of the metacarpus.

Metacarpus or Phalanges: Carpus proximally to the distal phalanges.

> ### ✎ TECHNICIAN NOTE
>
> The film cassette can be split to include both views on the image if the grid is not used. Make sure that the toes point in the same direction, collimate tightly, and place a lead shield on the side not being imaged to prevent scatter radiation from affecting the contrast.

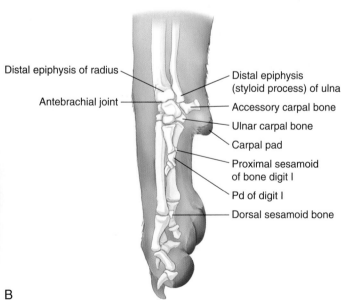

Distal epiphysis of radius

Antebrachial joint

Distal epiphysis (styloid process) of ulna

Accessory carpal bone

Ulnar carpal bone

Carpal pad

Proximal sesamoid of bone digit I

Pd of digit I

Dorsal sesamoid bone

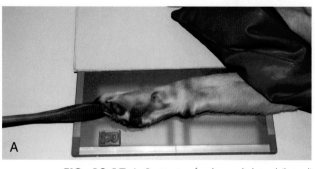

A   B

FIG. 18.17 A, Positioning for the mediolateral (lateral) projection of the canine carpus, metacarpus, and digits. Tape can also be used to secure the limb. **B,** Medial view of canine carpus, metacarpus, and digits.

Lateral (Mediolateral) View of the Foot—Routine—cont'd

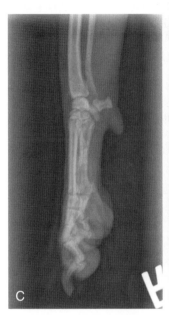
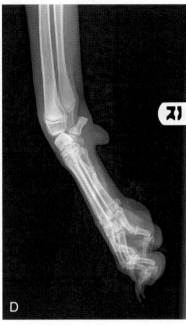

FIG. 18.17, cont'd C, Mediolateral (lateral) radiograph of the canine, metacarpus, and digits. **D**, Flexed lateral radiograph of the carpus when pressure is applied to the dorsal surface of the digits. (**B** and **C** courtesy Dana Greves and Jenn White, Mississauga Oakville Veterinary Emergency Hospital and Referral Group, Oakville, Ontario; **D** courtesy Rosedale Animal Hospital.)

Lateral (Mediolateral) Hyperextended View of the Foot—Ancillary

Hyperextended Lateral View of the Foot (Stressed View)[5]

- Position as for the lateral.
- Keep the carpus in a true lateral projection.
- Hyperextend the carpus by bending the toes upward.
- Apply tape at the radius and ulna, and secure to the table laterally (Fig. 18.18).
- Apply tape at the distal metacarpus/digits; extend the limb and secure the tape in the opposite direction of the tape on the radius/ulna.

- A wooden spoon can also be used to extend the toes dorsally provided that lateral counterpressure is placed on the radius/ulna.
- This view helps determine distribution of joint involvement and lesions that might not be visible if the joint is not stressed.

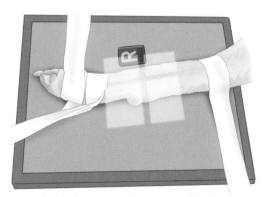

FIG. 18.18 Positioning for the hyperextended lateral view of the carpus.

Lateral (Mediolateral) Hyperflexed View of the Carpus—Ancillary

Positioning

Place In: Lateral recumbency with the affected limb down.

Head and Neck: Move dorsally, placing sandbags over the neck to keep it in position, taking care not to restrict breathing.

Hind Limbs: Leave in a natural position and support with sandbags if needed.

Forelimbs: Extend the contralateral limb caudally, and secure with a sandbag or tie. Extend the affected limb and hyperflex the carpus by either:

- Taping a figure-eight pattern around the metacarpus and radius and ulna (best).

- Keeping the carpus flexed by (1) bending the toes caudally toward the radius and ulna, (2) applying pressure with a wooden or plastic paddle at the phalanges, and (3) securing with a sandbag.

Comments and Tips

- Do not extend the carpus beyond the patient's available range of motion.
- This position helps evaluate the carpal articulation when joint laxity is noted.

MEASURE: At the carpus joint while in the flexed position.

CENTRAL RAY: On the middle row of carpal bones.

BORDERS: Distal third of the radius/ulna to proximal third of the metacarpus, including the digits if needed.

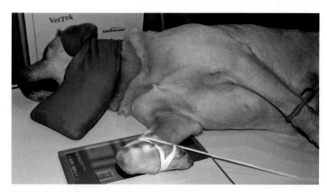

FIG. 18.19 Positioning for the flexed mediolateral projection of the canine carpus, metacarpus, and digits.

Dorsopalmar View of the Foot—Routine

Positioning

Place In: Sternal recumbency.

Head and Neck: Displace and support the head laterally with foam pads, sandbags, or tape away from the affected limb and the beam.

Hind Limbs: Extend in a natural position to keep the spine straight and support with sandbags if needed. A V-trough may be used for stability of the caudal half of the body.

Forelimbs: Extend both forward. Secure the affected forelimb with a sandbag at the proximal portion. Tie the metacarpus/digits at the distal portion and secure the limb to a sandbag.

MEASURE: At the site of interest:

Carpus: Carpus joint.

Metacarpus or Phalanges: Site of the phalangeal-metacarpal articulation at the level of the middle phalanx.

CENTRAL RAY: Centered on the area of interest:

Carpus: Middle row of carpal bones.

Phalanges: Third and fourth phalangeal-metacarpal articulations.

BORDERS:

Carpus: Distal third of the radius/ulna to proximal third of the metacarpals.

Metacarpus or Phalanges: Carpus proximally to the distal phalanges.

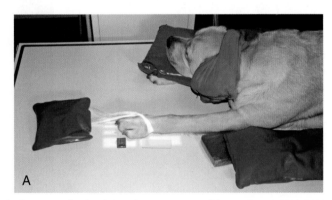

FIG. 18.20 A, Positioning for the dorsopalmar projection of the canine carpus, metacarpus, and digits.

Continued

Dorsopalmar View of the Foot—Routine—cont'd

Comments and Tips

- Abduct the affected elbow slightly to straighten the carpus.
- If joint laxity of the carpus is present and evaluation of the joint space is required:

- Stress can be put on the carpus by applying tape to the midradius/ulna and the distal metacarpus.
- Pull in opposite directions, as for the extended lateral view of the carpus (Fig. 18.21).[6]

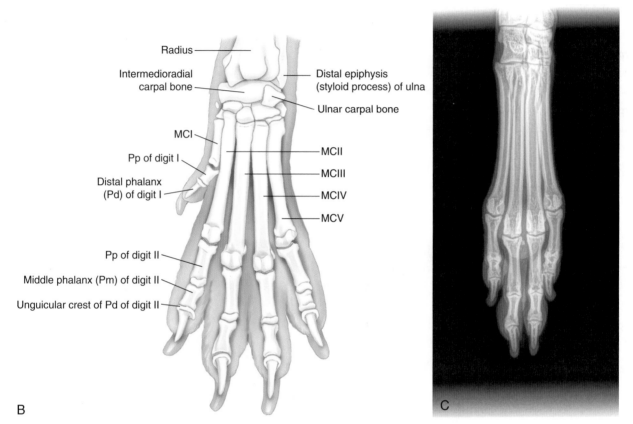

Radius

Intermedioradial carpal bone

Distal epiphysis (styloid process) of ulna

Ulnar carpal bone

MCI

Pp of digit I

Distal phalanx (Pd) of digit I

MCII

MCIII

MCIV

MCV

Pp of digit II

Middle phalanx (Pm) of digit II

Unguicular crest of Pd of digit II

B

C

FIG. 18.20, cont'd B, Dorsal view of the canine carpus, metacarpus, and digits. C, Dorsopalmar radiograph of the canine carpus, metacarpus, and digits. (C courtesy Jennifer White, Mississauga Oakville Veterinary Emergency Hospital and Referral Group, Oakville, Ontario.)

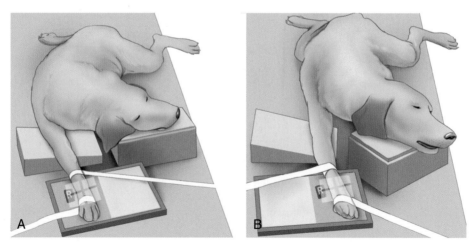

A

B

FIG. 18.21 Stress radiographs of the carpus may be completed if joint laxity is to be determined. The position and pulling of the tape change where pressure is applied on the carpus: A, Medial stress; B, lateral stress.

Oblique Views of the Foot—Ancillary

The two oblique views of the foot are the dorsolateral pal-maromedial oblique (DLPMO)–medial oblique view and the dorsomedial palmarolateral oblique (DMPLO)–lateral oblique view (Figs. 18.22 and 18.23).

Positioning
Place In: Sternal recumbency.
Head and Neck: Displace and support the head laterally, with foam pads, sandbags, or tape, away from the affected limb and beam.
Hind Limbs: Extend caudally in a natural position to keep the spine straight and support with sandbags if needed. A V-trough may be used for stability of the caudal half of the body.

Forelimbs: Extend both forward. Secure the affected distal metacarpus/digits and pull cranially.
- For the medial oblique view: rotate the elbow joint 45 degrees laterally and support it with tape and sandbag.
- For the lateral oblique view: rotate the elbow joint 45 degrees medially and support it with tape and sandbag.

Comments and Tips
- Rotate the elbow just enough so that the beam will enter the limb at about 45 degrees from the midsagittal plane either laterally or medially.

MEASURE: At the site of interest:

Carpus: Carpus joint.

Metacarpus or Phalanges: Site of phalangeal-metacarpal articulation at the level of the middle phalanx.

CENTRAL RAY: Centered on the area of interest:

Carpus: Middle row of the carpal bones.

Phalanges: Third and fourth phalangeal-metacarpal articulations.

Lateral Oblique View: Center the beam 45 degrees medially from the midsagittal plane (see Fig. 18.22).

Medial Oblique View: Center the beam 45 degrees laterally from the midsagittal plane (see Fig. 18.23).

BORDERS:

Carpus: Distal third of the radius/ulna to proximal third of the metacarpus.

Metacarpus or Phalanges: Carpus proximally to the distal phalanges.

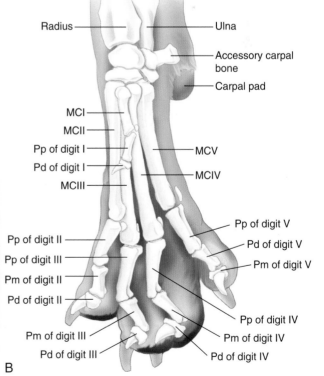

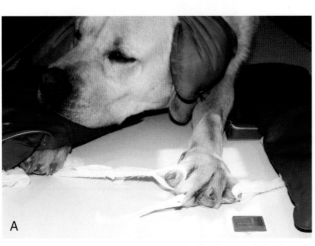

FIG. 18.22 A, Positioning for the dorsomedial-palmarolateral (lateral) oblique projection of the canine metacarpus and digits with the digits separated. B, Dorsomedial-palmarolateral (lateral) oblique view of the canine carpus, metacarpus, and digits.

Continued

Oblique Views of the Foot—Ancillary—cont'd

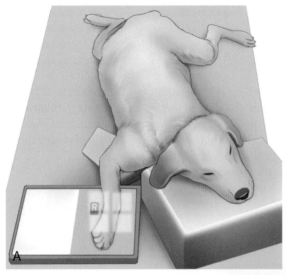

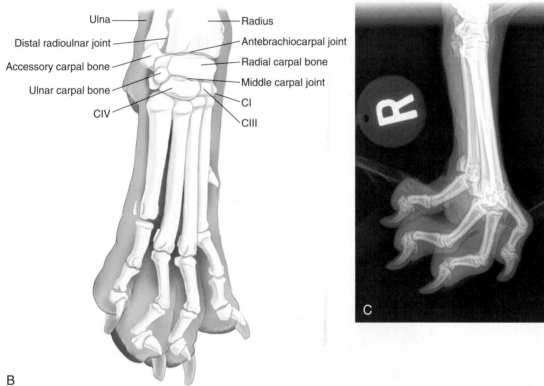

B

FIG. 18.23 **A,** Positioning for dorsolateral-palmaromedial (medial) oblique radiograph. **B,** Medial oblique radiographic anatomy of the canine carpus. **C,** Medial oblique radiograph of the metacarpus and digits. (**A** and **B** courtesy Joshua Schlote, BS, LVT, Northeast Community College; **C** courtesy Jennifer White, Mississauga Oakville Veterinary Emergency Hospital and Referral Group, Oakville, Ontario.)

Fig. 18.24 is a mystery radiograph. Review it and answer the question presented with it.

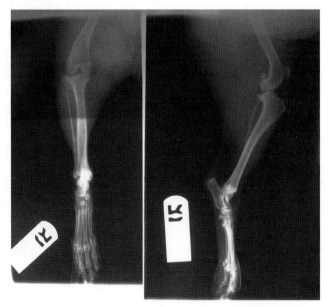

FIG. 18.24 Mystery radiograph. Other radiographs from the same source have a similar appearance, with the variation in contrast on one section of the radiograph. What could some of the causes be?

REVIEW QUESTIONS

1. A lateral radius/ulna radiograph of a Doberman is required. The marker should be placed at the:
   a. Cranial radius/ulna
   b. Lateral radius/ulna
   c. Caudal radius/ulna
   d. Medial radius/ulna

2. You are to radiograph the lateral shoulder joint of a feline patient. The field of view should include the:
   a. Shoulder joint itself
   b. Distal third of the humerus and proximal third of the scapula
   c. Proximal third of the scapula through the proximal third of the humerus
   d. Distal third of the humerus and proximal third of the scapula

3. The veterinarian requests that you complete images for the shoulder joint of a 6-month-old Great Dane who is limping on its right side, which worsens after exercise. He suspects osteochondrosis and wishes a lateral radiograph to confirm. It is best to complete the position so that:
   a. The shoulder joint is not superimposed over the trachea
   b. There is no pronation or supination of the affected limb
   c. Only a right lateral is taken as the left lateral is not needed
   d. The left lateral is taken to see the magnified lesion on the right limb

4. The caudocranial scapula radiograph of an Akita is best taken with the patient lying in:
   a. Dorsal recumbency
   b. Ventral recumbency
   c. A right lateral oblique position
   d. A left lateral oblique position

5. What is the primary disadvantage of the CrCd view of the humerus versus the CdCr view?
   a. The limb is positioned parallel to the image receptor.
   b. Superimposition over the ribs is likely.
   c. The limb must be abducted slightly from the thorax.
   d. Increased object-film distance can cause magnification.

6. For routine radiography of a Bichon Frise, the best views of the elbow are the lateral and the:
   a. Caudocranial
   b. Craniocaudal
   c. Palmarodorsal
   d. Dorsopalmar

7. To ensure proper symmetry for the elbow view of the Bichon Frise selected in the previous question, it is suggested to:
   a. Slightly raise the opposite limb
   b. Keep the opposite limb flat on the table
   c. Keep the patient on its back
   d. Position and raise the head toward the affected limb

8. The best view for evaluation of the ulnar anconeal process of a Bernese Mountain dog is a(an):
   a. Extended mediolateral view of the elbow
   b. Natural mediolateral view of the elbow
   c. Flexed mediolateral view of the elbow
   d. Craniocaudal view of the radius/ulna

9. The peripheral borders to evaluate the ulnar anconeal process of the Bernese Mountain dog elbow would be:
   a. Two thirds of the bones distal and proximal
   b. The carpus and the shoulder joint
   c. Proximal third of the tibia/fibula and distal third of the femur
   d. Proximal third of the radius/ulna and distal third of the humerus

10. It is important when radiographing either a lateral shoulder or humerus of a Boxer to:
    a. Keep the head and limbs in as natural position as possible
    b. Keep the patient in dorsal recumbency
    c. Raise the head and keep the affected and contralateral limbs in a natural position
    d. Raise the head and neck dorsally, and pull the affected limb cranially

11. You would measure a craniocaudal view of the radius and ulna of a Retriever at the:
    a. Proximal radius
    b. Distal humerus
    c. Distal radius
    d. Elbow joint

12. The veterinarian requires an orthogonal view of the right humerus of a Retriever who has a severe fracture with some thoracic pathology. In this case you are probably best to consider a radiograph of the:
    a. Caudocranial view with a vertical beam
    b. Right lateral decubitus view with a horizontal beam
    c. Left lateral decubitus view with a horizontal beam
    d. Right craniocaudal decubitus view with a horizontal beam.

13. The patient in the previous question requiring the orthogonal view of the humerus should be positioned:
    a. With the right limb uppermost on a large sponge
    b. With the right limb on the table on a small sponge
    c. In ventral recumbency
    d. In dorsal recumbency

14. Fractured toes are suspected in a German Shepherd. For a medial oblique view you should center on the:
    a. Dorsomedial aspect and place the lateral toes against the image receptor
    b. Palmarolateral aspect and place the medial toes against the image receptor
    c. Palmaromedial aspect and place the lateral toes against the image receptor
    d. Dorsolateral aspect and place the medial toes against the image receptor

15. For the medial oblique of the view in the previous question, you should include:
    a. Radius ulna to the distal digits
    b. Metacarpus to the distal digits
    c. From the carpus to the distal digits
    d. First to fifth digits

16. To prevent superimposition of the scapula and ribs in the caudocranial scapula of a Borzoi:
    a. Rotate the patient's sternum from the scapula about 40 degrees
    b. Rotate the patient's sternum from the scapula about 10 to 12 degrees
    c. Have the scapula perpendicular to the table and parallel to the sternum
    d. Have the forelimbs pulled caudally and separate the affected limb from the body

Answers to Review Questions can be found on the Evolve website.

References

1. Holloway A, McConnell F. *BSAVA Manual of Canine and Feline Radiography and Radiology: A Foundation Manual.* Suffolk: BSAVA; 2013:[Chapter 7].
2. Thrall DE. *Textbook of Veterinary Diagnostic Radiology.* 6th ed. St. Louis: Elsevier; 2013.
3. Aspinall V, Cappello M. *Introduction to Veterinary Anatomy.* London: Butterman-Heineman; 2009.
4. Muhlbauer MC, Kneller SK. *Radiography of the Dog and Cat: Guide to Making and Interpreting Radiographs.* Oxford: Wiley-Blackwell; 2013:[Chapter 2].
5. Sirois M, Anthony E, Mauragis D. *Handbook of Radiographic Positioning for Veterinary Technicians.* Clifton Park, NY: Delmar Cengage Learning; 2010.
6. Han C, Hurd C. *Practical Diagnostic Imaging for the Veterinary Technician.* ed 3. St. Louis: Mosby; 2005.
7. Orthopedic Foundation for Animals. Application for Hip/Elbow Dysplasia Database; 2016. http://www.offa.org/pdf/hdedapp_bw.pdf.

Bibliography

Ayers S. *Small Animal Radiographic Techniques and Positioning.* Oxford: Wiley-Blackwell; 2013.
Colville T, Bassert J. *Clinical Anatomy and Physiology for Veterinary Technicians.* 3rd ed. St. Louis: Mosby; 2015.
Done SH, Goody PC, Stickland NC, et al. *Color Atlas of Veterinary Anatomy, the Dog and Cat.* London: Mosby; 2009.
Dyce KM, Sack WO, Wensing CJG. *Textbook of Veterinary Anatomy.* 4th ed. St. Louis: Saunders; 2010.
Evans H, de Launta A. *Guide to the Dissection of the Dog.* 7th ed. St. Louis: Saunders; 2010.
Holloway A. *BSAVA Manual of Canine and Feline Radiography and Radiology: A Foundation Manual.* Suffolk: BSAVA; 2013.
Morgan JP. *Techniques of Veterinary Radiography.* Ames, IA: Iowa State University Press; 1993.
Owens JM, Biery DN. *Radiographic Interpretation for the Small Animal Clinician.* St. Louis: Ralston Purina; 1999.
Ryan G. *Radiographic Positioning of Small Animals.* Philadelphia: Lea & Febiger; 1981.
Tighe M, Brown M. *Mosby's Comprehensive Review for Veterinary Technicians.* 4th ed. St. Louis: Elsevier; 2015.

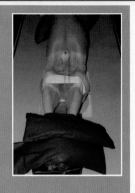

CHAPTER 19
Small Animal Pelvis and Pelvic Limb

Marg Brown, RVT, BEd Ad Ed

Adopt the pace of nature: her secret is patience.
—Ralph Waldo Emerson, American essayist and poet, 1803–1882

OUTLINE

LEARNING OBJECTIVES

When you have finished this chapter, you will be able to:

1. Properly and safely position a dog or cat for the various common positions of the pelvic limb with an emphasis on nonmanual restraint.
2. Correctly measure and center the patient to include the peripheral borders.
3. Ensure that the body part is parallel to the image receptor and the central ray is perpendicular to the field of view (FOV) and receptor.
4. Identify views that may need to be completed as an alternative.
5. Identify normal anatomy of the pelvis and hind limb found on a radiograph.

KEY TERMS

Abduction
Axial rotation
Cavitation
Congruence
Degenerative joint disease

Distraction index
Dysplasia
Frog-leg VD
Hip dysplasia
Laxity

Legg-Calve-Perthes (LCP)
   disease
Luxation
PennHIP
Positional terminology

Stance phase
Subluxation
Ventrodorsal extended leg
   view, OFA

TECHNICAL NOTE: To preserve space, the radiographs presented in this chapter do not show collimation. For safety, always collimate so that the beam is limited to within the image receptor edges. In film radiography, you should see a clear border of collimation (frame) on every radiograph. In some jurisdictions, evidence of collimation is required by law.

As indicated in the previous chapter, imaging of the appendicular skeleton is requisitioned to detect fractures, cause of pain, and/or lameness. Please review Chapter 18 for radiographic and patient concerns common to the pectoral and pelvic limbs because the same principles of proper imaging apply. See Box 18.1 for some terms relating to radiographic anatomy associated with bones.

Imaging of the pelvis is generally performed to evaluate dysplastic or degenerative changes of the coxofemoral joints (Box 19.1). Fractures, joint-associated neoplasia, and arthritis are further reasons for radiographing not only the pelvis but also the femur, stifle, tarsus, metatarsus, and phalanges, which make up the remaining portion of the hind limb of the appendicular skeleton.

A minimum of two perpendicular views of the pelvis and pelvic limbs, as with other body parts, is required in addition to the lateral (L) view (Table 19.1). The general rule for both pectoral and pelvic limbs is to have the patient in:

- Dorsal recumbency for the proximal portion of the pelvis and limb (pelvis and femur) (Fig. 19.1)
- Sternal recumbency for the distal portion (stifle, tibia/fibula, tarsus, metatarsus, and digits) (Fig. 19.2)
- If we keep this positioning in mind, it is easy to remember the proper names:
- The orthogonal view for the pelvis in dorsal recumbency is the ventrodorsal (VD).

- The femur in dorsal recumbency is termed craniocaudal (CrCd).
- The patient is in sternal recumbency for views of the limb distal to and including the stifle:
  - The stifle, tibia, and fibula are referred to as caudocranial (CdCr).
  - Views distal to and including the tarsus are plantarodorsal (PlD/PD).

As with the pectoral limb, a grid is not generally used because the tissue thickness is generally less than 10 cm. However, most canine pelvis views require a grid because of the greater thickness. The Orthopedic Foundation of Animals (OFA) requires that for radiographic submissions, "film contrast should be such that the microtrabecular pattern of the femoral head and neck are readily seen. The dorsal-lateral margin of the acetabulum must also be visible."[1]

Review the suggestions in Chapter 15 on techniques that can be used to assist in obtaining high-quality radiographs with the use of nonmanual restraint, including sandbags, tape, soft Velcro strapping, rope, etc. Try to give your patient the illusion it is being held without actually holding. Analgesia and chemical restraint are highly recommended.

BOX 19.1	Normal Coxofemoral Anatomy

Breed variations must be kept in mind, but generally:
- The cranial third of each coxofemoral joint space is equal in width.
- At least half of the femoral head should be positioned within the acetabulum.
- The angle of the femoral neck should be about 130 degrees.
- Femoral heads should be rounded and smooth; the fovea capitis is a normal flattened area on the femoral head.
- The femoral neck should be smooth with no proliferative remodeling changes.

TABLE 19.1	Protocol for the Pelvis and Pelvic Limb Radiography	
ANATOMICAL LOCATION	**ROUTINE VIEWS**	**ANCILLARY VIEWS**
Pelvis	Lateral, Ventrodorsal extended	Ventrodorsal: frog-leg PennHIP*: compression, distraction
Femur	Lateral, Craniocaudal	Caudocranial
Stifle	Lateral, Caudocranial	Proximodistal (skyline)
Tibia/fibula	Lateral, Caudocranial	
Foot: tarsus, metatarsus, and digits	Lateral, Plantarodorsal	Flexed and extended lateral, dorsoplantar, obliques

*Requires certification and training.

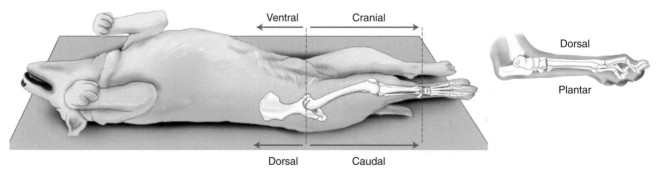

FIG. 19.1 Patient in dorsal recumbency for the proximal portion of the contralateral image of the pelvis, acetabulum, and femur. In this position the femur is the craniocaudal (CrCd) view and the pelvis is the ventrodorsal (VD) view. Although this view is not usually used for the foot, the digits would be termed dorsoplantar (DPl/DP) in this position.

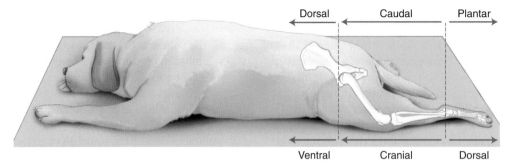

Dorsal   Caudal   Plantar

Ventral   Cranial   Dorsal

FIG. 19.2 For positioning of the distal rear limbs (patella, tibia, fibula, tarsus, metatarsus, and digits), the patient is generally in sternal recumbency. Note that the terminology changes at and including the tarsus. Thus in this position the patella would be referred to as caudocranial (CdCr) and the tarsus as plantarodorsal (PlD/PD).

✎ TECHNICIAN NOTES

For high-quality orthopedic radiographs:
- Low kV and high mAs technique
- Tabletop technique except for the pelvis and proximal limb of large dogs
- Small focal spot
- Measure at the thickest part of the area to be radiographed
- Measure the patient in the position in which it is to be imaged
- Minimize object-film distance (OFD)
- Center at the area of interest: either the center of the bone or at the joint
- Collimate and include only what is required
- Keep the bone parallel to the image receptor
- Keep the central ray perpendicular to the bone and image receptor
- No rotation
- Minimize superimposed structures
- Label correctly
- Place the label at the dorsal/cranial limb for the lateral views and laterally for orthogonal views
- Obtain orthogonal views
- Radiograph the contralateral limb for comparison when required

---

✎ TECHNICIAN NOTES

Mentally place the patient in sternal recumbency for the distal portion of the limb and in dorsal recumbency for the proximal portion, and the terms will be easier to remember. For long bones, the field of view includes the joints proximal and distal. For joints, the field of view includes one-third each of the bones proximal and distal.

BOX 19.2	Radiographic Signs of Hip Dysplasia as Evidenced on a Standard Ventrodorsal Extended-Leg View

- Subluxation or luxation occurs.
  - There is increased width of the joint space (only cranial portion is evaluated).
  - A shallow acetabulum is noted.
- Secondary degenerative joint disease is noted:
  - There is subchondral bone sclerosis and/or exostosis on the rim of the acetabulum (specifically the dorsal cranial margin).
  - Proliferative remodeling degenerative changes can be seen on the femoral neck at the site of the joint capsule attachment.
- The angle of the femoral neck is less than 130 degrees (coxa vara) or more than 130 degrees (coxa valga).

✎ TECHNICIAN NOTES

Collimate, ensuring that labels and markers are included and borders are visible for every film image.

✎ TECHNICIAN NOTES

Strategically used positioning aids give the patient the illusion that it is being held. A sandbag over the neck and limbs and/or the use of tape/Velcro is essential, especially if the patient is not properly sedated. Keep talking to your patient in a calm, low voice.

✎ TECHNICIAN NOTES

To be more efficient, ensure that the body parts that are not in the beam are positioned and secured first. Then position the area of interest.

Pelvis

The ventrodorsal extended-leg (hip-extended) and lateral views are the standard positions used to evaluate the small-animal pelvis, especially in suspected trauma. The most common view for diagnosis of hip dysplasia is the ventrodorsal extended-leg projection (Box 19.2), which has been adopted for coxofemoral joint certification by the OFA. PennHIP images also require a compression and distraction VD pelvis. The frog-leg VD position can be used when there is too much pain for the patient to tolerate a ventrodorsal extended-leg radiograph or for assessing the coxofemoral joint if there is suspicion of capital physeal or femoral neck fracture.[2]

Lateral View of the Pelvis—Routine

Positioning

Place In: Lateral recumbency with the affected leg down (Fig. 19.3).

Head: Keep in a natural position and, if needed, support appropriately with a sandbag over the neck. Be careful not to restrict breathing.

Forelimbs: Pull the forelimbs cranially, and secure with a sandbag, or tie to the table.

Hind Limbs: Slightly scissor the limbs so that the limb closest to the cassette is in a neutral position pulled slightly cranially with the stifle flexed (as if the patient was standing). Pull the upper limb caudally enough to differentiate the femurs. Place a foam pad under the uppermost stifle so the femur is parallel to the table and the tuber ischii are superimposed (Fig. 19.3B) and parallel. Place sandbags over the distal portion of the limbs to keep them in place.

Comments and Tips

- Keep the chest and abdomen in a true lateral position using positioning wedges as needed.
- To ensure symmetry, have the femoral heads, the iliac wings, and the transverse processes of the caudal lumbar vertebrae superimposed.
- The upper limb will be more magnified because of increased OFD (Fig. 19.3D).
- Separation of the limbs is particularly important if hip luxation is suspected.
- A lateral oblique view is required to visualize the hip joints without superimposition. The patient is positioned the same way and the x-ray tube head is angled cranially about 20 degrees to separate the hip joints on the image.[3]
- The pelvis consists of the paired ilia, acetabula, pubis, and ischia.

MEASURE: At the level of the trochanter or the thickest part.

CENTRAL RAY: Greater trochanter of the femur.

BORDERS: Slightly cranial to the wing of the ilium to include at least one lumbar vertebrae and caudally to the caudal ischium. Include one-third of the femur.

✎ TECHNICIAN NOTES

Have the thickest part of the pelvis toward the cathode to take advantage of the heel effect.

✎ TECHNICIAN NOTES

Remember to go through your mental checklist before pushing the exposure button: settings correct; image receptor/machine/grid in position; proper location of markers and ID (if using at this stage); correct body part and view; properly centered; borders correct and collimated; patient properly prepared, positioned, and restrained so that the pelvis or limb being imaged is perpendicular to the beam and parallel to the image receptor.

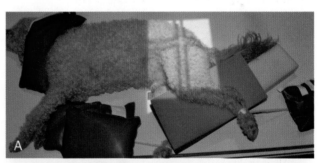

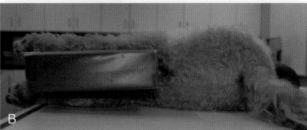

FIG. 19.3 A, Positioning for the canine lateral pelvis projection with the femurs slightly scissored. B, Make sure to place a foam wedge between the limbs to correct any rotation of the pelvis and to keep the wings of the ilia and the tuber ischii superimposed, and the femurs parallel to the table. (A and B courtesy Seneca College of Applied Arts and Technology, King City, Ontario.)

Continued

Lateral View of the Pelvis—Routine—cont'd

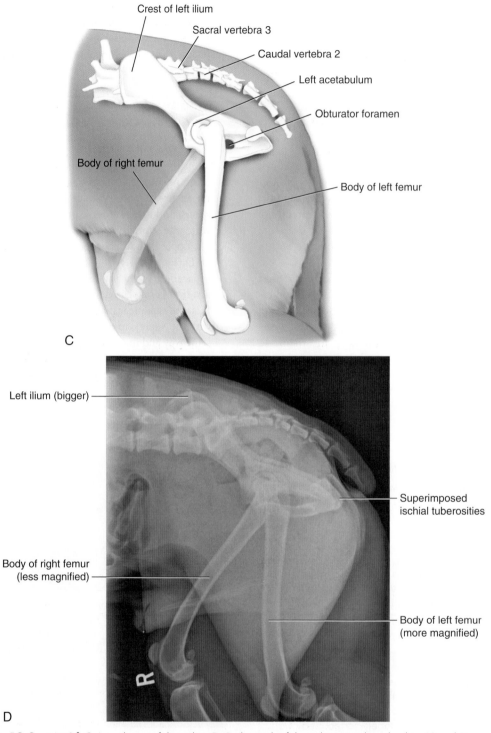

Crest of left ilium

Sacral vertebra 3

Caudal vertebra 2

Left acetabulum

Obturator foramen

Body of right femur

Body of left femur

C

Left ilium (bigger)

Superimposed ischial tuberosities

Body of right femur (less magnified)

Body of left femur (more magnified)

D

FIG. 19.3, cont'd C, Lateral view of the pelvis. D, Radiograph of the right canine lateral pelvis. (C and D courtesy Dana Greves and Jenn White, Mississauga Oakville Veterinary Emergency Hospital and Referral Group, Oakville, Ontario.)

Ventrodorsal Extended-Leg View of the Pelvis—Routine

Positioning

Place In: Dorsal recumbency.

A V-trough can be used for the cranial portion of the body (Fig. 19.4).

Head: Point forward and secure with a sandbag over the neck, if needed, being careful not to restrict breathing.

Forelimbs: Pull the forelimbs cranially, and secure with a sandbag, or tie to the table.

Hind Limbs: The hind limbs should be positioned as follows:

- Have one person grasp each hind limb at the level of the metatarsus so the thumbs face each other on the medial aspect of the patient's limb.
- The femurs are rotated inward so that the patellae lie over the trochlear groove of the stifle and the femurs are parallel to each other and the long axis of the spine and are level with the table.
- While rotating the femurs, have another person place a piece of tape long enough at the caudal proximal stifle, so the tape overlaps on the lateral aspect of the opposite femur.
- Take each end of the tape and forcibly pull to the opposite limb at the level of the proximal stifle to ensure that the femurs are maintained in a medial rotation.
- Additional tape can be placed around the pelvis just cranial to the acetabulae.
- Slowly lower the limbs until a point of resistance is felt. Place a pad underneath the tarsus to maintain this level.

- Each limb can be individually taped at the metatarsus. Extend the limbs and secure with tape caudally, so that the two digits are even with each other.
- Place a sandbag over the distal portion of the limbs to further keep them level with the table.

Comments and Tips

- If the pelvis is included in the V-trough, there will be magnification because of increased OFD.
- Sedation or anesthesia that permits muscle relaxation is required for proper positioning.
- To minimize any rotation of the body, make sure the nose is equidistant between the forelimbs and in line with the tail and that the sternum and vertebrae are superimposed.
- Palpate the greater trochanter of each femur to ensure the pelvis is symmetrical.
- Label appropriately. A positional marker should be included and placed at the cranial aspect of the pelvis.
- Keep the tail aligned with the spine.
- Any tilting of the pelvis will alter the perceived size and shape of the obturator foramina, iliac wings, and sacroiliac joints on the image.
  - If there is axial rotation, the side of the pelvis that is closest to the table will have the smaller obturator foramen and the larger iliac wing.
  - If one of the limbs appears shorter than the other, this limb is raised slightly and is not parallel to the table.

MEASURE: Thickest part of the pelvis.

CENTRAL RAY: Midline between the caudal ischia.

BORDERS: The tip of iliac wings (last two lumbar vertebrae) to the distal patella.

✎ TECHNICIAN NOTES

It is important to snugly secure the tape around the proximal stifles so that the femurs are parallel to each other and the patellae are superimposed over the centers of the femoral condyles. It is better to err on the side of having the tape too snug. Heavy sedation or general anesthesia is required.

✎ TECHNICIAN NOTES

If the image shows that the obturator foramina are of unequal size, for the subsequent image, slightly lower the side of the pelvis that has the larger circular obturator foramen (big is up). This repositioning will result in the more true oval shape of each obturator foramen on the radiograph.

✎ TECHNICIAN NOTES

For the pelvis radiograph to be evaluated, make sure that:

- The radiograph is legally labeled and positioning markers are included.
- The entire pelvis, femurs, and stifles are included.
- The femurs are extended, parallel to each other and to the ilia.
- The patellae are superimposed on the midline of each femur and positioned over the centers of the femoral condyles.
- There is no rotation, so that the wings of the ilia, the sacroiliac joints, and the obturator foramina are all equal in size and mirror images of each other.

Continued

Ventrodorsal Extended-Leg View of the Pelvis—Routine—cont'd

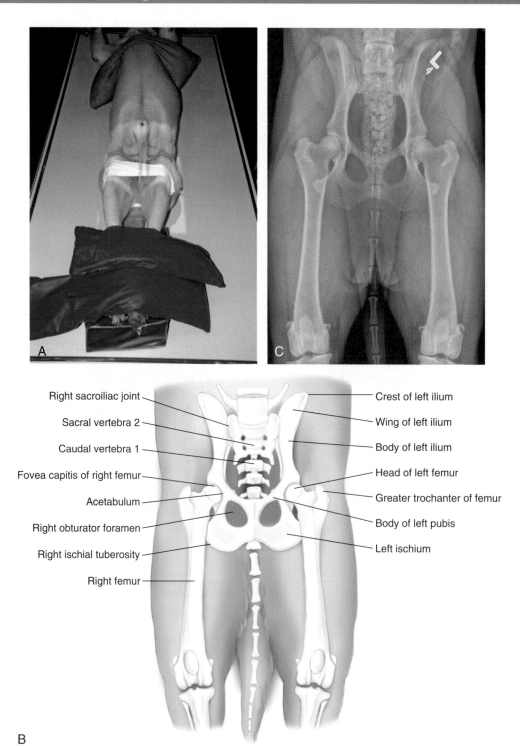

Right sacroiliac joint

Sacral vertebra 2

Caudal vertebra 1

Fovea capitis of right femur

Acetabulum

Right obturator foramen

Right ischial tuberosity

Right femur

Crest of left ilium

Wing of left ilium

Body of left ilium

Head of left femur

Greater trochanter of femur

Body of left pubis

Left ischium

FIG. 19.4 **A,** Positioning for the canine ventrodorsal extended-leg projection. Tape or gauze can be placed around the metatarsus and pulled caudally to keep the limbs as parallel to the table as possible. With enough support in the sandbag, tape may not be necessary. **B,** Ventral view of the canine pelvis. **C,** Radiograph of a standard ventrodorsal extended-leg projection. Note that the femurs are parallel to each other; the patellae are positioned over the center of the femoral condyles; there is no rotation; and the entire pelvis, femurs, and stifles are included. (**C** courtesy GK Smith, DVM, and Mandy Wallace, DVM, Veterinary School of the University of Pennsylvania.)

Ventrodorsal Frog-Leg View of the Pelvis—Ancillary

Positioning

Place In: Dorsal recumbency. A V-trough can be used for the cranial portion of the body, but avoid including the pelvis to prevent increased OFD. Keep sternum and spine superimposed.

Head: Keep in a natural position with the nose pointing forward. If needed, support appropriately with a sandbag over the neck, being careful not to restrict breathing.

Forelimbs: Pull the forelimbs cranially, and secure with a sandbag or tie to the table.

Hind Limbs: Leave the hind limbs in a naturally flexed position. For most patients the femur is positioned at 45 degrees to the spine. In some larger dogs, the femur may be 90 degrees to the spine. Place a sandbag over the tarsal joints (Fig. 19.5).

Comments and Tips

- Keep the limbs positioned identically to maintain symmetry.
- Locate the ischium by palpating for the right and left ischial tuberosity.
- Assesses acetabular depth and coxofemoral fit.[4]
- If the acetabular rim and femoral head are of interest, tilt the pelvis slightly toward the affected side, keeping the unaffected limb out of the field of view.[4,5]

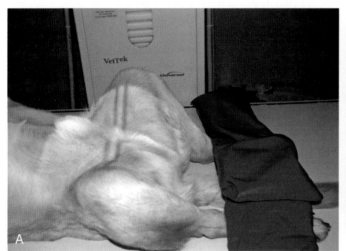

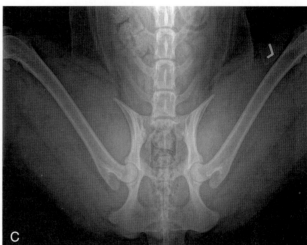

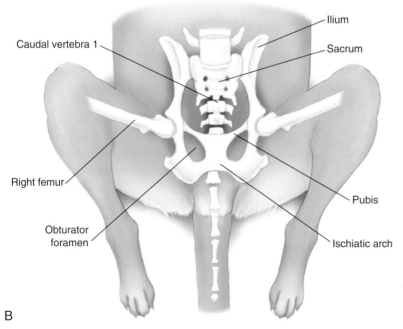

Caudal vertebra 1

Ilium

Sacrum

Right femur

Obturator foramen

Pubis

Ischiatic arch

MEASURE: Thickest part of the pelvis or over acetabulum.

CENTRAL RAY: Midline at the caudal portion of the pubis.

BORDERS: The wings of the ilia to the caudal border of the ischium. Include at least one-third of each femur.

FIG. 19.5 A, Positioning for the canine ventrodorsal frog-leg pelvis projection. **B,** Ventral view of the canine pelvis in a frog-leg position. **C,** Radiograph of the canine ventrodorsal frog-leg pelvis. (**B** and **C** courtesy Dana Greves and Jenn White, Mississauga Oakville Veterinary Emergency Hospital and Referral Group, Oakville, Ontario.)

OFA Evaluation of Hip Dysplasia

Hip dysplasia is the abnormal development of the femoral joint that results from a lack of conformity between the acetabulum and the femoral head. Hip dysplasia is a heritable disease manifested as hip joint laxity that leads to the development of osteoarthritis (OA). This polygenic and multifactorial disease is the most commonly inherited orthopedic disease in dogs. All breeds are affected, and in some cases more than 50% of the breed has canine hip dysplasia (CHD).

If exact duplicates are required for film radiography, two films can be placed in the cassette and the mAs increased. However, for optimum film quality, it is best to take two separate exposures.

In order for the radiographs to be eligible for OFA registration, there must be permanent patient identification on the film emulsion in film radiography. It could include lead letters, a darkroom imprinter, or radiopaque tape. The information required is the hospital or veterinarian's name, the date the radiograph was taken, and the registered name or number of the patient. Because of the Digital Imaging and Communications in Medicine (DICOM) standards, digital radiographs already include all of the identifying information.

Only dogs that are 24 months of age to the day or older at the time of radiography can qualify for an OFA hip number. A consultation report can be issued for younger dogs, but the hips are not certifiable. Toy and small breeds 12 months of age or older can register with the Legg-Calve-Perthes Database. Legg-Calve-Perthes (LCP) disease is a disorder of hip joint conformation most often seen in the miniature and toy breeds between the ages of 4 months and 1 year. Because there is a genetic component, it is recommended that dogs affected with LCP not be used in breeding programs.[1]

OFA recommends that the patient be in good physical condition and radiographs be taken 1 month after weaning puppies and before or after a heat cycle, because hormonal variations may cause increased joint laxity.[1]

Three board-certified radiologists independently evaluate the phenotype of the hips on a standard ventrodorsal extended-leg view.

The seven possible categories are normal (excellent, good, fair), borderline, and dysplastic (mild, moderate, severe).[1] Excellent, good, and fair hip grades are within normal limits and are given OFA numbers. This information is in the public domain and is accepted by the American Kennel Club and the Canadian Kennel Club for dogs with permanent identification (tattoo, microchip).

The radiograph is reviewed, and a report verifies the abnormal radiographic findings if radiographs reveal borderline, mild, moderate, or severe hip dysplasia grades. Dysplastic hip grades are not in the public domain, unless the owner has chosen the open database.

Alternative authorized identification, further information, and forms can be found on the OFA's website (www.offa.org).

Other hip registries are maintained by the Fédération Cynologique Internationale (FCI; European) in which the Norbert angle is used; British Veterinary Association/Kennel Club (BVA/KC; Britain, Ireland, Australia, and New Zealand), and the Verein für Deutsche Schäferhunde (SV; Germany); each has its own grading system.[1,4]

> **✎ TECHNICIAN NOTES**
>
> Patients must be 24 months of age to receive OFA hip registration and 16 weeks for PennHIP certification.

PennHIP Radiographs of the Pelvis—Ancillary

The ventrodorsal extended-leg view has been shown to tighten the joint capsule and the surrounding soft tissue, an effect that may mask evidence of joint laxity in mild-to-moderate hip dysplasia.[6] This finding has led to greater attention to dynamic pelvic radiographic studies such as the University of Pennsylvania School of Veterinary Medicine's Hip Improvement Program (PennHIP) to document the degree of laxity in coxofemoral joints.[2,7,8]

PennHIP is a radiographic screening method that quantitatively measures canine hip joint laxity through the use of stress radiographs to determine how likely a dog is to develop CHD and hip arthritis later in life.[9,10] The PennHIP method of evaluation is more accurate than the current standard in its ability to predict the onset of OA.[7,8,10] OA, also known as *degenerative joint disease (DJD)*, is the hallmark of hip dysplasia.

For quality assurance of the submissions to the database, veterinarians are required to be trained and certified. Qualified technical personnel are allowed to accompany the veterinarian to the training seminars or to take online seminars and, like the veterinarian, may become certified to perform the procedure. Alternatively, a PennHIP-certified veterinarian may train technical staff in his or her practice, who may then complete quality assurance radiographs for the certification process (Fig. 19.6).[10]

Conventional and digital PennHIP images are submitted for evaluation and storage in an ever-expanding database that collects information on the etiology, prediction, and genetic basis of CHD.

Dogs can be screened using PennHIP as early as 16 weeks of age, which can assist breeders, service or working dog organizations, and veterinarians to recommend appropriate strategies such as diet, medication, or activities to delay or minimize the disease.

The degree of laxity in an individual dog is ranked relative to others of the same breed, which allows the animals that have tighter hips within each breed to be identified and to be considered suitable for breeding.

A distraction index (DI) ranging from 0 to 1 compares the amount of laxity in each hip between the compression and distraction radiographs. The closer the DI is to 0, the less joint laxity is present and the less likelihood for predisposition to DJD or OA. Hips scoring close to 1 are considered to be very loose and thus highly likely to develop hip dysplasia.

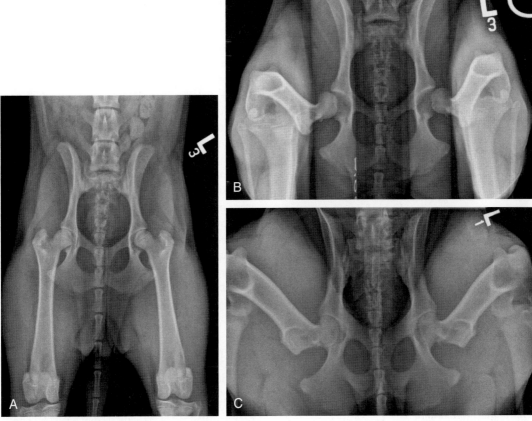

FIG. 19.6 **A,** Radiograph of a ventrodorsal extended-leg projection with an Orthopedic Foundation of Animals (OFA) rating of "good." **B,** Radiograph of a PennHIP distraction projection of the same dog with an index of 0.92 shows marked laxity that is not evident on the ventrodorsal extended-leg view. The dark lines are normal and caused by the air between the foam and acrylic rods. **C,** Radiograph of a PennHIP compression view of the same patient. (Courtesy GK Smith, DVM, and Mandy Wallace, DVM, Veterinary School of the Univerisity of Pennsylvania.)

Average DI does vary by breed. Dogs with hip laxity better than the respective breed average are considered appropriate for breeding. Generally dogs with DI values <0.3 have very low "risk" for development of OA later in life,[9,10,11] and conversely there is a direct relation when the DI is greater than 0.3 in breeds such as German Shepherds or 0.4 for Labrador retrievers and Rottweilers.[2]

Because the dog is anesthetized or deeply sedated and is not weight bearing, the laxity as determined by the DI is actually passive hip laxity, as opposed to functional hip laxity, which to date is not measurable.[9]

PennHIP recommends waiting 8 weeks postlactation or 16 weeks postwhelping before a PennHIP evaluation because relaxin and prolactin can increase hip laxity. The rise in hormone levels during the female heat cycle does not affect hip laxity as measured by PennHIP.[9,10]

Information regarding radiographic requirements for PennHIP can be found at http://info.antechimagingservices .com/pennhip/.

Other radiographic stress techniques described in the literature do not require certification, such as the ventrodorsal

view with limbs extended using fulcrum positioning and the ventrodorsal view with limbs flexed for the distraction positioning.[2,4,11] These are not discussed in this chapter.

Radiographs

Three radiographs are part of the PennHIP evaluation.

Ventrodorsal Extended-Leg View of the Pelvis

The first required image is the standard ventrodorsal extended-leg view, which has been described. The ventrodorsal extended-leg view is made so that secondary signs of hip dysplasia such as DJD and existence of OA of the hip joint can be evaluated.

Distraction View of the Pelvis

The second required submission is the distraction view, which requires specialized acrylic distractor rods to be placed between the hind limbs at the femoral heads (Figs. 19.6B and 19.7). The rods act as a fulcrum at the proximal femurs to lateralize the femoral heads when a small adduction force is applied, creating maximum lateral displacement of femoral heads.

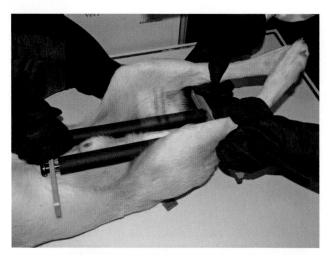

FIG. 19.7 Positioning for the distraction view, utilizing the distractor rods with the limbs in a natural stance.

Position the patient in dorsal recumbency. Position the limbs in a neutral stance such that the femurs are positioned between 10 degrees of flexion and 30 degrees of extension, 10 to 30 degrees of abduction, and 0 to 10 degrees of external rotation.[4] This neutral position avoids the main disadvantage of the extended hip projection, which is the spiral tensioning of the joint capsule that forces the femoral head into the acetabulum, reducing subluxation.[2]

This position is optimal for the measurement of hip joint laxity, which is the primary risk factor that predicts the development of DJD.

Cavitation occurs infrequently when the distractor device imposes a lateral distractive force on the hips, creating negative pressure that causes a void to form in the synovial fluid shown as an air bubble. Cavitation is not painful and does not cause short- or long-term damage to the joint. It resolves within 24 hours, and then the distraction image can be repeated. If cavitation occurs, that particular hip joint (if unilateral cavitation) or both (bilateral) cannot be evaluated.

Compression View of the Pelvis

The patient is also in dorsal recumbency and in a neutral or standing orientation referred to as the *"stance phase"* of weight bearing. Medial pressure is applied lateral to the greater trochanters to compress the coxofemoral joints and obtain an image at their most congruent position (see Fig. 19.6C). The femoral heads are fully seated in the acetabular fossae. Congruency is measured.

> ✎ **TECHNICIAN NOTES**
>
> All dogs have some degree of joint laxity—even Greyhounds and Borzois—so if you do not see any laxity, check the technique and the level of sedation.

Pelvic Limb Positions

Femur

Lateral (Mediolateral) View of the Femur—Routine

Positioning

Place In: Lateral recumbency with the affected leg down (Fig. 19.8).

Head: Keep the head in a natural position, and support the neck with a sandbag, being careful not to restrict breathing.

Forelimbs: Pull the forelimbs cranially, and support with a sandbag.

Hind Limbs: Flex the unaffected limb, abduct and pull laterally. Support the upper limb with a bungee cord or rope to the machine tube stand or to a stabilized IV pole beside the table. Extend the lower affected limb and secure with a sandbag over the distal limb. Place a thin foam pad under the proximal tibia to prevent rotation of the femur.

Comments and Tips

- The beam may have to be angled distoproximally if the upper limb is not out of the field of view.
- Be sure to palpate and include the femoral joint to ensure that the full affected femur will be radiographed.
- Abducting the affected limb eliminates superimposition of the proximal femur over the tuber ischium.
- Due to the difference in thickness at either end of the femur, especially in thickly muscled dogs, two views may need to be taken (measure accordingly at each end).
- If preferred, a fluid bag can be positioned over the distal end to emulate soft tissue. This may prevent overexposure to the distal aspect. Measure at the proximal femur.[12]
- Position the patient so that the femoral head is pointing toward the cathode of the x-ray tube.

MEASURE: Midshaft of the femur (to compensate for the difference in tissue thickness at either end of the femur).

CENTRAL RAY: Midshaft of the femur.

BORDERS: The coxofemoral joint to the stifle.

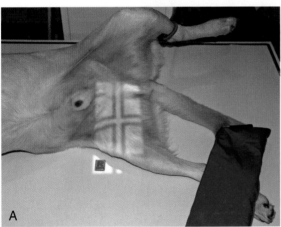

A

B

Acetabulum
Head of femur
Neck of femur
Lesser trochanter of femur
Body of femur
Patella
Tibial tuberosity
Sesamoid bones
Medial condyle of femur

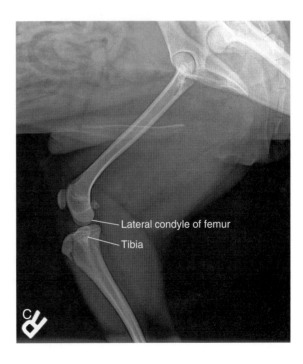

Lateral condyle of femur
Tibia

C

FIG. 19.8 **A,** Positioning for the mediolateral (lateral) view of the canine femur. **B,** Medial view of the femur. **C,** Radiograph of the right canine mediolateral (lateral) femur. (B and C courtesy Dana Greves and Jenn White, Mississauga Oakville Veterinary Emergency Hospital and Referral Group, Oakville, Ontario.)

Craniocaudal View of the Femur—Routine

Positioning

Place In: Dorsal recumbency in a V-trough or secure with the use of tape/Velcro or a sandbag if needed. To ensure symmetry, it is usually best if the patient can be positioned as for a ventrodorsal extended-leg view. Center on the affected limb (Fig. 19.9).

Head: Keep in a natural position and, if needed, support appropriately with a sandbag over the neck, being careful not to restrict breathing.

Forelimbs: Pull the forelimbs cranially and secure with a sandbag or tie to the table.

Hind Limbs: Rotate both femurs inward so that the patellae lie over the patellar grooves. Securing both limbs helps minimize rotation. Tape around the femurs just proximal to the stifle, keeping the femur parallel to the table and the patella between the femoral condyles. Place a sandbag over the distal portion of the limbs. Place a small sponge under the tarsus to prevent rotation of the stifle.

Comments and Tips

- Complete extension is required, so ensure that the affected limb is well secured.
- Measure only the femur itself.

MEASURE: Midshaft of the femur.

CENTRAL RAY: Midshaft of the femur.

BORDERS: The coxofemoral joint to the stifle.

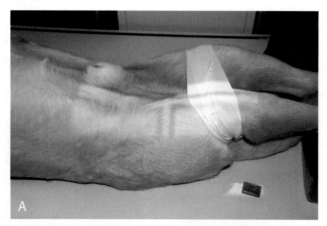

FIG. 19.9 A, Positioning for the craniocaudal view of canine femur. Securing limbs together as in a VD extended view assists in symmetry. Placing a sandbag over the tarsus will help straighten the limbs.

Craniocaudal View of the Femur—Routine—cont'd

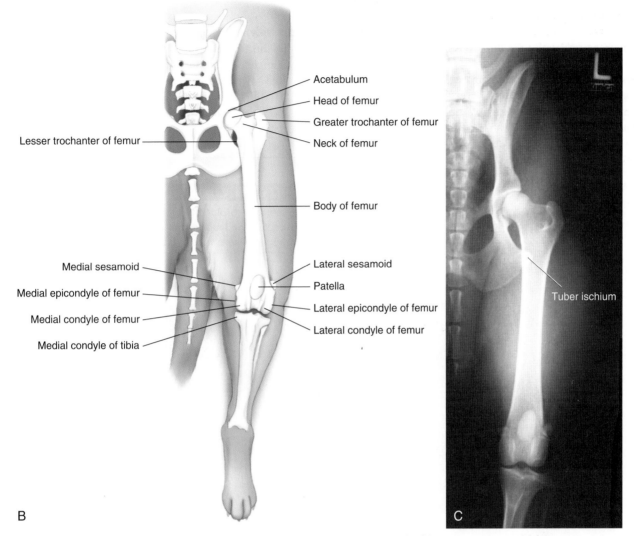

Lesser trochanter of femur

Acetabulum

Head of femur

Greater trochanter of femur

Neck of femur

Body of femur

Medial sesamoid

Medial epicondyle of femur

Medial condyle of femur

Medial condyle of tibia

Lateral sesamoid

Patella

Lateral epicondyle of femur

Lateral condyle of femur

Tuber ischium

B

C

FIG. 19.9, cont'd B, Cranial view of the canine femur. C, Radiograph of the canine craniocaudal femur. (B and C courtesy Dana Greves and Jenn White, Mississauga Oakville Veterinary Emergency Hospital and Referral Group, Oakville, Ontario.)

Caudocranial View (Horizontal View) of the Femur—Ancillary

Positioning

Place In: Lateral recumbency with the affected limb uppermost and supported on a sponge (Fig. 19.10).

Head: Keep in a natural position and, if needed, support appropriately with a sandbag over the neck. Be careful not to restrict breathing.

Forelimbs: Pull the forelimbs cranially and secure with a sandbag or tie to the table.

Hind Limbs: Position a cassette vertically against the cranial aspect of the affected limb. Extend the limb as much as possible and support with a sandbag or tie to a secure object.

Comments and Tips

- The horizontal beam is directed caudocranially.
- Complete extension is required. Ensure that the affected limb is well fastened.
- It is difficult to include the proximal portion of the femur and acetabulum with this position.

MEASURE: Midshaft of the femur.

CENTRAL RAY: Midshaft of the femur.

BORDERS: The coxofemoral joint to the stifle.

> ✐ **TECHNICIAN NOTES**
>
> Remember to place the label and markers on the cranial aspect of the limb for the lateral views and on the lateral aspect for the opposite views.

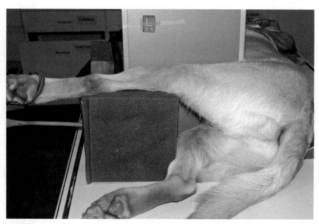

FIG. 19.10 Positioning for the caudocranial (horizontal) view of the canine femur.

Stifle

Lateral (Mediolateral) View of the Stifle—Routine

Positioning

Place In: Lateral recumbency with the affected leg down.

Head: Keep in a natural position and support appropriately with a sandbag over the neck, being careful not to restrict breathing.

Forelimbs: Pull the forelimbs cranially and secure with a sandbag or tie to the table.

Hind Limbs: Flex the unaffected limb, abduct, and pull laterally with a bungee cord or rope to the machine tube stand or to a stabilized IV pole beside the table. Extend the affected limb, keeping the stifle in a relatively natural position, so the patella is slightly rotated toward the cassette/detector. Avoid rotation. Secure with tape/Velcro or a sandbag over the distal limb (Fig. 19.11).

Comments and Tips

• The unaffected limb needs to be extended only dorsally enough to be out of the field of view.

• Place a sponge pad under the affected tarsus so the tibia is parallel to the image receptor.

• In a true lateral view, there will be superimposition of the femoral condyles.

• A flexed lateral radiograph (ancillary view) with tibial compression is used if interested in cranial drawer movement (to note cranial displacement of the proximal tibia in relation to the distal femur).

  • Flex the stifle 90 degrees and flex the tarsus as much as possible so the metatarsus is parallel to the humerus.

MEASURE: At the distal end of the femur.

CENTRAL RAY: Palpate and center on the indentation of the stifle joint (intercondylar fossa of the femur).

BORDERS: Proximal third of the tibia and distal third of the femur.

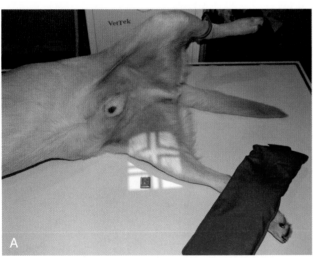

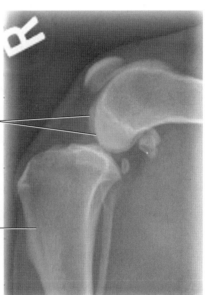

Medial and lateral condyles of femur

Cartilage between tibial tuberosity and body of tibia

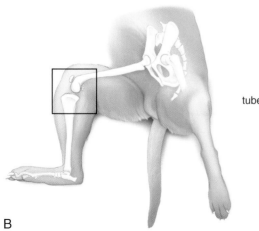

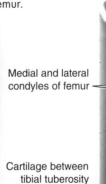

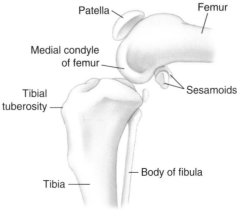

Patella

Femur

Medial condyle of femur

Tibial tuberosity

Sesamoids

Body of fibula

Tibia

FIG. 19.11 A, Positioning for the mediolateral view of the canine stifle. **B,** Medial view of the canine stifle joint. **C,** Radiograph of the canine mediolateral (lateral) stifle. (B and C courtesy Dana Greves and Jenn White, Mississauga Oakville Veterinary Emergency Hospital and Referral Group, Oakville, Ontario.)

Caudocranial View of the Stifle—Routine

Positioning

Place In: Sternal recumbency in a V-trough, or secure with sandbags if needed. (A feline patient will not likely need further support.)

Head: Keep in a natural position and support appropriately with a sandbag over the neck, being careful not to restrict breathing.

Forelimbs: Pull the forelimbs cranially and secure with a sandbag or tie to the table.

Hind Limbs: Allow the unaffected limb to lie flexed, next to the body, and raise with a foam pad (Fig. 19.12). Extend the affected limb and support with tape/Velcro or a sandbag. Place a small sponge under the tarsus to prevent rotation of the stifle.

Comments and Tips

- It is essential that the affected limb rests on the patella.
- Raising the unaffected limb will help image the affected patella in the patellar groove. The body will be slightly rotated.
- Palpate the femoral condyles to ensure proper placement in the patellar groove.
- The x-ray tube head may need to be angled cranially about 10 to 15 degrees to create a "tunnel" view of the distal femur.
- Ensure that the affected limb is pulled caudally and there is no rotation of the limb.

MEASURE: At the distal end of the femur.

CENTRAL RAY: On the stifle joint.

BORDERS: Distal third of the femur and proximal thirds of the tibia/fibula.

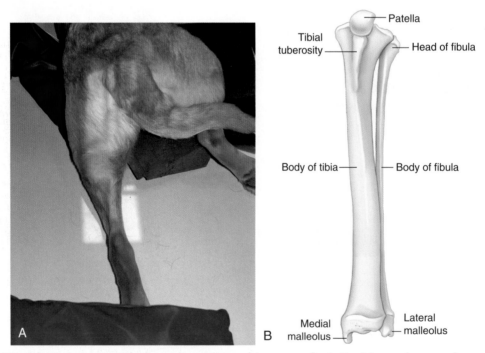

FIG. 19.12 A, Positioning for the caudocranial view of the canine stifle. B, Caudal view of canine stifle joint.

Caudocranial View of the Stifle—Routine—cont'd

Positioning With a Horizontal Beam for the Caudocranial Stifle Joint—Ancillary

Place In: Lateral recumbency with the affected limb uppermost and supported on a sponge.

Head: Keep in a natural position and, if needed, support with a sandbag over the neck, being careful not to restrict breathing.

Forelimbs: Pull the forelimbs cranially and secure with a sandbag or tie to the table.

Hind Limbs: Position a cassette vertically against the cranial aspect of the affected limb and extend the limb as much as possible. Support with a sandbag or tie to a secure object (see Fig. 19.10).

Comments and Tips

- The horizontal beam is directed in a caudocranial direction.
- This lateral decubitus view can be substituted if a true caudocranial view of the stifle is not possible.

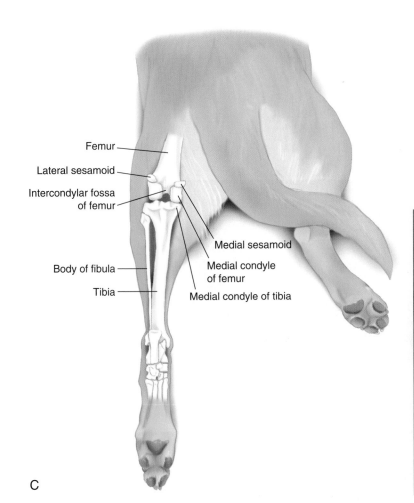

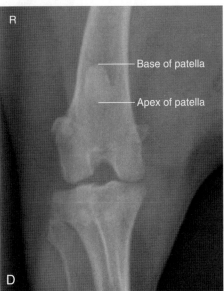

FIG. 19.12, cont'd C, Caudal view of tibia and fibula. D, Radiograph of the canine caudocranial stifle. (C and D courtesy Dana Greves and Jenn White, Mississauga Oakville Veterinary Emergency Hospital and Referral Group, Oakville, Ontario.)

Proximodistal (Cranioproximal-Craniodistal) or Skyline View of the Stifle—Ancillary

Positioning

Place In: Sternal recumbency in a V-trough or secure with sandbags if needed. (The feline patient will not likely need further support.)

Head: Keep in a natural position with the nose pointing forward and, if needed, support appropriately with a sandbag over the neck, being careful not to restrict breathing.

Forelimbs: Pull the forelimbs cranially and secure with a sandbag or tie to the table.

Hind Limbs: Allow the contralateral limb to flex partially and position itself laterally. Place a sandbag or sponge under the nonaffected limb to keep it slightly elevated (see Fig. 19.13A). Flex the affected pelvic limb lateral to the caudal abdomen, with the foot flexed, to slightly elevate the patella. Rotate the pelvis toward the affected limb, keeping the femur perpendicular to the image receptor.

Comments and Tips

- It is essential that the affected limb rest on the tibia.
- A small foam pad may be placed beneath the patella for more comfort, although there will be some OFD.
- Palpate the patella against the trochlea to determine the exact angle.
- The skyline is used to visualize trochlear groove and patellar alignment.
- Additional views, including the skyline, can assist in further diagnosis of osteochondrosis, fractures, neoplasia, or ligamentous instability.[2]

MEASURE: At the patella.

CENTRAL RAY: Over the patella angled 10 degrees in a craniocaudal direction.

BORDERS: Distal third of the femur and proximal thirds of the tibia/fibula.

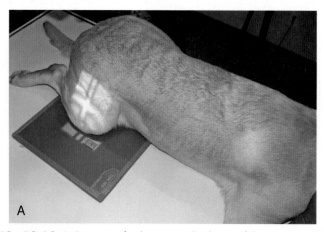

FIG. 19.13 A, Positioning for the proximodistal view of the canine patella.

Proximodistal (Cranioproximal-Craniodistal) or Skyline View of the Stifle—Ancillary—cont'd

Positioning With a Horizontal Beam for the Skyline Stifle Joint (Patella)—Ancillary

Place In: Lateral recumbency with the affected limb uppermost and supported on a sponge.

Head: Keep in a natural position and, if needed, support appropriately with a sandbag over the neck. Be careful not to restrict breathing.

Forelimbs: Pull the forelimbs cranially and secure with a sandbag or tie to the table.

Hind Limbs: Completely flex the affected limb as much as possible. Secure with a sandbag over the tarsus and pelvis, or tie a gauze or a cord around the metatarsus and fasten to the tube stand (see Fig. 19.13B). Alternatively tape a figure-of-eight–type bandage around the midtibia and femur to hold the stifle in place.

Comments and Tips

- Place the cassette against the cranial surface of the upper limb, and direct the beam in a caudocranial direction.
- Because of decreased tissue thickness, kV will be less than a regular caudocranial or proximodistal stifle view.
- Placing a 300-mL or greater saline bag against the cassette helps eliminate scatter and enhances contrast.
- This projection is technically called craniodistal-cranioproximal.

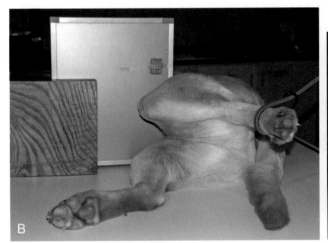
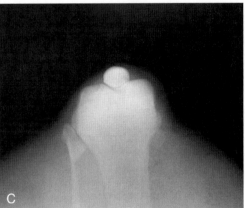

FIG. 19.13, cont'd B, Alternative positioning for the skyline view of the canine stifle joint (patella) using a horizontal beam. C, Radiograph of the canine proximodistal patella view or skyline view.

Tibia and Fibula

Lateral (Mediolateral) View of the Tibia/Fibula—Routine

Positioning

Place In: Lateral recumbency with the affected limb down.

Head: Keep in a natural position and, if needed, support appropriately with a sandbag over the neck. Be careful not to restrict breathing.

Forelimbs: Pull the forelimbs cranially and secure with a sandbag or tie to the table.

Hind Limbs: Flex the unaffected limb, abduct and pull laterally, supporting the limb with a bungee cord or rope to the machine tube stand. Extend the affected limb in a natural position, and either fasten the metatarsus with a sandbag or tie or tape/Velcro the metatarsus to the table or to a sandbag (Fig. 19.14).

Comments and Tips

- Place a sponge under the tarsus to elevate it and to prevent obliquity of the limb.
- If a cranial cruciate ligament tear is suspected and tibial plateau leveling osteotomy (TPLO) to be completed, both the stifle and tarsal joints are to be flexed 90 degrees.[5]

MEASURE: Midshaft of the tibia and fibula (to compensate for the difference in tissue thickness at either end).

CENTRAL RAY: Midshaft of the fibula and tibia.

BORDERS: The tarsus and the stifle.

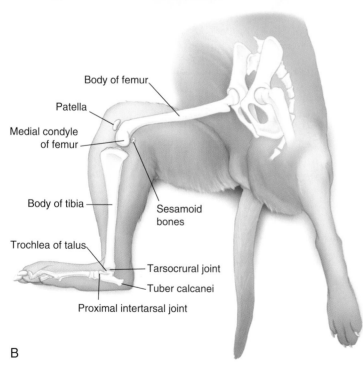

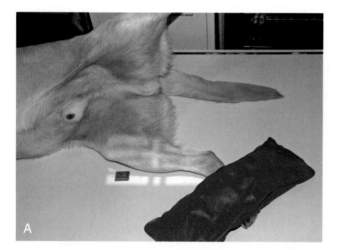

Body of femur

Patella

Medial condyle of femur

Body of tibia

Sesamoid bones

Trochlea of talus

Tarsocrural joint

Tuber calcanei

Proximal intertarsal joint

B

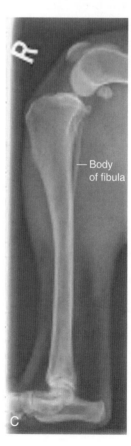

— Body of fibula

FIG. 19.14 A, Positioning for the mediolateral (lateral) view of the canine tibia and fibula. **B,** Medial view of canine tibia and fibula. **C,** Radiograph of the canine mediolateral (lateral) tibia and fibula. (**B** and **C** courtesy Dana Greves and Jenn White, Mississauga Oakville Veterinary Emergency Hospital and Referral Group, Oakville, Ontario.)

Caudocranial View of the Tibia/Fibula—Routine

Positioning

Place In: Sternal recumbency in a V-trough and secure with a sandbag or the use of tape/Velcro if needed. (The feline patient will not likely need further support.)

Head: Keep in a natural position and, if needed, support appropriately with a sandbag over the neck, being careful not to restrict breathing.

Forelimbs: Pull the forelimbs cranially and secure with a sandbag or tie to the table.

Hind Limbs: Allow the unaffected limb to lie flexed next to the body and slightly raise it with a foam pad. Secure the affected limb over the metatarsus with a sandbag, or tie or tape/Velcro the metatarsus to the table or to a sandbag. Place a small sponge under the tarsus to prevent rotation of the stifle (Fig. 19.15).

Comments and Tips

- It is essential that the affected limb rest on the patella.
  - If you place a foam pad under the unaffected stifle, the raised limb will help image the affected patella in the patellar groove.
  - The body will be slightly rotated.

Positioning With a Horizontal Projection for the Caudocranial Tibia and Fibula View—Ancillary

Place In: Lateral recumbency with the affected limb uppermost and supported on a sponge.

Head: Keep in a natural position and, if needed, support appropriately with a sandbag over the neck, being careful not to restrict breathing.

Forelimbs: Pull the forelimbs cranially and secure with a sandbag or tie to the table.

Hind Limbs: Position a cassette vertically against the cranial aspect of the affected limb and extend the limb as much as possible. Secure over the metatarsus with a sandbag, or tie or tape the metatarsus to a secure object.

Comments and Tips

- The horizontal beam is directed caudocranially.
- Complete extension is required, so ensure that the affected limb is well secured.
- This lateral decubitus view can be substituted if a true caudocranial view of the tibia/fibula is not possible.

MEASURE: Midshaft of the tibia and fibula (to compensate for the difference in tissue thickness at either end).

CENTRAL RAY: Midshaft of the tibia and fibula.

BORDERS: The tarsus and the stifle.

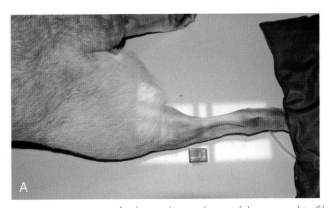

FIG. 19.15 A, Positioning for the caudocranial view of the canine tibia/fibula.

Continued

Caudocranial View of the Tibia/Fibula—Routine—cont'd

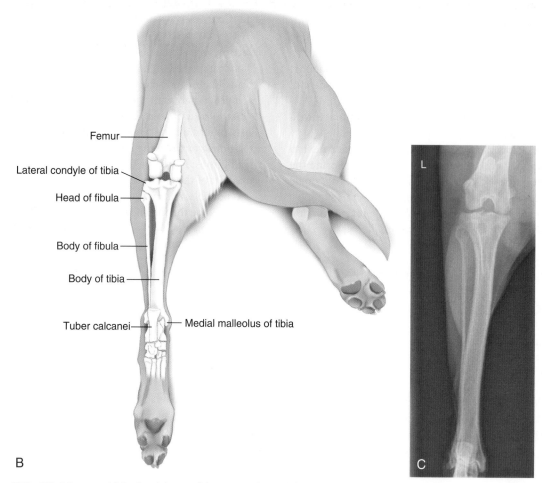

Femur

Lateral condyle of tibia

Head of fibula

Body of fibula

Body of tibia

Tuber calcanei

Medial malleolus of tibia

L

B

C

FIG. 19.15, cont'd B, Caudal view of the canine tibia and fibula. C, Radiograph of the canine caudocranial tibia/fibula. (B and C courtesy Dana Greves and Jenn White, Mississauga Oakville Veterinary Emergency Hospital and Referral Group, Oakville, Ontario.)

The Foot: Tarsus, Metatarsus, and Digits

The tarsus, metatarsus, and digits are typically radiographed in one view. If there is a particular area of interest, center and measure on this site.

Lateral (Mediolateral) Views of the Foot—Routine/Ancillary

Positioning

Place In: Lateral recumbency with the affected limb down.

Head: Keep in a natural position and, if needed, support appropriately with a sandbag over the neck, being careful not to restrict breathing.

Forelimbs: Pull the forelimbs cranially and secure with a sandbag or tie to the table.

Hind Limbs: Abduct the unaffected limb, pull dorsally, and either secure with tape/Velcro around the stifle and tarsus or support with a bungee cord to the x-ray tube stand.

Place a small foam pad or gauze under the calcaneus to keep the tibia parallel to the table. Minimize any rotation of the affected limb and secure in place, flexing as described in the next section.

Positioning for a Natural Lateral View of the Tarsus

- Place the affected limb in a natural position and secure with tape/Velcro, gauze, or a sandbag (Fig. 19.16).

MEASURE: At the site of interest:

Tarsus: At the tarsus joint.

Metatarsus or Phalanges: On the joint.

CENTRAL RAY: Center on the area of interest:

Tarsus: At the tarsus joint.

Metatarsus or Phalanges: On the central bone.

BORDERS:

Tarsus: Proximal third of metatarsus to distal third of the tibia and fibula.

Metatarsus or Phalanges: Tarsus proximally to the distal phalanges.

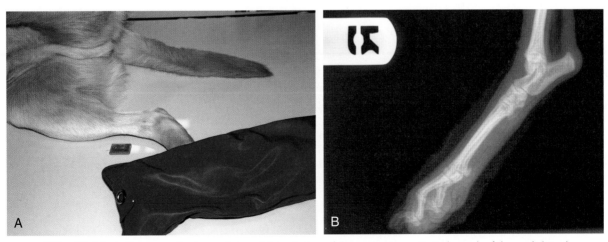

FIG. 19.16 A, Positioning for the mediolateral (lateral) view of the canine tarsus. **B,** Radiograph of the mediolateral (lateral) natural projection of the canine tarsus, metatarsus, and digits. A Robert Jones bandage has been applied. (B courtesy Dana Greves and Jenn White, Mississauga Oakville Veterinary Emergency Hospital and Referral Group, Oakville, Ontario.)

Continued

Lateral (Mediolateral) Views of the Foot—Routine/Ancillary—cont'd

Positioning for an Extended Lateral View of the Tarsus—Routine

- Extend the affected limb fully by pulling away from the body and secure with tape/Velcro, gauze, or a sandbag (Fig. 19.17).

Positioning for a Flexed Lateral View of the Tarsus—Ancillary

- Flex the affected foot at 90 degrees, and support with a paddle or sandbag.
- Alternatively, place a figure-of-eight tape around the distal tibia and proximal metatarsus to achieve full flexion of the tarsus.
- Place tape at the distal metatarsus, and pull slightly cranially and laterally (Fig. 19.18).

Positioning for a Lateral View of the Digits—Routine

- Separate the digits to prevent superimposition.
- This is best completed by separately taping around the toenail of the lateral (fifth) phalanx and the medial (second) phalanx.
- Pull the lateral phalanx slightly cranially and laterally, and the medial phalanx slightly caudally and laterally.
- Tape can also be put around the digit itself.
- Cotton or manicure pads can be placed between the toes, although this alone does not separate the phalanges as effectively.

Comments and Tips

- As for all lateral limb positions, keep the label cranial to the joint or bone.

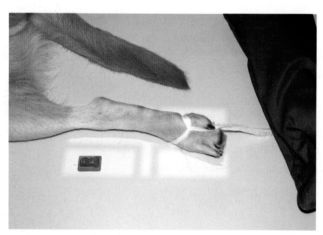

FIG. 19.17 Positioning for the mediolateral (lateral) extended view of the canine tarsus, metatarsus, and digits. The digits should be separated if they are of interest.

Lateral (Mediolateral) Views of the Foot—Routine/Ancillary—cont'd

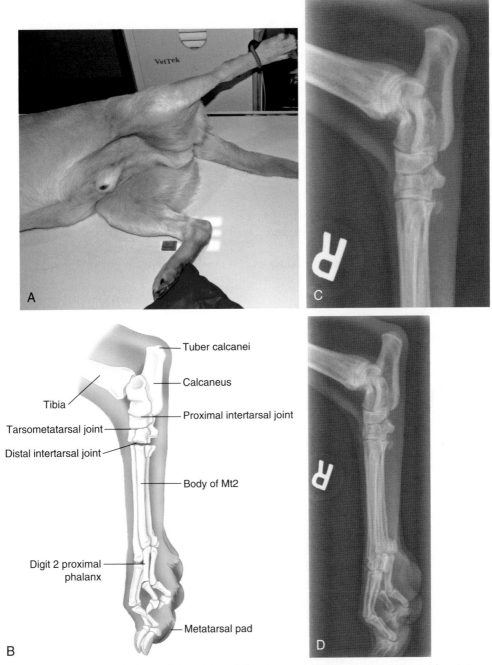

Tuber calcanei

Calcaneus

Tibia

Proximal intertarsal joint

Tarsometatarsal joint

Distal intertarsal joint

Body of Mt2

Digit 2 proximal phalanx

Metatarsal pad

FIG. 19.18 **A,** Positioning for the mediolateral (lateral) flexed view of the canine tarsus. **B,** Medial flexed view of the canine foot. **C,** Radiograph of the mediolateral (lateral) flexed canine tarsus view. **D,** Radiograph of the mediolateral (lateral) canine flexed tarsus, metatarsus, and digits. (*B, C,* and *D* courtesy Dana Greves and Jenn White, Mississauga Oakville Veterinary Emergency Hospital and Referral Group, Oakville, Ontario.)

Plantarodorsal View of the Foot—Routine/Ancillary

Positioning

Place In: The patient is placed in sternal recumbency in a V-trough or secured with the use of a sandbag if needed. (The feline patient will not likely need further support.)

Head and Forelimbs: Secure the head and forelimbs with a sandbag or tie the limbs to the table.

Hind Limbs: Allow the unaffected limb to lie flexed next to the body. Extend the affected foot and support with a sandbag, or tie at the metatarsus/digits and secure to the table or a sandbag (Fig. 19.19). Keep the femur, stifle, and tibia in true alignment and the calcaneus vertical for true plantardorsal tarsus.

Comments and Tips

- If you place a foam pad under the unaffected stifle, the raised limb will assist in keeping the calcaneus image more centered. The body is slightly rotated.
- Palpate for the tibial tuberosity to obtain a true plantarodorsal view.

- A dorsoplantar view is not routinely completed. If this view is required, the patient can be in either dorsal recumbency with the limb extended or in sternal recumbency with the plantar aspect of the foot against the image receptor (see Fig. 19.19D).

Flexed Dorsopalmar (Skyline) of the Tarsus—Ancillary

- The purpose of this view is to detect osteochondrosis lesions by better visualizing the tibiotarsul joint. Place the patient in dorsal recumbency with the tarsus of interest on a wooden or cardboard box with the detector underneath the foot.
- Flex the tarsus so the foot is perpendicular to the cassette and parallel with the x-ray beam.
- This prevents superimposition of the tuber calcis.
- Exposure factors may need to be modified due to the variation in source image distance.

MEASURE: At the site of interest:

Tarsus: Tarsus joint.

Metatarsus or Phalanges: On the joint.

CENTRAL RAY: Center on the area of interest:

Tarsus: Tarsal joint.

Metatarsus or Phalanges: On the central bone.

BORDERS:

Tarsus: Proximal third of metatarsus to distal third of tibia and fibula.

Metatarsus or Phalanges: Tarsus proximally to distal phalanges.

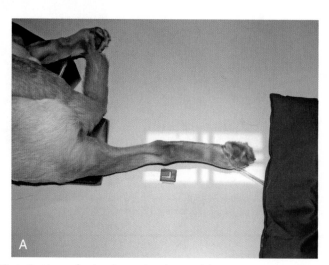

FIG. 19.19 A, Positioning for the plantarodorsal view of the canine tarsus, metatarsus, and digits.

Plantarodorsal View of the Foot—Routine/Ancillary—cont'd

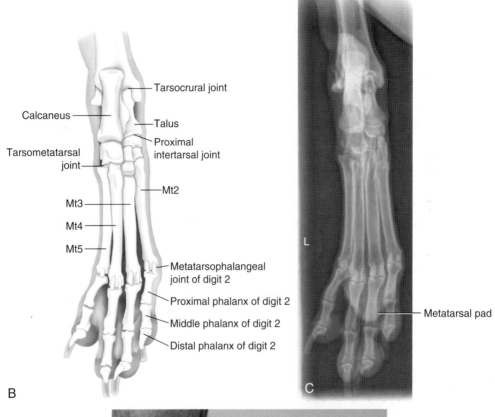

B, Plantar view

Tarsocrural joint

Calcaneus

Talus

Proximal intertarsal joint

Tarsometatarsal joint

Mt2

Mt3

Mt4

Mt5

Metatarsophalangeal joint of digit 2

Proximal phalanx of digit 2

Middle phalanx of digit 2

Distal phalanx of digit 2

L

Metatarsal pad

C

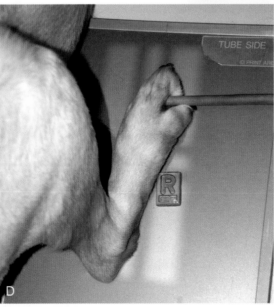

D

FIG. 19.19, cont'd B, Plantar view of tarsus, metatarsus, and digits. C, Radiograph of the plantarodorsal view of the canine tarsus, metatarsus, and digits. D, Positioning for the dorsoplantar view of the canine metatarsus and digits. A dorsoplanar view taken in this position has less object-film distance than that with the patient in dorsal recumbency. This view can also be used for the skyline of the calcaneus. (B and C courtesy Dana Greves and Jenn White, Mississauga Oakville Veterinary Emergency Hospital and Referral Group, Oakville, Ontario.)

Oblique Views of the Foot—Ancillary

The oblique views of the hind foot are the plantarolateral-dorsomedial (PLDMO)–medial oblique view and the plantaromedial-dorsolateral (PMDLO)–lateral oblique view (Fig. 19.20).

Positioning

Place In: Sternal recumbency. A V-trough may be used for stability.

Head: Keep in a natural position and, if needed, support appropriately with a sandbag over the neck, being careful not to restrict breathing.

Forelimbs: Pull the forelimbs cranially and secure with a sandbag or tie to the table if needed.

Hind Limbs: Keep the unaffected limb in a natural position. Tie and secure the affected metatarsus/digits as far caudally as possible.

For the medial oblique view: No rotation of the pelvis or padding is needed under the unaffected limb because the foot is in an oblique position naturally.

For the lateral oblique view: Rotate and elevate the unaffected pelvic limb with a large sponge.

Comments and Tips

- If the machine is capable, the patient can be placed in a true plantarodorsal position and the tube head angled 10 to 15 degrees toward the medial side of the tarsus for the lateral oblique view, or 10 to 15 degrees toward the lateral side of the tarsus for the medial oblique view.

✎ TECHNICIAN NOTES

The beam is always described as "point of entrance to point of exit." For the PMDLO the beam enters at the plantar aspect on the medial side and exits dorsally on the lateral side. The "point of exit" is where the image receptor is placed, which in this case is next to the dorsal surface. Because the beam does not exit perpendicular to the midline, the view is called an *oblique*. Thus in this case it is a lateral oblique because the beam exits laterally. (This concept is further described in Chapter 24.)

MEASURE: At the site of interest. Generally this view is for the tarsus.

Tarsus: Tarsal joint.

Metatarsus or Phalanges: Site of phalangeal metatarsal articulation at level of middle phalanx.

CENTRAL RAY: Center on the area of interest:

Tarsus: Tarsal joint.

Phalanges: Third and fourth phalangeal metatarsal articulations. For the medial oblique view: center the beam 45 degrees laterally. For the lateral oblique view: center the beam 45 degrees medially.

BORDERS:

Tarsus: Proximal third of metatarsus to distal thirds of the tibia and fibula.

Metatarsus or Phalanges: Tarsus proximally to the distal phalanges.

Oblique Views of the Foot—Ancillary—cont'd

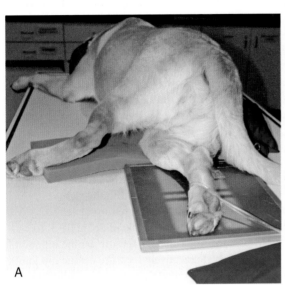

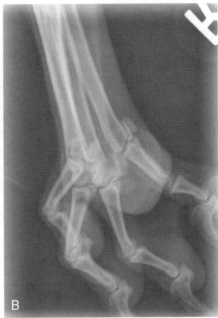

FIG. 19.20 A, Positioning for the plantaromedial-dorsolateral (lateral) oblique view of the canine tarsus, metatarsus, and digits. **B,** Radiograph of an oblique metatarsus and digits. (**B** courtesy Jenn White, Mississauga Oakville Veterinary Emergency Hospital and Referral Group, Oakville, Ontario.)

Fig. 19.21 is a mystery radiograph. Review it and answer the question presented with it.

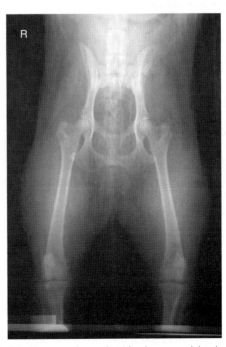

FIG. 19.21 Mystery radiograph. What has caused the density issues in this radiograph?

✳ KEY POINTS

1. For views perpendicular to the midsagittal plane, the dog or cat generally lies in dorsal recumbency for the pelvis and the proximal limb (femur), and in sternal recumbency for the distal limb (stifle, tibia and fibula, and foot).

2. Correct positioning and technique are required for proper interpretation. This includes where to measure and center the beam, what to include, and how to ensure that the positioning shows proper symmetry.

3. The label is placed lateral to the limb for the perpendicular projections and at the cranial aspect for the lateral projections.

4. For joints, include one-third each of the limbs proximal and distal. For long bones, include the joints proximal and distal.

5. Keep patient considerations in mind and utilize high-quality radiographic techniques.

REVIEW QUESTIONS

1. You are positioning for a right lateral pelvis of a Belgian Sheepdog. The femur that will be more magnified on the image is:
   a. The right, because of increased object-film distance
   b. The left, because of increased source-image distance
   c. The left, because of increased object-film distance
   d. Neither, because object-film distance does not affect image size

2. When positioning for this right lateral pelvis of the Belgian Sheepdog, you should position the hind limbs so that:
   a. The right limb is pulled slightly cranially and the left slightly caudally
   b. The left limb is pulled slightly cranially and the right slightly caudally
   c. Both limbs are superimposed and pulled cranially
   d. Both limbs are superimposed and pulled caudally

3. A Poodle is exhibiting severe pain and trauma in the pelvis. Using a vertical beam, you should position so that your patient is in:
   a. Lateral recumbency with the limbs superimposed
   b. Dorsal recumbency with the hind limbs in a frog-leg position
   c. Dorsal recumbency in a VD extended-leg view
   d. Sternal recumbency with the hind limbs in a frog-leg position

4. Center the VD frog-leg view of the Poodle:
   a. Midline at the caudal pubis
   b. Between the obturator foraminae
   c. Midline at the caudal portion of the ischium
   d. On the greater trochanters

5. The hind limbs of this VD frog-leg view of the Poodle should be:
   a. Pulled so that the femur is about 90 degrees from the spine
   b. Left in a natural position
   c. Extended as much as possible
   d. Raised and placed in a neutral stance

6. When positioning for a VD extended-leg pelvic radiograph in a German Shepherd, it is best to place the stifles:
   a. At an angle to the table
   b. Toward either the cathode or the anode
   c. Toward the cathode
   d. Toward the anode

7. The right marker for this VD extended-leg pelvis will be placed beside the:
   a. Left patella
   b. Right patella
   c. Wing of the left ilium
   d. Wing of the right ilium

8. The OFA label requirements for evaluation of hip dysplasia must include:
   a. Only the owner's name
   b. The name of the person taking the radiograph
   c. Only the positional marker
   d. All required identification to be permanent

9. The field of view for this VD extended-leg pelvis will be from the:
   a. Tip of the ilia to include the ischia
   b. Body of the ilia to the ischial tuberosities
   c. Tip of the ilia to the distal patella
   d. Body of the ilia to the distal patella

10. The obturator foramina on this radiograph are not of equal size. This means that for the next radiograph, you should raise the side of the pelvis with the:
    a. Larger circular obturator foramen
    b. Narrower obturator foramen

11. You also notice on this VD extended-leg radiograph of the German Shepherd that the right femur appears shorter than the left. This is because the:
    a. Left limb is slightly raised and not parallel to the table
    b. Right limb is slightly raised and not parallel to the table
    c. Patient is shifted to the right
    d. Patient has shifted to the left

12. The main principle of PennHIP is to:
    a. Subjectively measure canine hip joint laxity
    b. Subjectively measure canine hip joint irregularities
    c. Quantitatively measure canine hip joint irregularities
    d. Quantitatively measure canine hip joint laxity

13. A horizontal beam is being used for the proximodistal patella of a Retriever. The patient should be placed in:
    a. Lateral recumbency with the affected limb closer to the table
    b. Lateral recumbency with the affected limb uppermost
    c. Sternal recumbency with the image receptor underneath the patella
    d. Dorsal recumbency with the image receptor laterally to the patella

14. The field of view for the stifle joint of a feline is the:
    a. Stifle joint
    b. Proximal third of the femur to the distal third of the tibia
    c. Proximal third of the tibia to the distal third of the femur
    d. Femur, tibia, and digits

15. Measurement for the tibia and fibula of a cat should be taken at the:
    a. Center of the tibia/fibula
    b. Stifle joint
    c. Tarsal joint
    d. Distal femur

16. In a plantarodorsal view of the right tarsus of an Irish Terrier, the patient is routinely placed in:
    a. Dorsal recumbency
    b. Ventral recumbency
    c. Right lateral recumbency
    d. Left lateral recumbency

Answers to Review Questions can be found on the Evolve website.

References

1. Keller G. *The Use of Health Databases and Selective Breeding: A Guide for Dog and Cat Breeders and Owners.* ed 7. Columbus, MO: Orthopedic Foundation of America; 2012. http://www.offa.org/pdf/monograph_2012_web.pdf.
2. Thrall DE. *Textbook of Veterinary Diagnostic Radiology.* ed 6. St. Louis: Elsevier; 2013.
3. Holloway A. *BSAVA Manual of Canine and Feline Radiography and Radiology: A Foundation Manual.* Suffolk: BSAVA; 2013 [Chapter 7].
4. Muhlbauer MC, Kneller SK. *Radiography of the Dog and Cat: Guide to Making and Interpreting Radiographs.* Oxford: Wiley-Blackwell; 2013 [Chapter 4].
5. Ayers S. *Small Animal Radiographic Techniques and Positioning.* Oxford: Wiley-Blackwell; 2013 [Chapter 10].
6. Smith GK, Karbe GT, Agnello KA, et al. Pathogenesis, diagnosis, and control of canine hip dysplasia. In: Tobias KM, Johnston SA, eds. *Veterinary Surgery: Small Animal.* St. Louis: Elsevier; 2011:824-848.
7. Powers MY, Karbe GT, Gregor TP, et al. Evaluation of the relationship between Orthopedic Foundation for Animals' hip joint scores and PennHIP distraction index values in dogs. *J Am Vet Med Assoc.* 2010;237:532-541.
8. Verhoeven GEC, Fortrie RR, Duchateau L, et al. The effect of a technical quality assessment of hip-extended radiographs on interobserver agreement in the diagnosis of canine hip dysplasia. *Vet Radiol Ultrasound.* 2010;51:498-503.
9. PennHIP—The University of Pennsylvania Hip Improvement Program: home page. http://info.antechimagingservices.com/pennhip/index.html.
10. PennHIP information courtesy of Drs. GK Smith and M Wallace, University of Pennsylvania.
11. Morgan JP. *Techniques of Veterinary Radiography.* Ames, Iowa: Iowa State University Press; 1993.
12. Sirois M, Anthony E, Mauragis D. *Handbook of Radiographic Positioning for Veterinary Technicians.* Clifton Park, NY: Delmar Cengage Learning; 2010.

Bibliography

American College of Veterinary Radiology (ACVR). Radiology 2—equine, 2016, ACVR.
Aspinall V, Cappello M. *Introduction to Veterinary Anatomy.* 3rd ed. London: Butterworth-Heinemann; 2013.
Colville T, Bassert J. *Clinical Anatomy and Physiology for Veterinary Technicians.* ed 3. St. Louis: Mosby; 2016.
Done SH, Goody PC, Stickland NC, et al. *Color Atlas of Veterinary Anatomy, the Dog and Cat.* London: Mosby; 2009.
Douglas SW. *Principles of Veterinary Radiography.* London: Bailliere Tindall; 1980.
Dyce KM, Sack WO, Wensing CJG. *Textbook of Veterinary Anatomy.* ed 4. St. Louis: Saunders; 2010.
Evans H, de Launta A. *Guide to the Dissection of the Dog.* ed 7. St. Louis: Saunders; 2010.
Faber TL. *Radiographic Imaging and Exposure.* St. Louis: Elsevier; 2009.
Han C, Hurd C. *Practical Diagnostic Imaging for the Veterinary Technician.* ed 3. St. Louis: Mosby; 2005.
Orthopedic Foundation for Animals. An examination of hip grading. 2010. http://www.offa.org/hd_grades.html.
Orthopedic Foundation for Animals. Application for Hip/Elbow Dysplasia Database. 2010. http://www.offa.org/pdf/hdedapp_bw.pdf.
Owens JM, Biery DN. *Radiographic Interpretation for the Small Animal Clinician.* ed 2. Baltimore: Williams & Wilkins; 1999.
Romich J. *An Illustrated Guide to Veterinary Medical Terminology.* ed 4. Stamford, CT: Cengage Learning; 2015.
Sirois M. *Principles and Practice of Veterinary Technology.* ed 3. St. Louis: Mosby; 2011.
Smallwood JE, Shively MJ, Rendano VT, et al. A standardized nomenclature for radiographic projections used in veterinary medicine. *Vet Radiol.* 1985;26:2-9.
Ticer J. *Radiographic Technique in Small Animal Practice.* Philadelphia: WB Saunders; 1984.
Tighe M, Brown M. *Mosby's Comprehensive Review for Veterinary Technicians.* ed 4. St. Louis: Elsevier; 2015.

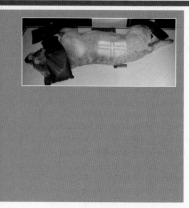

CHAPTER 20
Small Animal Vertebral Column

Marg Brown, RVT, BEd Ad Ed

The best lightning rod for your protection is your own spine.
— Ralph Waldo Emerson, American essayist and poet, 1803–1882

OUTLINE

LEARNING OBJECTIVES

When you have finished this chapter, you will be able to:

1. Describe the common positions and principles used to radiograph the small-animal vertebral column.
2. Properly and safely position a dog or cat for the various common positions of the vertebral column with an emphasis on nonmanual restraint.
3. Correctly measure and center the patient to include the peripheral borders.
4. Ensure that the body part is parallel to the image receptor and the central ray is perpendicular to both the field of view (FOV) and receptor.
5. Identify other views that may need to be completed as an alternative.
6. Identify normal spinal anatomy found on a radiograph.

KEY TERMS

Key terms are defined in the Glossary on the Evolve website.

Coned-down view	Flexed lateral	Kyphosis	Survey
Diverge	Hyperextension	Orthogonal	Vertebral formula
Dynamic	Hyperflexion	Positioning terminology	

TECHNICAL NOTE: To preserve space, the radiographs presented in this chapter do not show collimation. For safety, always collimate so that the beam is limited within the image receptor edges. In film radiography, you should see a clear border of collimation (frame) on every radiograph. In some jurisdictions, evidence of collimation is required by law.

Survey axial skeletal imaging does have limited diagnostic value in neurological disease and may be insufficient in conditions of the vertebral column, such as trauma. Definitive evidence may need to be obtained by myelography, computerized tomography (CT), or magnetic resonance imaging (MRI).[1,2] When these modalities are available, they have largely replaced radiography for spinal disease/trauma diagnosis in referral practices.

However, in spite of the limitations, proper survey vertebral radiographs are a valuable tool for those patients who have suffered spinal injuries and present with paresis or paralysis, either partial or complete. In addition, survey radiographs can demonstrate many of the signs consistent with intervertebral disk protrusion. Common intervertebral disk protrusion sites are T12 to T13, T13 to L1, C2 to C3, and C3 to C4.[1]

High-quality images are needed to see subtle changes in bone opacity, shape, and angulation of the vertebrae or vertebral column[1,2] (Table 20.1). The common views of this portion of the axial skeleton are the lateral (L) and ventrodorsal (VD) views of the cervical, thoracic, thoracolumbar, lumbar, lumbosacral, sacral, and caudal vertebrae. Depending on the size of the patient, a full survey study is either four or five images of each orthogonal view.

- Survey radiographs of a large dog center at C3 to C4, T6 to T7, thoracolumbar, L4, and lumbosacral
- Small dog survey radiographs center at C3 to C4, T6 to T7, L4, and lumbosacral

Cat survey studies of the vertebrae are often part of the whole-body view. For both the dog and the cat, coned-down views are important for areas of interest. Dynamic views of the vertebrae are not common in cats but can be completed.

See Appendix D on the Evolve website for information on the vertebral number and characteristics of the vertebrae of some common species.

Radiographic Concerns

- Each of the vertebral segments and adjacent intervertebral disks generally need to be examined, so correct positioning and attention to detail are essential to produce images of diagnostic value. This means centering the primary beam on the particular area of interest and tightly collimating immediately adjacent to the spine to increase the detail and contrast.
- Remember that the x-ray beam diverges from the central ray, so it is important to use smaller cassettes and take multiple views. Limit the number of vertebrae examined so that the intervertebral disk spaces are more perpendicular to the central beam. The farther away the area of interest is from the central beam, the greater the geometrical variation and the more inaccurate the interpretation of that area. Intervertebral spaces at the periphery of radiographs often appear falsely narrowed.[3] Coned-down views give further high-quality images.
- Having the anatomy parallel to the image receptor and perpendicular to the center of the beam is also essential for accurate diagnosis.
  - Tape placed along the spine may assist in proper alignment[4] (Fig. 20.1).
  - Use sponges or cotton padding between the limbs and under the sternum to keep the spine parallel to the tabletop, avoid any sagging, and prevent axial rotation.

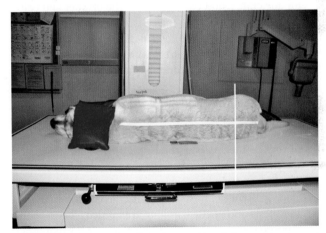

FIG. 20.1 Placing tape along the vertebrae helps maintain correct alignment and position. A small foam pad under the nose may be required. A line drawn between the greater trochanters should be perpendicular to the table.

TABLE 20.1	Protocol for Spinal Radiography	
ANATOMICAL LOCATION	**ROUTINE VIEWS**	**ANCILLARY VIEWS**
Cervical vertebrae	Lateral, Ventrodorsal Center at C3–C4	Hyperextended or hyperflexed lateral, open-mouth ventrodorsal, coned-down views, oblique
Thoracic vertebrae	Lateral, Ventrodorsal Center at T6–T7	Oblique, dorsoventral Coned down (T6–T7)
Thoracolumbar vertebrae	Lateral, Ventrodorsal Center at thoracolumbar junction	Oblique
Lumbar vertebrae	Lateral, Ventrodorsal Center at L3–L4	Oblique
Lumbosacral vertebrae	Lateral, Ventrodorsal Center at lumbosacral junction	Hyperextended or flexed lateral

- Sandbags can also be used for positioning on areas that will not be in the field of view.
  - For patients without spinal cord injuries, pulling and supporting the front and hind limbs in opposite directions keeps the thoracolumbar vertebral column extended to a near-parallel position, as well as opening the intervertebral spaces.[1-3]
- Choose a high-detail cassette/film combination if film is used. Low kilovoltage (kV) and high milliampere-seconds (mAs) provide better radiographic contrast, and the use of a grid further increases the contrast. Ensure there is enough kV for penetration and mAs for film darkening or signal (digital film).
- If using digital imaging, utilize appropriate algorithms to process raw data to prevent a sudden transition between bone and soft tissue that can create an artificial dark halo around the vertebrae.[2]
- The directional and identification labels should be in the field of view, but be conscious of overlapping the label on important anatomy, especially in VD views.
  - For lateral views, place the label along the dorsum.
  - In the VD views, the label may have to be taped to the patient in lieu of being placed on the image receptor.
- The hair coat should be clean and dry. Remove the collar for any cranial and cervical views. The bladder and colon should be emptied, as material within the colon or a distended bladder can create multiple superimposed shadows that might interfere with diagnosis.
- Generally it is more comfortable for right-handed radiographers to place the dog or cat in right lateral recumbency, but either side can be dependent.
- General anesthesia should be used to achieve accurate positioning with muscle relaxation; otherwise false narrowing of the intervertebral disk spaces due to muscle spasm may occur.[1,2,5]
- Because most feline patients requiring vertebral radiography likely present with spinal injury, sedation or general anesthesia and gentle handling are needed.
- If trauma is suspected, ensure that any concurrent issues such as thoracic pathology are addressed before obtaining the radiography.
- If the patient is compromised, VD views can also be made using the horizontal cross-table beam with the patient in lateral recumbency. This is especially useful if vertebral body fractures are suspected.
- Dorsoventral (DV) views (ancillary view) are not as accurate because of the increase in object-film distance (OFD). Also, it may be more difficult to obtain a parallel technique if the animal is in the DV position.
- Hyperflexion and hyperextension views (ancillary views) can further evaluate the caudal aspect of the lateral cervical and the lumbosacral vertebrae if the patient is chemically restrained and will not be traumatized by such handling. Be extremely gentle with handling.

TECHNICIAN NOTES

To understand the importance of and to demonstrate the optical illusion of variation in spacing that occurs farther from the central beam, evenly place a row of pennies on a 5-cm sponge about half an inch (1.5 mm) apart along the center length of the image receptor. Take an x-ray (suggested technique of 50 kV and 2 mAs) and look at the image. On the resulting image notice how the spacing between the pennies appears to distort as they progress toward the outside edges of the film.

TECHNICIAN NOTES

In general, each vertebra is made up of a body (the denser ventral portion, which is separated from the bodies of adjacent vertebra by intervertebral disks), vertebral arch (located dorsal to the body), and various processes (the cranial and caudal articular processes, the dorsal spinous process, and the lateral transverse process) (see Figs. 20.3, 20.9, 20.16, and 20.17).

The first letter designating each group, followed by the number of vertebrae in each group, is the vertebral formula. The vertebral formula for a dog and cat is $C_7T_{13}L_7S_3Cd_{6-20}$.

TECHNICIAN NOTES

The vertebral column is divided into five regions: cervical (neck), thoracic (chest), lumbar (abdomen), sacral (pelvis), and caudal (tail). To refer to a particular vertebra, use abbreviations for the region followed by the number within the region, beginning at the cranial end. For example, T12 is the twelfth thoracic vertebra. The abbreviation for caudal vertebrae is Cd (although sometimes the tail vertebrae are referred to as coccygeal and the abbreviation is Cy).

TECHNICIAN NOTES

Note that the positioning itself is fairly similar for most of the lateral and ventrodorsal views of the vertebrae. Keep important principles in mind.

TECHNICIAN NOTES

Remember to collimate tightly to the vertebrae. Place the label/marker on the dorsal aspect for the lateral views. For VD views, tape the marker on the body or place it on the table in an area that will not obscure important anatomy.

Cervical Vertebrae

Lateral View of the Cervical Vertebrae—Routine

Positioning

Place In: Lateral recumbency.

Hind Limbs: Superimpose and place the pelvic limbs caudally; secure with a sandbag.

Forelimbs: Position and superimpose the forelimbs caudally; secure with a sandbag.

A small foam pad can be placed between the limbs.

Head/Neck/Sternum: Extend the head and elevate the nose using a sponge. Keep the head in a true lateral position.

To see if the head is in a true lateral, draw an imaginary line between the medial canthi, and make sure this line is perpendicular to the table. Place a flat positioning device under the midcervical area if it is sagging. Support the cranial area of the head with a sandbag, or secure it with tape/Velcro strapping. Place sponges under the sternum to achieve true alignment with the vertebrae.

Vertebrae: Use foam pads or cotton beneath the cervical vertebrae to keep them parallel to the table.

MEASURE: Across the shoulder at the level of C6 to ensure adequate penetration of the caudal cervical vertebrae. Overexposure may occur with the cranial cervical vertebrae. Coned-down views can be made of these areas.

CENTRAL RAY: C3 to C4.

BORDERS: Base of the skull to the spine of the scapula (just past the shoulder joint, about T2, to include the cervical vertebrae). Collimate tightly to the edge of the wings of the atlas and the center of the spine of the scapula.

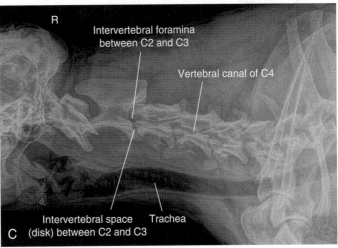

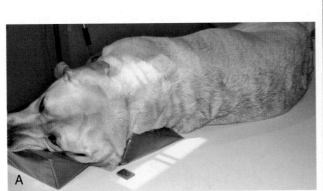

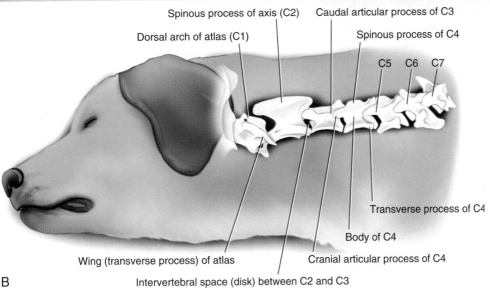

FIG. 20.2 A, Positioning for the lateral view of the cervical vertebrae. **B,** Left-to-right lateral anatomy of the cervical vertebrae. **C,** Lateral radiograph of cervical vertebrae. (**A** from Evans H, de Lahunta A. *Guide to the Dissection of the Dog,* 7th ed. St Louis: Saunders; 2010; **C** courtesy Vetel Diagnostics, San Luis Obispo, California, and Seth Wallack, DVM, DACVR, AAVR, Director and CEO of Veterinary Imaging Centre of San Diego.)

Continued

Lateral View of the Cervical Vertebrae—Routine—cont'd

Comments and Tips

- Keep the spine parallel to the table—the transverse processes of each vertebra should be superimposed on the image.
  - A separate image of the cervicothoracic junction may be required to better evaluate this region.[1]
- The head must be in a true lateral position because any obliquity of the head can change the position of the cranial cervical vertebrae.
- Try to keep true lateral positioning of the entire body even if radiographing only the cervical area.
  - Too much or too little padding can cause false narrowing of the intervertebral disks.
- Do not overextend the limbs because doing so might cause rotation of the spine.

- Do not flex or extend the head.
- To help align the cervical vertebrae with the long axis of the image receptor, position the pelvis region dorsally in a line with the head.
- Larger canine patients may have to be radiographed in two sections for the lateral and ventrodorsal cervical vertebrae:
  - *Radiograph 1:* Central ray at C2 to C3; include from the base of the skull to C4; measure at C2 to C3.
  - *Radiograph 2:* Central ray at C5 to C6; include from C4 to the center of the spine of the scapula; measure at the level of C6 to C7.

✎ TECHNICIAN NOTES

Strategically used positioning aids give the patient the illusion that it is being held.

✎ TECHNICIAN NOTES

Pulling the front limbs caudally prevents shoulder soft tissue from overlapping the spine.

✎ TECHNICIAN NOTES

Be extra careful when manipulating small-breed dogs that present with apparent neck pain.

✎ TECHNICIAN NOTES

Quickly go through your mental checklist *before* pushing the exposure button: settings correct; image receptor/machine/grid in position; proper location of markers and ID (if using at this stage); correct body part and view; properly centered; borders correct and collimated; patient properly prepared, positioned, and restrained so the vertebrae are in the same horizontal plane as the sternum for the lateral and superimposed for the VD, and parallel to the image receptor. The central ray is perpendicular to the field of view and the receptor.

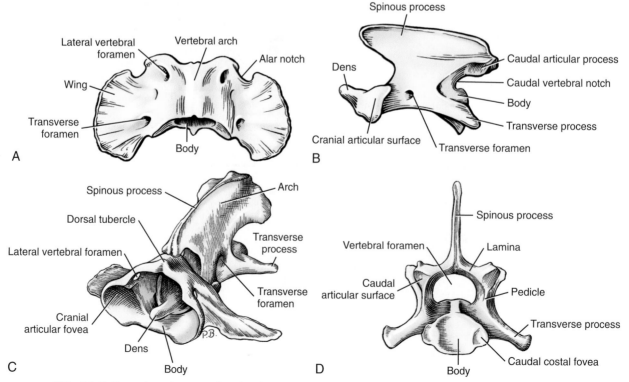

FIG. 20.3 Cervical vertebrae. A, Atlas, dorsal view. B, Axis, left lateral view. C, Atlas and axis articulated, craniolateral aspect. D, Seventh cervical vertebrae, caudal aspect.

Ventrodorsal View of the Cervical Vertebrae

Positioning

Place In: Dorsal recumbency in a V-trough or supported by tape/Velcro strapping or sandbag if needed.

Hind Limbs: Place the pelvic limbs in a neutral position and secure with sandbags.

Forelimbs: Evenly position the forelimbs caudally and secure with a sandbag.

Head/Neck/Sternum: Keep the head in a natural position with the nose slightly up to minimize the curvature of the cervical spine. Secure with padding lateral to the head and neck. Keep the sternum superimposed over the vertebrae.

Vertebrae: Use padding beneath the rostral neck to keep the cervical vertebrae parallel to the table.

Comments and Tips

- If possible, angle the beam in a slight caudocranial direction (20 degrees) between the intervertebral spaces to improve visualization of the disk spaces because they slope caudally in the VD position.
- Make sure that the sternum and vertebrae are superimposed and perpendicular to the image receptor to minimize rotation.
- The nose should be in line with the base of the tail with the limbs positioned evenly.
- If there is an interest in the occipital bone, point the nose upward and secure with sandbags lateral to the head and neck so that there is no bone superimposition of C1 to C2 with the occipital bone.
- As this is often the last view made, the endotracheal tube may need to be removed before the image is taken to avoid artifacts that might interfere with diagnosis.
- An open-mouth view of the odontoid process can be made as described in Chapter 21.

MEASURE: Level of C6 near the manubrium.

CENTRAL RAY: C3 to C4.

BORDERS: Base of the skull to just past the shoulder joint to about T2, with tight collimation laterally.

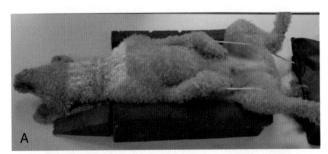

FIG. 20.4 A, Positioning for the ventrodorsal view of the cervical vertebrae. (**A** courtesy Seneca College of Applied Arts and Technology, King City, Ontario.)

Continued

Ventrodorsal View of the Cervical Vertebrae—cont'd

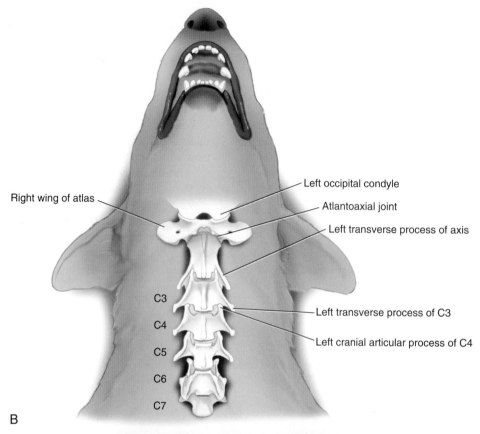

Right wing of atlas

Left occipital condyle

Atlantoaxial joint

Left transverse process of axis

C3

Left transverse process of C3

C4

Left cranial articular process of C4

C5

C6

C7

B

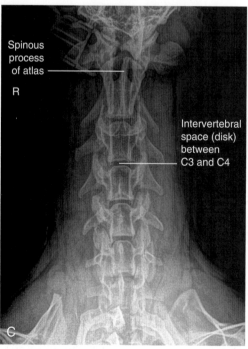

Spinous process of atlas

R

Intervertebral space (disk) between C3 and C4

C

FIG. 20.4, cont'd B, Ventrodorsal radiographic anatomy of the canine cervical vertebrae. C, Ventrodorsal radiograph of the cervical vertebrae. (C courtesy Vetel Diagnostics, San Luis Obispo, California, and Seth Wallack, DVM, DACVR, AAVR, Director and CEO of Veterinary Imaging Centre of San Diego.)

Hyperextended Lateral View of the Cervical Vertebrae—Ancillary

Positioning

Place In: Lateral recumbency.

Hind Limbs: Superimpose and place the pelvic limbs caudally; secure with a sandbag.

Forelimbs: Position and superimpose the forelimbs caudally; secure with a sandbag. A small foam pad may be placed between the limbs.

Head/Neck/Sternum: Elevate and keep the nose level to the table, using a foam pad. To see if the head is in a true lateral, draw an imaginary line between the medial canthi, and make sure this line is perpendicular to the table. Hyperextend the neck and head dorsally and caudally until resistance is met. Support the cranial area of the head with a sandbag, or secure with tape/Velcro strapping. Place foam pads under the sternum to achieve true alignment with the vertebrae.

Vertebrae: Use a foam pad or cotton beneath the cervical vertebrae as needed to keep each vertebra parallel to the table.

Comments and Tips

- For true hyperextension, all cervical vertebrae need to be extended dorsally.
- As with other cervical laterals, the head must be in a true lateral position; keep true lateral positioning of the entire body using proper padding, and do not overextend the limbs.
- Collimate tightly so that a coned-down view is obtained.
- If an endotracheal tube is present, be careful that the patient's breathing is not restricted at any point.
- The hyperextended view is usually completed before the flexion to determine if the latter is required.
- The hyperextended and hyperflexed views are referred to as *dynamic views* and are usually completed after myelography to note any spinal cord impingement due to extradural changes associated with vertebral instability.[2] Be very cautious with the procedures to prevent further injury.

MEASURE: C3 to C4 intervertebral space across the neck.

CENTRAL RAY: C3 to C4 intervertebral space.

BORDERS: Base of the skull to the spine of the scapula (just past the shoulder joint). Collimate tightly to the edge of the wings of the atlas and the center of the spine of the scapula.

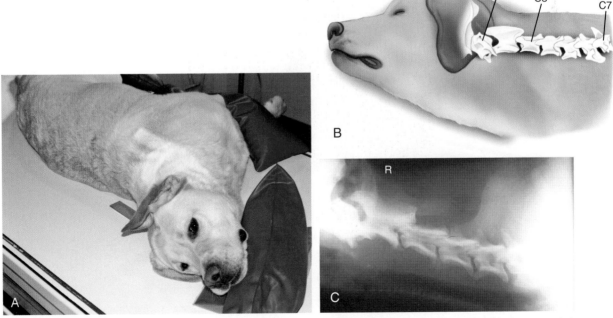

FIG. 20.5 **A,** Positioning for the lateral hyperextended cervical vertebrae. **B,** Left-to-right lateral anatomy of the hyperextended cervical vertebrae. **C,** Lateral radiograph of the hyperextended cervical vertebrae. (**C** courtesy Joshua Schlote, BS, LVT, Northeast Community College.)

Flexed Lateral View of the Cervical Vertebrae—Ancillary

Positioning

Place In: Lateral recumbency.

Hind Limbs: Superimpose and position the pelvic limbs caudally; secure with sandbags.

Forelimbs: Position and superimpose the forelimbs ventrally and caudally, and secure with a sandbag. A small foam pad can be placed between the limbs.

Head/Neck/Sternum: Place tape or thin rope around the nose or canine teeth, and gently apply traction on the end so the neck and head are flexed. Pull the tape caudally between the forelimbs close to the body, and secure to a sandbag. If needed, elevate the nose using a sponge so the head is in true lateral. Draw an imaginary line between the medial canthi, and make sure this line is perpendicular to the table. A sandbag can be placed dorsal to the nose to maintain the hyperflexed position. Place sponges under the sternum to achieve true alignment with the vertebrae.

Vertebrae: If needed, use sponges beneath the cervical vertebrae to keep the spine parallel to the table and at the same plane as the thoracic vertebrae.

Comments and Tips

- For true flexion, all cervical vertebrae need to be flexed.
- As with other cervical laterals, the head must be in a true lateral position; keep true lateral positioning of the entire body using proper padding, and do not overextend the limbs.
- The flexed lateral dynamic view is generally used to assess small-breed dogs with suspected subluxation.[2]
- Begin with the mildest extension that will demonstrate instability, as marked flexion may further damage the spinal cord.
- Collimate tightly so that a coned-down view is obtained for less distortion and better contrast.
- The radiographs should only be taken with the patient under general anesthesia and placement of an endotracheal tube. Be careful with hyperflexing the neck so as not to cause tracheal trauma or constriction of the endotracheal tube.

MEASURE: C3 to C4 intervertebral space across the neck.

CENTRAL RAY: C3 to C4 intervertebral space.

BORDERS: Base of the skull to the spine of the scapula (just past the shoulder joint). Collimate tightly to the edge of the wings of the atlas and the center of the scapular spine.

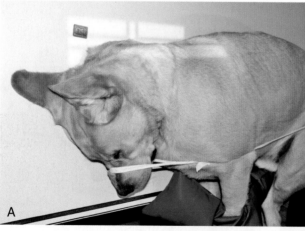

FIG. 20.6 A, Positioning for the lateral flexed cervical vertebrae. **B,** Lateral anatomy of the flexed cervical vertebrae. **C,** Lateral radiograph of the flexed cervical vertebrae. (**C** courtesy Joshua Schlote, BS, LVT, Northeast Community College.)

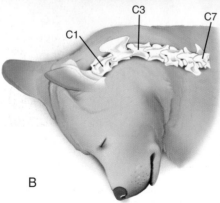

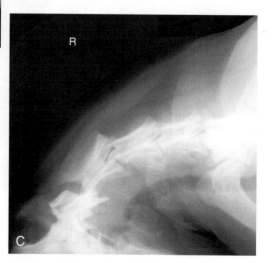

Lateral Oblique View for the Odontoid Process—Ancillary

Positioning

Place In: Lateral recumbency.

Hind Limbs: Superimpose and place the pelvic limbs caudally; secure with a sandbag.

Forelimbs: Position and superimpose the forelimbs caudally; secure with a sandbag. A small foam pad can be placed between the limbs.

Head/Neck/Sternum: Use tape/Velcro strapping to keep the head in its natural oblique position.[6] Place sponges under the sternum so it is on the same plane as the thoracic vertebrae.

Vertebrae: Use padding to keep the cervical vertebrae lateral and the head and C1 oblique.

Comments and Tips

- Position the ear pinnae laterally, and pull the tongue to avoid shadows on the radiograph.
- Lateral oblique views of C1 to C2 are used to demonstrate the dens.

MEASURE: C1 (for odontoid process).

CENTRAL RAY: C1 (for odontoid process).

BORDERS: Midskull to C4.

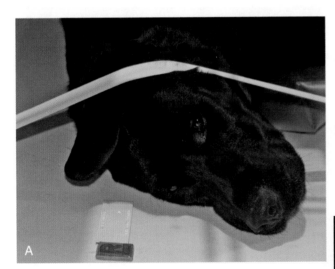

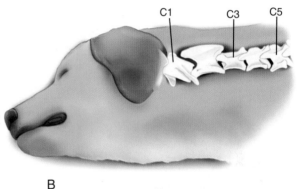

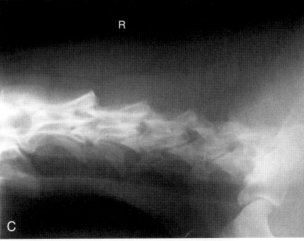

FIG. 20.7 A, Positioning for the lateral oblique view of the cervical vertebrae. The head is kept in a natural oblique position and a wedge is placed under the sternum. **B,** A lateral oblique view of the cervical vertebrae. **C,** Lateral oblique radiograph of all the cervical vertebrae. For the odontoid process, center at C1 and include from the midskull to C4.

Thoracic Vertebrae

Lateral View of the Thoracic Vertebrae—Routine

Positioning

Place In: Lateral recumbency with pelvis moved ventrally to straighten the thoracic spine.

Hind Limbs: Superimpose and place the pelvic limbs caudally; secure with a sandbag. A small foam pad can be placed between the limbs.

Forelimbs: Superimpose and cranially position the forelimbs slightly; secure with a sandbag. A small foam pad can be placed between the limbs.

Head/Neck/Sternum: Keep the head in a natural position, and support the neck with a sandbag. If needed, use sponges under the sternum and between the limbs to achieve true alignment of the sternum and vertebrae.

Vertebrae: Use padding if needed to keep each thoracic vertebra on the same horizontal plane as the sternum. Using tape as in Fig. 20.1 can assist with proper alignment.

MEASURE: Highest point of the midthorax.

CENTRAL RAY: T6 to T7 or the caudal border of the scapula.

BORDERS: From C7 to L1 inclusive (shoulder joint to past the origin of the last rib).

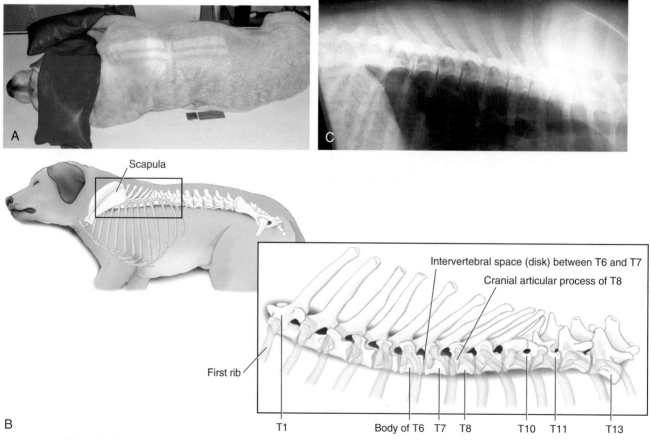

FIG. 20.8 A, Positioning for the lateral view of the thoracic vertebrae. **B,** Left-to-right lateral anatomy of the thoracic vertebrae. **C,** Lateral radiograph of the thoracic vertebrae. (**C** courtesy Joshua Schlote, BS, LVT, Northeast Community College.)

Lateral View of the Thoracic Vertebrae—Routine—cont'd

Comments and Tips

- Try to keep lateral positioning of the entire body even if radiographing only the thoracic area.
- Collimate tightly laterally.
- The pelvis should be positioned ventrally so that the thoracic vertebrae are aligned with the long axis of the image receptor. In the mid-to-caudal thoracic vertebrae region, dogs and cats have a natural area of kyphosis.[1]
- The ribs should be superimposed over each other so that the intervertebral spaces are better viewed, and the sternum should be on the same plane as the vertebrae. Use foam pads appropriately.
- Large dogs may require two separate views.

- Placing a lead mask or saline bag dorsal to the thoracic spine helps prevent scattered/secondary radiation from darkening the spinous processes in large dogs.

> ✎ **TECHNICIAN NOTES**
>
> Placing padding under the nose and the natural curvatures of the spine (neck and lumbar regions) and between the limbs for all lateral positions will keep the spine parallel and horizontal with the table/image receptor and perpendicular to the center ray.
>
> Keep a true lateral position of the entire body for each view, and keep the sternum and vertebrae on the same plane, parallel to the table and perpendicular to the x-y beam and receptor.

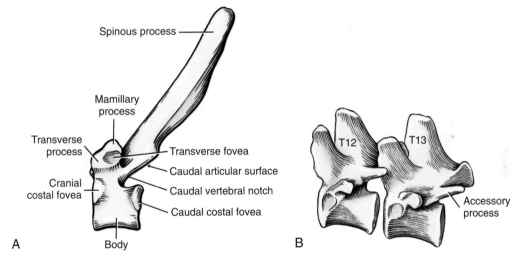

FIG. 20.9 A, Left lateral views of the sixth thoracic vertebra. B, Twelfth and thirteenth thoracic vertebrae.

Ventrodorsal View of the Thoracic Vertebrae—Routine

Positioning

Place In: Dorsal recumbency in a V-trough or use sandbags, if needed, to prevent rotation.

Hind Limbs: Equally place the pelvic limbs in a neutral position; secure with sandbags.

Forelimbs: Equally position the forelimbs cranially and tie or secure with sandbags.

Head/Neck/Sternum: The head and neck are best positioned with the nose parallel to the table and equidistant between the limbs. Support with ties or a sandbag, being careful not to restrict breathing.

Vertebrae: Superimpose the sternum and vertebrae to minimize any rotation.

Comments and Tips

- Ensure that there is a straight line from the tip of the nose to the base of the tail to achieve rib symmetry on the image.
- Large dogs may require two separate views.
- The symmetry of the normal patient is noted on an image when the spinous processes are evident on the midvertebral body and the sternum is superimposed over the vertebrae.

✎ TECHNICIAN NOTES

Image fewer vertebrae to prevent distortion due to the divergence of the x-ray beam.

MEASURE: T6 to T7 or the caudal border of the scapula.

CENTRAL RAY: T6 to T7 or the caudal border of the scapula.

BORDERS: C7 to L1 (shoulder joint to past the origin of the last rib).

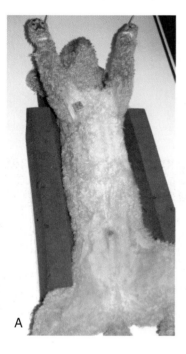

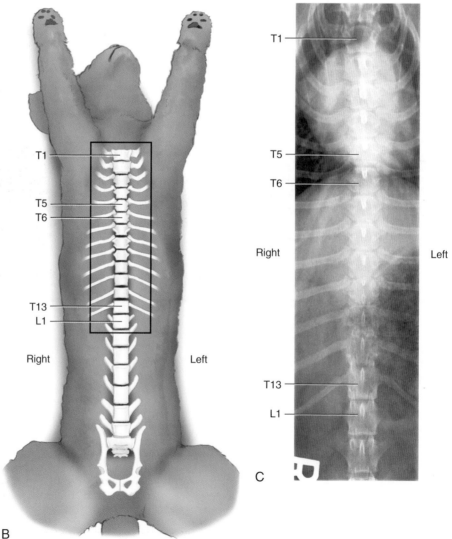

FIG. 20.10 A, Positioning for the ventrodorsal view of the thoracic vertebrae. **B,** Overlay of the ventrodorsal view of the thoracic vertebrae. **C,** Ventrodorsal radiograph of the thoracic vertebrae. (**C** courtesy Tara Wochesen, Ontario Veterinary College, Veterinary Teaching Hospital, Diagnostic Imaging at the University of Guelph.)

Thoracolumbar Vertebrae

Lateral View of the Thoracolumbar Vertebrae—Routine

Positioning

Place In: Lateral recumbency.

Hind Limbs: Superimpose and place the pelvic limbs caudally; secure with a sandbag.

A small foam pad can be placed between the limbs.

Forelimbs: Superimpose and cranially position the forelimbs slightly; secure with a sandbag. A small foam pad can be placed between the limbs.

Head/Neck/Sternum: If needed, use foam pads under the sternum to achieve true alignment with the vertebrae. Keep the head in a natural position and support the neck with a sandbag, being careful not to restrict breathing.

Vertebrae: Keep the thoracolumbar vertebrae on the same plane as the sternum. Using tape as in Fig. 20.1 can assist with proper alignment.

Comments and Tips

- Try to maintain true lateral positioning of the entire body even if radiographing only the thoracolumbar area.
- Collimate tightly. The vertebrae should be limited to four on either side of the thoracolumbar junction. If interested in both the thoracic and lumbar vertebrae, each area should be radiographed separately so that the number of vertebrae are limited.
- The ribs should be superimposed over each other so that the intervertebral spaces are better viewed, and the sternum should be at the same distance from the table as the vertebrae.
- On the image the intervertebral foramina should be superimposed, and they should be of equal sizes from the thoracolumbar junction toward the sacrum.

MEASURE: Highest point of the ribs.

CENTRAL RAY: T13 to L1 intervertebral space.

BORDERS: Xiphoid to most caudal portion of the last rib.

✎ TECHNICIAN NOTES

Keep these practical landmarks in mind as a general basis for the borders of all vertebrae:

- Base of the skull
- Shoulder
- Origin of the last rib
- Greater trochanter

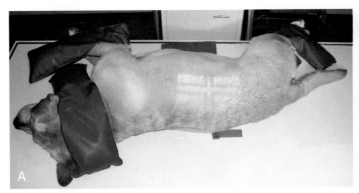

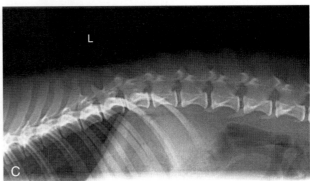

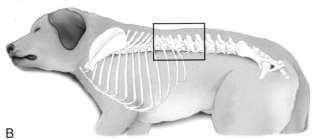

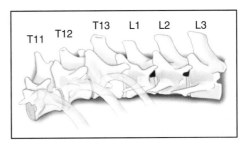

FIG. 20.11 **A,** Positioning for the lateral view of the thoracolumbar vertebrae. **B,** Right-to-left lateral radiographic anatomy of the thoracolumbar vertebrae. **C,** Lateral radiograph of the thoracolumbar vertebrae. Limit the number of vertebrae on either side of the thoracolumbar junction. (**C** courtesy Mount Pleasant Veterinary Hospital.)

Ventrodorsal View of the Thoracolumbar Vertebrae—Routine

Positioning

Place In: Dorsal recumbency in a V-trough or use sandbags, if needed, to prevent rotation.

Hind Limbs: Place the pelvic limbs in a neutral position; secure with sandbags if needed.

Forelimbs: Position the forelimbs cranially; tie or secure with sandbags.

Head/Neck/Sternum: The head and neck can be in a natural position. If needed, support with a sandbag, being careful not to restrict breathing. The nose should be equidistant between both front limbs.

Vertebrae: Have the sternum and vertebrae superimposed to minimize any rotation.

Comments and Tips

- Ensure that there is a straight line from the tip of the nose to the base of the tail.

- Collimate tightly. If interested in both the thoracic and lumbar vertebrae, each area should be radiographed separately so that the number of vertebrae are limited. See Box 20.1 to ensure you have proper symmetry on the image.

TECHNICIAN NOTES

Provide enough support with a V- trough, foam pads, or sandbags to prevent any axial rotation. The spine and sternum must be superimposed perpendicular to the table and plate for the ventrodorsal view; and on the same horizontal plane, parallel to the table and plate, for the lateral views.

TECHNICIAN NOTES

Collimate tightly to include the transverse process and muscle mass, but do not include the fat and skin.

MEASURE: Highest point of the midthorax.

CENTRAL RAY: T13 to L1 intervertebral space.

BORDERS: Xiphoid to the caudal portion of last rib (about T10–L3).

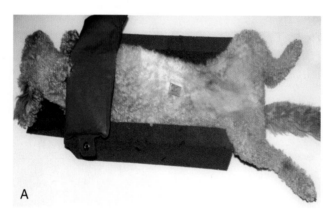

A

FIG. 20.12 A, Positioning for the ventrodorsal view of the thoracolumbar vertebrae.

Ventrodorsal View of the Thoracolumbar Vertebrae—Routine—cont'd

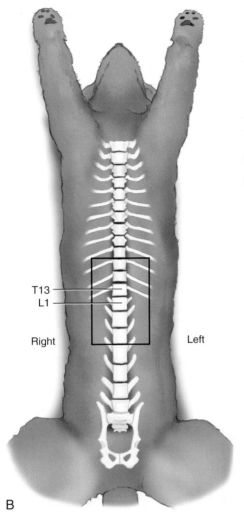

T13
L1

Right   Left

B

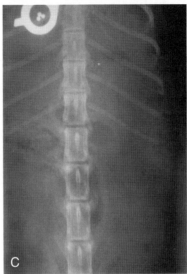

C

FIG. 20.12, cont'd B, Overlay of the ventrodorsal thoracolumbar vertebrae. C, Ventrodorsal radiograph of the thoracolumbar vertebrae. (C courtesy Joshua Schlote, BS, LVT, Northeast Community College.)

BOX 20.1 | Assessing Correct Positioning on a Vertebral Image

To assess correct positioning on a finished image.[1-3]
- Cervical and thoracic vertebrae:
  - Lateral view:
    - The wings of the atlas and individual transverse processes and rib heads superimposed.
    - The articular processes are parallel.
    - The intervertebral disks are of even thickness and regular shape.
  - VD view:
    - Equivalent anatomical features are symmetrical.
    - Spinous processes are on midvertebral body.
- Thoracolumbar vertebrae:
  - Lateral view:
    - The intervertebral foramina should be superimposed and should be of equal size and shape from the thoracolumbar junction toward the sacrum.
- Lumbar and sacral vertebrae:
  - Lateral view:
    - Transverse processes and wings of the ilia superimposed.
    - The lumbar transverse process superimposition has been described as a "Nike swoosh."[1]
    - The intervertebral foramina should be superimposed and of equal size and shape from the thoracolumbar junction to the sacrum.
  - VD view:
    - Spinous processes superimposed on the midvertebral body
    - Sacroiliac joints and equivalent anatomical features are symmetrical

Lumbar Vertebrae

Lateral View of the Lumbar Vertebrae—Routine

Positioning
Place In: Lateral recumbency.

Hind Limbs: Superimpose and place the pelvic limbs slightly caudally; secure with a sandbag. A small foam pad can be placed between the limbs.

Forelimbs: Superimpose and position the forelimbs slightly cranially; secure with a sandbag. A small foam pad can be placed between the limbs.

Head/Neck/Sternum: If needed, use foam pads under the sternum to achieve true alignment with the vertebrae. Keep the head in a natural position; support the neck with a sandbag, being careful not to restrict breathing.

Vertebrae: Keep each lumbar vertebra parallel to the table and image receptor and on the same horizontal plane as the sternum. Using tape as in Fig. 20.1 can assist with proper alignment.

Comments and Tips
- Try to maintain true lateral positioning of the entire body even if radiographing only the lumbar area.
- Collimate tightly.
- See Box 20.1 to ensure you have proper symmetry on the image.

MEASURE: Level of L1.

CENTRAL RAY: L3 to L4 (palpate).

BORDERS: T12 to S1 (Just cranial to origin of last rib to just before the greater trochanter).

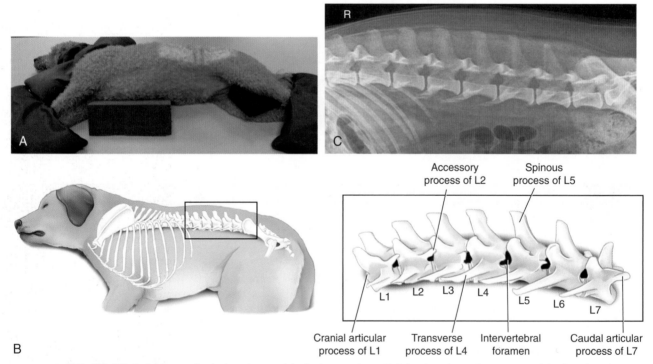

FIG. 20.13 A, Positioning for the lateral view of the lumbar vertebrae. **B,** Left-right radiographic anatomy of the lateral lumbar vertebrae. **C,** Lateral radiograph of the lumbar vertebrae of a 19-year-old male, neutered French Bulldog. Note the calcification at T12 to T13, L1 to L2, and L3 to L4. The transverse processes should be superimposed at their origins from the vertebral bodies, with each pair appearing as one. This appearance has been described as a "Nike swoosh." (**A** courtesy Seneca College of Applied Arts and Technology, King City, Ontario; **C** courtesy Jennifer White, Mississauga Oakville Veterinary Emergency Hospital and Referral Group, Oakville, Ontario.)

Ventrodorsal View of the Lumbar Vertebrae—Routine

Positioning

Place In: Dorsal recumbency in a V-trough or use sandbags, if needed, to prevent rotation.

Hind Limbs: Place the pelvic limbs in a neutral position; secure with sandbags if needed.

Forelimbs: Position the forelimbs cranially and secure with a sandbag if needed.

Head/Neck/Sternum: The head can be in a natural position.

Support with a sandbag, being careful not to restrict breathing. Position the nose equidistant between the forelimbs.

Vertebrae: Superimpose the sternum and vertebrae to prevent any rotation.

MEASURE: Level of L1.

CENTRAL RAY: Level of L4 (palpate).

BORDERS: T12 to S1 (Just cranial to both the origin of the last rib and acetabulum).

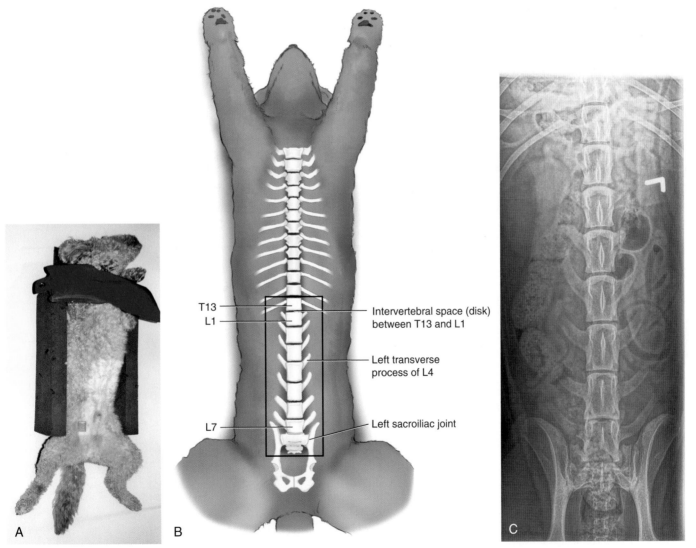

T13

L1

Intervertebral space (disk) between T13 and L1

Left transverse process of L4

L7

Left sacroiliac joint

A

B

C

FIG. 20.14 A, Positioning for the ventrodorsal view of the lumbar vertebrae. **B,** Overlay of the ventrodorsal lumbar vertebrae. **C,** Ventrodorsal radiograph of the lumbar vertebrae. (**A** from Evans H, de Lahunta A. *Guide to the Dissection of the Dog,* 7th ed. St Louis: Saunders; 2010; **B** and **C** courtesy Dana Greves and Jennifer White, Mississauga Oakville Veterinary Emergency Hospital and Referral Group, Oakville, Ontario.)

Continued

Ventrodorsal View of the Lumbar Vertebrae—Routine—cont'd

Comments and Tips

- Ensure that there is a straight line from the tip of the nose to the base of the tail.
- The transverse processes should be present and symmetrical on the image.
- Enemas are suggested before radiography of the lumbar and lumbosacral spine because feces can create artifacts.

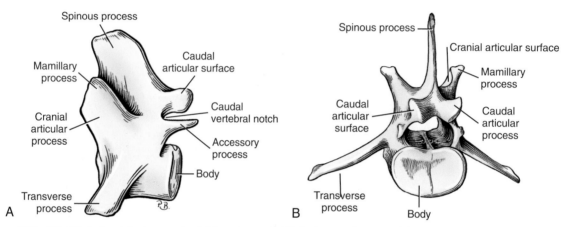

FIG. 20.15 **A,** Fourth lumbar vertebra left lateral view. **B,** Fifth lumbar vertebrae, caudolateral view. (From Evans H, de Lahunta A. *Guide to the Dissection of the Dog,* 8th ed. St Louis: Saunders; 2017.)

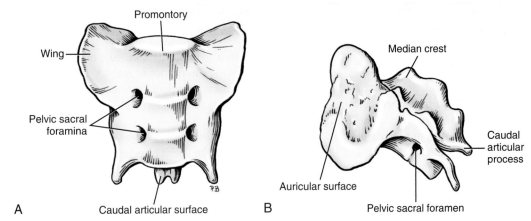

FIG. 20.16 Sacrum. **A,** Ventral view. **B,** Left lateral view. (From Evans H, de Lahunta A. *Guide to the Dissection of the Dog,* 8th ed. St Louis: Saunders; 2017.)

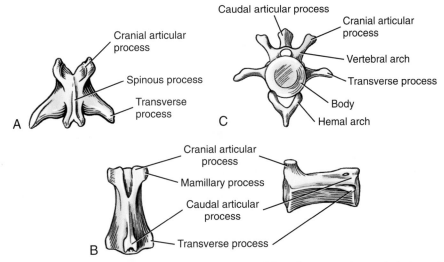

FIG. 20.17 A, Third caudal vertebrae, dorsal view. **B,** Fourth caudal vertebrae, cranial view. **C,** Sixth caudal vertebra, dorsal (*left*) and lateral (*right*) views. (From Evans H, de Lahunta A. *Guide to the Dissection of the Dog,* 8th ed. St Louis: Saunders; 2017.)

Lumbosacral Vertebrae

Lateral View of the Lumbosacral Vertebrae—Natural Positioning—Routine

Positioning

Place In: Lateral recumbency.

Hind Limbs: Superimpose and position the pelvic limbs slightly caudally, with a foam pad between them; secure with sandbags. Ensure that the wings of the ilia are superimposed and parallel to the image receptor by placing padding under the upper limb.

Forelimbs: Superimpose and cranially position the forelimbs slightly; secure with a sandbag. A small foam pad can be placed between the limbs.

Head/Neck/Sternum: Use foam pads under the sternum to achieve true alignment with the vertebrae. Keep the head in a natural position; support the neck with a sandbag, being careful not to restrict breathing.

Vertebrae: Use padding to keep each lumbar vertebra parallel to the table and the image receptor.

Comments and Tips

- Use the pelvis technique chart to ensure adequate penetration.
- See Box 20.1 to ensure you have proper symmetry on the image.
- Ancillary views of the lumbosacral include hyperextended and hyperflexed views of the vertebrae.

MEASURE: Level of the lumbosacral junction or the highest point of the wings of the ilia.

CENTRAL RAY: Level of the lumbosacral junction (just caudal to the wings of the ilia).

BORDERS: L4 to the most cranial caudal vertebra (just cranial to the wings of the ilia to the femoral head).

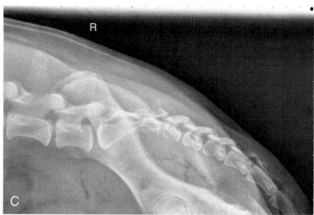

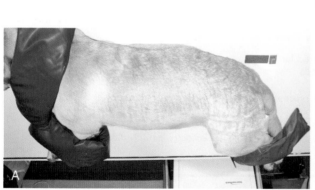

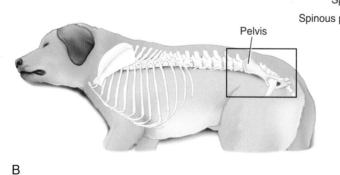

FIG. 20.18 A, Positioning for the lateral view of the lumbosacral vertebrae. B, Overlay and radiographic anatomy of the lateral lumbosacral vertebrae. C, Radiograph of the lateral lumbosacral vertebrae. (C courtesy Joshua Schlote, BS, LVT, Northeast Community College.)

Lateral View of the Lumbosacral Vertebrae—Ancillary

Comments and Tips

- These views are used to demonstrate lumbosacral instability.
- The measuring, centering, borders, and positioning is exactly the same as for the lateral view except for positioning of the hind limbs:

- For the hyperextended view (Fig. 20.19A): hyperextend the superimposed hind limbs as far caudally as possible, placing a sandbag over them to hold in position.
- For the hyperflexed view (Fig. 20.19B): position the superimposed hind limbs as far cranially as possible, placing a sandbag over them to hold in position.

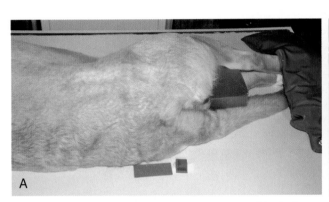 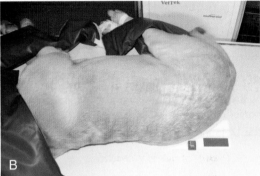

FIG. 20.19 A, Positioning for the lateral view of the lumbosacral vertebrae—hyperextended view. **B,** Positioning for the lateral view of the lumbosacral vertebrae—hyperflexed view.

> ### ✎ TECHNICIAN NOTES
> Collimate, ensuring that labels/markers are included and that borders are visible for every image.

Ventrodorsal View of the Lumbosacral Vertebrae—Routine

Positioning

Place In: Dorsal recumbency in a V-trough or use sandbags if needed.

Hind Limbs: Partially extend the pelvic limbs equally in a normal position, and secure with sandbags if needed. The pelvic limbs may be externally rotated.

Forelimbs: Position the forelimbs cranially and secure with a sandbag.

Head/Neck/Sternum: The head can be in a natural position. Support with a sandbag, being careful not to restrict breathing.

Vertebrae: Maintain the sternum and vertebrae in the same vertical plane.

Comments and Tips

- Ensure that the wings of the ilia are parallel to the table.
- A cleansing enema 1 to 2 hours before radiography should be considered to remove any feces in the colon that could obscure spinal lesions.

MEASURE: Wings of the ilia.

CENTRAL RAY: On the lumbosacral junction, caudal to the wings of the ilia, at an angle of 20 to 30 degrees in a caudocranial direction.

BORDERS: L4 to the most cranial-caudal vertebra (from just cranial to the wings of the ilia to the femoral head).

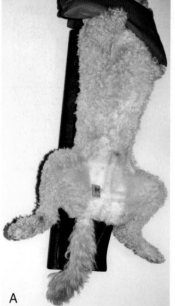

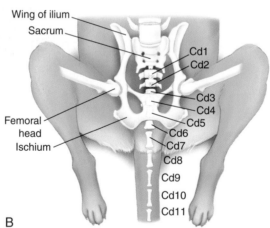

Wing of ilium
Sacrum
Cd1
Cd2
Femoral head
Ischium
Cd3
Cd4
Cd5
Cd6
Cd7
Cd8
Cd9
Cd10
Cd11

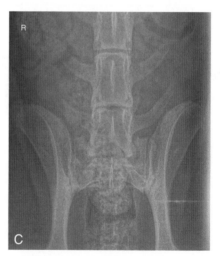

A   B   C

FIG. 20.20 A, Positioning for the ventrodorsal view of the lumbosacral vertebrae. **B,** Radiographic anatomy of the ventrodorsal lumbosacral vertebrae. **C,** Ventrodorsal radiograph of the lumbosacral vertebrae. (B and C courtesy Dana Greves and Jennifer White, Mississauga Oakville Veterinary Emergency Hospital and Referral Group, Oakville, Ontario.)

Caudal Vertebrae

Lateral View of the Caudal Vertebrae—Routine

Positioning

Place In: Lateral recumbency.

Hind Limbs: Superimpose and pull the pelvic limbs in a neutral position; secure with a sandbag.

Forelimbs: Superimpose and cranially position the forelimbs slightly; secure with a sandbag if needed.

Head and Neck: Keep the head in a natural position; support with a sandbag if needed.

Vertebrae: Place a foam pad to keep the vertebrae parallel to the table. A film cassette can be placed on the foam pad under the tail. Secure the tail to the cassette if needed.

Comments and Tips

- A grid is not used.
- If the cassette can be placed on the tabletop, divide the plate so that both views are on one cassette.

MEASURE: Thickest part of the tail.

CENTRAL RAY: Area of interest.

BORDERS: Four or five vertebrae on either side of the area of interest, or the full tail.

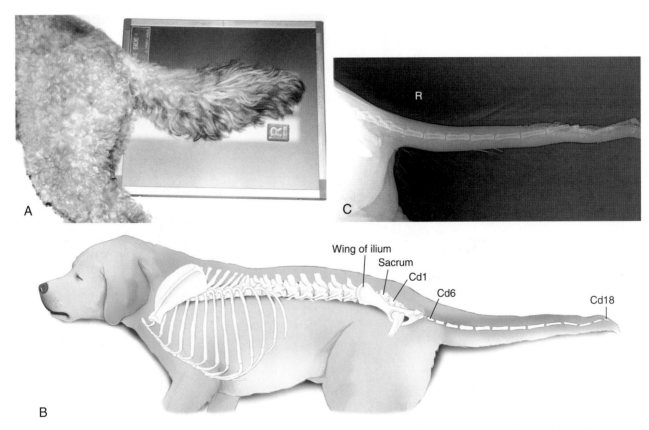

FIG. 20.21 A, Positioning of the lateral caudal (coccygeal) vertebrae. **B**, Radiographic anatomy of the lateral caudal vertebrae. **C**, Lateral radiograph of the caudal vertebrae that are fractured near the tip. (**C** courtesy Mount Pleasant Veterinary Hospital.)

Ventrodorsal View of the Caudal Vertebrae—Routine

Positioning

Place In: Dorsal recumbency in a V-trough or supported by tape/Velcro strapping or sandbag if needed.

Hind Limbs: Extend the pelvic limbs; secure with sandbags if needed.

Forelimbs: Position the forelimbs cranially; secure with sandbags if needed.

Head/Neck/Sternum: The head can be in a natural position. Secure if needed.

Vertebrae: Secure the tail with tape, if required, and keep it in a straight line with the body.

Comments and Tips

- A grid is not needed.

MEASURE: Thickest part of the tail.

CENTRAL RAY: Area of interest.

BORDERS: Four or five vertebrae on either side of the area of interest, or the full tail.

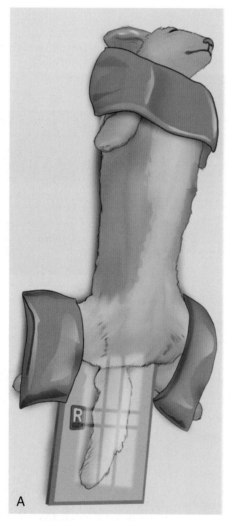
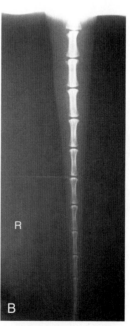

FIG. 20.22 A, Positioning for the ventrodorsal view of the caudal (coccygeal) vertebrae. B, Ventrodorsal radiograph of the caudal vertebrae.

Further Ancillary Views

- A VD view of the spinal column with a vertical beam may not always be feasible because of patient injury or other concerns.
- Alternatives include a lateral decubitus view, an oblique view, and a DV view (Fig. 20.23).
- Keep the principles of measuring, centering, and borders in mind for each of the positions described here.
- Center the beam on the area of interest and collimate.

Lateral Decubitus View of the Vertebrae (Ventrodorsal View With a Horizontal Beam)—Ancillary

- The VD view can also be achieved using a horizontal beam with the dog in lateral recumbency as described for the thoracic and abdominal views in Chapters 16 and 17.

Oblique View of the Vertebrae—Ancillary

- To help localize a lesion identified on the lateral or VD views that requires further examination, an oblique view may be requested.
- Place the patient in dorsal recumbency and rotate the body either to the right or to the left.

- Use padding under the mandible, cranial sternum, and pelvis to obtain a 30- to 45-degree oblique projection.
- Both the right and left oblique views should be compared.

Dorsoventral View of the Vertebrae—Ancillary

- A DV view with the dog in sternal recumbency can also be completed if an orthogonal view is required but the patient would be compromised in VD position or if the machine does not allow a lateral decubitus view. It is more difficult to maintain the vertebrae parallel to the table for a DV, and OFD—and thus magnification—will be increased.
- For completion of this view, keep a pad under the head so that all the vertebrae are parallel to the table (Fig. 20.23B).

Fig. 20.24 is a mystery radiograph. Review it and answer the question presented with it.

✳ KEY POINTS

1. General anesthesia or sedation should be considered for accurate positioning.
2. The common views are lateral and VD views of each spinal area. Ancillary views may further assist diagnosis.
3. It is essential that each vertebra being imaged is parallel to the table/image receptor and the central ray is perpendicular to both. This minimizes distortion that could lead to misdiagnosis.
4. Measure at the thickest part of the area of interest.
5. Collimate tightly to the vertebrae, being conscious of the placement of the labels and markers.
6. Multiple views are recommended. Limit the number of vertebrae on an image due to the divergence of the x-ray beam.
7. If the patient has a spinal column injury, manipulation of the limbs and spine may be contraindicated.

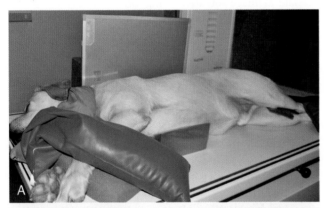

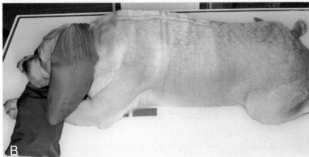

FIG. 20.23 A, Positioning for ventrodorsal views of the vertebrae with a horizontal beam. Tightly collimate the beam on the area of interest. **B,** A dorsoventral view can be obtained if it is difficult to obtain a ventrodorsal view. Object-film distance and magnification will be increased with the dorsoventral view, and the vertebrae are more difficult to keep parallel. Collimate the beam in tightly for spinal radiographs.

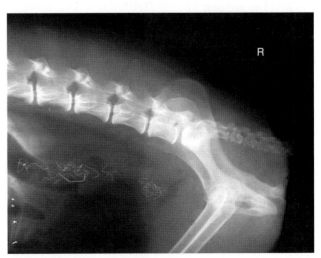

FIG. 20.24 Mystery radiograph. Identify the foreign images. (Courtesy Joshua Schlote, BS, LVT, Northeast Community College.)

REVIEW QUESTIONS

1. The ventrodorsal cervical vertebrae of a Doberman are to be radiographed. It is best to measure:
   a. And center at C6
   b. At C6 and center at C3-C4
   c. At C1 and center at C3-C4
   d. And center at C3-C4

2. For a radiograph of the lateral cervical vertebrae of the Doberman, sponges can be used to help ensure proper patient positioning. A sponge is not likely needed:
   a. Under the sternum
   b. Beneath the cervical vertebrae
   c. Between the rear limbs
   d. Under the nose

3. The front limbs of the Doberman for the lateral cervical vertebrae should be:
   a. Superimposed and positioned slightly caudally
   b. Superimposed and positioned slightly cranially
   c. Scissored and positioned slightly caudally
   d. Scissored and positioned slightly cranially

4. A flexed lateral view is required for the cervical vertebrae of this Doberman. The cervical vertebrae should be flexed, and:
   a. The head should be in a natural oblique position
   b. The head should be in a true lateral position
   c. The limbs should be extended as far cranial as possible
   d. No padding is required under the cervical vertebrae

5. A lateral view of the thoracolumbar vertebrae is required of a Dachshund. You should measure at the:
   a. T13 to L1 intervertebral space
   b. Cranial border of the scapula
   c. Highest point of the ribs
   d. Level of L4

6. The borders for this lateral view of the Dachshund thoracolumbar vertebrae should be at:
   a. The xiphoid to the most caudal portion of the last rib
   b. The cranial portion of C1 to T6
   c. T13 to caudal portion of L1
   d. T1 to just past L7

7. To ensure proper positioning for a ventrodorsal thoracolumbar view:
   a. Superimpose the ribs so that the intervertebral spaces are better viewed
   b. Place padding under the cervical vertebrae and sternum
   c. Place the pelvic limbs over each other in a neutral position, and secure with sandbags
   d. Superimpose the sternum over the vertebrae

8. In the lateral view of the TL junction, the label and positional markers should be placed:
   a. Ventral to the vertebrae being imaged
   b. Dorsal to the vertebrae being imaged
   c. At the cranial aspect of the vertebrae being imaged
   d. At the caudal aspect of the vertebrae being imaged

9. An Irish Setter is paralyzed. After it is stabilized and appropriate medication administered, the veterinarian wants you to take accurate orthogonal x-rays of the thoracic and lumbar vertebrae, as the veterinarian suspects compression fracture but is concerned about causing further injury. With film radiography you should complete a:
   a. Right lateral and right lateral decubitus view
   b. Right lateral only
   c. Right lateral and VD view
   d. Right and left lateral and DV view

10. In radiographing an Irish Wolfhound's thoracic and lumbar vertebrae for lateral and orthogonal views, you should measure and center at:
    a. T6/T7 and L4 to obtain four radiographs total
    b. T6/T7, TL junction, and L4 to obtain six radiographs total
    c. T6/T7 and L4 to obtain two radiographs total
    d. T6/T7, TL junction, and L4 to obtain three radiographs total

11. In radiographing the Irish Wolfhound's thoracolumbar vertebrae, you should include from:
    a. T1 to L3 on one image
    b. T4 to L3 on one image
    c. T10 to L3
    d. T1 to L7

12. You are checking the lateral lumbar radiographs of the Irish Wolfhound vertebrae to ensure that you are giving the veterinarian properly positioned radiographs. On the lateral image you are looking for:
    a. Superimposed intervertebral foramina and transverse processes
    b. Equal symmetry of the transverse processes
    c. A colon that does not contain any stool
    d. Spinous processes that are evident on the midvertebral body

13. To note symmetry on the VD lumbar radiograph of the Irish Wolfhound, you are looking for:
    a. Superimposed intervertebral foramina that are of equal size
    b. Superimposed pelvic limbs that are slightly positioned caudally
    c. Spinous processes that are evident on the midvertebral body
    d. A "Nike" swoosh created by the superimposition of transfer processes

14. A cleansing enema performed 1 to 2 hours before exposure is recommended for:
    a. The ventrodorsal lumbar and lumbosacral views
    b. Lateral and ventrodorsal lumbar and lumbosacral vertebrae views
    c. All ventrodorsal vertebrae views
    d. All ventrodorsal and lateral vertebrae views

15. Lumbosacral instability is suspected in a Greyhound. Along with the regular lateral the veterinarian will complete dynamic studies after a myelography study. The dynamic study is in reference to:
    a. VD and DV views
    b. Hyperextended only
    c. Hyperflexed only
    d. Both hyperextended and hyperflexed views

16. For a hyperextended lumbosacral view, a German Shepherd will be positioned in:
    a. Ventral recumbency with a horizontal beam aimed at the lumbosacral junction
    b. Lateral recumbency with the hind limbs superimposed and extended quite caudally
    c. Lateral recumbency with the hind limbs superimposed and extended quite cranially
    d. Dorsal recumbency with the hind limbs superimposed and extended quite cranially

17. Which chart should be used to determine the exposure factors for the lateral lumbosacral vertebrae?
    a. Spine
    b. Abdomen
    c. Pelvis
    d. Caudal vertebrae

18. If oblique views are to be taken of the vertebrae, the patient should be placed in:
    a. Lateral recumbency with 30 to 45 degrees rotation
    b. Sternal recumbency with 30 to 45 degrees rotation
    c. Dorsal recumbency with 30 to 45 degrees rotation
    d. Dorsal recumbency with 15 to 25 degrees rotation

19. A stabilized and paralyzed feline patient had been HBC (hit by car). The veterinarian suspects a complete fracture in the thoracic and lumbar region but wishes to take an initial radiograph to assist the owners to determine if treatment is an option. The veterinarian suggests that for now she would like you to obtain:
    a. Right and left lateral radiographs from C1 to S1
    b. Right lateral and VD radiographs from C1 to S1
    c. Three right lateral radiographs: C1 to L1, T10 to L3, and T12 to S1
    d. A right lateral radiograph from the shoulder joint to the pelvis

Answers to Review Questions can be found on the Evolve website.

References

1. Thrall DE. *Textbook of Veterinary Diagnostic Radiology*. 6th ed. St. Louis: Elsevier; 2013.
2. Holloway A. *BSAVA Manual of Canine and Feline Radiography and Radiology: A Foundation Manual*. Suffolk: BSAVA; 2013.
3. Muhlbauer MC, Kneller SK. *Radiography of the Dog and Cat: Guide to Making and Interpreting Radiographs*. Oxford: Wiley-Blackwell; 2013.
4. Sirois M, Anthony E, Mauragis D. *Handbook of Radiographic Positioning for Veterinary Technicians*. Clifton Park, NY: Delmar Cengage Learning; 2010.
5. Han C, Hurd C. *Practical Diagnostic Imaging for the Veterinary Technician*. 3rd ed. St. Louis: Mosby; 2005.
6. Morgan JP, Doval J, Samii V. *Radiographic Techniques: The Dog*. Schlutersche GmbH & Co. Hannover; 1998.

Bibliography

Ayers S. *Small Animal Radiographic Techniques and Positioning*. Oxford: Wiley-Blackwell; 2013.

Colville T, Bassert J. *Clinical Anatomy and Physiology for Veterinary technicians*. 3rd ed. St. Louis: Mosby; 2016.

Done SH, Goody PC, Stickland NC, et al. *Color Atlas of Veterinary Anatomy, the Dog and Cat*. London: Mosby; 2009.

Dyce KM, Sack WO, Wensing CJG. *Textbook of Veterinary Anatomy*. 4th ed. St. Louis: Saunders; 2010.

Evans H, de Lahunta A. *Guide to the Dissection of the Dog*. 7th ed. St. Louis: Saunders; 2010.

Muhlbauer MC, Kneller SK. *Radiography of the Dog and Cat: Guide to Making and Interpreting Radiographs*. Oxford: Wiley-Blackwell; 2013.

Owens JM. *Radiographic Interpretation for the Small Animal Clinician*. St. Louis: Ralston Purina; 1982.

Ryan G. *Radiographic Positioning of Small Animals*. Philadelphia: Lea & Febiger; 1981.

Tighe M, Brown M. *Mosby's Comprehensive Review for Veterinary Technicians*. 4th ed. St. Louis: Elsevier; 2015.

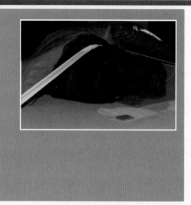

CHAPTER 21
Small Animal Skull

Marg Brown, RVT, BEd Ad Ed

"Life's true face is the skull."
—Nikos Kazantzakis, Greek author, 1883–1957

OUTLINE

LEARNING OBJECTIVES

When you have finished this chapter, you will be able to:

1. Identify the common positions and principles used to radiograph the small-animal skull.
2. Properly and safely position a dog or cat for the various common positions of the skull with an emphasis on nonmanual restraint.
3. Correctly measure and center the patient to include the peripheral borders.
4. Ensure that the body part is parallel to the image receptor and the central ray is perpendicular to both the field of view (FOV) and detector.
5. Recognize other views that may need to be completed as an alternative.
6. Identify normal skull anatomy found on a radiograph.

KEY TERMS

Key terms are defined in the Glossary on the Evolve website.

Brachycephalic
Canthi
Commissure
Dolicocephalic
Dorsal

Lateral oblique
Mesaticephalic
Positional terminology
Quadrant
Rostral

Rostrocaudal
Rostrodorsal-caudoventral oblique
Rostroventral-caudodorsal oblique

Skyline
Ventral

TECHNICAL NOTE: To preserve space, the radiographs presented in this chapter do not show collimation. For safety, always collimate so that the beam is limited to within the image receptor edges. In film radiography, you should see a clear border of collimation (frame) on every radiograph. In some jurisdictions, evidence of collimation is required by law.

The skull and the spine make up the axial skeleton. Proper imaging of the skull can be challenging because of complicated anatomy, superimposition of many of the structures, and the variation in size and shape of the various breeds. Images of the skull (Table 21.1) are often taken to evaluate trauma, congenital abnormalities, inflammatory lesions, tumors, or degenerative changes. Radiography may be inaccurate for detecting certain diseases and not as diagnostic as cross-sectional imaging modalities such as magnetic resonance imaging (MRI) and computerized tomography (CT). Alternative modalities might not always be available and are expensive, so radiography remains a primary diagnostic tool.[1]

TECHNICIAN NOTES

To be more efficient for any view, ensure that the body parts that are not in the beam are positioned and secured first. Position the area of interest last.

Radiographic Concerns and Anatomy

- Heavy sedation or general anesthesia will be required for most patients for views other than the routine lateral and dorsoventral survey to ensure that proper symmetry will be maintained. Consult an anesthesia text for suggested protocols and considerations.
- Recognize that the endotracheal tube, tongue, and pinnae could all cause dense shadows that may interfere with the diagnosis, so they should be repositioned or removed from the field of view when possible.
- Fortunately, the skull is relatively symmetrical and, in most small animals, approximately the same width in lateral and dorsoventral/ventrodorsal (DV/VD) dimensions. Both positions are measured at the widest area of the cranium. If air-filled sinus cavities are to be radiographed, measure just rostral to the thickest part of the cranium to avoid overexposure. Fig. 21.1 indicates the different skull types.

TABLE 21.1	Protocol for Skull Radiography
ANATOMICAL LOCATION	**VIEW(S)**
Routine Views	
Skull: routine or survey	Lateral (affected side down)
	Dorsoventral (DV) or Ventrodorsal (VD)
Ancillary Views	
Nasal cavity and frontal sinuses	Routine: DV/VD, Lateral
	Opposite lateral (L)
	Ventrodorsal open-mouth (rostroventral-Caudodorsal Oblique [R20-30V-CdDO] open-mouth)
	Rostrocaudal frontal sinus view (frontal 90-degree rostrocaudal-closed mouth view)
	Intraoral dorsoventral
Foramen magnum	Routine: DV/VD, Lateral
	Rostrocaudal closed-mouth view (rostral 30-degree dorsal-caudoventral) (fronto-occipital)
Tympanic bullae	Routine: DV/VD, Lateral
	Open-mouth rostrocaudal (rostral 10-degree ventral-caudodorsal) (R10-30V-CdD)
	Feline: Closed-mouth rostral 10-degree ventral-caudodorsal (R10V-CdD)
	Lateral oblique views: LeD-RtVO/RtD-LeVO, affected side up
	Lateral oblique (LeV-RtDO/RtV-LeDO), affected side down
Temporomandibular joint	Routine: DV and Lateral
	Lateral oblique (LeV-RtDO/RtV-LeDO), affected side down
	Lateral oblique [LeD-RtVO/RtD-LeVO], affected side up
Zygomatic bone and orbit	Routine: DV/VD, Lateral
Maxilla and dental extraoral studies*	Right or left open-mouth lateral
	Intraoral dorsoventral
	Lateral oblique (LeV-RtDO/RtV-LeDO)
Mandible and dental extraoral studies*	Right or left open-mouth lateral
	Intraoral ventrodorsal
	Lateral oblique views (LeD-RtVO/RtD-LeVO)

*For extraoral views, please see Chapter 22.

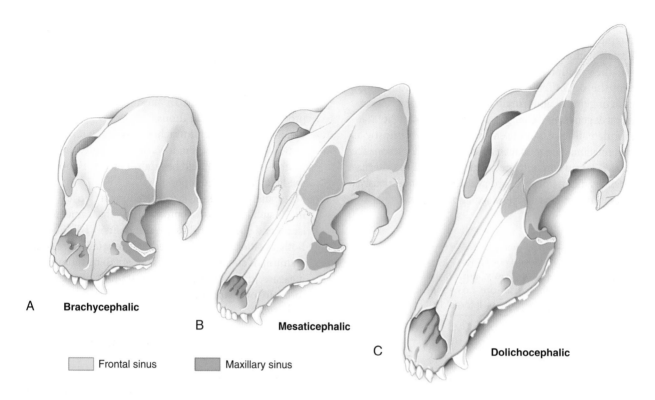

A   **Brachycephalic**

B   **Mesaticephalic**

C   **Dolichocephalic**

☐ Frontal sinus   ☐ Maxillary sinus

FIG. 21.1 The three basic shapes of the dog skull are the **(A)** brachycephalic, **(B)** mesaticephalic, and **(C)** dolichocephalic. The positions of the maxillary and frontal sinus on half of the skull are also shown. (From Aspinall V, Cappello M. *Introduction to Veterinary Anatomy.* London: Butterman Heineman, Elsevier; 2009.)

- High-contrast exposure is recommended. Use a grid for measurements over 10 cm, although with digital units, a grid may not be needed until 15 cm thickness. Use high mAs with a longer time station so that the lowest mA can be used that allows a small focal spot to improve geometrical sharpness. When possible, the radiograph should be tightly collimated to the primary area of interest to reduce scatter radiation and to improve the image quality.
- Keep the thickest part of the skull toward the cathode.
- No special preparation is required other than cleaning the hair coat and removing any collars or devices.
- Various-sized radiolucent wedges are required to properly and consistently position for extraoral oblique radiographs of the mandible and maxilla.
- Place the appropriate marker toward the nose. Correctly identifying the film with right and left markers is essential, especially for any oblique views. Both markers should be placed on the film for oblique images so that there is no confusion as to which is the dependent jaw. The markers also help identify the different quadrants of the teeth.
- The oblique mandible and maxilla views are further discussed in Chapter 22.
- For the lateral and DV/VD views, symmetry of the skull is essential to help identify asymmetrical structures and opacities, because most disease processes of the skull are not bilateral.[1]

> **✎ TECHNICIAN NOTES**
>
> Strategically use positioning aids to give the patient the illusion that it is being held. A sandbag over the neck and limbs and tape are essential if not properly sedated. Keep talking to your patient in a calm, low voice.

Routine Views

Lateral View of the Skull—Routine

The lateral view evaluates the nasal cavity, frontal sinuses, nasal margin and frontal bones, dorsal margin of the calvarium, and cribriform plate. It is the best view to examine the nasopharynx, retropharyngeal area, and hyoid apparatus. Because of superimposition, significant unilateral disease of the nasal cavity and bony margins may be missed.[1] Place the affected side on the table.

Positioning

Place In: Right or left lateral recumbency with the affected side to the image receptor (Fig. 21.2).

Hind Limbs: Leave in a natural position; support with a sandbag or ties if needed.

Forelimbs: Pull caudally, and support with a sandbag or ties.

Head and Neck: Position the head so that the mandible is parallel to the long edge of the image receptor. Put padding under the cranioventral cervical region. Place a foam pad under the ramus of the mandible to superimpose the rami and to prevent rotation of the skull. Tape the head or use Velcro straps over the nose and neck area so that the tape is extended across the table. A sandbag may be placed over the neck and against a foam pad at the dorsal aspect of the head to keep the head in position.

Comments and Tips

- Ensure that the pinnae of the ears and tape are not superimposed over areas of interest.
- Pulling the pectoral limbs caudally may help keep the skull in a true lateral position.
- To ensure that you have proper symmetry:
  - Viewing in a rostrocaudal direction (from the front), an imaginary line drawn through the medial canthi of the eyes and the hard palate should be perpendicular to the tabletop.
  - The midsagittal plane and nasal septum are parallel to the image receptor.
  - If you position your hand under the ventral mandible, it should be perpendicular to the table.
- The rami of the mandible and the tympanic bullae should be superimposed on the image.
- Because the skull in a brachycephalic breed is wider, geometrical distortion due to the divergent nature of the beam may not allow the appearance of symmetry of all structures.
- If either the mandible or maxilla are of particular interest, it may be beneficial to keep the mouth open with a speculum to minimize superimposition.

MEASURING, CENTERING, BORDERS: See Table 21.2.

✎ TECHNICIAN NOTES

Pads under the nose and neck will help keep the skull in a horizontal plane and minimize rotation. In the image, the wings of the atlas and all aspects of the skull should be even and superimposed.

✎ TECHNICIAN NOTES

Quickly go through your mental checklist *before* pushing the exposure button: settings correct; image receptor/machine/grid in position; proper location of markers and identification (if using at this stage); correct body part and view; properly centered; borders correct and collimated; patient properly prepared, positioned, and restrained so the part will be parallel to the image receptor and the central ray will be perpendicular to both.

✎ TECHNICIAN NOTES

True symmetry in a lateral view of a normal patient has been achieved if there appears to be only one structure on the image because the two sides are superimposed.

True symmetry in a DV/VD view of a normal patient has been achieved if the left and right sides are mirror images.

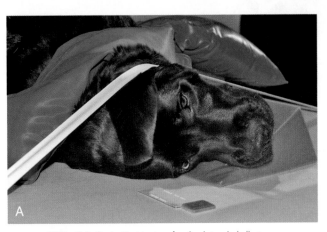

FIG. 21.2 A, Positioning for the lateral skull view.

Continued

Lateral View of the Skull—Routine—cont'd

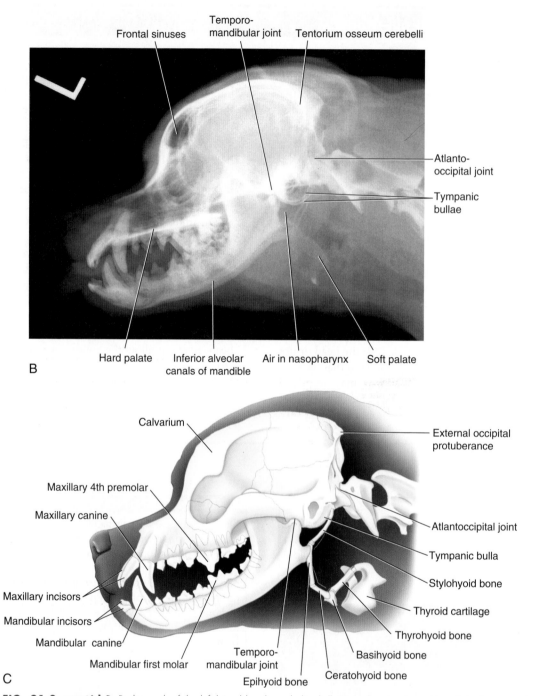

B

Frontal sinuses
Temporo-mandibular joint
Tentorium osseum cerebelli
Atlanto-occipital joint
Tympanic bullae
Hard palate
Inferior alveolar canals of mandible
Air in nasopharynx
Soft palate

C

Calvarium
External occipital protuberance
Maxillary 4th premolar
Maxillary canine
Atlantoccipital joint
Tympanic bulla
Stylohyoid bone
Maxillary incisors
Thyroid cartilage
Mandibular incisors
Thyrohyoid bone
Mandibular canine
Basihyoid bone
Mandibular first molar
Temporo-mandibular joint
Ceratohyoid bone
Epihyoid bone

FIG. 21.2, cont'd B, Radiograph of the left lateral brachycephalic skull. Note the superimposition of the bones and teeth in a true lateral view. C, Lateral left-to-right radiographic anatomy of the canine skull.

Lateral View of the Skull—Routine—cont'd

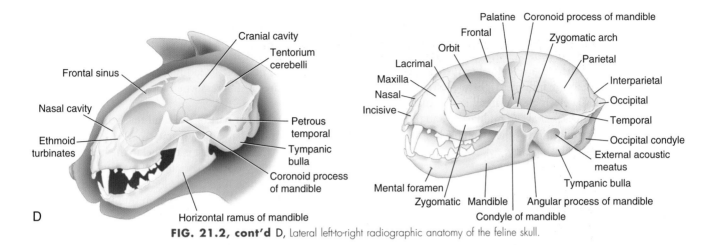

FIG. 21.2, cont'd D, Lateral left-to-right radiographic anatomy of the feline skull.

TABLE 21.2 | Lateral View of the Skull

	SURVEY	TEMPOROMANDIBULAR JOINT	TYMPANIC BULLAE	NARES/TEETH
Measure (on the area of interest)	Highest point of the zygomatic arch at the center of the cranium.	Highest point of the zygomatic arch over the joint.	Highest point of the zygomatic arch over the bullae.	Highest point of the zygomatic arch just rostral to the medial canthi.
Central ray (on the area of interest)	Lateral canthus of eye, midway between the eye and ear, or on area of interest.	Center just rostral to the ears.	Palpate and center on the base of the ear.	Just rostral to the lateral canthus.
Borders (depends on the area of interest)	Full skull: tip of the nose to the occipital protuberance.	Cranial and caudal to the joint.	Cranial and caudal to the ear.	Tip of the nose to the lateral canthi.

Dorsoventral View of the Skull—Routine

The DV is used for routine skull images and is often preferred over the VD, as it is easier to obtain true symmetry due to greater stability and less rotation when resting on the mandibles. Whatever view is chosen, it is important that the area of interest is close to the image receptor, geometrical distortion is reduced, and the image indicates right and left symmetry.

Both DV and VD views assess lateral and caudal aspects of the skull, external ear canal and middle ear, and the TMJs. There will be superimposition by the mandibles on the lateral nasal cavities and frontal sinuses.[2]

Positioning

Place In: Sternal recumbency in a V-trough if required.

Hind Limbs: Place in a natural position and support with a sandbag or ties.

Forelimbs: Pull caudally or leave in a natural position alongside the head, out of the field of view; support them with a sandbag or ties.

Head and Neck: Extend the neck and head. Place a sandbag over the neck for support, being careful not to restrict breathing. Tape across the nasal septum and the cranium to keep the sagittal plane of the head perpendicular to the image receptor. Make sure the ears are positioned laterally, equidistant from the head.

Comments and Tips

- To ensure symmetry: When viewing the skull in a rostro-caudal direction, an imaginary line drawn between the medial canthi should be parallel to the table.

- Slight downward pressure with positioning aids will assist in obtaining perfect positioning if the mandibles are symmetrical, as they will provide a flat and stable surface to support the head.[2]
- To prevent unwanted shadows, minimize the use of tape over the area of interest when lower exposure factors are used.
- Have the thickest part of the skull toward the cathode to help diminish changes in opacity.
- Make sure the hard palate is parallel to the image receptor.
- Place the marker on either side of the nose.
- The endotracheal tube can be left in place, with the possibility of causing a shadow kept in mind.

Intraoral Dorsoventral—Ancillary

- The nasal cavity can also be imaged with the plate in the mouth as will be described in Chapter 22 for the maxillary teeth.
- With the patient positioned as in the DV view, the image receptor is positioned in the mouth between the maxilla and endotracheal tube.
- The beam is centered on the dorsal aspect on the hard palate between the nasal planum and right and left orbits.

MEASURING, CENTERING, BORDERS: See Table 21.3.

> **TECHNICIAN NOTES**
>
> To maintain symmetry for the DV view, ensure that an imaginary line drawn between the medial canthi is parallel to the table. Look from the rostrocaudal direction. Keep the hard palate parallel to the table and image receptor.

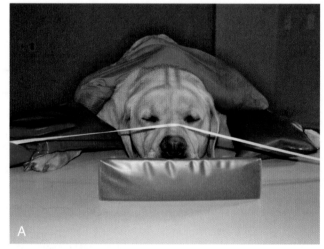

FIG. 21.3 A, Positioning for the dorsoventral skull view.

Dorsoventral View of the Skull—Routine—cont'd

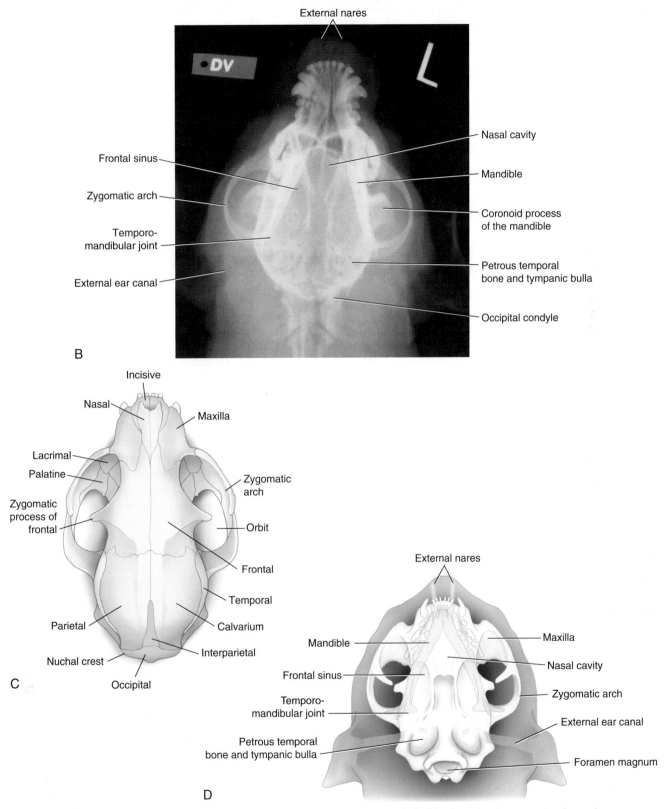

FIG. 21.3, cont'd B, Labeled radiograph of the dorsoventral skull. C, Skull of the dog, dorsal view. D, Overlay and radiographic anatomy of the ventrodorsal feline skull.

TABLE 21.3	Dorsoventral and Ventrodorsal Views of the Skull			
	SURVEY	**TEMPOROMANDIBULAR JOINT**	**TYMPANIC BULLAE**	**NARES/TEETH**
Measure (on the area of interest)	Highest point of the cranium just caudal to the lateral canthi.	Rostral to the ears on the dorsal (DV)/ventral (VD) midline of the skull.	Highest point of the cranium just caudal to the lateral canthi.	Rostral to the medial canthi.
Central ray (on the area of interest)	Between the two lateral canthi of the eyes on the sagittal crest(DV)/ventral midline(VD) or on the area of interest.	Center just rostral to the ears on the dorsal/ventral midline of the skull.	Palpate the base of the ear and center on the dorsal/ventral midline between the ears.	Center more rostral.
Borders (depends on the area of interest):	Full skull: tip of the nose to the occipital protuberance.	Cranial and caudal to the joint.	Cranial and caudal to the ear.	Tip of the nose to the lateral canthi.

Ventrodorsal View of the Skull—Routine

As described in the DV position, this view is used for a routine skull and other radiographs and for evaluation of the nasal sinus since the nasal passages are located dorsally.

Positioning
Place In: Dorsal recumbency in a V-trough, if required, and support with sandbags.
Hind Limbs: Leave the hind limbs in a natural position, and support with sandbags or ties.
Forelimbs: Pull the front limbs caudally, lateral to the chest, and support with sandbags or ties.
Head and Neck: Position a foam pad or sandbag under the neck so that the hard palate is parallel with the image receptor. Place a small foam pad under the nose and tape across the mandible to keep the head aligned with the table.

Comments and Tips
- Make sure the nose is parallel with the table.
- To ensure proper positioning, place your hands on either side of the skull and feel for the symmetry of the mandible and/or zygomatic arches. Your hands should be equidistant from the table on both sides.
- Move the tongue and endotracheal tube if present to minimize objectionable shadows on the area of interest. The endotracheal tube may have to be removed to prevent midline structures from being obscured.
- Ensure that there is symmetry of the head.
- The DV/VD views are compared in Fig. 21.5.
- A VD for a deep-chested dog may be easier to maintain proper skull symmetry rather than a DV view. See Fig. 21.1 for comparisons of the different skull types.

MEASURING, CENTERING, BORDERS: See Table 21.3.

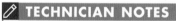

✎ TECHNICIAN NOTES
For the VD view, extend the neck so that the nose/hard palate are parallel with the table.

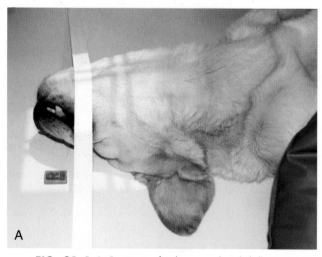

FIG. 21.4 A, Positioning for the ventrodorsal skull view.

Ventrodorsal View of the Skull—Routine—cont'd

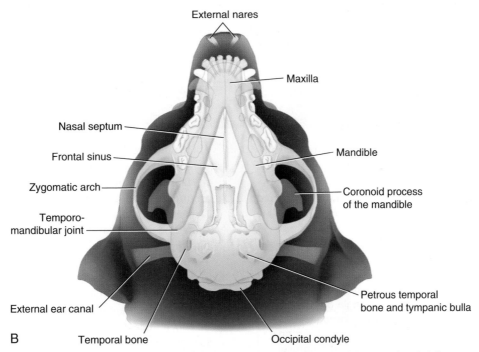

External nares

Maxilla

Nasal septum

Frontal sinus

Mandible

Zygomatic arch

Coronoid process
of the mandible

Temporo-
mandibular joint

Petrous temporal
bone and tympanic bulla

External ear canal

B Temporal bone Occipital condyle

FIG. 21.4, cont'd B, Overlay and radiographic anatomy of the ventrodorsal skull.

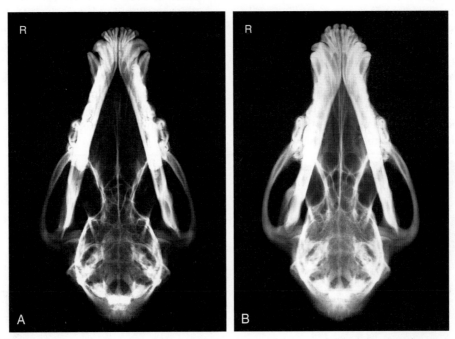

FIG. 21.5 A, Ventrodorsal radiograph of the skull. **B,** Comparison of the same skull in a dorsoventral position. Different exposure factors have been used in each case.

Ancillary Views

Because of the complexity of the skull, ancillary projections are used to assist in demonstrating certain regions. They are not used routinely, but are chosen based on the study required. Generally either the area of interest is at an angle to the primary beam or the x-ray beam is angled to the table. A moveable x-ray tube that can be rotated may be required. For any oblique views, proper identification, often with both the L and R markers, is essential.[3]

Ventrodorsal Open-Mouth (Rostroventral-Caudodorsal Oblique [R20-30V-CdDO] Open Mouth) View—Ancillary

- The ventrodorsal open-mouth view images the nasal sinus and ethmoid regions without superimposition of the mandible.[1-3]
- The patient is in a VD position with the mouth open and the tube angled. This position can be used only if the x-ray tube is movable or can rotate.

> ### ✎ TECHNICIAN NOTES
>
> "Rostroventral-caudodorsal oblique–(R20-30V-CdDO) (open-mouth)" means that the central ray enters the body from the nose (rostral) ventrally at an angle of 20 to 30 degrees and then exits obliquely toward the patient's back in a caudal direction. The patient is thus lying on its back in a VD position, with the nose almost parallel to the table, with its mouth open. The detector is under the dorsal aspect of the head.

Positioning

Place In: Dorsal recumbency in a V-trough, if required, and support with sandbags.

Hind Limbs: Leave in a natural position and sandbag or secure them to the table with ties.

Forelimbs: Pull the front limbs caudally, lateral to the chest, and support them with sandbags or ties.

Head and Neck: Place a small foam pad under the nose and have the hard palate parallel to the table. Position a strip of tape inside the mouth and securely adhere the ends to the table in a cranial direction so the maxilla is parallel to the table. Open the mouth wide by securing tape or gauze around the mandible and pulling caudally and ventrally. Depending on how wide the mouth is opened, the beam should be directed at 20 to 30 degrees from the vertical into the mouth and parallel to the mandible.[1,2,4]

Comments and Tips

- Decrease the kilovoltage (kV) slightly from that on the skull chart to account for decreased density of tissue to be penetrated.
- Keep the hard palate parallel to the cassette.
- The mouth can also be propped open with a modified tongue depressor, plastic speculum, or 1-mL syringe barrel placed between or over the canine teeth.
- The positioning device, tongue, and endotracheal tube may cause shadows, so move them away from the area of interest if possible. Keep the pinnae equally lateral to the head. Secure the endotracheal tube to the mandible to help prevent shadows on the area of interest.
- On a normal healthy patient, the nasal opacity and turbinate detail should be equal on both sides of the head.
- Feline patients will not likely require angulation of the beam.

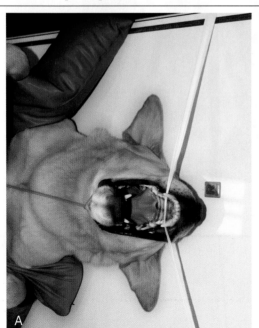

MEASURE: At the thickest area near the commissure of the lip (over the level of the third maxillary premolar).

CENTRAL RAY: On the nasal cavity—at the back of the palate about the level of the third premolar. Angle the x-ray tube rostrocaudally 20 to 30 degrees.

BORDERS: Tip of the maxilla to the pharyngeal region (all of the upper palate).

> ### ✎ TECHNICIAN NOTES
>
> If the tube can be tilted: Have the patient in a VD position with an open mouth for the nasal sinuses. Keep the maxilla parallel to the table, and tilt the x-ray tube. The collimator light should be on the hard palate back to the rear molars, and the image receptor must capture the primary beam at this area.

FIG. 21.6 A, Positioning for the ventrodorsal open-mouth view (rostroventral-caudodorsal oblique [R20-30V-CdDO] open-mouth) for the nasal sinuses.

Ventrodorsal Open-Mouth (Rostroventral-Caudodorsal Oblique [R20-30V-CdDO] Open Mouth) View—Ancillary—cont'd

Brachycephalic Breeds

- A better projection to image the nasal cavity of these breeds is a closed-mouth caudoventral-to-rostrodorsal oblique (CdV-RDO) projection with the nose (hard palate) tipped down toward the film approximately 30 degrees and the vertical beam centered 2 to 3 cm rostral to the angular processes of the mandible (Fig. 21.7).[2,3]
- See Fig. 21.1 for a comparison of the different skull types.

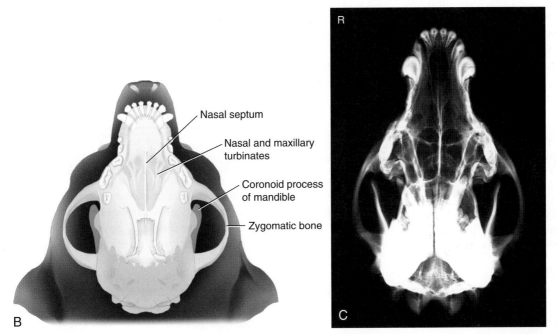

FIG. 21.6, cont'd B, Overlay and radiographic anatomy of the ventrodorsal open-mouth view. Tilt the x-ray tube about 20 to 30 degrees in relation to the table in a rostrocaudal direction. C, Open-mouth ventrodorsal radiograph of the skull (rostroventral-caudodorsal oblique [R20-30V-CdDO] open-mouth) view of the nasal sinuses. (Courtesy Susan McNeil, RVT, Georgian College.)

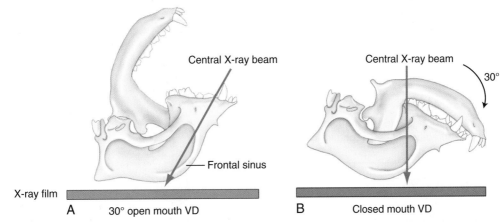

FIG. 21.7 A, The ventrodorsal open-mouth view (rostroventral-caudodorsal oblique) is not as effective at imaging the nasal cavity in brachycephalic breeds. B, The closed-mouth caudoventral-rostrodorsal oblique (CdV-RDO) projection is more satisfactory. The nose (hard palate) is tipped down toward the film about 30 degrees with the central beam 2 to 3 cm rostral to the angular processes of the mandible.

Rostrocaudal Views—Ancillary

Remember the rules of nomenclature if the full term or its abbreviations are used.[1,4–6] The first part of the term before the hyphen is where the central ray enters the body. This part of the body is closest to the x-ray tube. The part after the hyphen is where the central ray exits. This is the body part closest to the table or image receptor.

Thus a true rostrocaudal view means that the beam enters at the nose and exits at the back of the head. "Rostro" is derived from the Latin word "rostrum," which means beak, and emits from the head. To make it easier to remember, just think rostrocaudal means the nose is pointing up in some degree, so the dorsum is down.

To properly image different areas of the skull without superimposition, obliquity is required, so the oblique terminology is added. The mouth can be open or closed.

The descriptions are more accurate if the angle of either the beam or the position of the head away from the vertical plane is also included. Thus an open-mouth, rostral, 10-degree, ventral-caudodorsal oblique (R10V-CdDO) means that the patient is lying on its back with its mouth open and pointing to the x-ray tube. The head is positioned so that the central ray enters from the front of the patient inside the mouth (RV). The beam exits toward the back of the mouth and head (CdD) at an angle (O) 10 degrees ventral from the plane of the hard palate.

Rostrocaudal Frontal Sinus (90-Degree Rostrocaudal-Closed-Mouth) View—Ancillary

This frontal sinus view images the frontal sinuses, zygomatic bone, and orbits. The patient is in the VD position with the nose straight up and mouth closed. Another term for this view is *skyline view*.

Positioning

Place In: Dorsal recumbency in a V-trough if required; support with sandbags.
Hind Limbs: Leave in a natural position and secure with sandbag or ties.

Forelimbs: Pull the front limbs caudally, lateral to the chest, and support with a sandbag or ties.
Head and Neck: If needed, position a foam pad or sandbag under the neck so that the hard palate is perpendicular with the image receptor. Point the nose up so it is perpendicular to the image receptor and to the long axis of the body. Keep it in position by placing tape, tubing, Velcro, or gauze around the nose. Secure caudally, keeping the nose pointed up.

MEASURE: Over the site of the nasal sinuses (nasal stop). Found from medial canthus of eye to caudal part of the head.

CENTRAL RAY: Between the eyes (on the frontal sinuses).

BORDERS: Occipital crest to the dorsal aspect of the nasal planum (tip of nose).

> ### ✎ TECHNICIAN NOTES
> Keep the nose straight up and pointed at the x-ray tube for the frontal sinuses in medium- (mesaticephalic) and long-nosed (dolichocephalic) dogs.

> ### ✎ TECHNICIAN NOTES
> For any of the rostrocaudal ventrodorsal views, the patient will be in dorsal recumbency with the nose pointing at some angle toward the x-ray beam. The angle will depend on what is being imaged. The mouth may be open or closed.

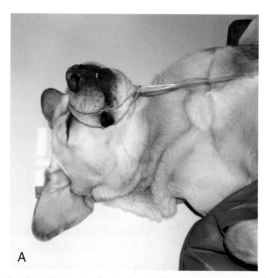

FIG. 21.8 A, Positioning for the frontal 90-degree rostrocaudal closed-mouth view of the skull for the frontal sinuses. The nose is pointing straight up, and the beam is centered between the eyes.

Rostrocaudal Frontal Sinus (90-Degree Rostrocaudal-Closed-Mouth) View—Ancillary—cont'd

Comments and Tips

- The hard palate and nose should be perpendicular to the table (nose points up). An imaginary line joining the medial canthi of the eyes should be parallel to the image receptor.
- If the nose is rotated too far dorsally or the beam centered too far ventrally, the nasal cavity will be superimposed over the frontal sinus.
- Be careful that the endotracheal tube is not kinked at the level of the oropharynx. Make sure the tongue does not create objectionable shadows on the area of interest.

- Reduce the kV because there is minimal tissue to penetrate.
- When positioned correctly, you should see two "bumps" (Fig. 21.8C) created by the shadow of the collimator light.
- Mesaticephalic and dolichocephalic breeds usually have a well-developed frontal sinus. A rostrocaudal image of the frontal sinuses in a brachycephalic breed that does not have a recognizable frontal sinus on a lateral radiograph will not be useful.[1,2]

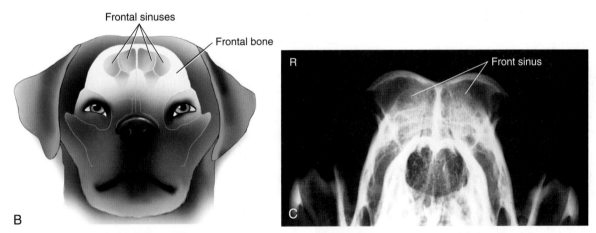

Frontal sinuses

Frontal bone

R

Front sinus

B

C

FIG. 21.8, cont'd B, Overlay and radiographic anatomy of the frontal 90-degree rostrocaudal closed-mouth view of the skull. C, A frontal 90-degreee rostrocaudal closed-mouth radiograph to show the frontal sinus. The nose is pointing straight up. (Courtesy Susan McNeil, RVT, Georgian College.)

Rostrocaudal Closed-Mouth (Rostral 20-30-Degree Dorsal-Caudodorsal Oblique) View—Ancillary

The rostrocaudal closed-mouth or fronto-occipital view demonstrates the foramen magnum, cranial vault, calvarium, and sagittal crest. This position is the same as the rostrocaudal frontal sinus view except that the nose is positioned caudally.

Positioning

Place In: Dorsal recumbency in a V-trough, if required, and support with sandbags.

Hind Limbs: Leave in a natural position; support with sandbags or tie if needed.

Forelimbs: Pull caudally, lateral to the chest; support with sandbags or ties.

Head and Neck: Point the nose upward and apply a long strip of tape or tubing to the nose. Angle the hard palate in a caudal direction toward the chest by pulling on the strip and securing it caudally (about 20 to 30 degrees).

Comments and Tips

- The central ray should intersect the bridge of the nose at an angle of 20 to 30 degrees to the dorsum of the nose or at an angle of 45 degrees to the hard palate.[1-3] The actual angle depends on the type of skull.
- The tongue and endotracheal tube may cause shadows. Try to keep the pinnae equally lateral to the head.
- The difference with this view from the regular rostrocaudal view is that the nose is pointing caudally 20 to 30 degrees for a view of the foramen magnum. Some sources suggest that the nose should be positioned down for an occipito-frontal projection with the beam centered at the junction of the right and left frontonasal sutures for dolichocephalic and mesaticephalic breeds, and about the top of the nasal fold for brachycephalic breeds.[4]

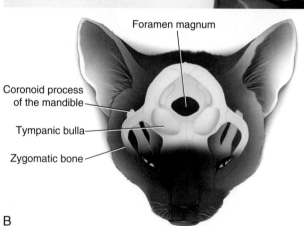

MEASURE: At the site of the frontal sinuses (from medial canthus of eye to caudal part of the head).

CENTRAL RAY: Midway between the eyes so that the cranium is centered and the beam intersects the bridge of the nose.

BORDERS: Entire cranium.

> ✎ **TECHNICIAN NOTES**
>
> The eyes are looking up at the x-ray tube for both the frontal sinuses and foramen magnum in the rostrocaudal views. The difference is that the nose is pointing caudally 20 to 30 degrees for a view of the foramen magnum.

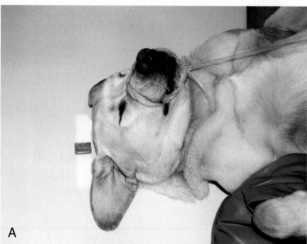

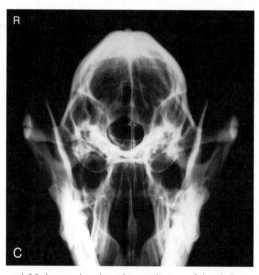

FIG. 21.9 A, Positioning for the rostrocaudal or fronto-occipital (rostral 30-degree dorsal-caudoventral) view of the skull to image the foramen magnum, cranial vault, calvarium, and sagittal crest. The nose is pulled more caudally than for the frontal 90-degree view. **B,** Overlay and radiographic anatomy of the rostrocaudal view (R30D-CdV) or fronto-occipital of the feline skull to view the foramen magnum. **C,** A skull radiograph of the rostrocaudal (R30D-CdV) or fronto-occipital view. Another term for when the nose points up is *rostrocaudal tangential*. (Courtesy Susan McNeil, RVT, Georgian College.)

Rostrocaudal Open-Mouth (Rostral 10-Degree Ventral-Caudodorsal Oblique) View—Ancillary

The rostrocaudal open-mouth view demonstrates the tympanic bullae, the base of the skull, and the odontoid process. This position is similar to the frontal sinus view, except that the mouth is opened for dogs. There is minimal superimposition of the petrous temporal bone.[7] This view is often referred to as the basilar view.

Positioning

Place In: Dorsal recumbency in a V-trough, if required, and support with sandbags.

Hind Limbs: Leave in a natural position; support with sandbags or ties if needed.

Forelimbs: Pull caudally, lateral to the chest, and support with sandbags or ties.

Head and Neck: A small amount of padding under the neck may help keep the head in position so the cervical spine is parallel to the tabletop. Avoid rotation. Point the nose upward, and apply a long strip of tape just below the maxillary canines. The commissures of the lip should be over C2. Pull the nose about 10 degrees cranially and secure. Apply tape or gauze to the mandibular canines, encompassing the endotracheal tube if used. Pull and secure the tape so that the mandible is about 10 degrees caudal from the perpendicular.

Comments and Tips

- The hard palate should be at about a 10-degree angle from the vertical for mesaticephalic breeds [1,2,5]
- The mouth can also be propped open with a tongue depressor, plastic speculum, or 1-mL syringe barrel placed between or over the canine teeth.
- The tongue and positioning devices may cause shadows. Try to keep the pinnae equilateral to the head.
- The beam should bisect the angle of the open mouth or at the junction of the hard palate and the horizontal rami of the mandible. The bullae should project freely.
- The angle of the beam varies with the patient and with how wide the mouth can be opened. Brachycephalic breeds likely require a larger palatial angle (21 degrees) and dolichocephalic breeds a smaller angle (4 degrees).[1,7]
- It may also be better in brachycephalic breeds to keep the mouth closed and position as for a cat with the hard palate at a 10-degree angle from the perpendicular (Fig. 21.11).[1]
- Slightly less kV is required because there is less tissue to penetrate.

MEASURE: At the commissure of the lips (level of maxillary third premolar).

CENTRAL RAY: At the commissure of the mouth just dorsal to the tongue from a rostroventral direction.

BORDERS: Entire nasopharyngeal region of the cranium.

> ### 🖉 TECHNICIAN NOTES
> To evaluate the tympanic bullae of dogs in the rostrocaudal open-mouth view, point the nose to the x-ray tube, open the mouth, and separate the mandible and maxilla, securing them slightly in each direction. Secure the tongue and endotracheal tube to the mandible or remove the endotracheal tube.

> ### 🖉 TECHNICIAN NOTES
> Collimate, ensuring that labels/markers are included and borders are visible for every image.

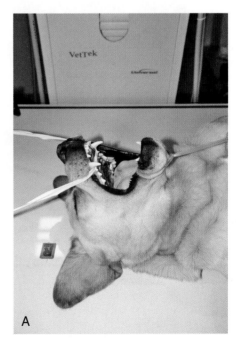

A

FIG. 21.10 A, Positioning for the rostrocaudal open-mouth (rostral 10- to 30-degree ventral-caudodorsal oblique) view. This rostrocaudal view demonstrates the tympanic bullae, the base of the skull, and the odontoid process. Measure and center at the level of the commissure of the lips.

Continued

Rostrocaudal Open-Mouth (Rostral 10-Degree Ventral-Caudodorsal Oblique) View—Ancillary—cont'd

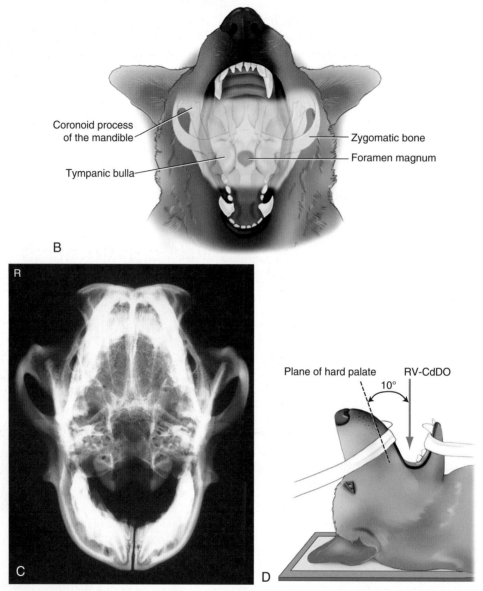

Coronoid process of the mandible

Zygomatic bone

Tympanic bulla

Foramen magnum

B

R

C

Plane of hard palate

RV-CdDO

10°

D

FIG. 21.10, cont'd B, Overlay and radiographic anatomy of the rostrocaudal open-mouth (RV-CdDO) view of the skull. **C,** An open-mouth R10V-CdDO radiograph of the skull demonstrating the tympanic bullae. **D,** RV-CdDO Open Mouth: Rostroventral-caudodorsal oblique view. The central ray enters from inside the mouth or the front and ventral aspect of the head (RV) and exits toward the back and top of the head (CdD) at an angle (O) 10 degrees ventral from the plane of the hard palate. (Courtesy Susan McNeil, RVT, Georgian College.)

Closed-Mouth Rostral 10-Degree Ventral-Caudodorsal Oblique View for Cat Tympanic Bullae—Ancillary

Comments and Tips

- Because the cat tympanic bullae are positioned anatomically more caudally than in a dog, keep the cat's mouth closed to view the tympanic bullae and odontoid process.
- Rest the dorsal aspect of the head on an angled foam wedge so that the hard palate is at an angle of 10 degrees from the vertical.
- Apply tape over the maxilla to secure.
- Center the beam at the level of the base of the mandibular body at the commissure of the mouth about 1 cm ventral to the external nares[5] (level of ears).

> ### TECHNICIAN NOTES
> Point the nose to the x-ray tube, keep the mouth closed, and pull slightly cranially for evaluation of the tympanic bullae of feline patients and possibly for brachycephalic breeds.

> ### TECHNICIAN NOTES
> Remember to apply the label appropriately in each image and to collimate the beam as tightly as possible.

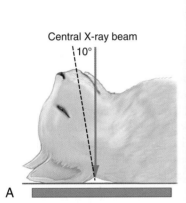

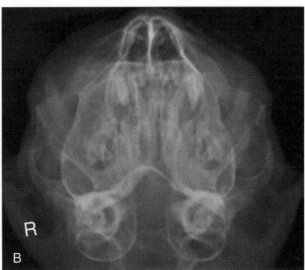

FIG. 21.11 A, Positioning for the rostrocaudal closed-mouth (rostral 10-degree ventral-caudodorsal) view of the skull for the cat tympanic bullae. The mouth is closed, and both mandible and maxilla are displaced dorsally 10 degrees. **B,** A rostrocaudal closed-mouth (R10V-CdDO) radiograph of the skull for the cat tympanic bullae. (**B** from Thrall DE: *Textbook of Veterinary Diagnostic Radiology*, 5th ed. St Louis: Saunders; 2007.)

Lateral Oblique Views—Ancillary

Lateral oblique views isolate the tympanic bulla, TMJs, frontal sinus, and maxillary or mandibular dentition depending on how the skull is rotated. The patient is lying in lateral recumbency, and the jaw is either pointed up or down.

To differentiate how the skull is obliqued, complete terminology is as follows using LeD-RtVO (left dorsal-right ventral oblique) view as an example:

- LeD—the beam enters the head from the patient's left side toward the dorsal aspect of the head.
- RtV—the right side is closest to the table; the beam exits from the ventral part of the head.
- O—indicates an angle.
- Thus in a LeD-RtVO the patient is lying in right lateral recumbency with the head in a dorsoventral oblique position.

- To help remember, temporarily ignore the left and right. A LeD-RtVO means the beam is coming from the top of the head. The jaw is pointing down in a modified dorsoventral oblique position ("dorsoventral down"—note the alliteration) (see Fig. 21.12C).
- The short form would be Right DVO.
- In this lateral oblique view the unaffected side is usually up. Have a system using both labels so that if the patient is positioned in right lateral recumbency, the right marker (unaffected bulla) will be dorsal to the skull and the left marker (affected bulla) ventral to the skull.

Lateral Oblique View (LeD-RtVO/RtD-LeVO)—Ancillary for the Tympanic Bullae

The lateral oblique or LeD-RtVO (modified dorsoventral oblique) view with the head lying in a natural position isolates the tympanic bullae. The view can also be used for mandibular dentition and frontal sinus.

Positioning

Place In: Right or left lateral recumbency with the unaffected side to the image receptor.

- Right lateral—to view the left oblique tympanic bulla
- Left lateral—to view the right oblique tympanic bulla

Hind Limbs: Leave the hind limbs in a natural position; support with sandbags or ties if needed.

Forelimbs: Position caudally and support with sandbags or ties.

Head and Neck: Position the head so that the mandible is initially parallel to the long edge of the table. Allow the

head to lie oblique naturally, with the jaw pointing to the table. If needed, tape the head over the nose and neck area, extending the tape across the table.

Comments and Tips

- The degree of rotation from the true lateral depends on the species and type of skull. Generally wider skulls require less rotation and narrower skulls more. There should be enough rotation to allow isolation of each tympanic bulla.
- Use both labels so that if the patient is positioned in right lateral recumbency, the right marker (unaffected bulla) will be dorsal and the left marker (affected bulla) ventral.
- This can also be used for an oblique view of the TMJ.

MEASURE: At the base of the ear over the tympanic bullae at the widest part of the cranium.

CENTRAL RAY: At the base of the ear over the tympanic bullae.

BORDERS: Cranial and caudal to the ear.

✎ TECHNICIAN NOTES

Have the patient lie in a natural oblique lateral position with the jaw and the unaffected tympanic bulla closest to the table. This could be considered a modified DV oblique view (the jaw is "down in a DV").

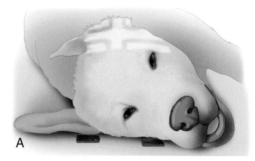

A

FIG. 21.12 A, A right lateral oblique (LeD-RtVO) view with the head lying naturally to show the affected left tympanic bullae in isolation. The unaffected right tympanic bullae is closer to the film. The dependent-side marker is placed dorsally, and the marker for the upper side is placed ventrally.

Lateral Oblique View (LeD-RtVO/RtD-LeVO)—Ancillary for the Tympanic Bullae—cont'd

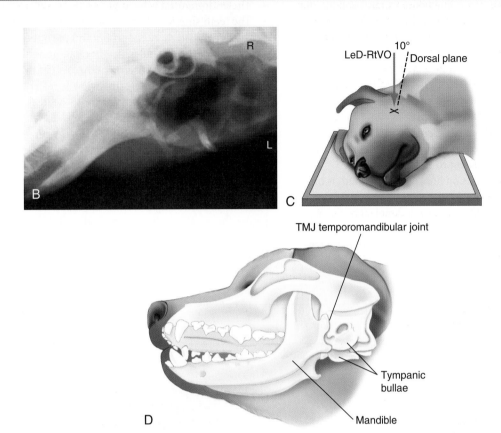

FIG. 21.12, cont'd B, Radiograph of the lateral oblique view of the tympanic bullae. The affected bulla is magnified and positioned ventrally. **C,** LeD-RtVO: Left dorsal–right ventral oblique view. The central beam enters the skull dorsally (from the top of the head) on the patient's left side (LeD) and exits the skull ventrally (toward the chin) on the patient's right side (RtV). Because the skull is not in a true lateral position, it is an oblique (O). The most accurate description is Le10D-RtVO. This locates the entrance angle at 10 degrees dorsal to the dorsal plane through the area of interest such as for the left temporomandibular joint. **D,** Overlay and radiographic anatomy of the lateral oblique or dorsoventral oblique view to visualize the tympanic bullae, temporomandibular joints, and maxilla.

Lateral Oblique View for the Mandible (LeD-RtVO/RtD-LeVO)—Ancillary

This lateral oblique view (modified dorsoventral oblique) for the mandible is used to radiograph the lower dental arcade or bony lesions of the nondependent mandible. The affected side will be down.

Comments and Tips

- The right side is down for visualizing the right mandibular teeth.
- A foam pad under the maxilla, creating a 20- to 45-degree angle of the mandible with the table, is required. (The affected mandible is closest to the table.)
- The actual angle depends on how wide the mouth is open and on the breed. There should be no superimposition of the affected mandibular premolars and molars by the other teeth.
- The mouth should be widely opened, and the beam centered over the fourth premolar.

- The endotracheal tube is tied to the maxilla.
- The teeth should be labeled with both positional markers, the dependent marker dorsally and the upper side marker ventrally. (The dependent teeth will be grayer because there is minimal superimposition of the rami of the mandibles.)
- Depending on the angle, this view is referred to as:
  - Le20-45°D-RtVO: left 20 to 45 degrees dorsal, right ventral oblique if the right side is down.
  - Rt20-45°D-LeVO: right 20 to 45 degrees dorsal, left ventral oblique view if the left side is down (Fig. 21.13).

> ### ✎ TECHNICIAN NOTES
>
> For the lateral oblique view of the mandibular teeth, raise the maxilla with a foam wedge. This is a modified DV oblique view because the beam enters at the top of the head and exits ventrally. The jaw is pointing down (DV is down). The affected mandible is on the film.

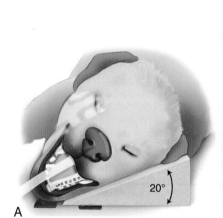

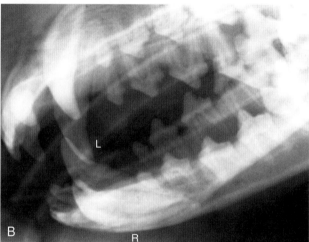

FIG. 21.13 A, Lateral oblique or dorsoventral oblique (Rt20D-LeVO) positioning for viewing the left mandibular dental arcade. The maxilla is raised from 20 to 45 degrees, depending on how wide the mouth is open or on the breed of the patient. **B,** Lateral oblique (or modified DVO, specifically the RtDLeVO) view for the left mandibular arcade. Note that the left mandibular teeth appear grayer because there is no superimposition with the mandible. The head angle also causes elongation, making the affected mandibular teeth appear more magnified. If the mouth is opened wider, there is less overlapping by the maxillary teeth.

Lateral Oblique (LeV-RtDO/RtV-LeDO)—Ancillary

- This lateral oblique or modified ventrodorsal oblique (jaw up) view can be used for the tympanic bullae, TMJ, and maxillary teeth.
- This provides a different view of the mandibular condyle than is projected on the lateral and DV/VD views.
- Another way to describe the view is laterorostral-laterocaudal oblique.

Positioning

Place In: Right or left lateral recumbency with the affected side to the image receptor.

Hind Limbs: Leave the hind limbs in a natural position; support with sandbags or ties if needed.

Forelimbs: Position caudally and support with sandbags or ties.

Head and Neck: Position the head initially so that the mandible is parallel to the long edge of the image receptor. Keep the skull in a straight lateral position. Place a foam pad under the mandible to raise the jaw from 10 to 30 degrees, depending on the breed of dog. The mouth can be partially opened. If needed, tape the head over the nose and neck area, extending the tape across the table. A sandbag may be placed over the neck and against a foam pad at the dorsal aspect of the head.

> **TECHNICIAN NOTES**
>
> For a lateral oblique view of the TMJ or maxillary teeth, position the jaw up on a foam pad and have the affected joint or teeth closer to the table.

> **TECHNICIAN NOTES**
>
> This view could also be called a *modified ventrodorsal oblique view* because the jaw is tipped up at an angle and the beam enters the head more from the ventrodorsal aspect. The maxilla is closer to the table than the mandible (jaw up).

MEASURE: Just caudal to the lateral canthus over the joint.

CENTRAL RAY: Between the caudal mandibular ramus and the base of the ear.

BORDERS: Cranial and caudal to the joint.

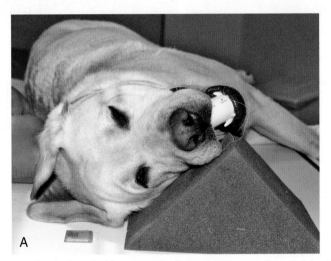

FIG. 21.14 A, Positioning for the lateral oblique (specifically LeV-RtDO) view of the skull for the maxillary teeth. The affected side is against the table. A smaller angle is used to visualize the tympanic bullae and temporomandibular joints. The left marker indicates that the left or nondependent side will be positioned more dorsally than the right maxilla when the head is rotated from the table. The R marker shows that the side closest to the film will be more ventral. It is under the foam pad nearer the right maxilla. The R and L marker in oblique cases do not show the side the animal is lying on. The markers only show the position of the jaws relative to each other.

Continued

Lateral Oblique (LeV-RtDO/RtV-LeDO)—Ancillary—cont'd

Comments and Tips

- This position displaces the nondependent bulla (upper) caudally and the dependent (down) bulla rostrally.
- The distance the mandible is raised depends on the breed. Dolichocephalic breeds require an angle of about 10 degrees, and mesaticephalic breeds about 15 degrees. Brachycephalic breeds generally require an angle of 25 to 30 degrees from the table.[1,4,6]
- Both right and left lateral oblique views should be taken for comparison.

- Ensure that the pinnae, tongue, and endotracheal tubes will not create objectionable shadows on the area of interest.
- The marker indicating the dependent side should be placed ventrally near the joint. The nondependent side marker should be placed dorsal to the nares to indicate that the raised joint is dorsal to the joint on the table.
- Use the skull technique chart, because more exposure is required to penetrate the cranium.

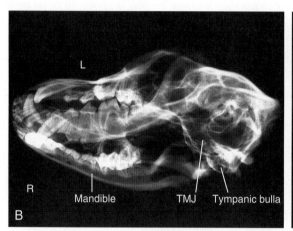

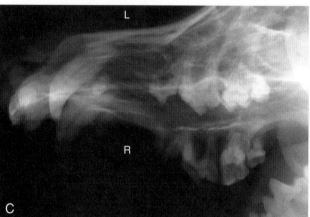

FIG. 21.14, con'd B, Radiograph of the lateral oblique (ventrodorsal oblique or LeV-RtDO) view of a skull in right lateral. **C,** Centering on the maxilla and opening the mouth wider in the open-mouth lateral oblique (LeV-RtDO open-mouth) radiograph provides this image of the maxillary dental arcade.

Lateral Oblique (LeV-RtDO/RtV-LeDO)—Ancillary—cont'd

Upper Dental Arcade

- This view can also be used to radiograph the upper dental arcade or bony lesions of the nondependent maxilla.
- A foam pad under the mandible, creating a 30- to 45-degree angle of the mandible with the table, is usually required (see Fig. 21.14A).
- The affected maxilla is closer to the table if imaging the teeth.

- The mouth should be widely opened, and the central ray is over the fourth premolar.
- The endotracheal tube should be tied to the mandible.
- The teeth should be marked with both positional markers—the dependent marker placed ventrally and the upper side marker dorsally. (The dependent teeth will be grayer because there is minimal superimposition of the palate.)

✎ TECHNICIAN NOTES

When placing the positional markers for an oblique view, consider the following:
- What quadrant are you attempting to image?
  - When that quadrant is in the correct position, look at which part of the jaw is touching the table.
  - Will it appear more ventral, or will it be displaced dorsally in relation to the opposite side of the jaw?
- If imaging the right mandible, the patient is lying on its right side and the jaw is pointed down.
  - When the maxilla is raised, the left or upper side of the mandible is tipped more ventrally than the right mandible, which, because of the sponge, is displaced dorsally.
  - Place the R marker near the tips of the right premolars and the L marker at the ramus of the left mandible.
- In these views, the markers do not indicate which side the patient is lying on, but rather the specific quadrant.[2]

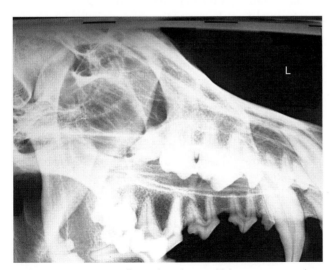

FIG. 21.15 Mystery radiograph. What would the correct terminology be for this view?

Fig. 21.15 is a mystery radiograph. Review it and answer the question presented with it.

✳ KEY POINTS

1. General anesthesia or sedation is required for accurate positioning for all skull views.
2. In order to achieve symmetry of the skull to minimize distortion and possibly misdiagnosis, the anatomical structures being examined must be parallel to the table/image receptor and perpendicular to the central ray:
   a. To help maintain symmetry for a lateral view, draw an imaginary line between the medial canthi. This line should be perpendicular to the table.
   b. To help maintain symmetry for a dorsoventral view, draw an imaginary line between the medial canthi. This imaginary line should be parallel to the table.
3. Collimate tightly to the area of interest, carefully placing the labels and markers.
4. Views imaged will depend on the suspected pathology.
5. In rostrocaudal projections, the angle of the central ray with the head varies because of breed variations. The patient will be in a VD position with the nose pointing to the x-ray beam with some angle variation.
6. When labeling oblique views, think of which part of the jaw is against the film and how the opposite side is positioned.

REVIEW QUESTIONS

1. A Rottweiler requires a lateral survey radiograph of the skull. You should measure at the highest point of the:
   a. Zygomatic arch just rostral to the lateral canthi of the eyes
   b. Zygomatic arch at the center of the cranium
   c. Cranium just caudal to the lateral canthi
   d. Occipital protuberance

2. In the lateral survey of the Rottweiler, peripheral borders are:
   a. From the tip of the nose to the occipital protuberance
   b. The rostral and caudal calvarium borders
   c. Cranial and caudal to the ears
   d. From the tip of the nose to the lateral canthi

3. You are also completing a survey dorsoventral radiograph of the Rottweiler. The central ray will be:
   a. Just rostral to the ears on the dorsal midline of the skull
   b. On the dorsal midline between the ears on the sagittal crest
   c. On the dorsal midline between the lateral canthi on the sagittal crest
   d. More rostral for this head type

4. In the survey dorsoventral radiograph of the Rottweiler, there will likely be:
   a. Even opacity of all of the tissues
   b. Overexposure of the cranium
   c. Overexposure of the nasal passages
   d. No overexposure of any part if the thickest part is toward the cathode

5. How can you determine whether there is likely to be symmetry on the final image of this dorsoventral skull of the Rottweiler?
   a. The nasal septum is parallel with the image receptor.
   b. An imaginary line drawn between the medial canthi should be perpendicular to the table.
   c. An imaginary line drawn between the medial canthi should be parallel to the table.
   d. The tongue will not obliterate any of the essential anatomy.

6. A Collie is to be imaged for frontal sinus view, and the veterinarian wishes a rostrocaudal position. This means that the patient is lying in:
   a. Ventral recumbency and the head is parallel to the table
   b. Ventral recumbency with the nose pointing to the x-ray tube and the mouth open
   c. Dorsal recumbency with the nose pointing to the x-ray tube and the mouth closed
   d. Dorsal recumbency with the nose pointing to the x-ray tube and the mouth open

7. The x-ray beam for the frontal view of the sinus in the Collie will be positioned:
   a. At the nasal cavity at the back of the palate
   b. At the lateral canthi of the eyes
   c. Rostral to the lateral canthi of the eyes
   d. Midway between the eyes so the cranium is centered

8. The veterinarian also requires a ventrodorsal open-mouth view of the nasal sinuses for the Collie. This is correctly referred to as:
   a. Rostroventral-caudodorsal oblique view
   b. Caudoventral-rostrodorsal oblique view
   c. 90-degree-rostrocaudal open-mouth view
   d. LeD-RtVO or RtD-LeVO depending on the side the patient is lying on

9. To position the VD open-mouth of the nasal sinuses of the Collie:
   a. The nose is parallel to the table and the beam directed 90 degrees inside the mouth
   b. The nose is pointed upward, with the hard palate angled in a caudal direction
   c. The mouth is opened wide and the x-ray tube tilted about 20 to 30 degrees in a rostrocaudal direction inside the mouth
   d. The mouth is opened wide and the x-ray tube tilted about 20 to 30 degrees to the table in a rostrocaudal direction on the mandible

10. The veterinarian would also like a foramen magnum view of the Collie. The patient is lying in dorsal recumbency and the nose is:
    a. Parallel to the table with the x-ray tube angled in a rostrocaudal direction
    b. Perpendicular to the table with the beam tilted 20 to 30 degrees
    c. Perpendicular to the table and the long axis of the body
    d. Pointed upward and pulled caudally 20 to 30 degrees

11. A complete evaluation of the tympanic bullae for a Boxer includes a lateral, DV/VD, and:
    a. Frontal 90-degree and two lateral oblique views
    b. Open-mouth rostrocaudal and two lateral oblique views
    c. Open- and closed-mouth rostrocaudal and two lateral oblique views
    d. Both dorsoventral oblique views

12. A LeD-RtVO radiograph is required for the tympanic bullae of the Boxer. This means that the patient is lying on its:
    a. Right side with the jaw pointing down
    b. Right side with the jaw pointing up
    c. Left side with the jaw pointing down
    d. Left side with the jaw pointing up

13. For this LeD-RtVO radiograph, the left marker should be placed:
    a. Dorsally with no right marker
    b. Dorsally alongside the right marker
    c. Ventrally and the right marker dorsally
    d. Ventrally with no right marker

14. The borders for the LeD-RtVO radiograph should include:
    a. The tip of the nose to the occipital-atlas junction
    b. Cranial and caudal to the ear
    c. The full cranium
    d. The occipital crest to the dorsal aspect of the nasal planum

15. The veterinarian requires a rostrocaudal view of a feline patient. Unlike in positioning for a normal canine skull, the mouth should be:
    a. Closed with the hard palate at 10° from the vertical
    b. Open with the hard palate at 10° from the vertical
    c. Closed and parallel to the table
    d. Closed and pulled caudally

Answers to Review Questions can be found on the Evolve website.

References

1. Holloway A. *BSAVA Manual of Canine and Feline Radiography And Radiology: A Foundation Manual.* Suffolk: BSAVA; 2013.
2. Thrall DE. *Textbook of Veterinary Diagnostic Radiology.* 6th ed. St. Louis: Elsevier; 2013.
3. Smallwood JE, Shively MJ, Rendano VT, et al. A standardized nomenclature for radiographic projections used in veterinary medicine. *Vet Radiol.* 1985;26:2-9.
4. Kus S, Morgan J. Radiography of the canine head: optimal positioning with respect to skull type. *Vet Radiol.* 1985;26:196-202.
5. Hammond Gawain J, Sullivan M, Weinrauch S, et al. A comparison of the rostrocaudal open mouth and rostro 10 degrees ventro-caudodorsal oblique radiographic views for imaging fluid in the feline tympanic bulla. *Vet Radiol Ultrasound.* 2005;46:205-209.
6. Morgan JP, Doval J, Samii V. *Radiographic Techniques: The Dog.* Schlutersche GmbH & Co. Hannover; 1998.
7. Han C, Hurd C. *Practical Diagnostic Imaging for the Veterinary Technician.* 3rd ed. St. Louis: Mosby; 2005.

Bibliography

Aspinall V, Cappello M. *Introduction to Veterinary Anatomy.* London: Butterworth-Heinemann; 2009.

Ayers S. *Small Animal Radiographic Techniques and Positioning.* Oxford: Wiley-Blackwell; 2013.

Colville T, Bassert J. *Clinical Anatomy and Physiology for Veterinary Technicians.* 3rd ed. St. Louis: Mosby; 2016.

Done SH, Goody PC, Stickland NC, et al. *Color Atlas of veterinary Anatomy, the Dog and Cat.* London: Mosby; 2009.

Douglas SW. *Principles of Veterinary Radiography.* London: Bailliere Tindall; 1980.

Dyce KM, Sack WO, Wensing CJG. *Textbook of Veterinary Anatomy.* 4th ed. St. Louis: Saunders; 2010.

Evans H, de Lahunta A. *Guide to the Dissection of the Dog.* 8th ed. St. Louis: Saunders; 2017.

Fauber TL. *Radiographic Imaging and Exposure.* 5th ed. St. Louis: Elsevier; 2017.

Muhlbauer MC, Kneller SK. *Radiography of the Dog and Cat: Guide to Making and Interpreting Radiographs.* Oxford: Wiley-Blackwell; 2013.

Owens JM. *Radiographic Interpretation for the Small Animal Clinician.* St. Louis: Ralston Purina; 1999.

Romich J. *An Illustrated Guide to Veterinary Medical Terminology.* Stamford, CT: Delmar Cengage Learning; 2015.

Ryan G. *Radiographic Positioning of Small Animals.* Philadelphia: Lea & Febiger; 1981.

Sirois M. *Principles and Practice of Veterinary Technology.* 3rd ed. St. Louis: Mosby; 2011.

Sirois M, Anthony E, Mauragis D. *Handbook of Radiographic Positioning for Veterinary Technicians.* Clifton Park, NY: Delmar Cengage Learning; 2010.

Smallwood JE, Shively MJ, Rendano VT, et al. A standardized nomenclature for radiographic projections used in veterinary medicine. *Vet Radiol.* 1985;26:2-9.

Thrall DE. *Textbook of Veterinary Diagnostic Radiology.* 6th ed. St. Louis: Elsevier; 2013.

Ticer J. *Radiographic Technique in Small Animal Practice.* Philadelphia: WB Saunders; 1984.

Tighe M, Brown M. *Mosby's Comprehensive Review for Veterinary Technicians.* 4th ed. St. Louis: Elsevier; 2015.

Wilson M, Mauragis D, Berry C, et al. Small Animal Skull & Nasofacial Radiography Including the Nasal Cavity & Frontal Sinuses. *Todays Vet Pract.* 2014;4(2):47-51.

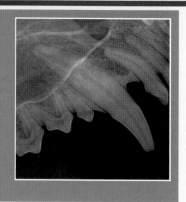

CHAPTER 22
Dental Radiography

Susan MacNeal, RVT, CVDT, BSc

A man begins cutting his wisdom teeth the first time he bites off more than he can chew.

—Herb Caen, San Francisco columnist, 1916–1997

OUTLINE

LEARNING OBJECTIVES

When you have finished this chapter, you will be able to:

1. Describe the dental x-ray unit and discuss its unique qualities.
2. Process dental x-ray film.
3. Understand dental radiography using film or digital systems, discussing the merits of each system.
4. Accurately identify dental anatomy, terminology, nomenclature, and formulas.
5. Produce diagnostic high-quality extraoral and intraoral dental radiographs of the dog and cat by properly measuring, centering, collimating, and positioning using either the parallel or bisecting angle.
6. Correctly view dental films.
7. Identify further concerns and idiosyncrasies, including the variations between dogs and cats.

KEY TERMS

Key terms are defined in the Glossary on the Evolve website.

Alveolar bone	Coronal surface	Incisal	Palatal surface
Apical	Cusp	Intraoral	Parallel technique
Arch	Direct digital radiography	Ipsilateral	Periapical
Bisecting angle	Distal	Labial	Position indicating device
Buccal	Distolateral oblique	Lamina dura	Processing chemicals
Carnassial tooth	Dorsal	Lateral (side)	Radicular groove
Caudal	Elongation	Lingual	Rostral
Cementoenamel junction	Enamel bulge	Malocclusion	Rostrocaudal oblique
(CEJ)	Extraoral	Mental foramina	Scissor arm
Chairside darkroom	Extension arm	Mesial	SLOB rule
Computed radiography	Facial	Mesiobuccal	Stationary anode
Concave	Foreshortening	Mesiolateral oblique	Source-image distance (SID)
Contralateral	Frenulum	Mesiolingual	Ventral
Convex	Furcation	Occlusion	

TECHNICAL NOTE: To preserve space, the radiographs presented in this chapter do not show collimation. For safety, always collimate so that the beam is limited to within the image receptor edges. In film radiography, you should see a clear border of collimation (frame) on every radiograph. In some jurisdictions, evidence of collimation is required by law.

Dental radiography has become a significant diagnostic tool in the veterinary clinic. Once the basic anatomy, terminology, and positioning principles are understood, dental radiographs are readily completed.

For true diagnostic radiographs of the canine and feline mouth, a dental x-ray machine should be used. The articulating arm on a dental x-ray machine enables one to obtain quality radiographs quickly and easily with minimal maneuvering of the patient. If there is no access to a dental x-ray unit, extraoral and intraoral radiographs can still be taken with a regular x-ray machine though the resulting images will not be as easily obtained or detailed depending on the position.

The Dental X-Ray Unit

Dental x-ray units used in veterinary practices are designed based on the similar technology used in human dental x-ray units. Many veterinary practices use refurbished human dental x-ray units, but a separate technique chart needs to be designed. To determine the settings in newer veterinary dental x-ray units, you simply press the selection button that applies to the tooth you are going to radiograph (Fig. 22.1).

Dental x-ray units all consist of the same parts: generator, extension arm, scissor arm, and the x-ray tube, which has the collimator cone (Fig. 22.2). The generator is a small box that is located on the wall of the dental operatory room and requires a standard 110-volt power outlet without any special wiring. Most dental x-ray units are preset with a kV of 70 or 80 and a mA of either 7 or 8, so the only variable is seconds. Some of the newer dental x-ray units are DC (direct current) units and have the ability to vary the kV.

The extension arm extends from the generator. It swings 180 degrees and is available in variable lengths. At the end of the extension arm is the scissor arm. The scissor arm and extension arm allow the dental x-ray machine to maneuver about the patient to allow ease of positioning.

The x-ray tube is a stationary anode tube (see Chapter 2) that is encased in the housing at the end of the scissor arm and will rotate around that stem. Because it is a stationary anode there is no rotor noise. The collimator cone or positioning indicator device (PID) is a projection from the tube housing. Cones are not interchangeable and are available in variable lengths and diameters depending on the manufacturer (Fig. 22.3). Most presets on the unit are based on a distance of 2 inches or 5(cm) from the tooth. Any variation does require a change in settings as based on the inverse square law stated in Chapter 5. There is no collimator light, thus the operator

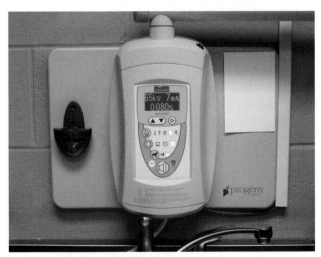

FIG. 22.1 Dental x-ray control panel.

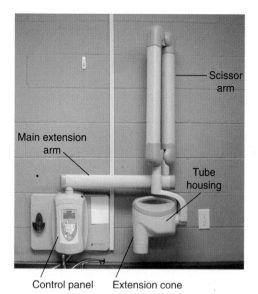

FIG. 22.2 A dental x-ray machine.

Labels: Scissor arm; Main extension arm; Tube housing; Control panel; Extension cone

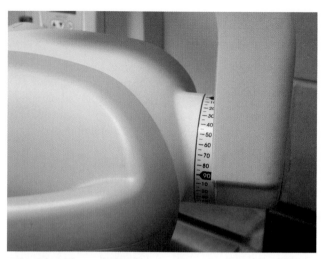

FIG. 22.4 The angle meter on the side of the dental x-ray tube. The angle meter is used for imaging canine teeth when the beam direction needs to be adjusted.

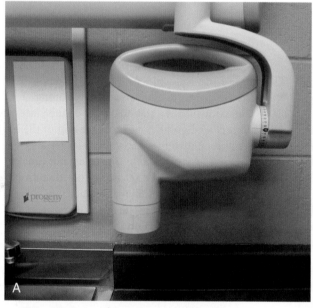

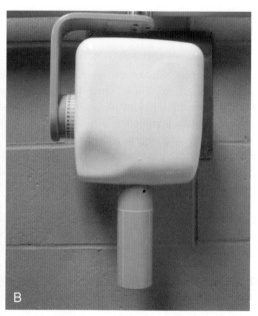

FIG. 22.3 A and B, Two examples of collimator cones on dental x-ray machines. The length of the cones, as well as the diameter of the cone, varies between machines.

must view the cone from different perspectives to best estimate the center of the beam.

On one side of the x-ray tube is an angle meter (Fig. 22.4). The angle meter is useful for setting up some dental x-ray views, depending on what technique is used. The angle meter is especially helpful for imaging canine teeth, as a "tilt" in the cone is required to prevent superimposition on the premolars distal to it.

Dental X-Ray Imaging

Three imaging choices are available. One is nonscreen dental film and the other two are digital systems. The digital systems are divided into computed radiography (CR), available as photostimulable plates (PSP), and direct digital receptors (DDR or DR).

Film

Due to the fact there are no intensifying screens, the kV required for imaging teeth is generally much higher than imaging a cat abdomen with a cassette-screen system.

Dental film is available in different speeds and brands. The common speed of film used in veterinary practice is D-speed (Fig. 22.5). An F-speed film is also available, under the brand name Insight, which is a faster-speed film allowing for a decreased radiation dose. It is not practical to switch between film speeds once the technique chart has been established. Film is available in four sizes (Table 22.1). The most common

TABLE 22.1	Dental X-Ray Film Sizes
FILM SIZE	**FILM DIMENSIONS**
0	1⅜ × ⅞ 35 mm × 22 mm
1	1⁹⁄₁₆ in × 1⁵⁄₁₆ in 40 mm × 24 mm
2	1⅝ in × 1¼ in 40.5 mm × 30.5 mm
4	3 in × 2¼ in 57 mm × 76 mm

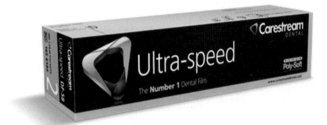

FIG. 22.5 Dental film, D-speed. This is the most common speed of film used in veterinary practice.

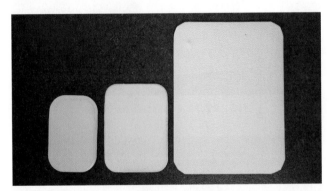

FIG. 22.6 Size 0, 2, and 4 dental x-ray film. These are the most common sizes used for imaging dog and cat teeth.

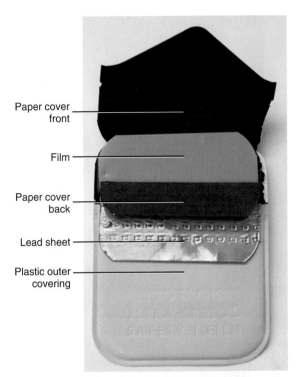

FIG. 22.7 An opened dental film packet.

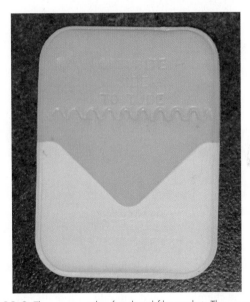

FIG. 22.8 The reverse side of a dental film packet. The reverse side should face away from the x-ray tube. It is a different color and has a tab used to open the film packet during processing.

sizes used are 2 and 4, as well as the 0 for small dogs and cats (Fig. 22.6).

The film packet has several layers (Fig. 22.7). The film is wrapped in a paper layer with a thin lead foil layer at the back of the packet, all enclosed in a plastic outer covering. The back of the film packet is clearly identified with a green or purple color, as well as a small tab for opening the packet (Fig. 22.8). The purpose of the lead layer in the film packet is to prevent x-rays from continuing through the packet, causing extra radiation exposure to the patient (Fig. 22.9). In many municipalities the lead is considered a hazardous substance and must be disposed of through an environmental control company or a lead recycling program.

On the front of the film packet is a convex dot with the same raised dot on the film inside the packet (Fig. 22.10). On the opposite side of the film the dot is concave. The purpose of the "dot" is to help determine left or right once the film is developed, as dental films are too small to put a left/right marker on them. The film is always positioned with the convex dot facing the tube and at the front of the mouth. If the dot is consistently kept toward the front of the mouth, it is easy to determine left or right based on the orientation of the teeth.

Film Processing

The x-ray film can be processed through a dental automatic processor or processed manually. In human dental offices that still use dental film, a dental automatic processor is

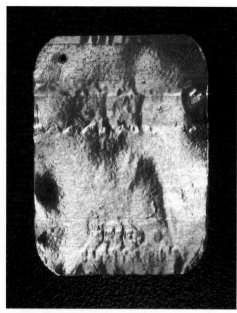

FIG. 22.9 The thin lead sheet enclosed in the dental film packet. The lead sheet should be disposed of with an environmental control company.

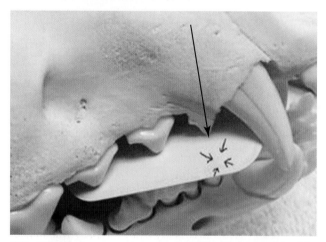

FIG. 22.10 The convex dot on the dental film. The convex side of the film should face the tube head, and the dot should be placed rostrally.

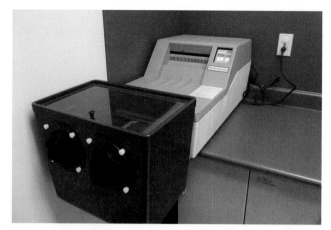

FIG. 22.11 An automatic dental film processor.

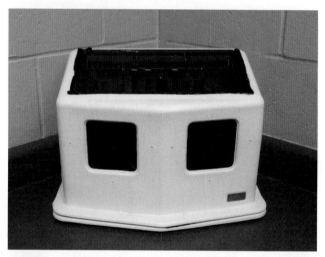

FIG. 22.12 A chairside darkroom.

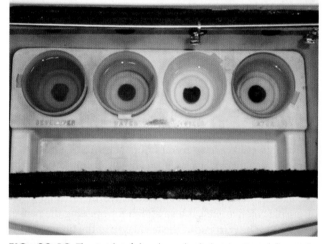

FIG. 22.13 The inside of the chairside darkroom. From left to right: developer, water, fixer, water.

common due to the high volume of films produced (Fig. 22.11). Although highly efficient, they can be costly if not used often. The chemicals would naturally evaporate and exhaust before the cost of the chemicals could be recovered.

Manual Processing

Manual processing is the most common way to process films in a veterinary hospital. This can be accomplished by using a chairside darkroom (Fig. 22.12) or by setting up four small jars with sealed lids in the regular darkroom. The chairside darkroom allows the operator to process the films in close proximity to where they are being exposed. The chairside darkroom has a red translucent cover and light-tight arm holes. Inside the chairside darkroom are four jars containing (left to right) developer, water (stop bath), fixer, and water (Fig. 22.13). The solutions should be at room temperature (70-76 °F [21-24 °C]).

Once the film is exposed, the technician takes the film to the chairside darkroom and inserts both hands into the light-tight sleeves, holding the film packet in one hand. The packet is opened and a film clip is attached to the film. The film clip allows the operator to move the film through the chemicals safely while keeping his or her hands out of the liquids

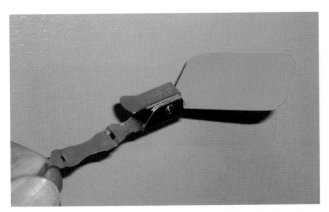

FIG. 22.14 A film clip attached to a dental film. The film clip is attached in the chairside darkroom to move the film through the processing chemicals.

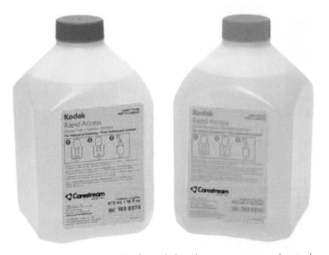

FIG. 22.15 An example of rapid dental x-ray processing chemicals.

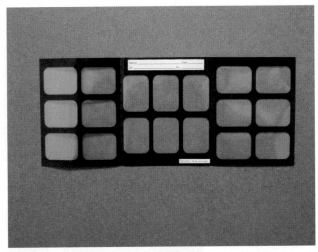

FIG. 22.16 A dental film mount. Dental radiographs are arranged as if you are looking at the animal.

(Fig. 22.14). The red translucent cover allows the technician to view the process without light fogging the film.

The times for processing vary with the brand of chemicals used, and it is best to consult the manufacturer's instructions. Kodak Rapid Access Dental Developer and Fixer by Carestream (Fig. 22.15) is an example of rapid dental processing solutions that are available. The instructions for these solutions state that their system is compatible with both Ultra-speed and Insight dental films. Ready-to-read radiographs are available by immersing for 15 seconds in developer, rinsing in water, then immersing for 15 seconds in fixer followed by a thorough rinse in water. If the films appear to have a yellow discoloration after drying, this indicates they were not thoroughly rinsed. If the radiographs are to be kept as part of the patient's record, they should be developed, put in the stop bath for 15 seconds (agitating constantly), then fixed for 2 to 4 minutes, and then washed in running water for 10 minutes.

Ideally the solutions should be used for the dental session and then disposed of. Watch for signs of chemical deterioration.

Labeling, Mounting, and Storing the Images

Each clinic should develop their own system for storing dental radiographs. Some veterinary governing bodies require the films to be permanently labeled. This can be accomplished by writing on the film with a fine-point permanent marker or using a film mount (Fig. 22.16), which is also considered acceptable. The film mount allows the films to be organized in a prearranged layout and filed for future reference. Digital systems also have templates built into the software to mount the digital radiographs.

A full-mouth set of dental radiographs should always be mounted as if you were looking directly at the animal's mouth. The animal's right side of the mouth should be on your left when viewing the full set of radiographs (Fig. 22.17).

Dental radiographs can be attached in an envelope to the dental chart, or if in a paperless clinic, a separate filing system can be used. The radiographs are part of the patient's medical record and must be saved for future reference.

Digital Dental Radiography

The advantage of any digital dental imaging system is the ease with which images can be processed, manipulated, and stored. Dental radiography is generally said to have a "steep learning curve," and if films need to be manually processed, it can become a very time-intensive procedure. Digital systems also allow the image to be easily manipulated with annotation tools (Fig. 22.18). For example, magnification, windowing and leveling for optimizing the image, labeling of the exact tooth, and emailing the image with the press of a button are all advantages of digital systems. The dental x-rays can easily be attached to the patient's file and incorporated into a discharge summary.

Computed Radiography

The computed radiography (CR) dental processor (Fig. 22.19) is similar in design to the standard CR unit used in whole-body radiographs described in Chapter 8.

Photostimulable Phosphor (PSP) plates are used as the image receptor. They are thin and flexible and are available in sizes 0, 1, 2, 3, and 4 (Fig. 22.20). Each plate has a small

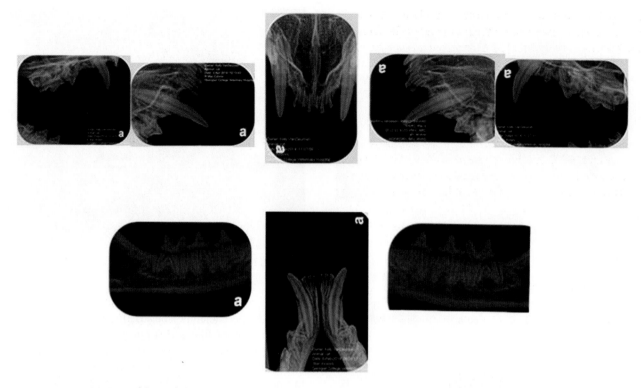

FIG. 22.17 A full set of dental x-ray films on a cat. The maxillary views are on the top and the mandibular views on the bottom. The cat's right is on your left and vice versa.

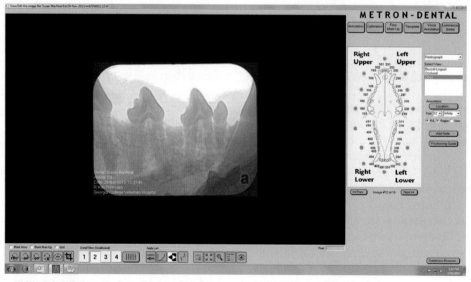

FIG. 22.18 Annotation tools on a digital x-ray system. The colors in this image have been inverted.

"a," which replaces the "dot" used in regular dental film. The PSP plates are light sensitive and must be protected from light. They are sealed in a barrier envelope for patient use (Fig. 22.21). The active side of the plate is light blue with the rear side of the plate containing the writing; it is easily viewed through the window of the barrier envelope. Once exposed the PSP plate is removed from the barrier envelope and put through the scanner, which converts it into an image viewed on the computer. As the plate is scanned, the plate is erased and is ready to use again once the scanning is complete.

Direct Digital Imaging

The image receptor for DR is a size 2 sensor (Fig. 22.22). Smaller sensors are available, but are not practical for veterinary use. The sensor is attached directly to the computer's universal serial bus (USB) port. Once the sensor is exposed, the software program immediately converts the information into an image. The sensor should be protected from fluids by using a barrier sleeve. A thin layer of plain Vetrap around the sensor, once covered with the plastic sleeve, enables the sensor to stay in place without slipping. DR sensors can be permanently damaged if dropped and are costly to replace. DR sensors have an inactive area around the perimeter of the sensor. A size 2 sensor is typically 30 by 43 mm, but has an active area of 26 by 36 mm (Fig. 22.23). Table 22.2 lists the advantages and disadvantages of the different types of image receptors.

Dental Exposures

For most dental x-ray machines, the choice of settings is simple because most of the machines have presets based on the tooth to be x-rayed. The majority of dental x-ray machines have a preset mA and kV, so the only variable is seconds, although newer machines also have variable kV. If using an older machine or a refurbished human dental x-ray machine, you will need to create your own technique chart. Table 22.3 is a suggested chart for imaging teeth.

Radiography Log

It is essential that all dental x-ray exposures are recorded in a log designated for your dental x-ray machine. If the

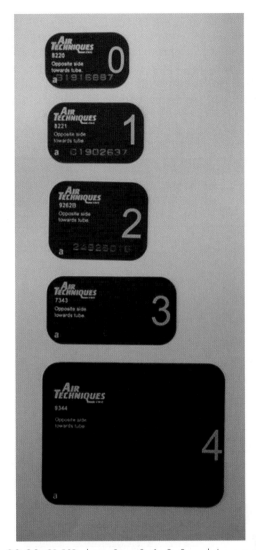

FIG. 22.20 CR PSP plates. Sizes 0, 1, 2, 3, and 4 are available. Shown here is the reverse side of the plate. Note the "a" acts as the dot in regular film and should be placed rostrally.

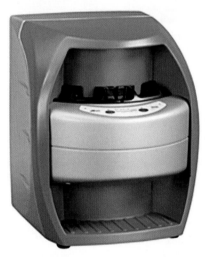

FIG. 22.19 An example of a computed radiography (CR) digital dental x-ray unit.

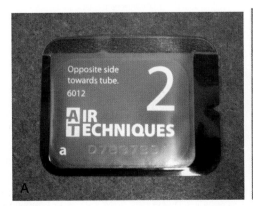
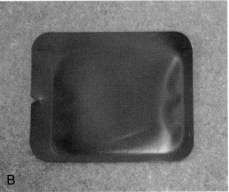

FIG. 22.21 CR plates are light sensitive and need to be protected from light and moisture. **A,** A size 2 plate enclosed in a barrier envelope showing the reverse side of the plate. **B,** This is the side of the CR plate that needs to face the x-ray tube.

dental x-ray machine has a preset mA and kV, you will need a column to record only seconds for each exposure as long as there is a statement at the beginning of the log stating the presets. The log requires an entry for each exposure, including patient, client, date, area imaged, and settings as discussed. This is a legal requirement from the radiation protection agency.

> **✎ TECHNICIAN NOTES**
>
> In this chapter the term *film* is used with the understanding that in digital radiography, the digital sensor or PSP plate is substituted for the film.

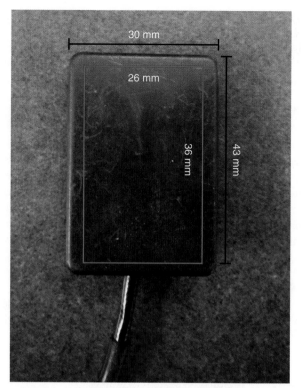

FIG. 22.23 A DR sensor. The active portion of the sensor is smaller than the dimensions of the sensor. The active portion of the sensor is outlined in red.

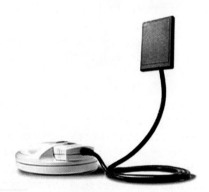

FIG. 22.22 An example of a direct digital radiography (DR) sensor. The sizes of the sensor are only available as size 1 or 2 (most common).

TABLE 22.2	A Comparison of Dental Image Receptors' Advantages and Disadvantages	
DENTAL RECEPTOR	**ADVANTAGES**	**DISADVANTAGES**
Film	Inexpensive for initial setup in comparison to digital systems Easy to use and store Different film sizes available: size 0, 1, 2, and 4 Switching between sizes is easily done Exceptionally high resolution	Time consuming—film must be manually processed Individual storage means that films can be lost or damaged Processing adds time and ongoing cost Must be viewed on a viewing box Radiation amounts may be higher as compared to digital systems (varies among dental x-ray machines)
Computed radiography (CR)	Different receptor sizes available: size 0, 1, 2, 3, and 4 PSP plates are thin and flexible, similar to regular film Scanning time is approximately 30 seconds Plates can be imaged hundreds of time and are inexpensive to replace	More expensive than DR systems Ongoing costs for barrier envelopes Intermediate step for processing takes time Plates can be damaged (scratched or bent) if used carelessly "Plate" is removed for processing, so it cannot be repositioned according to its previous position
Direct digital radiography	Less expensive than CR systems Sensor remains in position while radiograph is reviewed so adjustments are simplified if positioning is incorrect No intermediate step—image is displayed within seconds of the exposure	Size of the sensor is limited to #1 or #2, which necessitates multiple exposures for full-mouth radiographs The sensor is thick and inflexible, making sensor placement difficult for trickier areas; alternative techniques must be used Larger teeth must be imaged with two exposures after repositioning of sensor The sensor may be damaged by rough handling and is very expensive to replace Inactive area on sensor makes sensor smaller than it appears

TABLE 22.3	Suggested Exposure of Dental Equipment Supplied Without a Technique Chart	
	EXPOSURE(S) BASED ON 70-kV, 8-mA DENTAL X-RAY MACHINE REDUCE EXPOSURE BY 40% FOR DIGITAL	
	DOG (S)	DOG (M)
Maxillary PM/M	0.33	0.40
Maxillary canine tooth	0.41	0.50
Maxillary incisor	0.20	0.23
Mandibular PM/M	0.27	0.30
Mandibular canine tooth	0.33	0.40
Mandibular incisor	0.18	0.20
	CAT	
Maxillary teeth	0.30	
Mandibular teeth	0.20	

PM/M, premolar/molar.

Indications

In veterinary medicine it is essential to have dental radiographs as part of a comprehensive oral health examination. The visual inspection and tactile examination (probing) of the tooth is only a small part of the information required to make informed treatment decisions. Dental radiography is an essential component of a proper diagnosis, treatment planning, and monitoring.

Oral disease is common in dogs and cats. A particular challenge with these patients is their inability to communicate pain and discomfort until oral disease is well advanced. Even then, isolating the exact origin and extent of the disease is difficult. Dental radiographs enable us to thoroughly evaluate the entire tooth and surrounding tissues, including bone.

Full-mouth radiographs should be taken as part of a complete oral examination. Specific indications for radiographs include, but are not limited to, periodontal disease, missing teeth, resorptive lesions, oral tumors and gingival inflammation, malformed teeth, discolored teeth, dental extractions, and dental trauma.

Positional Terminology

Some of the terms you should be familiar with are those associated with the direction of the beam and the intraoral terminology (Fig. 22.24).

Tooth Anatomy and Dental Formula

Tooth Anatomy

In Fig. 22.25, the crown is above the gums (supragingival) and the root below the gums (subgingival). The apex is the tip of the root. At the tip of the root there are small openings

to allow the blood supply and nerves to enter the tooth; these openings are referred to as the *apical delta.*

On a radiograph, the pulp chamber is the darker inner content of the tooth extending throughout the crown and the root. The root portion of the pulp chamber is generally referred to as the *root canal.*

The dentin constitutes the bulk of the tooth and appears lighter than the pulp chamber on a radiograph. As a patient ages, secondary dentin is continuously produced. Over time, the pulp chamber decreases in size because of the secondary dentin. Fig. 22.26 illustrates how the size of the pulp chamber evident on a radiograph of the lower first molar can help with aging of an animal.

The enamel is the outer covering of the crown, and the cementum is the outer covering of the root. The area where they meet is termed *the cementoenamel junction (CEJ).* The enamel and cementum are difficult to distinguish from the dentin.

The periodontal ligament forms the attachment of the cementum to the alveolar bone. It appears as a thin gray line surrounding the roots.

The lamina dura is the wall of the alveolar socket that surrounds the tooth. It appears as a dense white line adjacent to the periodontal ligament space.

The four basic tooth types in dogs and cats are as follows:
1. Incisors (I or i) are used for grooming as well as grasping and cutting food. All incisor teeth are single rooted.
2. Canine teeth (C or c) are single-rooted teeth that are used for grasping and holding prey. The structure of feline canine teeth supports that cats are true carnivores. There are shallow longitudinal groves on the buccal surfaces of the canine teeth. These grooves "wick" away blood from held prey.
3. Premolar teeth (P or p) are designed for cutting and shearing meat. Premolar teeth have prominent sharp cusps and have one to three roots.
4. Molar teeth (M or m) generally have flattened occlusal surfaces with the exception of the mandibular first molar tooth in dogs, which does have a cutting edge on the mesial cusp. The first mandibular molar tooth in cats has no flattened occlusal table; instead it has two cutting edges. Molar teeth have two or three roots, but some roots appear to be fused together to give the appearance of being single rooted (feline maxillary first molar). Molar teeth in dogs are used for grinding food.

Dental Formula

The *dental formula* illustrates how many of each tooth type are present in half of a dog and cat's mouth. The short form for the type of tooth is followed by the number of that particular type. The formula is presented in a "fraction," with maxillary teeth shown above the teeth in the mandible, using the following conventions:

Tooth type: Refer to description given in former discussion of tooth anatomy
Permanent: Uppercase (I, C, P, M)
Deciduous: Lowercase (i, c, p, m)

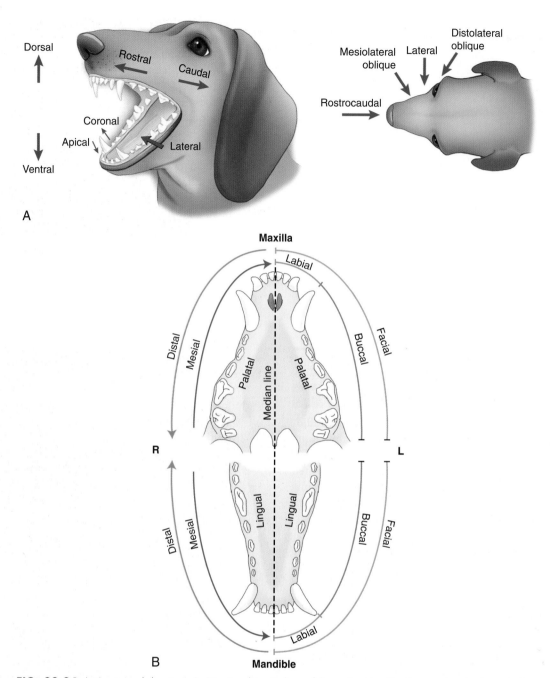

FIG. 22.24 A, Anatomical directions. **B,** Directional terminology of the oral cavity. Directions and terminology apply to both sides of the mouth.

Canine Dental Formula

Fig. 22.27 illustrates the canine dental formula, which is as follows:

$$\text{Deciduous teeth}: 2 \times \left(\frac{\text{i3c1p3m0}}{\text{i3c1p3m0}} \right) = 28 \text{ in total}$$

A shortened version to remember is 313/313.

$$\text{Permanent teeth}: 2 \times \left(\frac{\text{I3C1P4M2}}{\text{I3C1P4M3}} \right) = 42 \text{ in total}$$

A shortened version to remember is 3142/3143.

Feline Dental Formula

Fig. 22.28 illustrates the feline dental formula, which is as follows:

$$\text{Deciduous teeth}: 2 \times \left(\frac{\text{i3c1p3m0}}{\text{i3c1p2m0}} \right) = 24 \text{ in total}$$

A shortened version to remember is 313/312.

$$\text{Permanent teeth}: 2 \times \left(\frac{\text{I3C1P3M1}}{\text{I3C1P2M1}} \right) = 30 \text{ in total}$$

A shortened version to remember is 3131/3121.

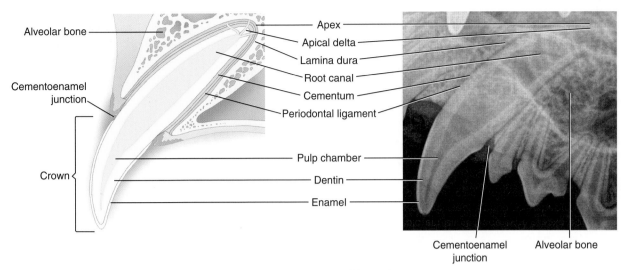

FIG. 22.25 Anatomy of the tooth.

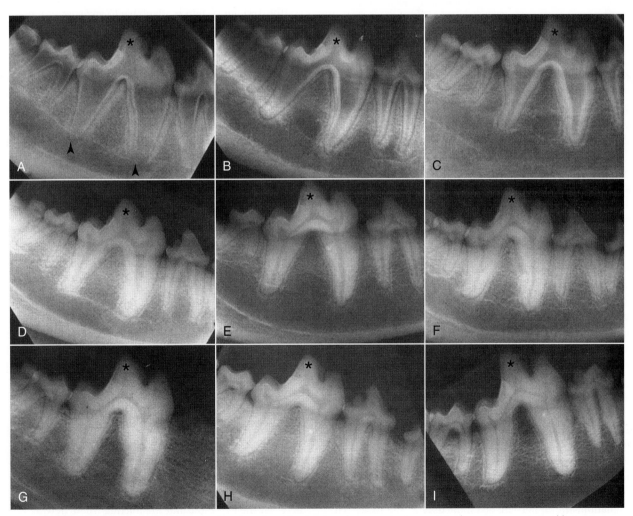

FIG. 22.26 A to I, Radiographs show how the pulp chamber decreases in size as animals age (youngest, A; oldest, I). A, 6 months, open apex (*arrowheads*); B, 9 months, apical closure; C, 16 months; D, 2 years; E, 3 years; F, 4 years; G, 6 years; H, 8 years; I, 12 years. (From Tutt C, Deeprose J, and Crossley DA. *BSAVA Manual of Canine and Feline Dentistry*, 3rd ed. Gloucester, UK: British Small Animal Veterinary Association; 2007.)

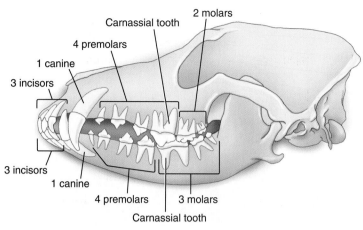

FIG. 22.27 Canine dental formula.

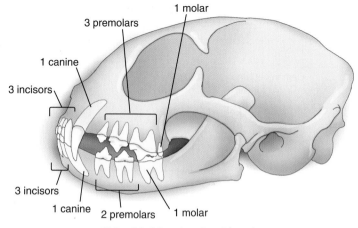

FIG. 22.28 Feline dental formula.

> ✎ **TECHNICIAN NOTES**
>
> There are no deciduous precursors for the first premolar of the adult dog. Cat and dog molar teeth never have deciduous precursors.

Nomenclature

Two types of numbering systems are used in veterinary medicine for identifying teeth. The anatomical system is an older system but is still used in veterinary clinics. The modified Triadan system is the current numbering system of choice. It is easily integrated into paperless records, and it is much faster to use than the anatomical system once it has been learned. Fig. 22.29 illustrates the anatomical orientation and structure of the teeth with each system illustrated.

Anatomical System for Notation

The anatomical system uses a combination of short forms for tooth type (I, C, P, M for permanent teeth or i, c, p, m for deciduous teeth) and the numbers of those teeth in their group (i.e., premolars 1-4) to designate a specific tooth. The number of the tooth is placed on the left for a left-sided tooth and the right for a right-sided tooth; the number is superscript for a maxillary tooth and subscript for a mandibular tooth. For example, I^2 designates the right maxillary second incisor (intermediate incisor).

Modified Triadan System

The modified Triadan system labels each tooth with a code of three numbers, starting at the midpoint of the arch in each quadrant. The first number designates the quadrant. The upper-right quadrant uses the number 1 as the quadrant designation, the upper-left quadrant uses 2, the lower-left quadrant uses 3, and the lower-right quadrant uses 4. Deciduous teeth use the series 5 through 8 for the quadrants.

The second two numbers are determined by the tooth position, counting back from the midline of the arch in each quadrant. Incisors are numbered 01, 02, and 03; the canine

tooth is 04; premolars are 05, 06, 07, and 08; and the molars are 09, 10, and 11. So, for example, the Triadan number for ^3I is 203.

The Triadan system is adaptable to any species regardless of how many teeth are normally present for that species. However, in order to assign the Triadan numbers to species that are normally missing teeth in the dental formula, you need to know the anatomical number designations, especially for the premolars. Because the cat is missing the upper first premolar, there is no 105 or 205 tooth in a cat. Likewise, for the mandibular premolars, because the cat is missing the first and second premolars, the numbers 305, 306, 405, and 406 are not used.

> ✎ **TECHNICIAN NOTES**
>
> The canine tooth always ends in a 04, and the first molar always ends in a 09. From there you can count forward or backward in the dental arch as needed.

Roots of the Various Teeth

It is very important to appreciate the structure and number of tooth roots (Fig. 22.30). The appreciation of this anatomy is vital to determine tooth angle and to decide when to change the direction of the x-ray beam to isolate the roots. It is also important in the interpretation of radiographs to recognize extra or malformed roots.

Normal Radiographic Anatomy in Dogs and Cats

The following radiographs illustrate normal findings of the areas listed here. It is important to be able to distinguish between the mandible and the maxilla when viewing radiographs. It is also important to become familiar with the orientation of the teeth and the anatomical differences in root and crown structure. The more familiar you are with these areas, the easier it will be to distinguish between teeth on a radiograph.

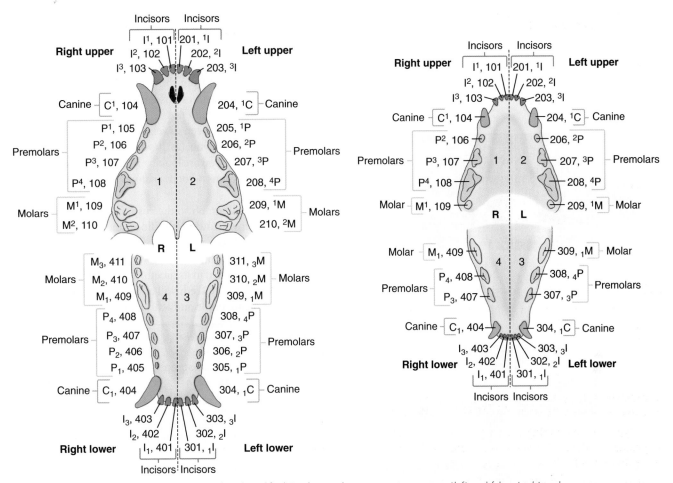

FIG. 22.29 Anatomical and modified Triadan numbering systems in canine (*left*) and feline (*right*) teeth.

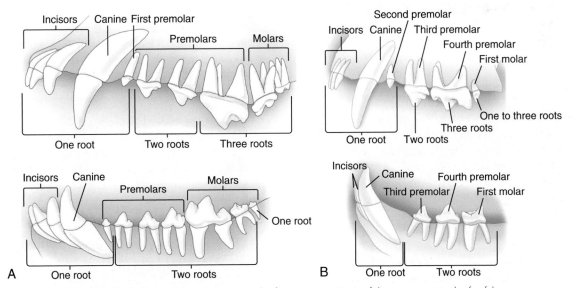

FIG. 22.30 A, Roots of the permanent teeth of a canine. **B,** Roots of the permanent teeth of a feline.

1. Normal adult maxillary incisors: Look for white space distal to incisors, with two oval (dark) spaces, which are the palatine fissures (Fig. 22.31).
2. Normal adult mandibular incisors: Look for a dark black line distal to incisors that separates mandibular rami (mandibular symphysis) (Fig. 22.32).
3. Normal adult maxillary premolars and molars: Look for the fine white line representing the maxillary recess apical to the roots (Fig. 22.33).
4. Normal adult mandibular premolars and molars: Look for dark black areas above and below the mandible (Fig. 22.34).

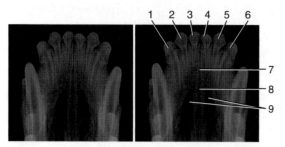

FIG. 22.31 Normal radiographic anatomy of the canine adult maxillary incisors. *1*, 203; *2*, 202; *3*, 201; *4*, 101; *5*, 102; *6*, 103; *7*, incisive canal; *8*, interincisive suture; *9*, palatine fissure.

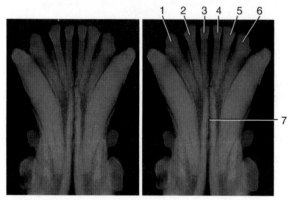

FIG. 22.32 Normal radiograph anatomy of the canine adult mandibular incisors. *1*, 403; *2*, 402; *3*, 401; *4*, 301; *5*, 302; *6*, 303; *7*, mandibular symphysis.

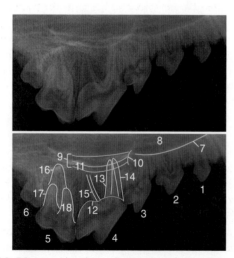

FIG. 22.33 Normal radiograph anatomy of the canine maxillary premolars and molars. *1*, 105; *2*, 106; *3*, 107; *4*, 108; *5*, 109; *6*, 110; *7*, nasal surface of the alveolar process of maxilla; *8*, nasal cavity; *9*, infraorbital canal; *10*, infraorbital foramen; *11*, palatine canal; *12*, palatal marginal enamel; *13*, mesiopalatal root; *14*, mesiobuccal root; *15*, radicular groove on distal root; *16*, palatal root; *17*, distobuccal root; *18*, mesiobuccal root.

Viewing Dental Radiographs

Film is always exposed with the convex dot at the rostral end of the mouth; therefore views on the right side have the dot in a different location from those on the left side. Fig. 22.35 demonstrates with digital films how the locations of the dot ("a" on digital plates) differ.

Once the film has been developed, hold it so the convex dot is raised toward you (as it was placed in the mouth). Determine whether you are looking at a maxilla or a mandible (see earlier discussions of tooth anatomy and normal anatomy radiographs).

Orient the radiograph so the cusps of the maxillary teeth are pointing down toward the floor and the cusps of the mandibular teeth are pointing up toward the ceiling (Fig. 22.36). Look at the film as if you were looking at the animal with the film positioned in its mouth. The anatomical structures and orientation of the teeth will allow you to determine if it is a maxilla or mandible and left or right (Fig. 22.37).

⟳ FIGURE IT OUT

Several films were imaged on a canine patient. When viewing one of the radiographs, the vet was unsure as to which teeth he was viewing. The technician says: "If the dot was placed toward the front of the mouth, then it makes sense for this to be a right maxillary premolar." Upon further explanation she says: "We are viewing it with the convex side of the dot facing us as it was placed in the mouth. The smaller teeth are at the rostral end of the mouth, which is where we placed the '"dot,"' and this radiograph agrees with our film placement, so this must be a right maxillary premolar."

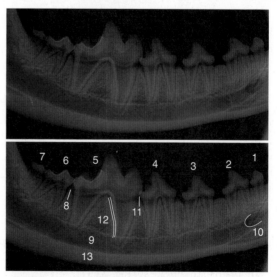

FIG. 22.34 Normal radiograph anatomy of the canine mandibular premolars and molars. *1*, 405; *2*, 406; *3*, 407; *4*, 408; *5*, 409; *6*, 410; *7*, 411; *8*, alveolar margin; *9*, mandibular canal; *10*, middle mental foramen; *11*, overlap of enamel; *12*, radicular groove; *13*, ventral mandibular cortex.

Right maxilla   Left maxilla

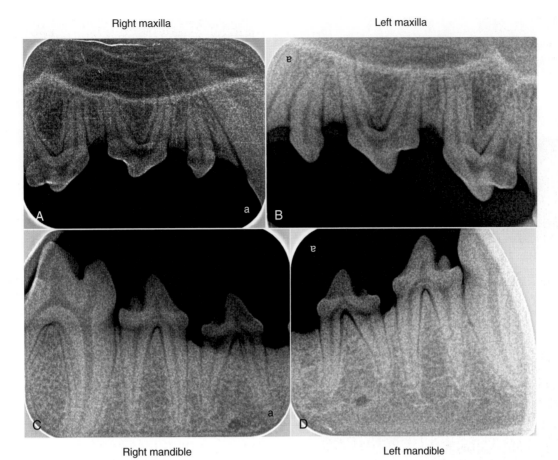

Right mandible   Left mandible

FIG. 22.35 A to D, Digital films showing how placement of dot (a) differs.

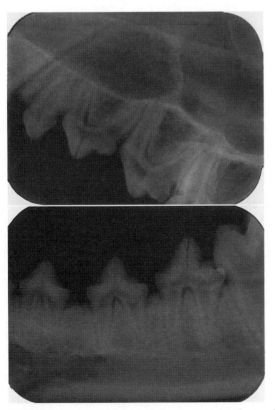

FIG. 22.36 Proper viewing of a radiograph. Note that the maxillary cusps are pointing down and the mandibular cusps are pointing up.

Projection Geometry

Parallel Technique

The parallel technique involves placing the dental film directly behind and parallel to the tooth and then directing the x-ray beam perpendicular to the film (Fig. 22.38A). The anatomy of dog and cat mouths allows the parallel technique to be used in only one area. This area encompasses the teeth distal to and including the mandibular third premolars ($_3P_3$ or 307/407).

Bisecting Angle Technique

Because of the anatomical structure of the mouths of dogs and cats, film cannot be placed directly behind most teeth. The bisecting angle technique is used to image these teeth. This technique is used on all maxillary teeth, all incisors and canines, and mandibular premolars 1 and 2.

The bisecting angle is formed by the intersection of the plane of the film and the long axis of the tooth. If the central ray is perpendicular to a line that bisects this angle, the resulting image is as accurate as possible (Fig. 22.38B).

In order to accurately visualize the long axis of the tooth, you should stand at the patient's front (premolar teeth) or the patient's side (incisor and canine teeth) to find the bisecting angle (Fig. 22.39).

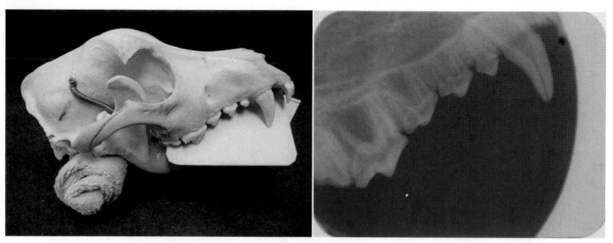

FIG. 22.37 Proper film placement in mouth and accompanying radiograph (right maxilla). Note the convex dot in the upper-right corner of the film.

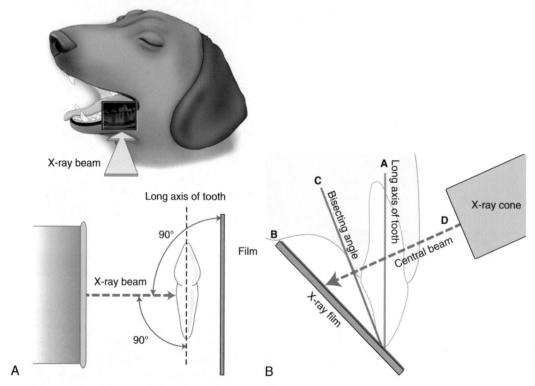

FIG. 22.38 A, Parallel technique. B, Bisecting angle.

✎ TECHNICIAN NOTES

Another way to think of the bisecting angle is to split the difference between pointing the beam at the tooth angle and the film angle. Simply speaking, the bisecting angle is aiming the cone halfway between the tooth and film.

Foreshortening and Elongation

If the x-ray beam is not aimed directly at the bisecting angle, the image will not be a true representation of the tooth. An artifact—elongation or foreshortening—will result.

The analogy of using the shadows created by the position of the sun overhead is one way to explain elongation and foreshortening. If you were standing in the middle of a field, the shadow created on the ground by the sun coming up on the horizon would create quite different shadows from those created by the sun directly overhead. When the sun is coming up on the horizon, a very long shadow is created; this effect is elongation. At noon the sun is overhead, and your shadow is smaller than you are; this effect is foreshortening.

Elongation results when the x-ray beam is aimed too directly at the long axis of the tooth instead of at the bisecting angle (the sun is lower on the horizon). Because the beam is directed at the angle of the tooth, the image will appear "stretched out," and the entire tooth may not have been captured on the film (Fig. 22.40).

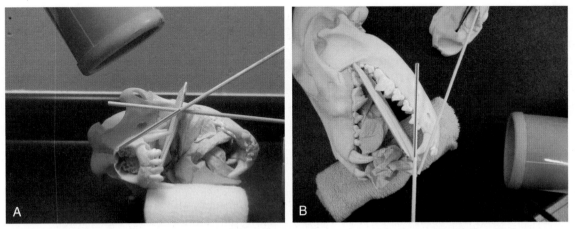

FIG. 22.39 Bisecting angle; the bisecting angle is shown in red. Note the x-ray beam is perpendicular to the bisecting angle. **A,** Radiograph setup for maxillary premolars (lateral recumbency). *Note:* You must be at the front of the patient to appreciate the angle that the tooth enters the skull. **B,** Radiograph setup for mandibular incisors (lateral recumbency). *Note:* You must be at the side of the patient (looking from overhead if patient is in lateral recumbency) to appreciate the angle that the tooth enters the skull.

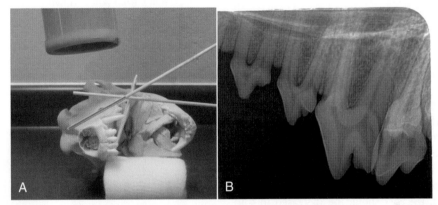

FIG. 22.40 Elongation. **A,** Radiograph setup. **B,** Resulting radiograph demonstrating elongation. The red line is the bisecting angle that the x-ray beam should be perpendicular to. In this setup, the x-ray beam is focused too much on the tooth angle.

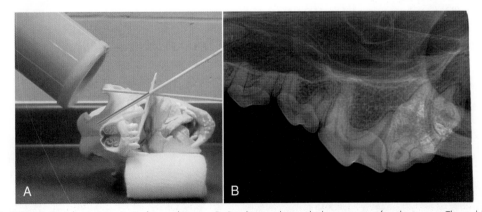

FIG. 22.41 Foreshortening. **A,** Radiograph setup. **B,** Resulting radiograph demonstrating foreshortening. The red line is the bisecting angle that the x-ray beam should be perpendicular to. In this setup the x-ray beam is focused too much on the film angle.

Foreshortening results when the x-ray beam is aimed too directly at the film instead of at the bisecting angle (the sun is directly overhead). Because the beam is directed at the angle of the film, the tooth will appear to have the crown overlapping on the root (Fig. 22.41).

✎ TECHNICIAN NOTES

If the beam is perpendicular to the film, the image is foreshortened. If the beam is perpendicular to the tooth, the image is elongated. If you split the difference, the image is truer. The bisecting angle is splitting the difference.

Intraoral Dental Radiography With a Dental X-Ray Machine

The size of film chosen for each view depends on the size of the animal and the tooth to be radiographed. In general, when choosing a film size for incisors and canine teeth, pick a film size where both of the patient's canine teeth can occlude with the film. This allows the film to sit evenly in the mouth and provides ample room for imaging the teeth. In many cases size 4 films are used for canine patients, except for small dogs. If performing full-mouth radiographs, choose a size 4 film, which allows multiple teeth to be taken with one exposure. Most views in cats utilize size 2 films, with the exception of the mandibular premolars and molar, where a size 0 works best. The following views are demonstrated with the patient in lateral recumbency. This is the recommended patient position because it greatly reduces moving the patient during anesthesia.

The mandible and maxilla should be kept parallel with the tabletop. A small roll or foam wedge can be used to accomplish this goal. The source of many issues with nondiagnostic radiographs is that the patient was not in true lateral, especially with views that require a degree of angulation of the cone (imaging the canine tooth). If maxillary views are taken, the endotracheal tube should be tied to the mandible. If views of mandibular teeth are to be taken, the endotracheal tube should be tied to the maxilla. A paper towel should be used to position the film in the mouth.

The distance between the cone and film depends on the size of film that is used. If using small film (sizes 0, 1, or 2), the standard SID of 2 inches will provide optimal density. If size 4 film is used, the SID should be increased to 4 to 6 inches to allow for a wider area of x-rays (Fig. 22.42). If any change in density is noted, alter the settings based on the SID changes suggested in Chapter 5.

The exposure will have to be increased if the SID is increased beyond 4 inches. Each machine varies, but generally, if the distance is approximately 6 inches from the film, the exposure will have to be increased by 1.5 times the normal exposure for that area. Remember the inverse square law from Chapter 5. Digital systems may not need an increase in exposure because of the greater sensitivity of digital plates.

Always center the cone on the tooth in question. This is often the source of many nondiagnostic radiographs. Dental x-ray machines have no collimator light; therefore you must view the cone from different perspectives to ensure the "imaginary crosshairs" are centered on the tooth in question (Fig. 22.43). Remember that once the beam leaves the collimator cone, it gets wider the farther it must travel.

Also remember in film imaging that the "dot" should be placed rostrally with the convex side of the film (white side) facing the tube head ("a" on digital plates).

✎ TECHNICIAN NOTES

To find the bisecting angle: If the cone is coming from the side (premolars), you should be standing at the patient's front (kneel down at the nose level to visualize the tooth angle). If the cone is coming from the patient's front (incisors and canines), you should be standing at the patient's side (look from overhead when the patient is in lateral). This gives you the "bird's eye view" to visualize the edge of the film and best estimate the tooth angle you should use when determining bisecting angle.

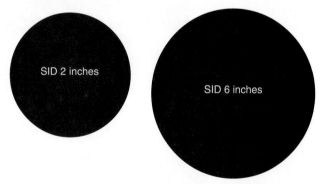

FIG. 22.42 Field of view illustrated as focal film distance differs.

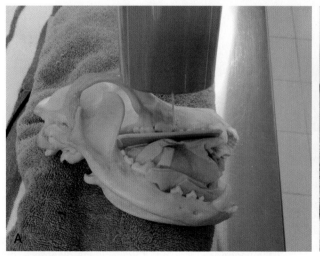

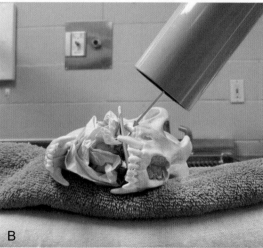

FIG. 22.43 The center of the cone must be visualized from the side **(A)** and the front **(B)** to accurately determine where the beam is directed.

Canine Radiographs With Dental X-Ray Units

Canine Maxillary Premolars and Molars

FILM: The opposite edge of the film should be touching the hard palate; if a size 4 film is used, the opposite edge will be resting against the palatal surface of the contralateral teeth. The tips of the premolar/molar should be at the edge of the film closest to the cone to allow ample space for the roots of the tooth to "fall onto" the film. A size 0 or 2 film is likely necessary to capture distal molars because of anatomical space constraints.

CENTRAL RAY: The cone is directed laterally and centered over the tooth in question. The SID depends on the size of film. For a size 4 film, the SID is 4 to 6 inches.

ANGLE: The bisecting angle is found by standing at the patient's front rostral aspect (Fig. 22.44).

> ### TECHNICIAN NOTES
> Superimposition of multirooted teeth is always a concern. Multiple radiographs may be necessary to isolate specific roots if required (see later).

> ### TECHNICIAN NOTES
> Capturing distal molars may be difficult due to space constraints with film placement. Fig. 22.45 illustrates film placement for distal molars if film placement as described earlier in this section is unsuccessful in capturing these teeth. If difficulty is still experienced, use the distolateral beam direction with the bisecting angle. Difficulty is generally experienced in small breeds and brachycephalics.

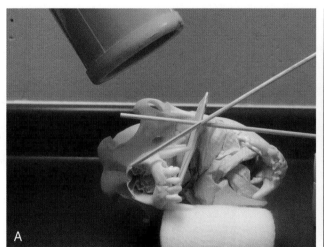

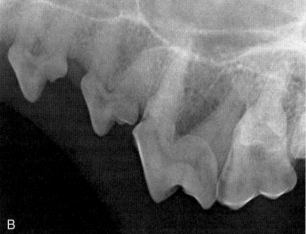

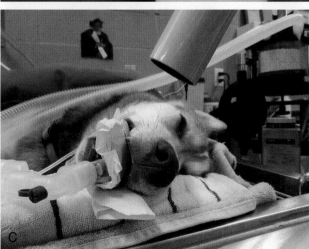

FIG. 22.44 Canine maxillary premolars and molars (lateral recumbency). **A,** Skull setup. **B,** Radiograph. **C,** Final setup.

Continued

Canine Maxillary Premolars and Molars—cont'd

Maxillary Premolars: SLOB Rule

The maxillary fourth premolar (108 [P⁴] or 208 [⁴P]) is a triple-rooted tooth that has one large distal root and two smaller mesial roots. The mesial roots superimpose over each other if the beam is directed from the lateral aspect. If a desired root needs to be isolated, the direction of the beam can be directed from the mesial or the distal aspect to "split" the roots on the film. This view is necessary if endodontics are to be performed and the diseased root needs to be isolated. The distolateral beam direction can also be used for capturing distal molars in patients where film placement is difficult.

The SLOB rule stands for "same lingual opposite buccal." This term is used to help identify the particular root when the beam is directed from the mesial or distal aspect. "Same lingual" means that the lingual-mesial root (which is actually the palatal root-maxilla) appears to move in the same direction as where the x-ray beam is being directed from. "Opposite buccal" means that the buccal-mesial root appears to move in the opposite direction from where the x-ray beam is coming from.

The SLOB rule can be illustrated using your hands as shown in Fig. 22.46. In this diagram the root structure of 208 or ⁴P

is depicted. In the first diagram, you can see the thumb and one finger. In the second diagram, you can see an additional finger. If the direction the beam is coming from is changed, you will be able to see objects that were superimposed on the initial view. In the second diagram, you can see that if the beam (your eyes) is directed from the distal aspect, the palatal root appears to move in the same direction as where the beam is being directed.

If the beam is directed from the distal aspect, the palatal root will appear as the middle of the three roots on the radiograph. If the beam is directed from the mesial aspect, the buccal root will appear as the middle of the three roots on the radiograph.

Technique

The same setup for the film, cone, and bisecting angle as described previously for maxillary premolars and molars is used as the starting point. Once the bisecting angle is found and the cone is aimed perpendicular to it from the lateral aspect, the cone can be directed from the mesial or distal aspect (Fig. 22.47).

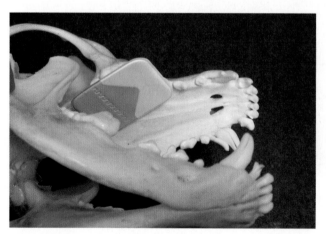

FIG. 22.45 Film placement for distal molars. Note the film is slightly turned to follow the natural curvature of the palate.

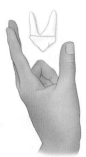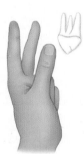

FIG. 22.46 SLOB rule: Left hand used to demonstrate root isolation of 208 by changing x-ray beam direction. The second image depicts beam direction from the distal aspect and the ability to visualize all roots.

Canine Maxillary Premolars and Molars—cont'd

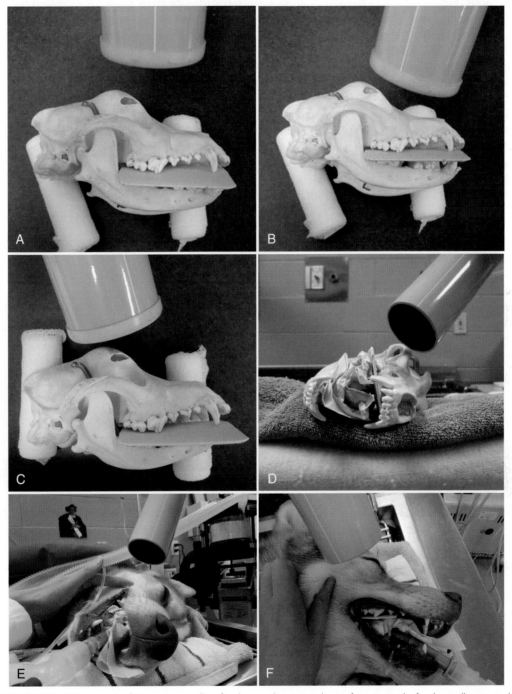

FIG. 22.47 Oblique angles for imaging maxillary fourth premolar. **A,** Initial setup for imaging the fourth maxillary premolar as viewed from the patient's side. **B,** Mesiolateral oblique radiograph setup of maxillary fourth premolar (lateral recumbency) showing final oblique x-ray cone with the beam 30 degrees from the initial setup. **C,** Distolateral oblique radiograph setup of maxillary fourth premolar (lateral recumbency) showing final oblique x-ray cone with the beam 30 degrees from the initial setup. **D,** Distolateral as viewed from front. **E,** Final preparation for distolateral on canine patient as viewed from front. **F,** Final preparation for distolateral on canine patient as viewed from side.

Continued

Canine Maxillary Premolars and Molars—cont'd

Mesiolateral Oblique View

For the mesiolateral oblique view, the cone is directed from the mesial aspect (mesial to distal), approximately 30 degrees from the initial position. Fig. 22.48 shows the mesial roots isolated on the radiograph. However, the distal root will superimpose over the first maxillary molar tooth.

Distolateral Oblique View

For the distolateral oblique view, the cone is directed from the distal aspect (distal to mesial), approximately 30 degrees from the initial position. Fig. 22.49 shows the mesial roots separated on the radiograph. However, the mesial roots may superimpose over the third maxillary premolar tooth.

Comments and Tips

- The distolateral oblique view should be used for the distal molars if roots are not properly imaged using a direct bisecting angle. The cone direction sends the image of the molars forward in the mouth onto the film.

> **TECHNICIAN NOTES**
>
> The SLOB rule states that if the beam is directed from the distal aspect, the palatal root will appear as the middle of the three roots on the radiograph. If the beam is directed from the mesial aspect, the buccal root will appear as the middle of the three roots on the radiograph.

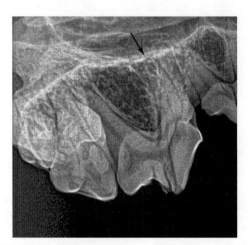

FIG. 22.48 Mesiolateral oblique radiograph; the central root is the mesial-buccal root.

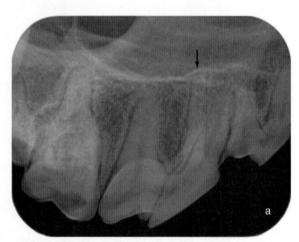

FIG. 22.49 Distolateral oblique radiograph; the central root is the mesial-palatal root.

Maxillary Canine Teeth

The radiograph of the maxillary canine tooth is set up using the long axis of the tooth, which can be visualized from the side of the patient while the x-ray cone is tilted at 30 degrees (use the angle meter on the tube head). This change in beam angle helps prevent superimposition of the canine tooth over the premolar teeth. The 30-degree tilt only works if the animal is in true lateral. The canine tooth curves distally, with its apex typically over the root of the second premolar; always use the root of the tooth to find the bisecting angle, not the crown. This view can also be used to visualize the ipsilateral incisors (Fig. 22.50).

Imaging Maxillary Canine Teeth in Large Dogs With a DR Sensor

Canine teeth in larger dogs will likely require two exposures due to the size of the tooth and the limitation of a size 2 sensor. The same technique as described earlier (bisecting angle while cone is at a 30-degree tilt) is used, but the placement of the size 2 sensor will differ. The first image is set up as described for maxillary canine tooth with sensor placement as shown in Fig. 22.51. This image will capture the crown and most of the root. If the radiograph doesn't capture the entire root, reposition the sensor until it is flat against the palate (Fig. 22.52). Keep the same tilt and angle but center more distally over the apex of the root with the cone.

FILM: Choose a film size where both canine teeth are touching the film ("biting on it"). Size 4 is used for most dogs. The film should be placed sufficiently rostral to evaluate the ipsilateral incisors as well.

CENTRAL RAY: The film-to-cone distance should be about 4 to 6 inches for a dog's canine tooth. Ensure the animal is in true lateral and adjust the cone until the angle meter reads 30 degrees. Center the middle of the cone on the maxillary canine tooth.

ANGLE: The bisecting angle of the tooth is found by standing at the patient's side using the long axis of the tooth. Canine teeth curve distally. Visualize the curvature of the root to accurately reflect the long axis of the tooth. If root cutoff occurs and both canine teeth are "biting" on film, you need to foreshorten the angle slightly. To foreshorten the angle, focus more on the film.

> ✎ **TECHNICIAN NOTES**
>
> Remember that the same parallel and bisecting angle techniques are used for digital radiography as for the film system. For DR systems, the digital sensor replaces the film. For CR systems, PSP plates replace the film. Because of the smaller, bulkier DR sensors, modifications need to be made for imaging incisors and canine teeth in larger dogs. See additional notes for imaging incisors and canine teeth.

> ✎ **TECHNICIAN NOTES**
>
> If you are having difficulty accurately determining the bisecting angle while the cone is tilted 30 degrees, you can line up the bisecting angle at 0 degrees and then perform the 30-degree tilt. It is essential that the animal is in true lateral. Difficulty with this approach is ensuring you continue to aim at the bisecting angle while the cone is maneuvered toward the final 30-degree tilt.

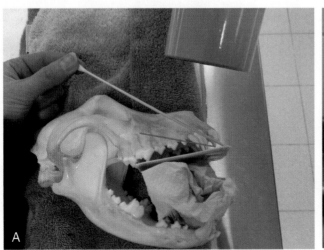 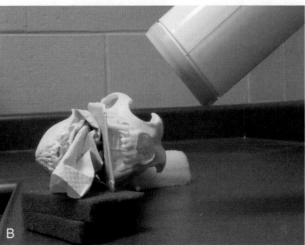

FIG. 22.50 Intraoral technique radiograph setup of the maxillary canine tooth (lateral recumbency). **A,** View from the patient's side to aim at the bisecting angle. **B,** View from the front while finding the bisecting angle (angle meter should be at 30 degrees).

Continued

Maxillary Canine Teeth—cont'd

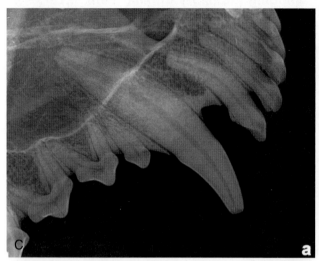

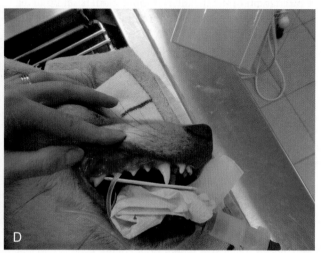

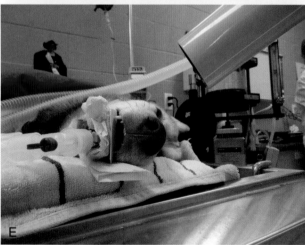

FIG. 22.50, cont'd C, Radiograph of the maxillary canine tooth. Note: Ipsilateral incisors can be imaged as well. D, Final preparation for view from patient's side on a canine patient. E, View from patient's front on a canine patient demonstrating 30-degree tilt.

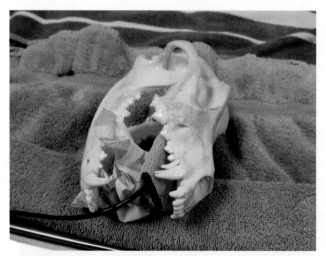

FIG. 22.51 Placement of DR sensor for imaging a maxillary canine tooth. The crown is on the corner of the sensor, and the rest of the sensor is against the palate. Note: Sensor is wrapped in Vetrap, which prevents the sensor from slipping once positioned.

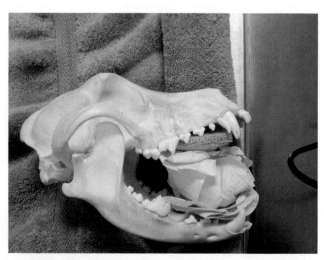

FIG. 22.52 Placement of DR sensor for imaging the apex of the maxillary canine tooth. In larger patients it may be necessary to take two radiographs to image the entire tooth. The sensor is flat against the palate.

Maxillary Incisors

The typical rostrocaudal view can capture all the incisors on one film. Elongation is a common artifact for this view. Dog incisors have long roots that curve distally, like the root(s) of a canine tooth.

FILM: The tips of the incisor teeth should be at the rostral edge of the film to allow ample space for the roots of the incisors. Choose a film size where both canine teeth are touching the film ("biting on it"). Size 4 film is used for most medium to large dogs.

CONE: The cone is directed in a rostrocaudal direction and centered over the nose. If the patient is in true lateral, the angle meter is at 0. It is imperative that the cone is centered between all six incisors (Fig. 22.53).

ANGLE: The bisecting angle is found by standing at the patient's side. Remember that the incisor teeth in dogs curve distally (Fig. 22.54).

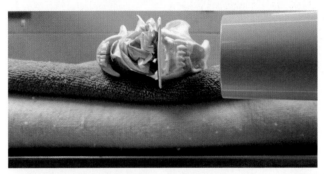

FIG. 22.53 For imaging maxillary incisors, the cone must be low enough to center between all six incisors. It may be necessary to have a towel under the patient's head to raise the head up high enough to allow this.

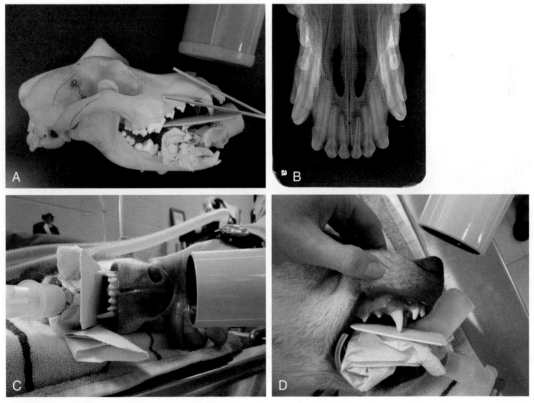

FIG. 22.54 Canine maxillary incisors. **A,** Skull setup showing the bisecting angle viewed from the patient's side. **B,** Radiograph of the maxillary incisors. **C,** Maxillary incisors on a canine patient as viewed from the front. Note: The cone is low enough to be centered between all six incisors. **D,** Maxillary incisors on a canine patient as viewed from the side prior to taking the image.

Continued

Maxillary Incisors—cont'd

Imaging Maxillary Incisors in Large Dogs With a DR Sensor

For larger dogs all six incisors should be imaged three at a time. If the patient's size allows the sensor to fit evenly between the canine teeth, the lateral edge of 103 and 203 will be cut off. This is due to the inactive perimeter on the sensor. To avoid this, image three incisors at a time. The sensor is positioned with a slight tilt toward the ipsilateral canine tooth (Fig. 22.55). Have the cone at 15 degrees (patient in true lateral) and direct the beam at the bisecting angle. Ensure the cone is centered on the three ipsilateral incisors (Fig. 22.56).

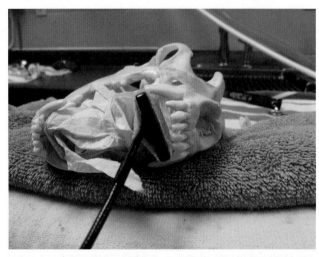

FIG. 22.55 DR sensor placement for imaging maxillary incisors in larger patients. Note: The sensor is angled toward the canine.

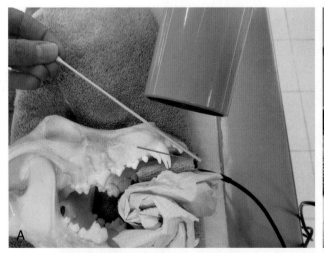
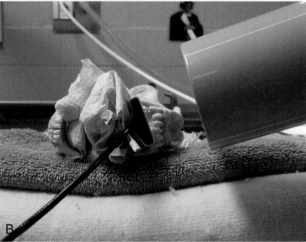

FIG. 22.56 Canine maxillary incisors with a DR sensor. **A,** The bisecting angle is visualized from the side. **B,** View from the front showing the 15-degree tilt with the cone centered on the three incisors that are up.

Mandibular Incisors

The typical rostrocaudal view can capture all the incisors on one film. Because they converge at the midline, the roots cannot always be isolated because they will overlap slightly. In some instances, if a specific incisor needs to be isolated, the x-ray cone can be directed obliquely from the left or right side so its root is more isolated (see the technique used to image incisors with the DR sensor). Elongation is a common artifact for this view. Dog incisors have long roots that curve distally like the root(s) of a canine tooth.

FILM: The tips of the incisor teeth should be at the rostral edge of the film to allow ample space for the roots of the incisors. Choose a film size where both canine teeth are touching the film ("biting on it"). Size 4 film is used for most medium to large dogs.

CENTRAL RAY: The cone is directed in a rostrocaudal direction and centered over the chin. If the patient is in true lateral, the angle meter is at 0. It is imperative that the cone is centered between all six incisors (Fig. 22.57).

ANGLE: The bisecting angle is found by standing at the patient's side. Remember that the incisor teeth in dogs curve distally (Fig. 22.58).

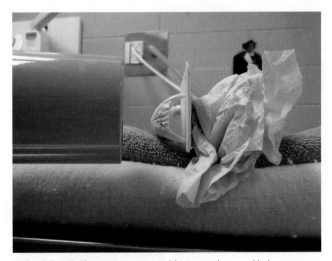

FIG. 22.57 The cone is centered between the mandibular incisors.

Continued

Mandibular Incisors—cont'd

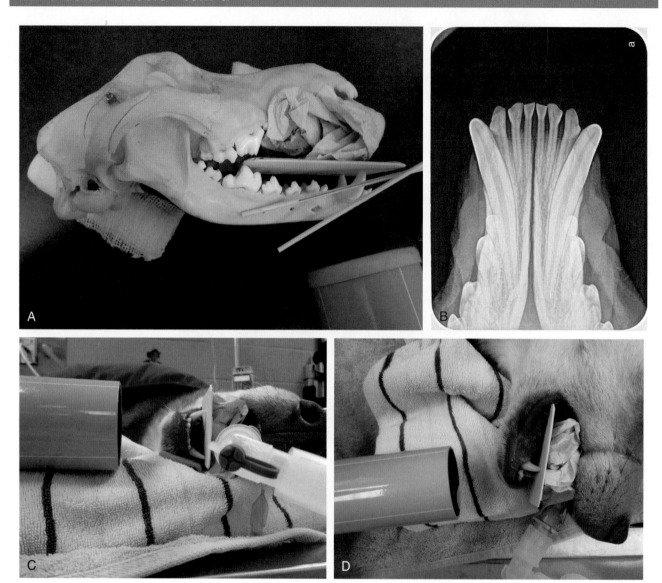

FIG. 22.58 Canine mandibular incisors. **A,** Skull setup showing the bisecting angle from the patient's side. **B,** Radiograph of mandibular incisors. **C,** Canine patient showing the cone low enough that it is centered between all six incisors. **D,** Canine patient showing the final setup from the side.

Mandibular Incisors—cont'd

Imaging Mandibular Incisors in Large Dogs With a DR Sensor

For larger dogs, all six incisors should be imaged three at a time. If the patient's size allows the sensor to fit evenly between the canine teeth, the lateral edge of 303 and 403 will be cut off. This is due to the inactive perimeter on the sensor. To avoid this, image three incisors at a time. The sensor is positioned with a slight tilt toward the ipsilateral canine tooth (Fig. 22.59). Have the cone at 15 degrees (patient in true lateral) and direct the beam at the bisecting angle. Ensure you are centered on the three ipsilateral incisors (Fig. 22.60B).

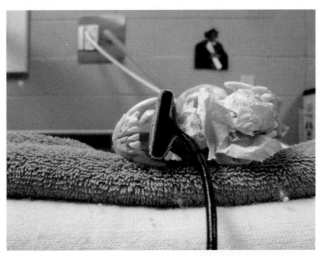

FIG. 22.59 DR sensor placement for imaging mandibular incisors in larger patients. Note: The sensor is angled toward the affected canine.

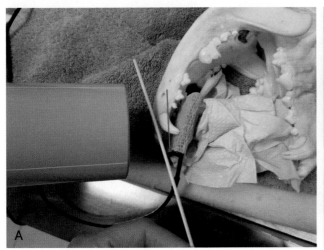
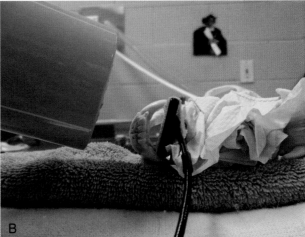

FIG. 22.60 Canine mandibular incisors with a DR sensor. **A,** The bisecting angle is visualized from the side. **B,** View from the front showing the 15-degree tilt with the cone centered on the three incisors that are uppermost in this lateral position.

Mandibular Canine Teeth

The radiograph of the mandibular canine tooth is set up using the long axis of the tooth, which can be visualized from the side of the patient while the x-ray cone is tilted at 15 degrees (use the angle meter on the tube head). This change in beam angle helps prevent superimposition of the canine tooth over the premolar teeth. The 15-degree tilt only works if the animal is in true lateral. Always use the root of the tooth to find the bisecting angle, not the crown. Mandibular canine teeth converge toward midline; therefore the angulation toward midline is less than required for the maxillary canine tooth.

Imaging Mandibular Canine Teeth in Large Dogs With a DR Sensor

Canine teeth in larger dogs will likely require two exposures due to the size of the tooth and the limitation of a size 2 sensor. The same technique as described earlier (bisecting angle from the side while cone is at 15-degree tilt) is used, but the placement of the size 2 sensor will differ. The first image is set up as described for the mandibular canine tooth, with sensor placement as shown in Fig. 22.62. This image will capture the crown and most of the root. If the radiograph doesn't capture the entire root, reposition the sensor until it is flat against the floor of the mandible (Fig. 22.63). Center over the apex of the root with the cone.

FILM: Choose a film size where both canine teeth are touching the film ("biting on it"). Size 4 film is used for most canine teeth. The tongue is positioned on the opposite side of the film. The film should be placed sufficiently rostral to evaluate the ipsilateral incisors as well.

CENTRAL RAY: The film-to-cone distance should be about 4 to 6 inches for a dog's canine tooth. Ensure the animal is in true lateral and adjust the cone until the angle meter reads 15 degrees. Center the middle of the cone on the maxillary canine tooth.

ANGLE: The bisecting angle of the tooth is found by standing at the patient's side using the long axis of the tooth. If root cutoff occurs and both canine teeth are "biting" on the film, you need to foreshorten the angle slightly. To foreshorten the angle, focus more on the film (Fig. 22.61A-C).

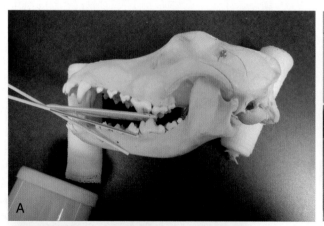

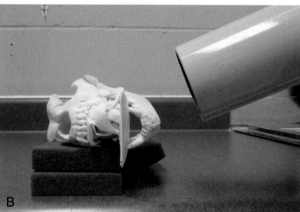

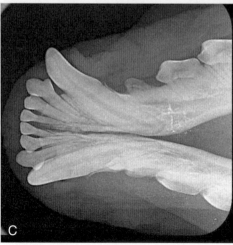

FIG. 22.61 Mandibular canine. **A,** Skull setup with bisecting angle viewed from the side. **B,** Skull setup showing 15-degree tilt as viewed from the front. **C,** Radiograph of mandibular canine.

Mandibular Canine Teeth—cont'd

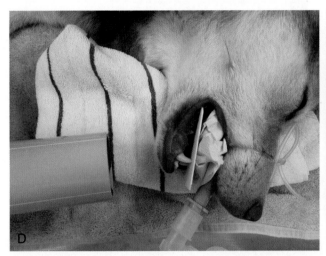

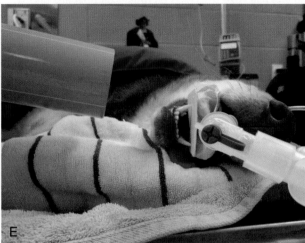

FIG. 22.61, cont'd D, Canine patient final setup as viewed from the side. E, Canine patient final setup showing 15-degree tilt.

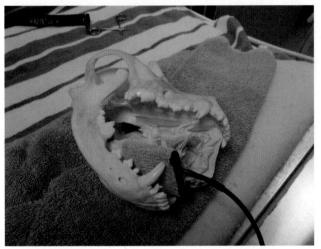

FIG. 22.62 Placement of DR sensor for imaging mandibular canine tooth. The crown is in the corner of the sensor, and the rest of the sensor is against the floor of the mandible. Note: The sensor is wrapped in Vetrap (barrier sleeve should be used under Vetrap to protect from moisture), which prevents the sensor from slipping once positioned.

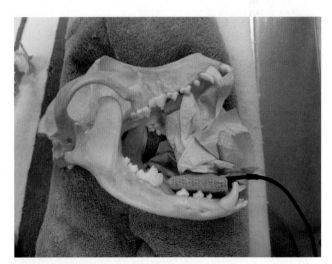

FIG. 22.63 Placement of DR sensor for imaging the apex of the mandibular canine tooth. In larger patients it may be necessary to take two radiographs to image the entire tooth. The sensor is flat against the floor of the mandible.

Mandibular Premolars 1 and 2

FILM: The film (size 2) should be resting on both first and second premolars (left and right), behind the canine teeth, facing the floor of the mandible. The tips of the premolars to be radiographed should be at the edge of film closest to you (lateral) to allow ample space for the roots of the tooth to "fall onto" the film.

CENTRAL RAY: The cone is directed laterally and centered at the tooth to be radiographed.

ANGLE: The bisecting angle is found by standing at the patient's front (Fig. 22.64).

> ### ✎ TECHNICIAN NOTES
>
> The parallel technique cannot be used on mandibular premolars 1 and 2. Dogs have an elongated mandibular symphysis, which makes correct film placement impossible. The bisecting angle technique must be used on these teeth.

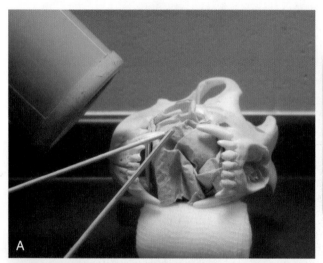

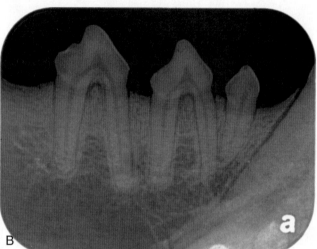

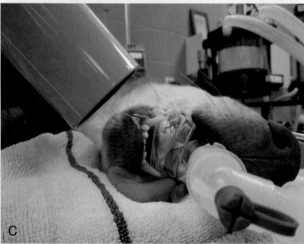

FIG. 22.64 Canine mandibular premolar 1 and 2 require a bisecting angle technique due to an elongated mandibular symphysis in dogs. **A,** Skull setup with the bisecting angle viewed from the front. **B,** Radiograph of mandibular premolar 1,2 and 3. **C,** Canine patient showing final setup.

Mandibular Premolars 3 and 4 and Molars

FILM: The film is placed between the tongue and the mandible, parallel to the long axis of the teeth. It is necessary to push the film down until you can feel the film pop out under the ventral mandible. This maneuver ensures that the entire tooth is captured. A paper towel can be used to keep the film pushed down. The film can be gently bent to accommodate placement, and if a larger film is used, it can be placed behind the tooth diagonally so it fits.

CENTRAL RAY: The cone is directed laterally and centered on the tooth to be radiographed, perpendicular to the film.

ANGLE: Parallel technique (Fig. 22.65).

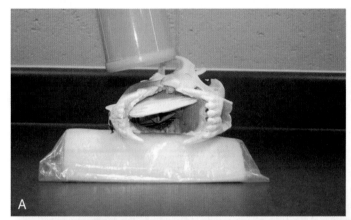

> ✎ **TECHNICIAN NOTES**
>
> The parallel technique can be used for the mandibular premolars 3 and 4 and the mandibular molars because there is no hard palate to interfere with film placement behind the roots of these teeth.

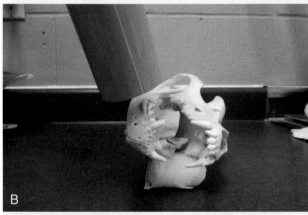

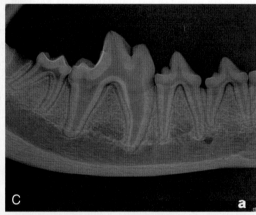

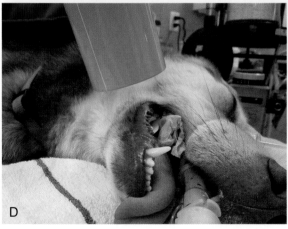

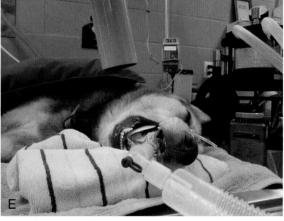

FIG. 22.65 Canine mandibular premolar 3, 4, and molars. **A,** Skull setup with size 4 film; the beam is directed perpendicular to the film. **B,** Skull setup with size 2 film. **C,** Radiograph of mandibular premolar 3, 4, and molars. Note: 411 is missing. **D,** Canine patient showing final setup with a size 2 film. **E,** Canine patient showing final setup with a size 4 film.

Feline Radiographs

Anatomical differences between dogs and cats allow for some modifications to the views. Maxillary canine and incisor teeth are more upright in cats than in dogs. This is important when estimating the long axis of the tooth for the bisecting angle technique. Follow the crown when estimating the long axis of the tooth, as the root follows the same angle. Mandibular canine teeth in cats do curve distally, and the curvature of the root should be used when estimating the long axis of the tooth. Cats are missing mandibular premolar 1 and 2, which allows the mandibular incisors and canine teeth to be imaged together. Maxillary premolars and molars in cats is the most difficult area to image due to a very prominent zygomatic arch. If a standard bisecting angle technique is used, the zygomatic arch will superimpose over the teeth, negating any diagnostic value to the radiograph. The cat should be positioned in true lateral for all views. It is often difficult to get the cone low enough to the table to image the incisors and canines due to the design of the tube head. In order to avoid this, raise the cat's head up on a small towel.

TECHNICIAN NOTES

CR PSP plates are enclosed in a barrier envelope. For some views it is necessary to tape the excess envelope behind the plate to ensure the actual plate is as close as possible to the desired area. This approach is necessary for imaging maxillary premolars and molar (intraoral technique: tape edge that will be against the palate) as well as mandibular premolars and molar (parallel technique: tape edge closest to the mandibular symphysis).

Feline Maxillary Premolars: Intraoral Technique

FILM: The endotracheal tube should be carefully secured to the mandible for this view. The top edge of the film (size 2) is resting against the palatal aspect of the maxillary premolar teeth on the side of the mouth opposite to the teeth you are imaging (tape excess envelope behind the plate if using CR PSP plates). The bottom edge of the film rests against the lingual aspect of the mandibular canine tooth on the side of the mouth you are radiographing. The tongue should be behind the film on the mandible. The maxillary arcade should be parallel to the tabletop.

CENTRAL RAY: The x-ray cone is directed perpendicular to the film visualized from the front and ventral aspect of the patient. The center of the cone should be on the roots.

ANGLE: The angle is referred to as a *modified parallel technique*. It is very important that the beam is perpendicular to the film from the front and side. Note: If root cutoff occurs, the beam must be centered more on the roots of the teeth (Fig. 22.66). If there is too much zygomatic interference, center more on the crown.

TECHNICIAN NOTES

The standard bisecting angle that is traditionally used for maxillary premolars in a dog cannot be used for feline teeth because the zygomatic arch will be superimposed on these teeth. A "modified parallel technique" is used to minimize this superimposition.

Feline Maxillary Premolars: Intraoral Technique—cont'd

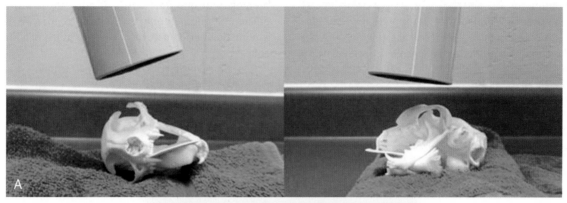

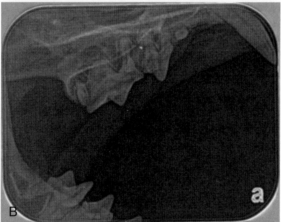

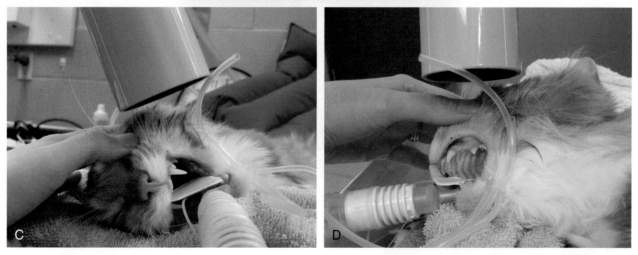

FIG. 22.66 Feline maxillary premolars and molar (intraoral technique) viewed from the front and side. **A,** Skull setup showing film placement; top edge of film is against palatal aspect of teeth on opposite side; bottom edge of film is resting against lingual aspect of the mandibular canine on the same side. The beam is directed perpendicular to the film. **B,** Radiograph of feline maxillary premolars and molar. Note: The zygomatic arch is present but the teeth can still be assessed. **C,** Feline patient showing final setup as viewed from the front. Note: The endotracheal tube is carefully tied to the mandible. **D,** Feline patient showing final setup as viewed from the side prior to exposure.

Feline Maxillary Premolars: Extraoral Technique

Another option for imaging the maxillary premolars in cats is to use an extraoral technique. This is the preferred technique if a DR sensor is used, because film placement using the standard technique with the bulky sensors is problematic.

Comments and Tips

On the radiograph, you will see the premolars on the opposite side, but they should not be superimposing on the maxillary premolars in question. If the arcades are superimposed, a greater tilt in the cone is required. If there is too much zygomatic interference, there was too much of a tilt with the cone.

The film will need to be identified properly because the extraoral technique was used.

POSITION: The cat should be positioned in lateral recumbency with the mouth propped open. A 1-mL syringe (cut down) can be used to prop the mouth open. The endotracheal tube should be gently pulled ventrally so it is not superimposed over the premolars.

FILM: Size 2 film is positioned extraorally under the side to be radiographed. The cusps of the premolars should be at the edge of the film, allowing ample space for the roots of the teeth to be imaged (most of the maxilla should be on the film) (Fig. 22.67).

CENTRAL RAY: As a starting point, with the patient in lateral recumbency, the cone is aimed at both maxillary arcades as if to superimpose them on the radiograph. Then the cone is directed toward the film, centering at the roots of the premolars near the film and bypassing the opposite arcade (Fig. 22.68).

ANGLE: The beam is aimed at the film in a "near-parallel" technique. From the starting point it is about a 20- to 25-degree tilt to bypass the opposite arcade.

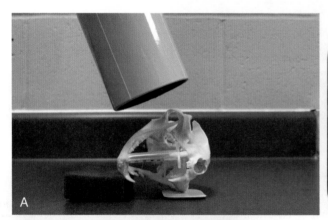

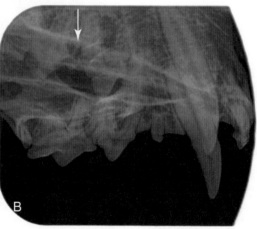

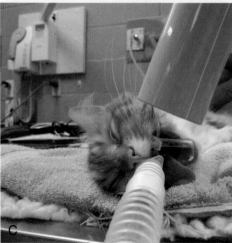

FIG. 22.67 Feline maxillary premolars and molar (extraoral technique). **A,** Skull setup showing film placement under maxilla with beam directed at arcade that is closest to the table. **B,** Radiograph. Note the contralateral premolars at the top of the film edge (*arrow*). **C,** Feline patient showing final setup.

Feline Maxillary Canine Teeth

The radiograph of a maxillary canine tooth in a cat is set up using the long axis of the tooth, which can be visualized from the side of the patient while the x-ray cone is tilted 30 degrees (use the angle meter on the tube head). This change in beam angle helps prevent superimposition of the canine tooth over the premolar teeth. The 30-degree tilt only works if the animal is in true lateral. The canine tooth tilts distally but not in as pronounced a way as the same tooth in a dog.

Comments and Tips

The ipsilateral maxillary incisors cannot be captured in one image as those of dogs can because of anatomical differences between these species in tooth placement and the rostral maxilla.

FILM: Size 2 film is used. Both canine teeth should be touching the film ("biting on it"). The tip of the canine tooth desired should be at the lateral edge of the film to allow ample space for the root of the canine tooth.

CENTRAL RAY: The tube head is tilted 30 degrees so that the canine tooth does not superimpose over the premolars distal to it (Fig. 22.69). Center the beam on the canine tooth.

ANGLE: The bisecting angle of the tooth is found by standing at the patient's side using the long axis of the tooth (follow the crown as the root follows the same axis). If root cutoff occurs even though both canine teeth were "biting on" the film, you should ensure that the beam is centered on the film, and you may need to foreshorten the angle slightly. To foreshorten the angle, focus more on the film.

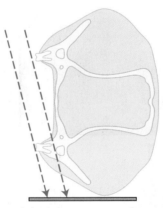

FIG. 22.68 Labeled extraoral sketch for imaging maxillary premolars and molar in a cat.

Continued

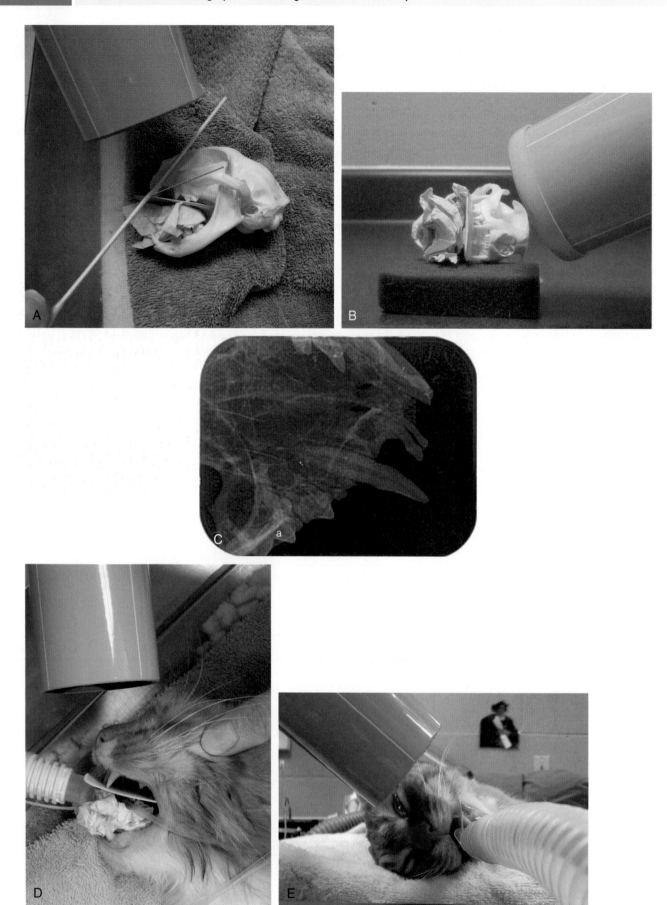

FIG. 22.69 Feline maxillary canine tooth. **A,** Skull setup showing bisecting angle from the side. **B,** Skull setup showing 30-degree tilt from the front. **C,** Radiograph of maxillary canine tooth. **D,** Feline patient showing final setup from the side. **E,** Feline patient showing final setup with 30-degree tilt from the front.

Feline Maxillary Incisors

FILM: Size 2 film is used for the maxillary incisors. The tips of the incisor teeth should be at the edge of the film closest to you (rostral) to allow ample space for the roots of the incisors to "fall onto" the film.

CENTRAL RAY: The cone is directed in a rostrocaudal direction and centered over the nose. (Fig. 22.70).

ANGLE: The bisecting angle is found by standing at the patient's side.

> ✎ **TECHNICIAN NOTES**
>
> The typical rostrocaudal view can capture all the maxillary incisors on one film. Feline maxillary incisors are similar to little "pegs"; they curve slightly distally and do not converge in the middle like dog incisors.

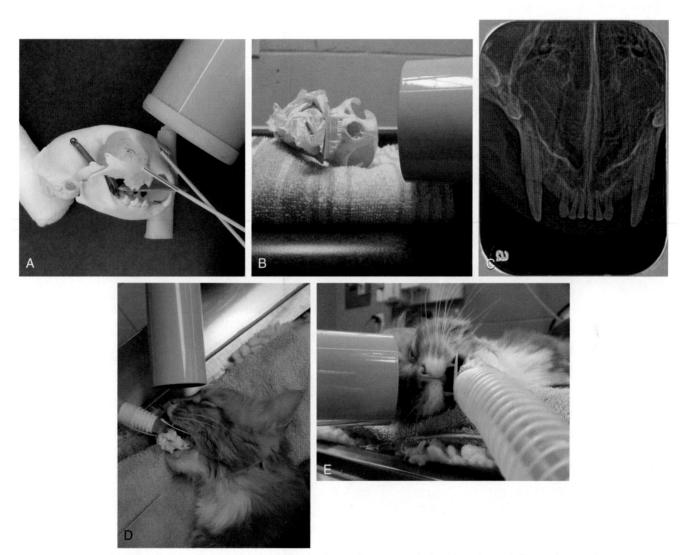

FIG. 22.70 Feline maxillary incisors. **A,** Skull setup showing bisecting angle from the side. **B,** Skull setup showing the cone centered between all six incisors. **C,** Radiograph of maxillary incisors. **D,** Final setup on a feline patient as viewed from the side. **E,** Final setup on a feline patient as viewed from the front.

Feline Mandibular Canines and Incisors

FILM: Size 2 film is used. Both canine teeth should be touching the film ("biting on it"). The tongue should be pushed out of the way, ideally on the opposite side of the film.

CENTRAL RAY: The cone is directed in a rostrocaudal direction and centered over the patient's chin.

ANGLE: The bisecting angle is found by standing at the patient's side. The long axis of the canine tooth, not the incisors, should be used to find the bisecting angle. Remember that the canine tooth has a large root that curves in distally (Fig. 22.71).

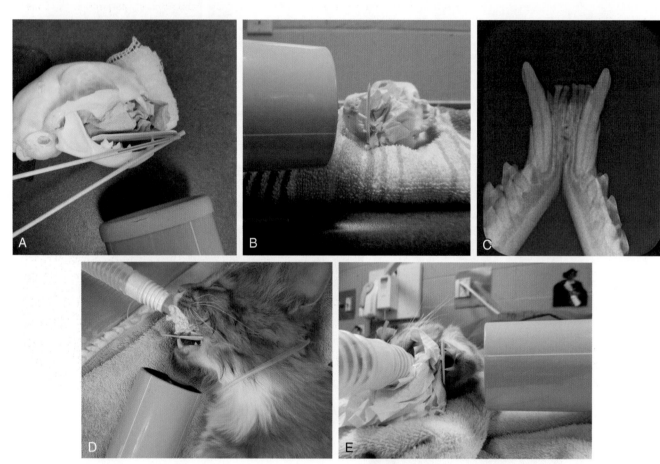

FIG. 22.71 Feline mandibular incisors and canines. **A,** Skull setup showing bisecting angle from the side. **B,** Skull setup showing the cone centered between all six incisors and canines. **C,** Radiograph of mandibular incisors and canines. **D,** Final setup on a feline patient as viewed from the side. **E,** Final setup on a feline patient as viewed from the front.

Feline Mandibular Premolars and Molar: Parallel Technique

The parallel technique can be used to image the mandibular premolars and molar of the cat because there is no hard palate to interfere with film placement behind the roots of these teeth. The mesial root of premolar 3 can be difficult to capture due to interference with film placement and the mandibular symphysis. A bisecting angle technique can be used to image these teeth if this problem occurs.

FILM: The film (size 0 works best) is placed behind the teeth parallel to the long axis of the teeth. It is necessary to push the film down until you can feel it pop out under the ventral mandible, and it is imperative that the film is positioned as close as possible to the mandibular symphysis (tape excess envelope behind plate if using CR PSP plates). A paper towel can be used to keep the film pushed down. The film can be gently bent to accommodate placement, and if a larger film is used, it can be placed behind the tooth diagonally to fit behind it (this increases the chance that the mesial root of the third premolar will be cut off).

CENTRAL RAY: The cone is directed in a lateral direction and centered at the tooth to be radiographed, perpendicular to the film (Fig. 22.72).

ANGLE: Parallel technique.

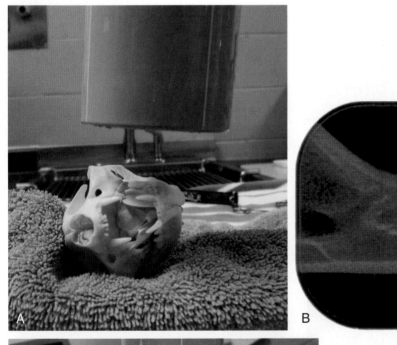

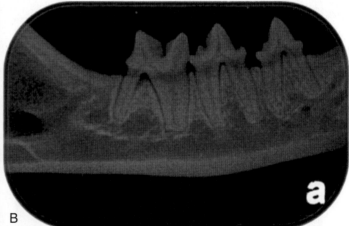

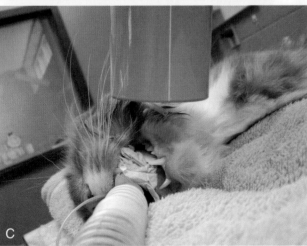

FIG. 22.72 Feline mandibular premolars and molar (parallel technique). **A,** Skull setup showing parallel technique; the x-ray cone is perpendicular to the film (size 0). **B,** Radiograph of mandibular premolar 3, 4, and molar. **C,** Final setup on a feline patient as viewed from the front.

Feline Mandibular Premolars and Molar: Bisecting Angle Technique

If the mesial root of the third premolar continues to be cut off and the film is placed as rostral as possible, then a bisecting angle technique can also be used to image these teeth. If a DR sensor is used, this is the preferred technique because film placement using the standard technique with the bulky sensors is problematic.

> ✎ **TECHNICIAN NOTE**
>
> A combination of parallel and bisecting angle technique may be necessary to image the mandibular premolars and molar in cats, especially with DR sensors.

FILM: The film (size 2) should be resting on the floor of the mandible, preferably with the tongue on the opposite side of the film. If this is not possible, the tongue can be left between the film and the teeth. If the film is not pushed far enough back in the mouth, the molar will be cut off (use the parallel technique for the molar if this is problematic).

CENTRAL RAY: The cone is directed in a lateral direction at the tooth to be radiographed.

ANGLE: The bisecting angle is found by standing at the patient's front. The x-ray beam is angled through the floor of the mandible (Fig. 22.73).

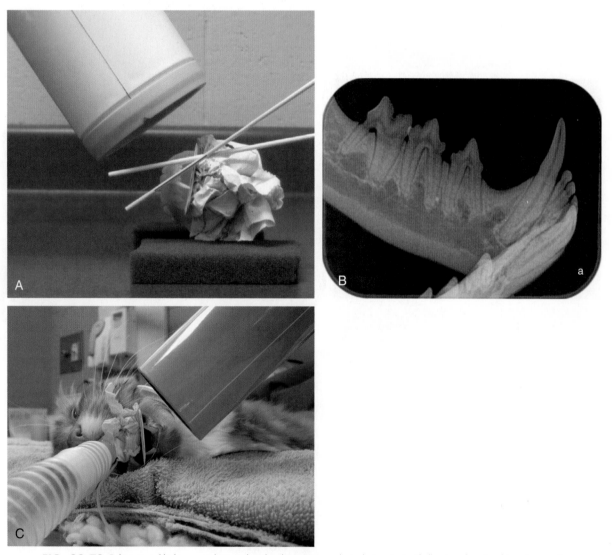

FIG. 22.73 Feline mandibular premolars and molar (bisecting angle technique). **A,** Skull setup showing bisecting angle technique as viewed from the front. **B,** Radiograph of mandibular premolar 3, 4, and molar. **C,** Final setup on a feline patient as viewed from the front.

Canine and Feline Nasal Sinus Radiographs

Indications for radiographs of the nasal sinus cavity in either the dog or cat include evaluation of disease, such as neoplasia, as well as the detection of foreign bodies.

POSITION: The patient should be in sternal recumbency with the maxilla parallel to the tabletop.

FILM: For dogs, size 4 film is inserted as far as possible into the patient's mouth between the maxilla and the endotracheal tube. For cats, the film may need to be placed in on an angle or a size 2 film may be used.

CENTRAL RAY: The cone is 6 to 8 inches away from the film and centered on the nasal cavity. Use settings for a maxillary canine tooth, and adjust for the distance from the film.

ANGLE: The cone is directed perpendicular to the film (Fig. 22.74).

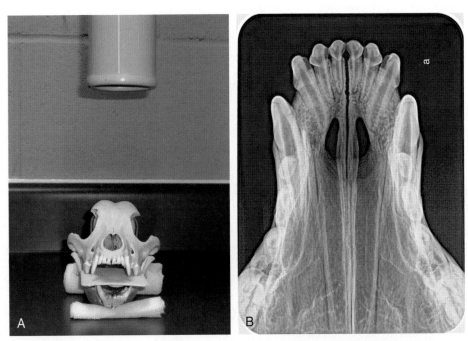

FIG. 22.74 Setup for radiograph of nasal sinus. A, Skull setup. B, Radiograph.

Dental Radiography With Conventional Cassette: Common Views

The use of conventional cassettes is not the ideal way to image teeth, but if there is no dental x-ray machine or nonscreen film, it is the only option. Screened cassettes and radiolucent positioning devices are required.

Difficulties expected include positioning of the cassettes in the mouth because of the general characteristics of cassettes (size, thickness, weight). Teeth in the distal aspect of the mouth may be difficult to image due to superimposition of the contralateral arch.

See further discussion of intraoral radiography with a conventional machine elsewhere in this chapter.

Maxillary Premolars and Molars: Ventrodorsal Oblique Extraoral Views

Positioning

Position the patient in lateral (side) recumbency, affected side down on the cassette; then rotate the patient so it is placed midway onto its back, in an oblique between the lateral and ventral-dorsal (ventrodorsal [VD]) positions. Ensure the patient is in true lateral by placing a foam wedge or roll under the nose. Place the mandible on a foam wedge, rotating the mandible at a 45-degree angle to the table surface. The mouth should be propped wide open with a radiolucent mouth gag in place (Fig. 22.75).

Comments and Tips

- Make sure the contralateral maxillary teeth and roots do not superimpose against interested maxilla premolars and molars.

MEASURE: Caudal hard palate at commissure of lips.
CENTRAL RAY: Maxillary third premolar.
INCLUDE: Maxillary premolars and molars.

> ✎ **TECHNICIAN NOTES**
>
> The contralateral maxillary premolars and molars appear whiter because of bone superimposition. The affected side's premolars and molars appear magnified because of the angle of the head, causing elongation.

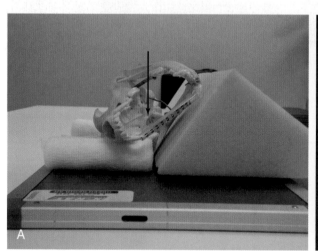 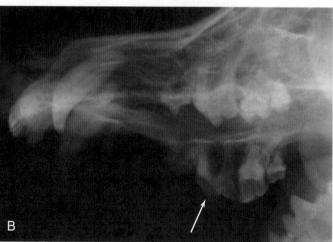

FIG. 22.75 Extraoral technique of maxillary premolars and molars. **A,** Setup. **B,** Radiograph.

Mandibular Premolars and Molars: Dorsoventral Oblique Extraoral Views

Positioning

Position the patient in lateral recumbency with the affected side down on the cassette.

Place the maxilla on a foam wedge, raising the maxilla to a 20-degree angle to the table surface. The mouth should be wide open with a radiolucent mouth gag (Fig. 22.76).

Comments and Tips

- Make sure the contralateral mandibular teeth and roots do not superimpose over the areas of interest, which are the mandibular premolars and molars.

- The contralateral mandibular premolars and molars appear whiter because of the bone superimposition.
- The affected side's premolars and molars appear magnified because of the angle of the head, causing elongation.

MEASURE: Thickness of mandible at the commissure of lips.
CENTRAL RAY: Site of interest.
INCLUDE: Mandibular premolars and molars.

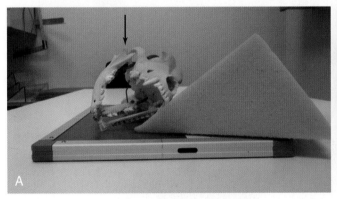
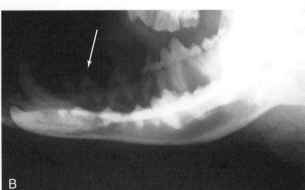

FIG. 22.76 Extraoral technique of mandibular premolars and molars. **A,** Setup. **B,** radiograph.

Maxilla Incisors and Canine: Dorsoventral Intraoral/Occlusal View

Positioning

Position the patient in sternal recumbency. A foam sponge should be placed under the mandible and cassette to keep it parallel to the tabletop. Place one corner of the film cassette into the mouth as far as possible (Fig. 22.77).

Comments and Tips

- Source-image distance (SID) will have to be adjusted because of the raised cassette.

- The roots of the canine teeth will be superimposed over the premolars distal to the canine tooth.
- The rostral nasal sinus cavity can be assessed with this view.

MEASURE: At the level of the commissure of the lips (maxilla thickness).

CENTRAL RAY: Site of interest.

INCLUDE: All incisors and canines, including roots.

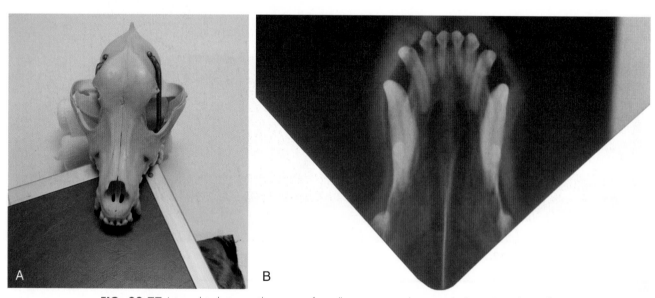

FIG. 22.77 Intraoral technique with cassette of maxillary incisors and canine. **A,** Setup. **B,** radiograph.

Mandibular Incisors and Canine: Ventrodorsal Intraoral/Occlusal View

Positioning
The patient should be positioned in dorsal recumbency with a foam sponge placed under the nose and cervical spine to keep the mandible and cassette parallel to the tabletop. Place one corner of the film cassette into the mouth as far as possible (Fig. 22.78).

Comments and Tips
- Raise the tube head because the SID has decreased.
- The mandibular canine tooth will be slightly superimposed over the first premolar.

MEASURE: At the level of the commissure of the lips (mandible thickness, which is $_1M_1$ in dogs).

CENTRAL RAY: Site of interest.

INCLUDE: All incisors and canines, including roots.

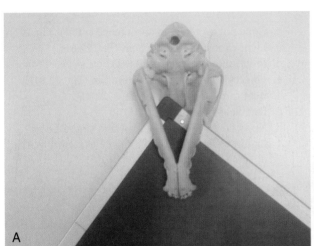
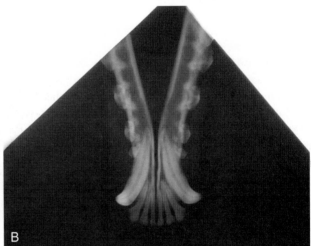

FIG. 22.78 Intraoral technique with cassette of mandibular incisors and canine. A, Setup. B, radiograph.

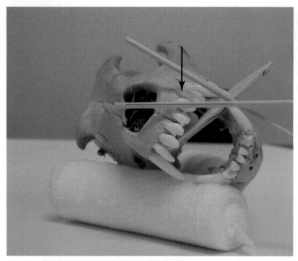

FIG. 22.79 Setup for a radiograph of the canine maxillary premolars using a conventional x-ray machine. Note: Beam comes from straight above.

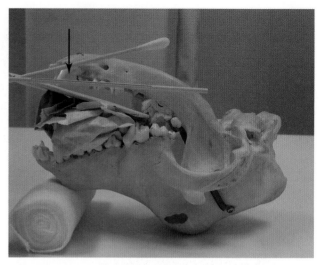

FIG. 22.80 Setup for a radiograph of the canine mandibular incisors using a conventional x-ray machine. Note: Beam comes from straight above.

Intraoral Dental Radiography With a Conventional Machine

If a dental radiography machine is not available, the intraoral radiographs previously described can be accomplished with a conventional machine. In the descriptions of the intraoral views, the x-ray cone was maneuvered to focus on the bisecting angle or film where indicated. With use of a conventional x-ray machine, the patient's body position and skull must be rotated so the previously described angles will line up with the vertical central ray.

The following procedure and supplies are used with this technique:

- Nonscreen dental film
- Foam wedges or rolls (assortment of sizes)
- SID should be 15 inches from the tabletop
- Settings: 60 to 70 kilovolts (kV), 100 milliamperage (mA), 1.6 milliamperes-seconds (mAs)
- If SID cannot be reduced, the following settings should be used: 40 inches SID, 60 to 70 kV, 100 mA, 3.2 mAs

Any of the previously described views can be accomplished with this technique, as illustrated by two examples. Fig. 22.79 shows a radiographic setup for imaging the maxillary premolars with a conventional machine. The bisecting angle is found as previously described (see Fig. 22.39), but note that in the setup shown, the skull is rotated ventrally so that the vertical central ray is aimed at the bisecting angle. In Fig. 22.80, the mandibular incisors are imaged with a conventional machine. The patient is in dorsal recumbency with a small foam wedge placed under the nose. This positioning allows the central ray to be directed at the bisecting angle.

Errors in Film Placement and Artifacts

Some common errors in film placement (not including previously described elongation and foreshortening) are as follows:

a. Not pushing film in far enough (root cutoff) (Fig. 22.81A)

b. Cone not centered on tooth (cone cutoff) (Fig. 22.81B)
c. Light exposure in darkroom (Fig. 22.81C)
d. Processing errors (Fig. 22.81D)
e. Fingerprints and scratches on film (Fig. 22.81E)
f. Bent film (crescent line) (Fig. 22.81F)
g. Double exposure (Fig. 22.81G)
h. X-ray taken through back of film (Fig. 22.81H)
i. Light exposure on CR PSP plate (haze on top half of image) (Fig. 22.81I)

Radiographs of Abnormal Dental Pathology

Examples of common abnormal pathology found in dogs or cats include the following:

a. Horizontal bone loss (Fig. 22.82A)
b. Vertical bone loss (Fig. 22.82B)
c. Periapical lucency (Fig. 22.82C)
d. Resorptive lesions (Fig. 22.82D)
e. Ankylosis (Fig. 22.82E)
f. Missing teeth (Fig. 22.82F)
g. Unerupted teeth (Fig. 22.82G)
h. Supernumerary teeth (Fig. 22.82H)
i. Complete extraction (Fig. 22.82I)
j. Retained root tip (Fig. 22.82J)

✳ KEY POINTS

1. Dental radiography is essential for a proper assessment of the oral cavity in dog and cat mouths.
2. Dental radiographs can be accomplished in any veterinary hospital, even those without a dental x-ray unit.
3. The bisecting angle technique is used in most areas of dog and cat mouths.
4. Manual processing of films can be a source of many errors.
5. The SLOB rule helps identify specific roots when the x-ray cone is directed obliquely.

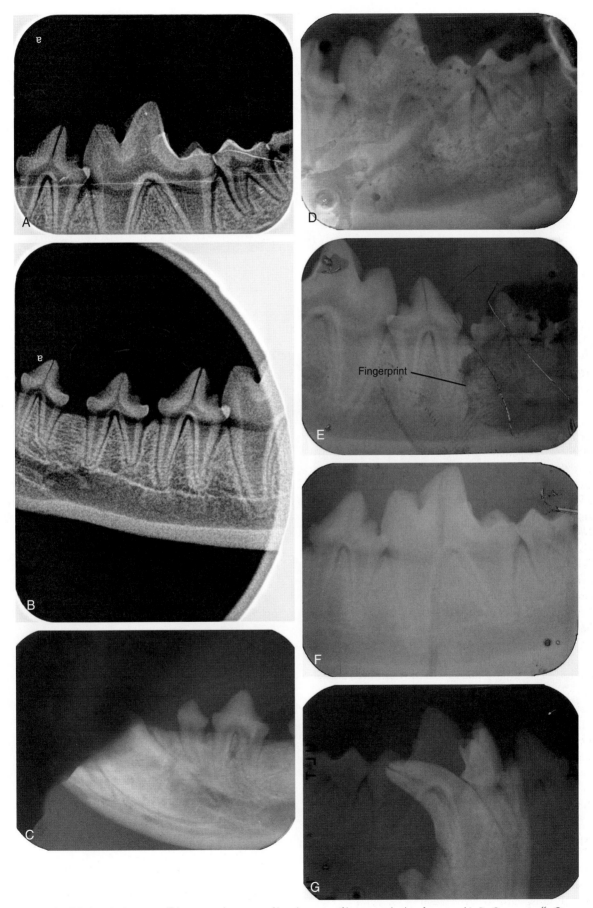

FIG. 22.81 A, Root cut off because of improper film placement (film not pushed in far enough). B, Cone cut off. C, Light exposure in chairside darkroom. D, Film processing error: fixer not rinsed off film. E, Black fingerprints and scratches on film. F, Bent film (crescent line). G, Double exposure.

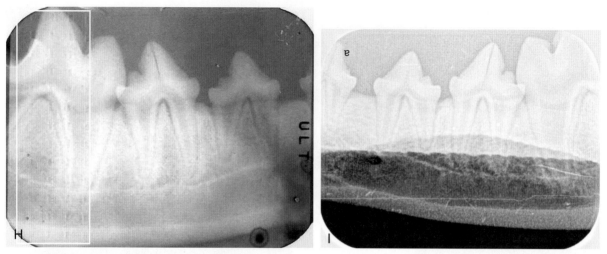

FIG. 22.81, cont'd H, X-ray taken through back of film (note faint checkerboard pattern on left side). **I,** light exposure on CR PSP plate (grey haze).

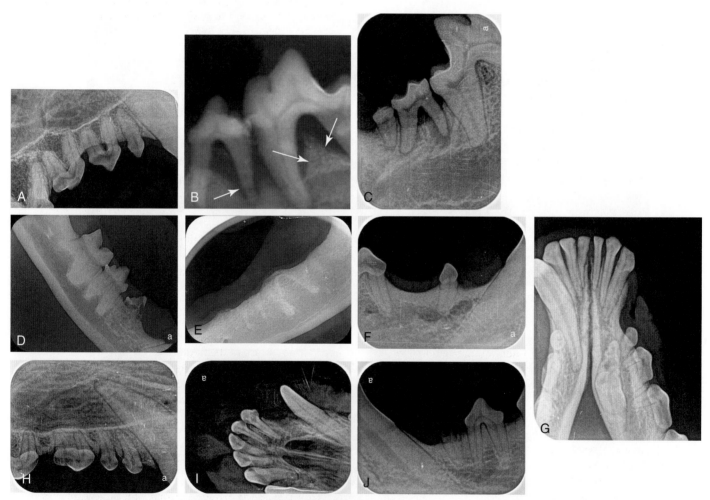

FIG. 22.82 A, Horizontal bone loss evident on 106. **B,** Vertical bone loss (*arrows*). **C,** Periapical lucency on 410. **D,** Feline resorptive lesion 407. **E,** Ankylosis of canine mandibular premolar and molars. **F,** Congenitally missing tooth 406. **G,** Unerupted canine tooth 304. **H,** Supernumerary 105. **I,** Complete extraction of 103. **J,** Retained root tip 305. (Courtesy Dental Vet, Weston, Florida.)

REVIEW QUESTIONS

1. If one used a conventional unit to image a mandible, the kV is likely 45 to 50, yet when using the dental unit for mandibular teeth, the settings are generally preset at 70 or 80. More exposure is required:
   a. Because dental units are high-frequency units
   b. For teeth as compared to the mandible itself
   c. Because there are no intensifying screens in dental film
   d. Because the SID is increased in dental radiography

2. Your clinic has ordered a dental radiography unit, and the veterinarian wishes you to investigate what extra electricity is required. You report that the dental unit requires:
   a. A 110-volt line with no special wiring
   b. A 110 volt-line with special grounding
   c. A 220-volt line with a ground wire
   d. A 220-volt line without special wiring

3. Which part of your new dental x-ray machine can swing 180 degrees?
   a. Scissor arm
   b. X-ray tube
   c. Extension arm
   d. Control panel

4. Direct digital dental radiography in dentistry:
   a. Requires an intermediate step for processing
   b. Is more expensive to buy compared with the other digital system
   c. Generally utilizes a smaller sensor
   d. Utilizes thin and flexible plates similar to regular film

5. CR PSP plates are available in the following size, which is not available in film:
   a. 0
   b. 2
   c. 3
   d. 4

6. You are getting a patient file for the veterinarian to review about a month after dental films were processed. You notice that the films, which were perfectly diagnostic at the time, now appear foggy and have a coffee color appearance with poor density and contrast. You realized that you:
   a. Fixed the film for 15 seconds and dabbed the film in the water jar
   b. Fixed the film for 2 to 4 minutes and washed in running water
   c. Developed for 15 seconds and fixed for 2 to 4 minutes
   d. Used fresh chemicals for processing these films

7. The dental formula for the permanent teeth in the cat is
   a. (3121/3131) = 30
   b. (3131/3121) = 30
   c. (3133/3142 = 42
   d. (3142/3143) = 42

8. A dog has the following three rooted teeth:
   a. 108, 109, 110, 208, 209, 210
   b. 308, 309, 310, 408, 409, 410
   c. $_4^4 P_4^4, _{1,2}^{1,2} M_{1,2}^{1,2}$
   d. 208 and 108 only

9. The area on the periphery of the tooth where the crown and root meet is the:
   a. Dentin
   b. Enamodental junction
   c. Cementoenamel junction
   d. Cementum

10. When x-raying a maxillary canine tooth, what is the angle in which the tube head is moved up vertically to prevent superimposition of the canine tooth over the premolars distal to it?
    a. 20
    b. 30
    c. 15
    d. 45

11. The bisecting angle technique in a dog is used on all of the following areas except:
    a. 303
    b. 409
    c. 204
    d. 105

12. The veterinarian suspects damage of tooth 104 in a Border Collie. You are best to position the patient in:
    a. Right lateral recumbency
    b. Left lateral recumbency
    c. Dorsal recumbency
    d. Ventral recumbency

13. You should utilize the bisecting angle with the long axis of the maxillary canine tooth. This is best visualized from the:
    a. Side of the patient with a 30-degree tilt of the x-ray cone
    b. Side of the patient with a 45-degree tilt of the x-ray cone
    c. Front of the patient with a 30-degree tilt of the x-ray cone
    d. Front of the patient with a 45-degree tilt of the x-ray cone

14. The tips of the teeth should be situated on this size 4 film on the:
    a. Center of the film
    b. Convex side of the film
    c. Away from the convex dot side of the film
    d. Concave side of the film

15. As you are setting up for tooth 104 you notice that the central ray is angled more on the film instead of the bisecting angle. You alter the angle because otherwise you will have:
    a. Foreshortening
    b. Elongation
    c. Magnification
    d. A blurred image

16. You are using the extraoral technique for a mandible of the Lhasa Apso. To isolate the maxillary premolars, you will need to angle the mandible:
    a. 60 degrees
    b. 40 degrees
    c. 20 degrees
    d. 45 degrees

17. A modified x-ray technique is used to x-ray the maxillary premolars in a cat because of interference of which structure?
    a. Palatine fissure
    b. Mandibular symphysis
    c. Zygomatic arch
    d. Nasal sinus

18. The extraoral x-ray technique for a feline's patient tooth 208 (left maxillary premolar) that is preferred is with the patient lying in lateral recumbency and the DR sensor placed:
    a. In the mouth under the right maxillary premolar
    b. In the mouth under the left maxillary premolar
    c. Under the right side of the patient because it is in right lateral recumbency
    d. Under the left side of the patient because it is in left lateral recumbency

19. The beam for this modified x-ray technique of the maxillary premolar should be aimed:
    a. In a parallel technique with the beam 90 degrees to the film
    b. Perpendicular to the film visualized from the front and ventral aspect of the patient
    c. Laterally and the bisecting angle found by standing at the patient's front
    d. In a near-parallel technique with a 20- to 25-degree tilt to bypass the opposite arcade

20. If the x-ray cone is directed from the distal aspect of tooth 108, the root that will appear in the middle on the radiograph is:
    a. The distal root
    b. The mesial-palatal root
    c. The mesial-buccal root
    d. Neither as they will be superimposed

Answers to Review Questions can be found on the Evolve website.

Bibliography

Bellows J. *The Practice of Veterinary Dentistry: A Team Effort.* Iowa City: Iowa State Press; 1999.

Bellows J. *Small Animal Dental Equipment, Materials and Techniques: A Primer.* Iowa City: Blackwell Publishing; 2004.

Derbyshire G. *Veterinary Dentistry for the Nurse and Technician.* St. Louis: Elsevier; 2005.

Emily PP. *Handbook of Small Animal Dentistry.* New York: Pergamon Press; 1990.

Hale F. Veterinary dentistry. Presented at 28th Ontario Association of Veterinary Technicians Conference, Toronto; 2006.

Han C, Hurd C. *Practical Diagnostic Imaging for the Veterinary Technician.* 3rd ed. St. Louis: Mosby; 2005.

Harvey CE. *Small Animal Dentistry.* St Louis: Mosby; 1993.

Holmstrom SE. *Veterinary Dentistry for the Technician and Office Staff.* St. Louis: Saunders; 2000.

Holmstrom SE, ed. *Veterinary Clinics of North America.* Vol. 35, Issue 4. St. Louis: Elsevier; 2005.

Iannucci J, Howerton LJ. *Dental Radiography: Principles and Techniques.* St. Louis: Saunders; 2012.

Mulligan TA. *Atlas of Canine and Dental Radiography.* Yardley, PA: Veterinary Learning Systems; 1998.

Niemic BA. *A Color Handbook of Small Animal Dental, Oral and Maxillofacial Disease.* London: Manson Publishing; 2010.

Piasentin W. Techniques of veterinary dental radiography. *Vet Tech.* 1996;17:419-424.

Tutt D. *BSAVA Manual of Canine and Feline Dentistry.* 3rd ed. Gloucester, UK: British Small Animal Veterinary Association; 2007.

CHAPTER 23

Small Animal Special Procedures*

Marg Brown, RVT, BEd Ad Ed

Do not go where the path may lead, go instead where there is no path and leave a trail.

—Ralph Waldo Emerson, American essayist and poet, 1803–1882

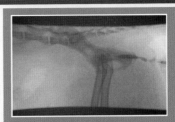

(Courtesy Tara Wochesen, Ontario Veterinary College, Veterinary Teaching Hospital, Diagnostic Imaging at the University of Guelph.)

OUTLINE

LEARNING OBJECTIVES

When you have finished this chapter, you will be able to:

1. Recognize the types of contrast media, including the differences between positive- and negative-contrast media, the physiological effects, the appearances on a radiograph, the indications, and the contraindications.
2. Comprehend the value of proper survey radiographs and patient preparation before the performance of contrast studies.
3. Summarize the procedures and protocols for common contrast studies.

4. Explain other radiographic contrast studies that may be used in practice.
5. Appreciate the other modalities used in addition to or in lieu of contrast studies.
6. Identify normal contrast study anatomy found on a radiograph.

KEY TERMS

Key terms are defined in the Glossary on the Evolve website.

Angiocardiography
Angiography
Antegrade
Arthrography
Barium sulfate
BIPS
Cathartic

Celiography
Contrast medium
Cystography
Dimer
Double contrast
Dyschezia
Esophagography

Excretory urography
Filling defects
Fistulography
Functional study
Gastrography
Granuloma
Iatrogenesis

Inert
Ionic iodine
Lower gastrointestinal (LGI) study
Monomer
Morphological studies
Myelography

---

*Special thanks to Evelyn Kelly, RTR, ACR, RN, BSc, MSc, for her assistance with this chapter in the previous edition.

Negative-contrast agents
Nephrogram
Nonionic iodine
Osmolality
Parasympatholytic agents

Pneumocystogram
Pneumoperitoneography
Positive-contrast agents
Pyelogram
Radiolucent

Radiopaque
Reflux
Retrograde
Tenesmus
Triiodinated compounds

Upper gastrointestinal
  (UGI) study
Urethrography
Vaginocystourethrography
Viscosity

TECHNICAL NOTE: To preserve space, the radiographs presented in this chapter do not show collimation. For safety, always collimate so that the beam is limited to within the image receptor edges. In film radiography, you should see a clear border of collimation (frame) on every radiograph. In some jurisdictions, evidence of collimation is required by law.

Organs or soft tissue structures are often difficult or impossible to identify on plain or survey abdominal radiographs because the tissue densities and atomic numbers of many organs are similar and thus have no natural contrast. Contrast medium introduced into the body changes the density, or atomic number within an organ, to make the tissue or organ visible upon imaging. The introduction of radiolucent or radiopaque media differentiates these structures from the surrounding tissues.

Contrast studies can use either a positive or a negative medium that can be administered to increase the radiographic contrast within an organ or system. In normal radiographic imaging, positive-contrast agents appear white, or radiopaque, on the completed radiograph, whereas negative-contrast agents appear black, or radiolucent.

The desired effect of any contrast substance injected into the body is to cause a difference in density and organ visibility yet still be harmless to the patient.

The agents are administered so that they will either demonstrate the anatomy, by outlining or filling a cavity or organ such as the stomach or urinary bladder, or demonstrate the physiology, by being excreted through an organ such as the kidney. They can be useful in determining the anatomy, such as size, shape, location, position, and contour; defects in the mucosal surface of an organ; the luminal contents; or the presence of extramural lesions. Functional assessment of the organ can be obtained through determining transit time after giving a contrast meal or by injecting a water-soluble organic iodide; however, this is more time consuming and detailed.

With any procedure there are contraindications. To minimize risks, certain questions must be asked before administration of a contrast agent. Depending on the procedure, the veterinarian needs to determine whether the contrast study will be useful, whether it is the best diagnostic tool, and whether it will furnish sufficient information to be worthwhile. Risks may be involved, and it has to be determined whether the procedure could harm the patient. The patient may not tolerate fasting, which is usually required, or may not be a good anesthetic risk if anesthesia is recommended. Also, because of the time and costs involved, other diagnostic procedures may be more useful.

Patient preparation, equipment, and technique vary depending on the special procedure.

A contrast study should never replace routine survey radiographs. Survey radiographs performed before the contrast study help determine proper exposure and patient preparation for the contrast study. Settings may need to be increased for positive-contrast studies and decreased for negative-contrast studies from the survey radiograph. The need for contrast media may also be eliminated if a diagnosis can be achieved with a survey radiograph.

These special contrast studies are used to provide information that might not otherwise be available to make a diagnosis, further evaluate the character of a suspected lesion, or determine appropriate treatment.

Endoscopy, ultrasound, and other imaging modalities, when available and feasible, have replaced contrast radiography for many evaluations. Some of these modalities use similar contrast agents.

TECHNICIAN NOTES

- Strategically used positioning aids give the patient the *illusion* that it is being held. A sandbag over the neck and limbs and/or the use of tape/Velcro/ties is essential if the patient is not sedated. Keep talking to your patient while taking the images, gradually stepping back from the primary beam. Be safety conscious at all times.
- Collimate, ensuring that labels/markers are included and borders are visible for every image.
- Quickly go through your mental checklist *before* pushing the exposure button: settings correct; image receptor/machine/grid in position; proper location of markers and identification (if using at this stage); survey radiographs taken, proper preparation; agent administered; correct body part and view; properly centered; borders correct and collimated; thickest part to the cathode; patient properly positioned and restrained so the body part will be parallel to the image receptor and the central ray is perpendicular to both; correct timing; full expiration for abdomen views.

Contrast Media Used for Radiographic Imaging

Positive-Contrast Media

Barium sulfate and water-soluble organic iodides—both ionic and nonionic—are the agents used to produce a positive-contrast image (Fig. 23.1; Table 23.1).

The atomic numbers of barium (56) and iodine (53) are higher than that of tissues and bones. Calcium, an element of bone, has an atomic number of 20.

Barium sulfate is used exclusively for radiographic examination of the gastrointestinal (GI) tract and can be administered orally or rectally. It is an insoluble, white, crystalline substance that is available commercially as a powder, colloid suspension, or paste. When first manufactured, barium separated easily, like chalk in water. Barium is currently refined so that each molecule is covered with a wetting agent to keep the barium in suspension.[1] Proper viscosity is required for the specific area being studied. Esophageal studies require a paste, whereas a thin mixture is needed for a single-contrast enema.

Barium is chemically inert and does not alter normal physiological function. If there is a suspected bowel perforation, the contrast agent of choice is a water-soluble organic iodide.

Water-soluble organic iodides are generally used in intravascular studies or injected into other body cavities. Iodides mix readily with blood or other body fluids and are excreted through the kidneys. The iodine atoms in the contrast medium molecule are the primary attenuators of the x-ray beam, so the concentration of the iodine in the contrast agent is important. A higher iodine concentration shows more contrast on an image.

The two major types of iodinated contrast media are ionic and nonionic. The media whose molecules dissociate and cause changes in osmolality are termed *ionic,* and the media whose molecules remain whole in solution are termed *nonionic.*[1]

Water-soluble organic ionic iodides are triiodinated compounds derived from the benzoic acid ring structure. (See further images on the website.) These compounds are called *ionic* because an anion (negative) and cation (positive) make up each compound; when they dissociate, the ions are dispersed, changing the osmolality of the solution they are in.

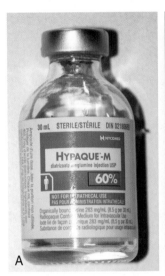
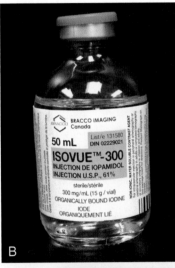
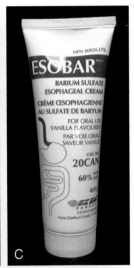
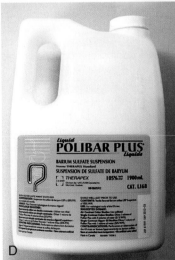
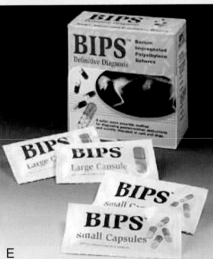

FIG. 23.1 Positive contrast media: A, Ionic iodine. B, Nonionic iodine. C, Barium paste. D, Barium suspension E, Barium-impregnated polyurethane spheres (BIPS).

TECHNICIAN NOTES

- Osmosis is the movement of water through a semipermeable membrane from a liquid of low concentration to one of a higher concentration until the two concentrations are equal.
- Osmotic pressure is the pressure of a solution against a semipermeable membrane to prevent water from flowing inward across that membrane. It is determined solely by the concentration of dissolved particles.
- An osmole is the unit of measurement that refers to the number of moles of a compound that contributes to this osmotic pressure of a solution.
- Osmolality is the number of osmoles of solute per kilogram of solvent and is usually expressed as mOsmol/kg (milliosmoles/kg). (Osmolarity is the concentration of the osmotic solution and is expressed as mOsm/L.)
- Tonicity is the measure of this osmotic pressure.

- A solution can be described as having an osmotic pressure or equilibrium that does not cause osmosis between the blood vessels and the surrounding fluids. This is an isosmolar fluid, and it has the same osmolality as the plasma, so there will be no water exchange.
- A hyperosmolar or hypertonic fluid will have a higher osmolality than the plasma, and thus liquid will be pulled into the plasma.
- A hypotonic or hyposmolar fluid will have a lower osmotic pressure than plasma, so water will leave the plasma.
- A centipoise (cPs) is the unit used to describe the viscosity of a solution. It is one hundredth of a poise and is the amount of force needed to move one layer of liquid in relation to another liquid.

TABLE 23.1	Positive Contrast Agents for Gastrointestinal (GI) Studies in Animals[4-7]		
CONTRAST AGENT	**USES**	**ADVANTAGES**	**DISADVANTAGES**
Barium Sulfate Suspensions			
Trade name(s): • Liquid Polibar Plus • Esobar esophageal cream (60% w/w)	Routine GI contrast studies—use only rectally or orally. Do not use if a GI perforation is suspected.	Low cost Palatable Delineates the mucosal walls well Excellent opacity Remains in suspension Does not become diluted with secretions Not absorbed through the intestines Good density	Slow to be transmitted Insoluble—cannot use with perforation Aspiration in lung can be fatal, although small amounts are usually benign Very irritating to the peritoneum Can hide mucosal surfaces during surgical or endoscopic procedures Blocks ultrasound waves
• Barium sulfate USP powder	Not recommended.	Inexpensive	Flocculates, poor mucosal detail
Characteristics of or Concerns or Comments About Barium			
• Radiodense • Physiologically inert • Resists dilution • Completely insoluble • If leaked into peritoneal cavity, may induce granulomas or adhesions • Hygroscopic nature absorbs water from the bowel, so may cause a bowel obstruction from barium impaction in debilitated patients			
Ionic Iodine			
Oral Organic Iodine—Ionic Solution			
Type, trade name(s) • Common oral forms: meglumine diatrizoate and sodium diatrizoate (Gastrografin)	Suspected intestinal perforation or obstructions	Rapid transit time Nonirritating to serosal surfaces and peritoneum Readily absorbed from peritoneal cavity if leakage Can be absorbed across the mucosa and excreted by the urinary tract	Has a bitter taste Expensive in comparison with barium suspension Hypertonicity can cause: • Fluid movement into the lumen (osmotic diarrhea) • Dilution of the contrast medium • Electrolyte imbalance • Dehydration • Nausea, vomiting • Decreased blood pressure

TABLE 23.1	Positive Contrast Agents for Gastrointestinal (GI) Studies in Animals[4-7]—cont'd		
CONTRAST AGENT	**USES**	**ADVANTAGES**	**DISADVANTAGES**
Injectable Organic Iodine—Ionic Solution			
Type, trade name(s) • IV: Sodium diatrizoate (Hypaque); meglumine diatrizoate (Hypaque M) • Iothalamate meglumine (Conray)	Intravenous (IV) injections for urinary radiography, infusion in hollow organs	Less viscous	The hypertonicity effects listed earlier are more likely to occur after rapid IV bolus, causing peripheral vasodilation and bradycardia due to increased parasympathetic activity Irritating to the brain and spinal cord Can cause toxicity and tissue irritability (e.g., in kidney, bladder)
Characteristics of or Concerns or Comments About Ionic Iodine			
• Diatrizoates provide opacification for excretory urography. Because they are water soluble and absorbed into the bloodstream, hypertonicity is a real concern, especially with sodium diatrizoate. They cannot be used for pyelography. • Rapid IV administration is more likely to initiate the vasovagal response that can cause nausea and brief retching or vomiting.[5]			
Injectable Organic Iodine—Nonionic Solution			
Type, trade name(s) • Iohexol (Omnipaque) • Iopamidol (Isovue) • Ioversol (Optiray) • Iopromide (Ultravist) • Iotrolan (Isovist, Osmovist) • Ioxilan (Oxilan) • Nonionic dimer iodixanol (Visipaque)	Myelography. Can be used IV, especially for young or debilitated patient	Fewer side effects than with ionic form—rapid transit time Nonirritating Resorbed after extraluminal leakage Does not become increasingly dilute Endoscopy and ultrasonography will not be impaired if a contrast study is first completed	Expensive
Characteristics of or Concerns or Comments About Nonionic Iodine			
• Low osmolarity and chemical nature • Nonionic dimer contrast media is virtually isotonic with blood and cerebrospinal fluid			
Radiopaque Markers			
Trade name • BIPS	Determine orocolic transit rate Note obstructive disease	Easy to administer Not likely to be aspirated or to cause peritonitis Can be given with food Time frame for radiographs not as important Do not obscure abdominal detail More likely to detect motility disorders	Cannot visualize mucosal detail or luminal margins Expensive in comparison with barium suspension Studies can take longer
Characteristics of or Concerns or Comments About BIPS			
• If delayed emptying occurs, the cause will not be known • Do not use barium-impregnated spheres (BIPS) for 24-48 hours after barium suspension			

The cation is a salt, usually sodium (Hypaque) or meglumine (Conray), or a combination of the two. Sodium is slightly more toxic than either the meglumine or the combination. The salts increase the solubility of the compound.

The cation is combined with a negatively charged component called an *anion*. The benzene ring with three iodine atoms attached, plus other chemical components (side chains),

makes up the anion. Diatrizoate and iothalamate are common anions.

In an ionic contrast medium, there are three iodine atoms to two particles in the solution, which will give a 3:2 ratio (3 components of the iodine: 1 positive cation + 1 negative ion), resulting in higher osmolality. These are referred to as *high-osmolar contrast agents (HOCAs)*. The higher the osmolality, the greater the risk of anaphylactic reactions. These contrast agents can have an osmolality above 1500 mOsm/kg water, whereas normal serum or plasma osmolality is between 290 and 330 mOsm/kg water. The normal osmolalities of the sera of humans and dogs are relatively equivalent.

In the water-soluble organic nonionic iodide contrast agent, the ionizing carboxyl group is replaced with a group such as amide or glucose that does not dissociate into ions. This lack of dissociation differentiates ionic from nonionic iodide contrast agents.

When dissolved in water, a nonionic compound forms with each molecule containing three iodine atoms, for a ratio of 3:1 (3 iodine: 1 nondissociating molecule). Due to their nonionizing nature, these contrast media are referred to as *low-osmolality contrast agents (LOCAs),* and therefore they do not increase the osmolality of the blood plasma. The nonionic contrast agent is closer to being isotonic and is therefore better tolerated by the body, causing fewer anaphylactic reactions, although it is more viscous and more expensive to purchase.

Intravascular contrast media molecules are also classified according to a second characteristic—monomer versus dimer. Both ionic and nonionic contrast agents come in a monomer form (one benzene ring) and a dimer form (two benzene rings). The osmolality is reduced when there are more iodine molecules.

The ionic monomer has the highest osmolality, and the nonionic dimer has the lowest osmolality (280 mOsm/kg water). When low-osmolar agents are administered intravenously (IV), they cannot cross an intact blood–brain barrier and are excreted via glomerular filtration through the kidneys, causing fewer side effects.[2] Fewer side effects mean greater patient comfort.

See Table 23.2 for further comparisons among positive-contrast media used for radiographic imaging. Trade names and concentrations constantly vary.

✎ TECHNICIAN NOTES

The most isotonic iodine contrast media currently on the market are the water-soluble organic nonionic dimers.

Physiological Effects of Intravenous Contrast Media

If the contrast medium has a high osmolality, water will move into the vessels, both from the extravascular tissues and from the red blood cells. The red blood cells begin to shrink, or crenate. With crenation, circulating blood volume and peripheral blood flow increase; systemic vascular resistance and blood pressure decrease.

All of this happens because of the introduction of a solution such as organic ionic iodine that has a higher concentration (hyperosmolar) than blood. Peripheral vasodilation due to increased parasympathetic activity, produced by the injection of a contrast medium, is thought to be the primary cause of the accompanying pain, discomfort, and flushing.

Many of the side effects of using ionic and nonionic contrast media have been alleviated with the introduction of the ionic and nonionic dimers, which have lowered the osmolality of contrast media to an almost isosmolar level. When an isotonic contrast agent is used, the discomfort and flushing are reduced. *Isotonic* means that the osmolalities or concentrations of the two fluids (contrast media and blood) are the same relative to each other.

Many of the adverse physiological effects of contrast media can be related to osmolality, but there are other factors to consider as well, such as viscosity. *Viscosity* refers to the resistance of fluid to flow. This influences the injectability or delivery of the contrast agent. Nonionic dimers such as iodixanol (Visipaque) have the lowest osmolality but the highest viscosity of the water-soluble organic iodides. This means that the solution will pass slowly through the syringe. Warming the solution decreases the viscosity. The thinner the liquid, the lower the viscosity and cPs (water at 21 °C [70 °F] is about 1cPs) (see Table 23.2).

The clearance or elimination of the molecules of injectable contrast media occurs primarily by glomerular filtration and renal clearance. The speed of elimination depends on the glomerular filtration rate, but virtually 100% of the contrast agent will be out of the body in 24 hours. None of the molecules are reabsorbed or secreted by the renal tubules.

In the case of complete cessation of renal function, breakdown and elimination take place through the liver and gut

---

TABLE 23.2	Chemical Structure and Physiochemical Properties of Iodine-Based Contrast Agents					
CHEMICAL STRUCTURE	**OSMOTIC CLASS**	**REPRESENTATIVE COMPOUNDS**	**OSMOLALITY (mOsm/kg)**	**VISCOSITY (cPS*AT 20 °C)**	**VISCOSITY (cPS AT 37 °C)**
Ionic					
Monomer	High osmolality	Diatrizoate, meglumine, metrizoate (Renografin, Conray, Hypaque, Isopaque)	1400-1800	6	4
Dimer	Low osmolality	Ioxaglate (Hexabrix)	600	15	8
Nonionic					
Monomer	Low osmolality	Iohexol (Omnipaque), iopamidol (Isovue), Ioversol (Optiray), iopromide (Ultravist)	600-850	9-21	5-10
Dimer	Iso-osmolality	Iodixanol (Visipaque)	280	27	12

*cPS, centipoise is a unit to describe the viscosity of a solution.

at a much slower rate. The thyroid and liver retain about 1.5% of the contrast media, which can result in elevation of blood values after a procedure.

Nuclear medicine scans of the thyroid should not be attempted after a contrast medium injection because the results will be inaccurate.

Negative- and Double-Contrast Media
Negative-Contrast Media

Negative-contrast media are the low–atomic number or low-density agents such as air, nitrous oxide, oxygen, and carbon dioxide. These substances absorb fewer x-rays than soft tissue and appear dark or radiolucent on the radiograph. This effect enhances the contrast between the soft tissues. There is less mucosal detail with the use of negative-contrast than with positive-contrast media, but double-contrast media does assist in mucosal detail.

Oxygen and carbon dioxide are more soluble than water. Be careful not to overinflate organs such as the bladder, especially if using room air, because air embolism leading to cardiac arrest can result if an organ ruptures or if there are ulcerative lesions.[3-5] Symptoms will develop immediately, and severity depends on volume and extent of embolism. If any unexplained symptoms are noted, place the patient in left lateral recumbency and elevate the caudal portion of the body immediately to trap the gas in the right ventricle. Further treatments will likely be required.

Double-Contrast Procedures

Double-contrast procedures utilize both positive-contrast and negative-contrast agents to image an organ, commonly the urinary bladder, stomach, or colon. To avoid air bubbles in an organ such as the bladder, which can be misinterpreted as lesions, the negative-contrast medium is generally administered first, followed by the positive-contrast agent.

Gastrointestinal Tract Studies
Patient and Other Preparation

1. Patient preparation is essential.
2. Actual preparation does vary slightly according to the procedure, but generally the area that is being radiographed should not have any radiodense artifacts, such as food, bowel contents, and gas, that could be misdiagnosed as lesions or abnormalities.
   a. The patient should be fasted so that the GI tract is emptied.
   b. A cathartic or enema should be administered in a timely manner to minimize gas production.
3. Make sure the hair coat is clean and dry with no mats.
4. Any sedation or anesthetics given need to be taken into account if transit time for the contrast agent through the GI tract is of concern. Anticholinergics such as atropine decrease GI time.
5. It is essential to take a survey radiograph before giving contrast media to ensure that the procedure is still necessary and that the proper radiation techniques are utilized.

6. Along with proper preparation of the patient, it is important to give the correct amount of contrast medium to properly coat or distend the organ as required.
7. Another error is not taking enough radiographs in the proper sequence. Imagine judging a book by reading the front and back covers and perhaps a few pages in the middle. For accurate diagnosis of the stomach, all four views (ventrodorsal [VD], dorsoventral [DV], and right and left lateral views) should be imaged. Depending on the study, oblique views or abdominal compression may be required. The views must be properly positioned and centered and must include the appropriate landmarks.
   See Chapter 16 to review the positions of the abdomen and common anatomy.

Indications for Gastrointestinal Studies

Special studies of the GI tract are usually completed when there are concerns about vomiting, diarrhea, constipation, hematochezia, melena, abdominal mass, abdominal pain, foreign bodies, or postabdominal trauma. In the study, the barium is administered, and the GI tract is generally evaluated for morphological changes, blockages, and functional changes such as the rate of gastric emptying or small bowel transit time.

Contraindications

Special studies should not be completed if the patient has a fluid-filled, distended esophagus (Fig. 23.2) or stomach or if the bowel is atonic. Patients with ileus due to torsion (Fig. 23.3) or other conditions are not good candidates.

Contrast Agents

The suspension form of barium is the positive-contrast agent generally used because its particles do not flocculate or separate. The barium sulfate does settle upon standing, so the suspension should be shaken before use.

Barium sulfate is not hypertonic and does not increase the intraluminal fluid.

A disadvantage is the slow transit time through the small bowel. Chilling the barium sulfate for an upper gastrointestinal (UGI) study does speed up the transit time; however, for a

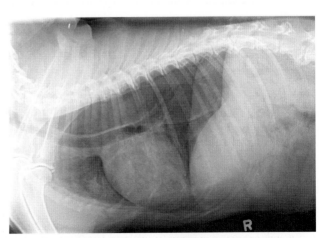

FIG. 23.2 Lateral thorax showing megaesophagus. If megaesophagus is to be evaluated, the esophagus should be emptied before administration of a contrast agent. (Courtesy Mount Pleasant Veterinary Hospital.)

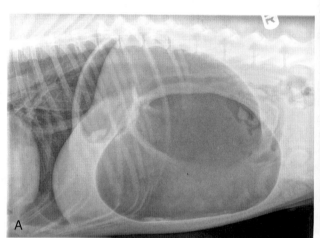
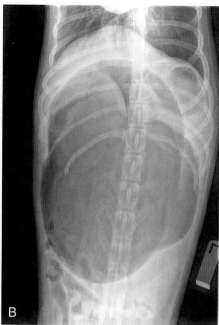

FIG. 23.3 Gastric torsion. Note the characteristic double bubble. **A,** Right lateral abdomen. **B,** Ventrodorsal abdomen. (Courtesy Secord Animal Hospital.)

lower gastrointestinal (LGI) study, it is more comfortable for the patient if barium temperature is between room and body temperature.

Barium is not sterilely produced, and once the container is open, there is a possibility for contamination to occur. Any equipment that is reused, such as a reservoir-type container, enema tube, or syringes, must be thoroughly cleaned and sterilized before use.

If there is a perforation of the bowel, a combination of diatrizoate meglumine and diatrizoate sodium (Gastrografin) iodinated water-soluble organic iodine can be used.

Nonionic compounds are safer than ionic agents because they are more isosmolar, so they draw less fluid into the bowel with minimal dilution of the contrast agents. The hyperosmolality of the solution and the resulting complications that could arise with use in dehydrated patients or those with severe electrolyte imbalance need to be considered. The high cost of nonionic compounds limits their use to mostly small patients.

> **✎ TECHNICIAN NOTES**
>
> - To decrease the viscosity of organic nonionic dimer iodine solutions such as iodixanol, warm the solution before use.
> - Chill barium to quicken the transit time in UGI studies.
> - For LGI studies, have the solution at room to body temperature for patient comfort.

Esophagram

Contrast radiography of the esophagus, or esophagography, is often needed to accurately identify lesions or further characterize survey radiographic findings (Box 23.1). It is

> **✎ TECHNICIAN NOTES**
>
> To convert kg to lb, multiply by 2.2. Thus 10 kg is basically 22 lb and 40 kg is 88 lb.
>
> For dilution of contrast medium, saline is best, especially for barium studies. To calculate the dilution, it is easiest to use either a ratio and proportion method or a fraction method.
>
> For example: You need to use 120 mL of a final dilution of 20% barium. The initial barium sulfate comes as a 60% concentrated solution. How much of the concentrated barium will you use, and how much diluent will you need?
>
> *Ratio and proportion method:*
>
> Final diluted percentage : Initial concentration
> = Volume needed : Final volume administered
>
> $$20\% : 60\% = X : 120 \text{ mL}$$
>
> *Fraction method:*
>
> $$\frac{\text{Final diluted percentage}}{\text{Initial concentration}} = \frac{\text{Volume needed}}{\text{Final volume administered}}$$
>
> $$\frac{20\%}{60\%} = \frac{X}{120 \text{ mL}}$$
>
> In both cases, now continue as:
>
> $$(20)(120) = X(60)$$
>
> $$60X = 2400$$
>
> $$X = 40 \text{ mL of the concentrated barium needed}$$
>
> Because you will use 120 mL total volume with 40 mL of concentrated solution, you need 80 mL of diluent (120 − 40 = 80).

BOX 23.1 | Esophagram Contrast Study Procedure

Indications

- Dysphagia, regurgitation of undigested food, acute gagging or retching, excessive salivation, megaesophagus (see Fig. 23.2), abnormal swallowing, esophageal dysfunction, and foreign bodies are all indications for esophagography.
- The double-contrast study evaluates morphological abnormalities such as mucosal abnormalities, intraluminal foreign bodies, and partial strictures or stenosis.

Precautions or Contraindications

- Patients with dysphagia may aspirate the contrast agent.
- It may not be necessary to add contrast media to a dilated, fluid-filled, or food-filled esophagus because enough contrast may be present for visualization of lesions or abnormalities.
- If asphyxiation is a concern, barium sulfate paste should not be used.
  - Consider the use of organic iodine preparation in cases of perforation.
  - Do not use if known allergy or sensitivity to contrast agents.

Contrast Media and Dosage

- The dosage is 5-20 mL 60% w/v barium sulfate suspension liquid or paste (preferred), depending on the size of the patient to induce several swallows.[6]
- A barium meal can be used by mixing 1 cup dry kibble with 20 mL barium sulfate suspension for dog and half of each for cats.[6]
- For oral aqueous iodine solution (Gastrografin): mix 1:2 and give 5-15 mL depending on the patient size.

Equipment and Supplies

- Large-dose syringe
- Optional—canned food or kibble

Patient Preparation

- Remove collar, clean hair coat.
- Fast if further GI studies to be completed.

Positions

- Generally lateral, pulling downward limb more cranial and upper limb caudal (minimize brachium musculature over thoracic inlet).
- VD or VD oblique optional.

Borders

- Full length of esophagus (atlantooccipital junction (oropharynx) to T12 (cranial portion of stomach).

Procedure for Positive-Contrast Esophagram

1. Expose survey radiographs—lateral and VD.
2. Position the patient in lateral recumbency on the x-ray table.
3. Place paper towels on tabletop or towels around the patient's mouth and neck.
4. Slowly infuse the barium into the buccal pouch. Close the mouth and wait for the patient to swallow.
5. Take serial radiographs of the patient in lateral recumbency—the right is usually easier for the positioner.
6. Administer additional barium or barium-soaked kibble in the buccal pouch. Close the mouth and wait for the patient to swallow.
7. Obtain further lateral radiographs if required, or place the patient in ventral recumbency for VD or oblique views as required. The oblique projections avoid superimposition of the esophagus over the spine (see Chapter 16 for positioning).
8. If a lesion has been noted by esophagoscope or with the passage of a tube, a partial esophagram can be made: gently pass the tube until the point of the abnormality, and administer barium sulfate at the site.

Procedure for Double-Contrast Study Esophagram

1. Obtain survey radiographs and perform an esophageal study using liquid barium suspension as described previously.
2. Pass a stomach tube through an oral speculum if required. Avoid forcing the tube through partial obstructions.
3. Perform a lateral radiograph to confirm the placement of the tube in case the tip of the tube needs to be readjusted for study of a specific portion of the esophagus.
4. Attach a syringe and inject barium sulfate, 3-5 mL for a small dog or cat and 8-10 mL for a large dog.
5. Keeping the patient in lateral recumbency, attach an air syringe and inject 20-30 mL of air for a small dog or cat and 40-50 mL of air for a large dog.
6. Immediately radiograph the dorsal thorax.
7. Reposition the patient in sternal recumbency. Repeat the air injection and radiograph immediately.

Comments and Tips

- Avoid getting contrast medium on the patient, image receptor, and table, as the artifacts may interfere with the diagnosis.
- Iodine should be used if endoscopy is to follow, as the barium will obscure the mucosa.
- The patient is usually sedated or anesthetized for the double-contrast study.
- This is usually completed after gastrography, after the stomach tube is retracted to the esophagus.
- If there is gastroesophageal reflux, further barium sulfate suspension is not needed. Administer only the air.
- A very small amount of aspirated barium sulfate is generally well tolerated in healthy lungs and cleared from the airways within 24 hours.[4]
- Oropharyngeal issues are best evaluated in the midst of a swallow and during a pause after completion of the swallow.
- Oblique views may eliminate superimposition of the spine and sternum for better visualization of the esophagus.

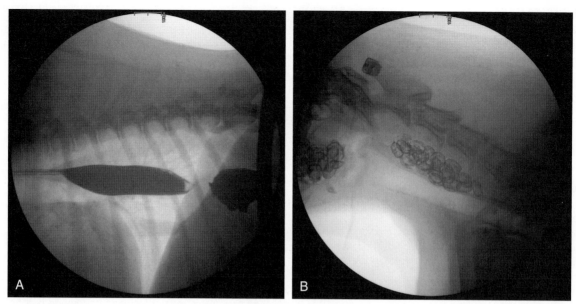

FIG. 23.4 A barium swallow during an esophageal study utilizing fluoroscopy. Note the reversal of the densities from regular radiography. The barium is darkest, and the bones are also black. The trachea is white, as is the spinal cord. **A,** Liquid barium swallow. **B,** Barium meal swallow. (Courtesy of Carolyn Bennet, OVC.)

best used to evaluate morphological or structural alterations of the esophagus. Dynamic imaging such as fluoroscopy is recommended for specific evaluation of functional abnormalities (Fig. 23.4).

Upper Gastrointestinal Study

The patient is given the contrast medium orally, and images are taken during the transit of the contrast medium through the stomach and small bowel and into the colon as required.

See Box 23.2 and Table 23.3 for the full procedure, although actual timing and centering depend on the patient's condition.

Morphological studies of the stomach and intestines are made to examine (1) the size, shape, and position of the organs; (2) the character of the stomach wall and the stomach contents; or (3) extramural, mural, or intramural lesions of the GI tract. Gastric motility and pyloric and intestinal function can be determined by noting gastric and intestinal emptying, keeping in mind that the times vary, depending on the size and nature of the test meal. Functional studies are performed slightly differently from morphological ones. Sedation or anesthesia affects transit time in functional studies.

Barium food mixture studies have also been completed to further evaluate gastric function. There appears to be evidence that there is a wide range of normal gastric emptying times. Unless there are gross abnormalities, a barium solid food meal is not useful. Barium-impregnated polyethylene spheres (BIPS, Chemstock Animal Health Ltd., Christchurch, New Zealand) have been used as an alternative to evaluate the emptying of solids in dogs and cats (see Fig. 23.1E).

Endoscopy is an alternative modality that can be used, although it is difficult to adequately access the mesenteric small intestine with the endoscope. Ultrasonography can often provide diagnostic information about the small bowel, negating the need for a contrast radiographic study.

✎ TECHNICIAN NOTES

- To minimize artifacts, always make sure that the patient has a clean, dry hair coat, with no traces of contrast medium. Remove the collar if cranial body radiographic views are to be taken.
- Make sure to give the complete volume for proper distention of the lumen for a diagnostic barium study.
- Before administering the barium, have everything ready, such as the image receptors in position, technique set, protective gear, patient near the table, etc. Make sure to minimize barium spillage, and thus artifacts, if administering the barium with the patient on the table.
- When using an orogastric tube, make sure that placement in the esophagus has been verified. Before removing the tube, clear it with a small amount of air, and kink the tube to minimize aspiration into the lungs.
- The UGI is complete when the barium is in the colon. To avoid technical errors, make sure you take survey radiographs, properly prepare the patient, use the correct exposures, center the beam correctly, place the tube in the stomach, use the correct volume, and take the required number and proper sequence of radiographs.

TABLE 23.3	Upper Gastrointestinal Tract Positive-Contrast Film Sequence and Typical Structures in Normal Canine and Feline[4-7]

BARIUM	IONIC AND NONIONIC ORGANIC IODINE	STRUCTURES TYPICALLY OPACIFIED IN NORMAL ANIMALS*
Dog		
Immediate	Immediate	Stomach
15 minutes		Stomach begins to empty, duodenum fills
30 minutes	15 minutes	Stomach small amount, duodenum, jejunum
1 hour		Stomach vestigial, duodenum, jejunum filled and reach ileum
1½ -2 hours	30 minutes	Stomach mostly empty, complete small intestine, ileocecal junction
4 hours	1 hour	Small and large intestine
1-4 hours		Stomach empty
3-5 hours		Small intestines empty
Cat		
Immediate	Immediate	Stomach
5-10 minutes	5 minutes	Stomach emptying, duodenum fills
15-20 min		Reach jejunum
30-60 minutes	30 -60 minutes	Complete small intestine, cecum fills
1 hour	1 hour	Small and large intestine
30-60 minutes		Stomach empty
1-3 hours		Small intestines empty

*These are only approximations of the components of the gastrointestinal tract visible at these times, as individual transit times vary greatly.

BOX 23.2	Upper Gastrointestinal Study Procedures[4-7]

Indications
- Recurrent unresponsive vomiting, diarrhea, hematemesis, anorexia, melena, mass lesions, suspected foreign body or obstruction, wall distortions, wall lesions, abdominal organ displacement, chronic weight loss, persistent abdominal pain, and inconclusive results on a survey radiograph.

Precautions or Contraindications
- If rupture or perforation is suspected, use water-soluble organic iodides. In dehydrated patients, avoid the use of such agents.
- Endoscopy or ultrasonography should be considered if available or feasible, especially in compromised patients.
  - Avoid barium if endoscopy or surgery is possible.
- Delay the study if the stomach is filled with ingesta.
- The use of barium in gastric dilatation/volvulus, chronic obstructive bowel disease, and paralytic ileus cases is complicating.
- Gastric distention is not recommended immediately after gastric surgery or deep biopsy.
- Prior use of tranquilizers or other drugs affects the transit time.
  - Avoid parasympatholytic agents and drugs used for treatment in gastrointestinal disorders, which may cause gaseous distention or decrease motility before the contrast study.
  - Use of anticholinergics should be suspended at least 24 hours, though preferably 48-72 hours, before the administration of contrast media.[6]

Contrast Media and Dosage
- Barium sulfate suspension, 60%: dosages vary depending on source. The following tends to be common[4,5]:
  - 8-10 mL/kg for dogs less than 10 kg and cats
  - 5-7 mL/kg for medium-sized dogs, 10-40 kg
  - 3-5 mL/kg for dogs heavier than 40 kg
- Iodine (less than 300 mg/mL)[4]:
  - Dogs 2.0-3.0 mL/kg
  - Cats 1.0- 2.0 mL/kg
- For double-contrast or negative-contrast study:
  - 20 mL/kg via orogastric tube[5]
- Effervescent granules (Baros, E-Z-Gas II)

Equipment/Supplies
- Gastric tube
- Oral speculum
- 50-mL syringe
- Towels

Patient Preparation
- The gastrointestinal tract should be empty so that it does not interfere with interpretation of transit time.
  - Foreign bodies or small gastric and intestinal lesions may be obscured by ingesta.
  - If the patient is not anorectic or vomiting, fast at least 12 hours before administration of the contrast meal.
  - Twenty-four hour fasting is best if mucosal disease of the small intestine is being evaluated.

Continued

BOX 23.2 Upper Gastrointestinal Study Procedures[4-7]—cont'd

- Take lateral and VD radiographs before the administration of an enema.
- If an enema is required, as indicated by the survey radiograph, administer at least 2-4 hours before the procedure to minimize gas artifacts.
- If the patient has severe abdominal stress, fasting, enemas or laxatives are not suggested.
- Perform without sedation, if possible, as motility-altering drugs may affect interpretation.
  - If sedation is required, consider acepromazine in dogs and ketamine/diazepam in cats.[5]

Measure, Center, and Peripheral Borders

- Measure at the thickest part (liver), at the thoracolumbar (TL) junction.
- Center over caudal aspect of 13th rib at level of L2-L3 or over umbilicus for the canine and two to three finger widths caudal to 13th rib for the feline.
- Include about an inch cranial to xiphoid and caudally to the acetabulum.
  - For gastrography and cranial abdomen just include to L5-L6 distally.

Procedure for Positive-Contrast Upper Gastrointestinal Study

1. Using either the buccal pouch and syringe or a gastric tube, administer barium sulfate.
   a. An orogastric tube is preferred with the patient lying on the x-ray table ready for exposure (especially for gastrogram).
2. If completing a gastrogram, immediately take four radiographs centering over the cranial abdomen: ventrodorsal, right and left lateral, and dorsoventral views (Fig. 23.5).
3. 15 minutes after administration: ventrodorsal and right lateral views (Fig. 23.6).
4. 30 minutes after administration: ventrodorsal and right lateral views (Fig. 23.7).
5. 60 minutes after administration: ventrodorsal and right lateral views (Fig. 23.8).
6. Hourly after administration: ventrodorsal and right lateral views until the study is completed (see Fig. 23.9 for a canine image and Fig. 23.10 for a feline image).
7. See Table 23.3 for barium GI times.

Comments and Tips

- The 15-minute radiographs may be eliminated in dogs, depending on the nature of the study, but are highly recommended in cats because of the rapid GI transit time.
- An extra radiograph at 90 minutes may also reveal further information for the cat.
- If gastric and intestinal emptying time is of concern, perform the study early enough in the day to be able to properly complete the procedure.
- If an orogastric tube is not used, barium may leave the stomach before all the agent is administered, meaning that the stomach will not have optimal distention. It is important to give sufficient volume of barium sulfate suspension.
- The gastrogram is finished when the majority of the barium is no longer visible in the stomach. The small bowel study ends when there is little evidence of barium left in the small intestine.

- If the pylorus is of interest, oblique views may be required.
- The rugal folds are best seen on gastric emptying.

Procedure for Double-Contrast Upper Gastrointestinal Study

1. Double-contrast imaging may provide further information primarily for the stomach wall and by allowing further visualization of the gastric location or extramural gastric lesion.
   a. Evaluation of mural and intraluminal gastric lesions may also benefit by the ability to "see through" the stomach.
2. A double-contrast study does not evaluate motility or emptying.
   a. It should not be performed if the patient is not fasted.
3. The patient is best chemically restrained.
4. Complete a routine noncontrast survey.
5. Administer barium sulfate using a gastric tube.
   a. For small dogs use 2 mL/kg; large dogs 1 mL/kg, and cats 6 mL/kg.[5]
2. Attach an air-filled syringe, and administer air until the stomach is distended.
3. Withdraw the tip of the tube into the caudal esophagus or remove completely.
4. Gently rotate the patient to coat the gastric mucosa.
5. Immediately take required views of the stomach: right and left laterals, ventrodorsal, and dorsoventral (Fig. 23.11) if gastrogram is desired; otherwise, a right lateral and VD.
6. Center the beam over the cranial abdomen.
7. Administer further negative-contrast medium if air has been lost by regurgitation or has passed into the small bowel, and repeat the radiographs.

Comments and Tips

- It is difficult to determine the exact dosage. Judge the amount required by noting the resistance to injection of air as well as palpating for the distended stomach.
- Make sure stomach is distended so that the gastric wall will appear thin and uniform.
- Negative-contrast gastrography or a pneumogastrogram can be substituted for a positive-contrast study or a double-contrast study.
  - Follow the same procedure as for the double-contrast study, omitting the barium sulfate.
- If required, the study can be continued as a double-contrast or negative-contrast morphological study of the small intestine:
  - Take lateral and ventrodorsal radiographs at 15 minutes, 30 minutes, 60 minutes, and hourly as required.
  - The distended small bowel can be easily evaluated.
- If inserting a gastric tube is not practical, carbon dioxide–producing granules or spansules that cause effervescence, such as Baros, or E-Z-Gas II, can be substituted for the air in both the double-contrast and negative-contrast studies.
- Place the granules/spansules in the patient's buccal pouch and close the mouth to prevent foam from dissipating before it reaches the stomach.
- Radiograph immediately because the gas produced may be belched.[4,5]
- The procedure in the cat is the same for a double-contrast or negative-contrast morphological study.

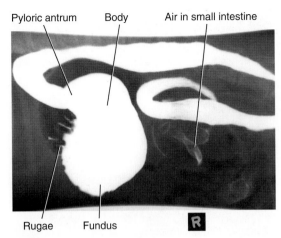

Pyloric antrum   Body   Air in small intestine

Rugae   Fundus

FIG. 23.5 An upper gastrointestinal radiograph taken within minutes of the administration of barium. This is an inverted fluoroscopic image. (Courtesy Tara Wochesen, Ontario Veterinary College, Veterinary Teaching Hospital, Diagnostic Imaging at the University of Guelph.)

Lower Gastrointestinal Study

This procedure is less common due to other modalities such as endoscopy and the low yield of diagnostic information with contrast enema (Box 23.3). The radiographic examination of the cecum, colon, and rectum through retrograde administration of contrast medium generally evaluates extramural masses, mural or larger mucosal lesions, and intraluminal lesions. Smaller mucosal lesions are better determined endoscopically. Disease in the area of ileocolic valves and the ascending and transverse processes is better examined with contrast studies.

For visualization of the entire large bowel and small lesions such as mucosal irregularities, full distention of the area and removal of feces are required. Oral administration of a positive-contrast medium does not fully distend the large bowel, so rectal administration of contrast media is required for certain procedures. Chemical restraint is usually needed, as many patients will not otherwise tolerate rectal infusion (Box 23.3).

Text continued on p. 464

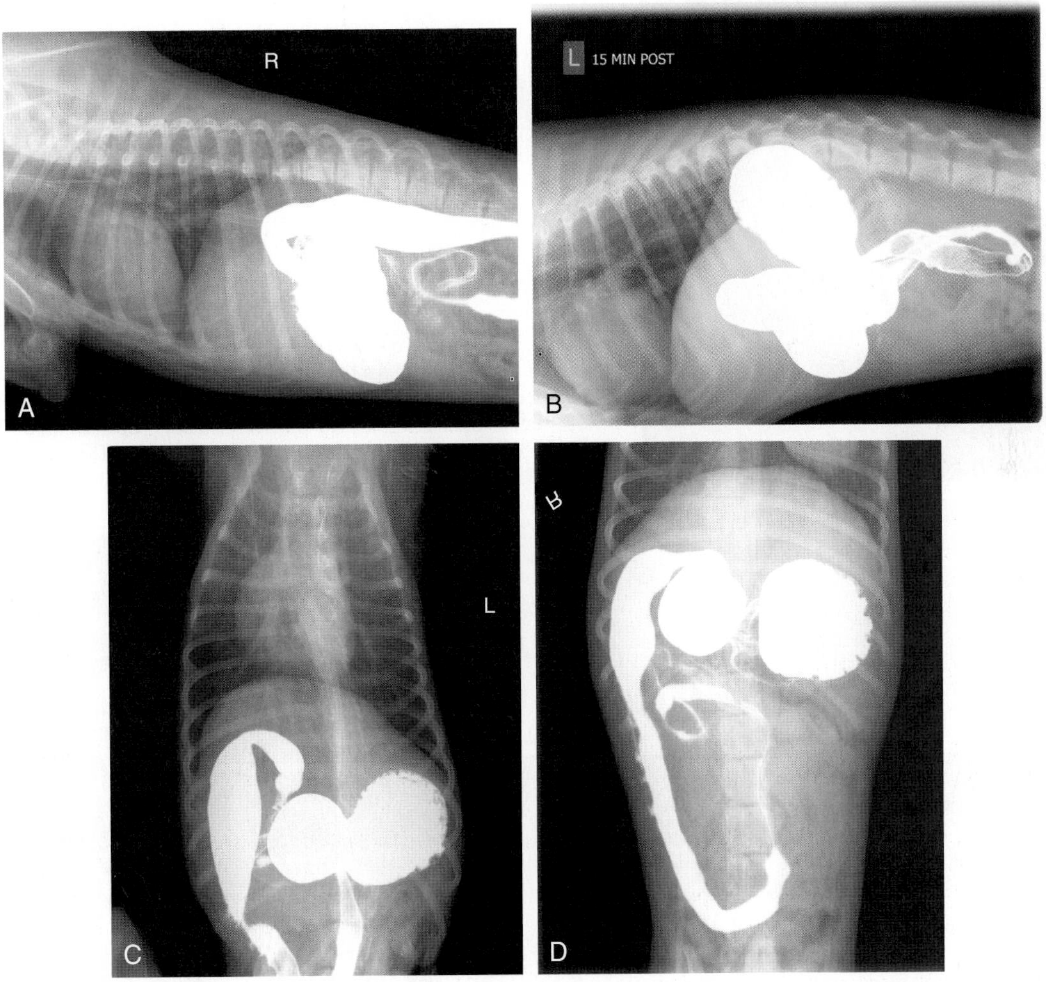

FIG. 23.6 15 minutes after administration of barium in a dog. **A,** Right lateral abdomen. Note that there is gas in the fundus and barium in part of the body and the duodenum. **B,** Left lateral abdomen. There is more gas in the pyloric portion and duodenum in comparison with the right lateral 15-minute exposure. The heart is also more slightly rounded than in the right lateral. **C,** Ventrodorsal abdomen. The gas is in part of the body and pyloric antrum. **D,** Dorsoventral abdomen. The gas rises to the cardia and fundus. The diaphragm has a slightly "bumpier" appearance than in the ventrodorsal view because the trilobed crura are lateral to the central cupula. (Courtesy Tara Wochesen, Ontario Veterinary College, Veterinary Teaching Hospital, Diagnostic Imaging at the University of Guelph.)

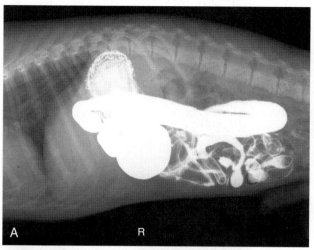

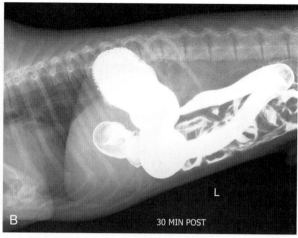

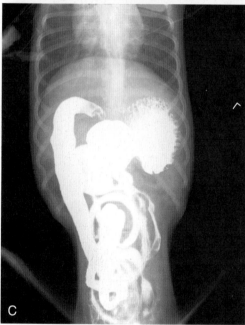

FIG. 23.7 30 minutes after the administration of barium. **A,** Right lateral abdomen. The gas is more evident in the fundus than in the left lateral. **B,** Left lateral abdomen. Gas is more evident in the pyloric antrum. **C,** Ventrodorsal abdomen. Gas is more evident in the pyloric antrum and part of the body. (Courtesy Tara Wochesen, Ontario Veterinary College, Veterinary Teaching Hospital, Diagnostic Imaging at the University of Guelph.)

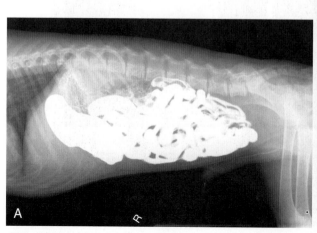

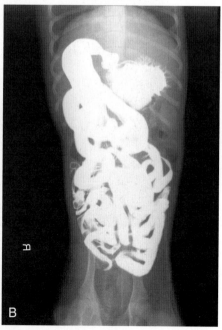

FIG. 23.8 60 minutes after the administration of barium. **A,** Right lateral abdomen. **B,** Ventrodorsal abdomen. (Courtesy Tara Wochesen, Ontario Veterinary College, Veterinary Teaching Hospital, Diagnostic Imaging at the University of Guelph.)

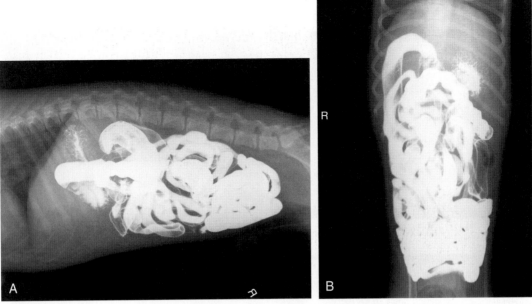

FIG. 23.9 2 hours after the administration of barium. **A,** Right lateral abdomen. **B,** Ventrodorsal abdomen. See the Image Gallery at the end of this chapter for 3 to 6 hours postadministration. (Courtesy Tara Wochesen, Ontario Veterinary College, Veterinary Teaching Hospital, Diagnostic Imaging at the University of Guelph.)

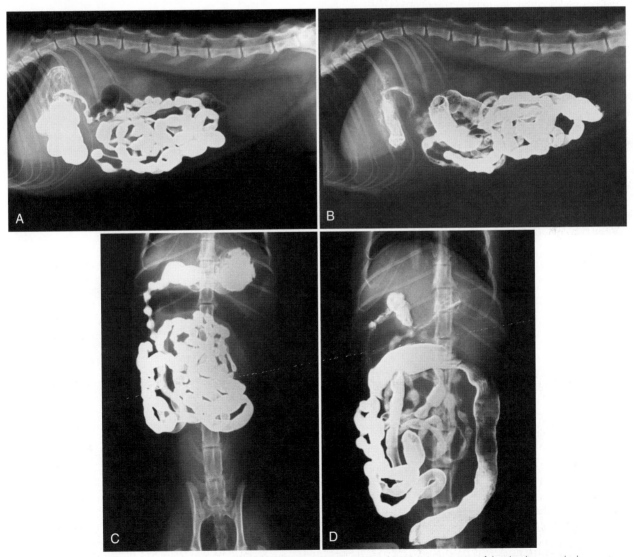

FIG. 23.10 Normal feline upper gastrointestinal series. Note the "string-of-pearls" appearance of the duodenum, which is not uncommon in cats. **A** and **B,** Lateral views made 15 minutes after barium administration. **C** and **D,** Ventrodorsal views made 3 hours after barium administration. (From Han C, Hurd C: *Practical Diagnostic Imaging for the Veterinary Technician,* 3rd ed. St Louis: Mosby; 2005.)

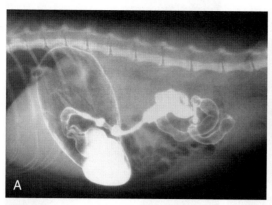
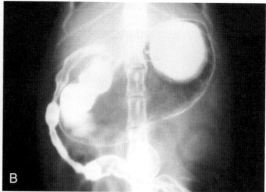

FIG. 23.11 Double-contrast gastrogram. **A,** Lateral view. **B,** Ventrodorsal view.

BOX 23.3 | Lower Gastrointestinal Study Procedures[4-7]

Indications

- Abnormal defecation, especially in combination with excessive mucus or bright red stool, stricture, tenesmus, colonic obstruction, dyschezia, colonic or rectal neoplasia, colitis, and ileocolic intussusception are all indications to complete a barium enema study (Fig. 23.12).
- The barium enema is most indicated when narrowing of the lumen prevents passage of an endoscope, a mural or extramural lesion is suspected, or the mucus is found to be normal endoscopically.

Precautions

- Do not complete a retrograde administration or barium enema if perforation or a known allergy is suspected.
- Barium enemas are not recommended if the patient has had proctoscopy within 12 hours because the wall may be weakened.
- Reflux into the distal small bowel may occur without overdistention.
- Transient spasm may occur if the agent is cold, the wall is irritated by the tube, or narcotic premedication is used.[4]

Contrast Media and Dosage

- 20% barium sulfate brought between room and body temperature.
- Approximate dosage to fill the large intestine administered rectally[4]:
  - 10-20 mL total in a small dog or cat; 30 mL in medium-sized dogs (10-40 kg); 60 mL for dogs heavier than 40 kg.
  - Another source quotes 7-15 mL/kg.[6]
  - Use half the dosage to evaluate the rectum or to partially fill the colon.
- Dosage for double-contrast technique:
  - Dog: 5-10 mL of barium sulfate and 50-200 mL of air.
  - Cat: 2-3 mL of barium sulfate suspension and 25-50 mL of air.
- Dosage for negative-contrast technique:
  - Dog: 60-100 mL of air; cat: 20-30 mL of air.

Equipment/Supplies

- Bardex or Foley catheter for the inflatable cuff
- Syringe/enema bag/can/commercial enema set
- Three-way stopcock valve
- Lubricant
- Compression paddle

Patient Preparation

- The colon should be absent of fecal material if mucosal disease is being studied.
  - No food for 24-36 hours.
  - Water up to 4 hours before the procedure, but make sure the patient is properly hydrated.
- Administer both cathartic and warm-water enemas the previous evening if the disease process has not emptied the gastrointestinal tract. Consider using a low nonsoap enema to stimulate defecation if stool is present. Just before the study, confirm with a warm-water enema that the effluent is clear. Unlike for endoscopy, the colon does not need to be washed clean, but any feces or ingesta in the colon could create confusing artifacts.
- Take survey lateral and VD radiographs of the abdomen if not done so previously. This is best completed 2-4 hours before the procedure.
- Sedate or anesthetize the patient.
- For patients with acute abdominal pain, acute persistent vomiting, or palpable, enlarged, fluid- or gas-filled bowels, no preparation is needed. The gas or fluid may be helpful in diagnosis.
- Endoscopy will likely be more diagnostic than radiographic contrast for this study.

Measure, Center, and Include

- Measure, center, and include as for the small intestinal study.

Procedure for Positive Contrast Barium Enema for Both Dogs and Cats

1. Have the chemically restrained patient on the table.
2. Insert the Foley catheter rectally and inflate the cuff to prevent leakage.
3. Keep the reservoir bag slightly above the tabletop to maximize gravity or use minimum pressure on the syringe.
4. Clamp the tube, stopping the infusion if there is resistance to the flow of the contrast agent.
5. Close off the three-way stopcock.
6. Take ventrodorsal and both right and left lateral radiographs.

BOX 23.3 | Lower Gastrointestinal Study Procedures[4-7]—cont'd

7. Oblique views may be required, especially in males (see Chapter 16 for technique).

8. Process the films, and if no additional contrast agent or radiographs are required, remove as much of the contrast medium as possible before removal of the catheter.

    a. Placing the patient in left lateral recumbency, raising the cranial part of the body, and allowing the barium to drain into the bag placed on the floor may assist removal.

9. Further radiographs may be obtained if desired once the barium is removed.

Comments and Tips

- The catheter should be removed from the rectum away from the x-ray table, preferably above a container near a floor drain.

- Compression of the large bowel may further show the presence of a lesion.

- It is best to give small increments of the barium until the desired effect is seen on the radiographs.

- Soapy water enemas too close to the imaging could irritate the large bowel mucosa, leading to spasms or gas accumulations that could cause radiographic artifacts during a barium enema study.

Procedure for Double-Contrast Large Intestinal Study for Both Dogs and Cats

1. Have the chemically restrained patient on the table.

2. Insert the catheter rectally and inflate the cuff to prevent leakage. Place a three-way stopcock valve at the end of the catheter.

3. Infuse the barium sulfate suspension (2-10 mL; see dosages listed earlier) through the three-way stopcock valve and close the valve.

4. Open the valve, infuse the air, and close the valve.

5. Take ventrodorsal and right and left lateral radiographs.

6. View the images and determine whether additional contrast agents or radiographs are required.

7. Release the stopcock valve. Gently remove as much air and barium as possible before removing the catheter.

    a. Place the patient in left lateral recumbency to minimize effects of air embolism.

    b. Gentle massage of abdomen with catheter in place may aid in removing air from colon.

8. Further images may be obtained if desired, once the barium is removed.

Comments and Tips

- Move the patient to an appropriate location for defecation.

- The amount of air infused can be decreased if distention is not required.

Pneumocolon

- This large intestine negative-contrast study can be used if the colon is not emptied.

- The same procedure is followed as for the double-contrast large intestinal study without barium sulfate.

- Infuse 20-100 mL of air according to the weight of the patient as previously outlined.

Double-Contrast Technique of Ileocecum in Connection With UGI

1. Indicated if the patient is unable to tolerate a conventional barium enema study or if a view of the ileocecal region is required.

2. When the swallowed barium reaches the right ileocolic junction, insufflate the calculated amount of air through a small catheter inserted into the rectum.

3. Inflate the cuff and use a three-way stopcock valve to infuse the air and keep it in the colon.

4. Open the stopcock valve and remove the catheter.

5. Continue the study if required.

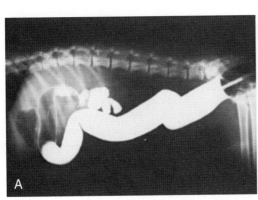
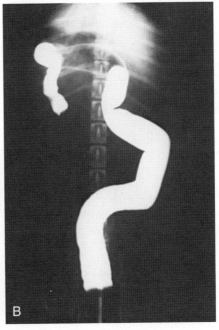

FIG. 23.12 Barium enema. **A,** Lateral view. **B,** Ventrodorsal view.

Use of Barium-Impregnated Polyethylene Spheres

Barium-impregnated polyethylene spheres (BIPS) are inert, low-density, radiopaque spheres designed for evaluation of gastric dysmotility and intestinal transit time in dogs and cats (Box 23.4). The spheres are a mixture of plastic and barium sulfate and come in two diameters: 5-mm spheres to evaluate partial and complete obstruction and 1.5-mm spheres meant to mimic food passage. The number and size of the spheres, fasting period, and type and amount of food will affect the gastric emptying time and orocolic transit. Strict adherence to the manufacturer's suggestions should be followed for a proper functional study. Their advantages and disadvantages in comparison with barium suspension are mentioned in Table 23.1.

✎ TECHNICIAN NOTES

Formula for gastric emptying with use of BIPS
1. Count the number of BIPS that have left the stomach.
2. Calculate as follows:

$$\frac{\text{Number of BIPS that have left stomach}}{\text{Total number of BIPS seen on image}} \times 100 = \%\text{ of BIPS that have left stomach}$$

Formula for orocolic transit rate
1. Count the number of BIPS that are in the colon and calculate as follows:

$$\frac{\text{Number of BIPS in colon}}{\text{Total number of BIPS seen on radiograph}} \times 100 = \%\text{ of BIPS in the colon}$$

BOX 23.4	Use of BIPS[8–11]

Dosage
- The inert spheres are available in capsules of two sizes that can be purchased as 5- or 10-dose packs.
- Give either 1 large orange capsule or 4 small blue capsules (see Fig. 23.1E) (contains 10 large spheres and 30 small spheres).

Patient Preparation
- No food if gastrointestinal obstruction is suspected or there are acute gastrointestinal concerns.
- For chronic gastric emptying or orocolic transit problems, feed with an intestinal diet following the BIPS package insert.
- Sedatives and drugs influence gastrointestinal motility.

Procedure for Use of BIPS
1. Right lateral and a ventrodorsal simultaneously at each time period.
2. Follow standard abdominal protocol to include the complete abdomen.
3. Generally imaging is 6-24 hours after administration, if the capsules are given on an empty stomach, to rule out pyloric and small intestinal blockage (Fig. 23.13).
4. For chronic vomiting or diarrhea, generally image 8 hours after food and the capsules are administered to detect delayed gastric emptying.
5. Actual times are not crucial, but it is essential to note on the images the time that has elapsed after administration of the spheres so the reference can be properly consulted.
6. If gastric dumping is suspected, take one set of radiographs within 1-2 hours after BIPS administration.[11]
7. Continue the study until the BIPS are in the colon.
8. Large bowel transit can be assessed:
   a. An enema or cathartic should be given to remove the retained feces.
   b. Give the BIPS with recommended diet, and radiograph at 24, 48, and 72 hours.

Comments and Tips
- A separate reference interval for gastric transit if acetylpromazine is administered is provided. Check the reference intervals to make sure to follow the time suggestions.[11]
- The gastric emptying rate and orocolic transit rate are determined by applying a formula separately to the large and small spheres (see Technician Note).
- Generally small BIPS are used to determine the gastric emptying for motility disorders, as they more closely mimic food.
- The gastric emptying rate of the large BIPS is best considered for partial obstructions of the pylorus or intestine.[11]
- Compare the results based on the size of the sphere, whether food is given, or the type of food eaten, with a standardized chart indicating average and mean emptying rate/transit times probable at that time after administration.
- Times are quicker if the capsules are given without food.
- The total number seen on the image will be a maximum of 10 large or 30 small spheres.
- If the location of a sphere cannot be accurately determined, it is not included in the formula calculation.
- If obstruction is noted, it is not necessary to calculate the formula, as the large spheres are trapped at the orad aspect of an obstructing lesion, giving the appearance of dumping.
- Both views are required to determine exactly where the spheres are, because parts of the large intestine are superimposed over the cardia of the stomach and over the stomach just caudal to the left crus of the diaphragm in some animals in the lateral view (see Chapter 16).
- Also, on a VD, BIPS in the transverse colon can be mistaken for BIPS bunched in the small intestine if only a lateral abdominal view is taken.
- Because of the limited use of BIPS, the procedure is not common.

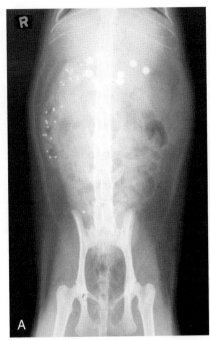
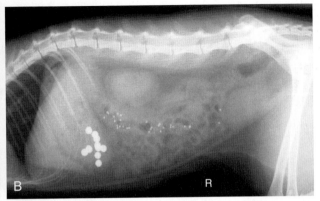

FIG. 23.13 A, Ventrodorsal abdomen 4 hours after administration of BIPS. All of the small BIPS have left the stomach, but the majority of large BIPS are still present. None of the BIPS are in the colon, so the orocolic rate is 0% for both the small and large BIPS. **B,** Right lateral abdomen BIPS study 4 hours after administration. Both views are required to determine the actual location of the BIPS.

Normal Radiographic Anatomy of the Gastrointestinal Tract

Normal Radiographic Appearance of the Esophagus With Contrast Media

The normal oropharyngeal region shows coating of the mucosa with no significant retention of the contrast agent. A small amount of medium may sometimes stay in the esophageal lumen immediately caudal to the cranial esophageal sphincter.

The normal canine esophageal mucosa appears as a series of longitudinal folds with its lines close together throughout, except at the thoracic inlet, where the esophagus passes along the left lateral side of the trachea. The normal feline esophagus also has parallel lines at the level of the heart base, with the caudal third of the esophagus being described as having a herringbone pattern. It consists of obliquely directed folds that correspond to the smooth muscle segment.[6] The esophagus is best evaluated on a lateral radiograph of the neck and on lateral and DV views of the thorax.

Normal Radiographic Stomach and Small Bowel Anatomy

Please review the anatomy in Chapter 16 and Appendix C on the Evolve website to view what is generally visualized on a survey radiograph and normal canine and feline stomach diagram (also see Fig. 16.13). Table 16.1 gives an overview of the anatomy in the various positions, and Fig. 23.14 shows normal variations in fluid and gas distribution depending on patient position. Box 23.1 indicates the image sequence for the positive-contrast UGI study.

The gastric emptying time of normal animals varies greatly. Factors such as the effect of medication and the type or volume of meal given also alter times. Low dosages of barium may delay emptying and transit time because the stomach empties slower when there is less volume in it. Delay may also occur in nervous animals or in a stressful environment.

On a UGI barium sulfate study without any food, delayed gastric emptying is diagnosed when gastric emptying is not completed after 3 hours in dogs and 1 hour in cats. Gastric emptying time longer than 8 hours for barium mixed with solid food is considered abnormal.[7]

Abnormal gastric emptying may be seen with incomplete pyloric obstruction. This can be associated with a pyloric tumor, congenital or acquired pyloric stenosis, or a gastric or duodenal foreign body.

The rugal folds are best seen at the periphery as the stomach begins to empty (see Fig. 23.14B and D). They are also more evident with negative contrast, but if the stomach is too distended in a double-contrast study, the folds may disappear. The rugae should be uniform, linear, or slightly tortuous and parallel.

In about a third of cats, the duodenum has a "string-of-pearls" appearance during a positive-contrast study (see Fig. 23.10). This is due to the peristaltic contractions.

In dogs, transient peristaltic contractions may be noted in the body of the stomach, pyloric canal, and antrum. Pseudoulcers or square outpockets may also be noted on the nonmesenteric descending duodenum of the dog but not in the cat.[6]

The cecum in a cat appears pointed, whereas in a dog it has a corkscrew appearance. On VD or DV views, the cecum appears just to the right of midline in both species.

Variations do exist in the appearance of the normal stomach, when the patient changes position, and as the amount and

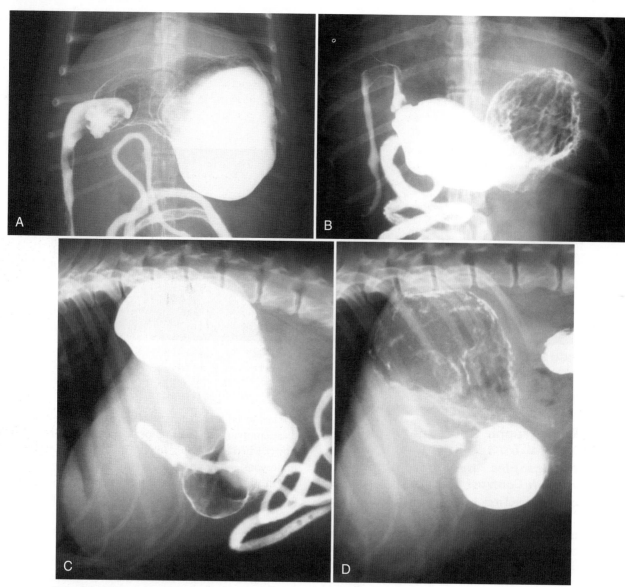

FIG. 23.14 Normal variations in barium (fluid) and gas distribution within the stomach with different patient positions. *A,* Ventrodorsal view. Gas is located in the body and pyloric antrum. Fluid settles dependently to fill the fundus, body, and pyloric portions. *B,* Dorsoventral view. Gas rises to the cardia and fundus, and fluid settles dependently to fill pyloric portions and part of the body. *C,* Left recumbent lateral view. Gas rises to the pyloric portion, and fluid settles dependently to fill the fundus and body. *D,* Right recumbent lateral view. Gas rises to the fundus and dorsal body, which are coated with barium. Fluid settles dependently to fill the pyloric portion and part of the body. (From Thrall DE. *Textbook of Veterinary Diagnostic Radiology,* 6th ed. St Louis: Elsevier; 2013.)

percentage of fluid and gas change. See the table in the Technician Notes box for a simplified version of where gas and fluid can be found as the position of the patient changes.

> ✎ **TECHNICIAN NOTES**
>
> The following box summarizes how positioning with the use of a vertical beam affects the distribution of gas and liquid[6]:
>
> | VIEW | LOCATION OF GAS | LOCATION OF FLUID |
> |------|-----------------|-------------------|
> | Dorsoventral | Fundus | Body/pylorus |
> | Ventrodorsal | Body (± pylorus) | Fundus |
> | Left lateral | Pylorus (± body) | Fundus |
> | Right lateral | Fundus dorsal body | Pylorus |

In the normal dog and cat, the rest of the small intestine should appear smooth. In dogs, barium between the intestinal villi may show up as a fine brush pattern.[6] Short lengths of the bowel may reveal peristalsis.

The colon wall is generally smooth and the lumen uniform in width. Barium adhering to mucus or feces may create artifacts.

Lymph follicles that are present in the mucosa of both the dog and the cat colon and in the cecum of the dog may appear as spicules on a barium enema study or as pinpoint radiopacities if viewed head on in a double-contrast study.[6]

Upon removal of the positive-contrast medium, longitudinal folds are visible that are made more detailed with the infusion of air. The VD or DV view of the colon shows a question-mark configuration.

Delayed gastric or intestinal emptying can be evaluated by means of a simple or double-contrast radiographic study, BIPS, scintigraphy, ultrasonography, or endoscopy. In some cases, gastric outflow obstruction may be documented only with food or with BIPS. Scintigraphy, using a radioactive meal, is the ideal modality to study gastric emptying because the study is very close to natural conditions and gives a quantitative index.[6,7] Scintigraphic evaluation of gastric emptying can be completed in 4 to 5 hours and is more consistent than gastric emptying times as measured by BIPS.[6,8,9] Magnetic resonance imaging (MRI) has not yet been applied for assessment of gastric emptying in small animals. Ultrasonography for determining gastric emptying can be subjective. Further methods are not practical outside the laboratory.[10]

Contrast Studies of the Urinary System

Contrast studies of the urinary system evaluate the kidneys, urinary bladder, ureters, prostate gland, and urethra. Survey radiographs of the kidneys may provide external anatomical information such as size, shape, and radiographic opacity if existing radiographic contrast is adequate. However, when kidneys cannot be assessed by survey radiographs or when qualitative functional urography is needed, excretory urography or ultrasonography may provide better information than survey radiographs.[6] Survey radiographs may also indicate that contrast studies are not necessary or would obliterate lesions (Figs. 23.15 and 23.16).

There are different ways of evaluating the urinary system, as well as different dosages and techniques. The method chosen is dictated by the clinical signs of the patient and the clinician.

Studies performed through contrast radiography have limitations, and with the advent of ultrasonography, a safer and more accurate method for evaluating the kidneys and prostate is available; however, the combination of the two methods may provide the greatest information.

> ### TECHNICIAN NOTES
> Never use barium for any urinary studies, including cystography.

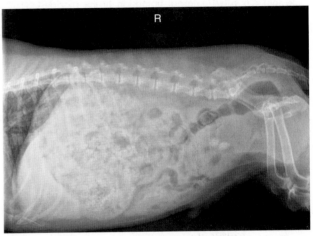

FIG. 23.15 Lateral survey of the abdomen of a diabetic patient. Positive-contrast studies would obliterate the bladder stones. (Courtesy Secord Animal Hospital.)

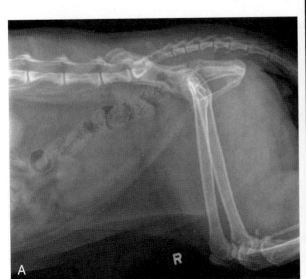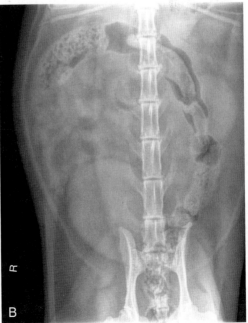

FIG. 23.16 A, Right lateral survey before a cystogram. Note the presence of stool, which could mask lesions. B, Ventrodorsal abdomen survey before a cystogram.

Retrograde Cystography

Cystography is the study of the bladder via the retrograde infusion of contrast media through a urinary catheter. Positive-, negative-, or double-contrast studies can be performed, with or without an excretory urogram. The actual study used is dictated by clinical history, clinical signs, radiographic signs, and character of the urine obtained with bladder catheterization (Box 23.5). Ultrasonography, if available and feasible, is preferred.

> **TECHNICIAN NOTES**
>
> While inserting contrast medium into the bladder, stop the infusion when external palpation of the bladder shows that it is moderately distended, if reflux occurs around the catheter, or if you feel back-pressure on the syringe.

> **TECHNICIAN NOTES**
>
> To calculate the concentration of contrast medium needed, use the following formula:
>
> $$\frac{\text{Final diluted percentage}}{\text{Initial concentration}} = \frac{\text{Volume needed}}{\text{Final volume administered}}$$
>
> A 15-kg dog requires 60 mL of a 10% iodinated contrast medium for a urinary study. If the stock bottle is 50%, what is the amount in mL taken from the bottle?
>
> $$\frac{10\%}{50\%} = \frac{X}{60\ \text{mL}}$$
>
> $$\left(\frac{1}{5}\right)(60\ \text{mL}) = X\ \text{mL}$$
>
> $X = 12$ mL that should be taken from the bottle
>
> *Note:* The sterile diluent required will be 60 mL − 12 mL = 48 mL.

BOX 23.5 Retrograde Cystography[4–7]

Indications for Cystography

- Clinical indications for retrograde cystography include unresponsive clinical signs due to abnormal urine (hematuria, crystalluria, and bacteriuria), abnormal urination (dysuria, pollakiuria), trauma, and abnormalities noted on survey radiographs such as abdominal masses, a change in bladder opacity or wall, or a change in location.
- Retrograde positive-contrast cystography is used to evaluate the bladder wall character in a trauma patient or to locate the bladder after trauma or herniation (Fig. 23.17).
- Retrograde negative-contrast cystography (pneumocystogram) is used to identify the integrity of the bladder wall after trauma or to locate the bladder. A pneumocystogram is best for cystic calculi.
- Double-contrast cystography is best for assessing bladder wall lesions and intraluminal filling defects (Fig. 23.18).
- In the absence of ultrasound, the studies can help determine caudal abdominal masses.

Precautions

- Iatrogenesis due to catheterization and cystographic procedures—trauma, bacterial infections, kinked or knotted urethral catheters—can occur.
- Intramural or subserosal accumulation of contrast media occurs more frequently in cats and usually does not cause a clinical problem.
- Mucosal ulceration, inflammation, and granulomata reactions are usually transitory with no serious clinical problems.
- Fatal, although rare, complications can occur with the introduction of a gas embolism after administration of negative-contrast media.
  - Nitrous oxide or carbon dioxide should be used, especially in patients with hematuria, because blood in the urine may be evidence of communication between the bladder lumen and vascular system.
  - Nitrous oxide or carbon dioxide is 20 times more soluble in serum than air or oxygen.
  - Left lateral recumbency may decrease the chance for any emboli to reach the lungs.[4]

Contrast Media and Dosage*

- Volume depends on body weight, species, and pathological process.
- Positive-contrast media:
  - Water-soluble nonionic organic iodide: 240 mg/mL or 300 mg/mL
  - Dogs 5-10 mL/kg; cats 2-5 mL/kg (maximum 25 mL in cats)[12,13]
- Negative-contrast media:
  - Nitrous oxide, carbon dioxide, air
  - Volume varies: 3-12 mL/kg.
- Double-contrast media:
  - Total: Positive nonionic contrast media: 0.5-6 mL, depending on species and weight.

Equipment/Supplies

- Sterile male or female urinary catheter.
- Vaginal speculum or adapted otoscope for female dogs.
- Skin prep, gauze, sterile gloves, sterile lubricating jelly.
- Light source.
- 20- to 50-mL syringe.
- 2% lidocaine jelly.
- Three-way stopcock.
- Source to deposit urine.
- 2-5 mL total of 2% lidocaine without epinephrine (optional).
- Broad-spectrum antibiotics (optional).

Patient Preparation

- Sedation is suggested, as urinary bladder distention can be uncomfortable, especially in patients with cystitis.

BOX 23.5   Retrograde Cystography[4-7]—cont'd

- Withhold food for 24 hours if possible, and administer an enema 4 hours before the study to avoid superimposition of fecal matter and to minimize gas artifacts.
- Take survey radiographs.
- Proper sterile technique is required.
  - If a catheter was inserted to collect urine for an excretory urogram, leave it aseptically inserted.
- If urine samples are required for examination, they should be collected before infusion of the agent.
  - Contrast agents increase specific gravity, cause a false-positive increase in protein as detected by sulfosalicylic acid, and may inhibit bacterial growth.

Measure and Center
- Measure and center over the bladder (cranial to the crest of the ilium).

Procedure for Negative-Contrast Study (Pneumocystogram) or Positive-Contrast Cystography
1. Take ventrodorsal and lateral survey radiographs of the full urinary tract.
2. Apply sterile 2% lidocaine jelly on the tip of a premeasured urethral catheter and aseptically and atraumatically insert until the catheter tip is within the urinary bladder.
3. Gently empty the bladder, and note the volume of urine removed.
4. Apply a syringe and three-way stopcock, and infuse with 2-5 mL total of 2% lidocaine without epinephrine to reduce bladder pain and spasm.
5. Carefully infuse the medium; stop when bladder feels firm and adequately distend through external palpation or back pressure of syringe plunger.
6. Close the stopcock valve when adequate distention is reached.
7. Take radiographs: right and left lateral and ventrodorsal views.
8. An oblique view is optional but is suggested for evaluation of prostate or urethral problems in a male.
9. If further distention of the bladder is required, inject additional contrast agent and repeat the radiographs.
10. Carefully remove the contrast medium.
11. Flush with a broad-spectrum antibiotic if the patient is not receiving systemic antibiotics as per the veterinarian.
12. Remove the catheter.

Procedure for Double-Contrast Retrograde Cystography
1. Follow the preparation and procedures infusing the negative-contrast medium first.
2. Take the required radiographs.
3. Infuse the organic water-soluble iodine into the bladder, gently rotating the patient from side to side to coat the bladder wall with iodine.
4. Take the required radiographs as noted earlier.
5. Complete the process as noted earlier.

Comments and Tips
- Both lateral views are suggested because a change in position may define a lesion more accurately; an oblique may also be suggested.

- Ensure that the catheter has been premeasured and just within the urinary bladder.
- If urine is removed from a relatively full bladder, infusing the same amount of contrast medium is a good guide for volume required.
- It is best if the small bowel is empty and the colon is void of fecal material.
- Using lidocaine without epinephrine helps decrease the possibility of spasm and helps obtain complete bladder distention.
- Moderate distention is preferred because full distention may hide subtle mucosal and mural lesions if the bladder wall is stretched.
- A diseased bladder may only hold a fraction of the anticipated volume (as little as 1 mL/kg)[5] of air or positive-contrast medium. Palpate carefully, note resistance in the syringe, and watch for leakage.
- If the catheter has an inflatable cuff, deflate after the radiographs have been taken.
- Any urine leakage with positive-contrast medium should be cleaned from the table, image receptor, or patient to minimize artifacts on the image.
- A decrease in exposure factors may be required for the pneumocystogram because of inherent contrast.
- Compression through the use of a paddle will help move the contrast pool for better evaluation of the integrity of the bladder wall.
- After taking the positive-contrast cystography radiographs, the catheter tip can be repositioned into the urethra to perform an urethrogram. This will better evaluate the bladder neck.
- Urethral reflux of positive-contrast agent may be a normal finding.
- If a ruptured bladder is suspected, contrast agent can be used without dilution to better visualize the agent in the peritoneal cavity.
- Extravasation of the positive-contrast agent in the extraperitoneal soft tissues or peritoneal cavity is well tolerated.[4]

Cystography via Cystocentesis in the Dog and Cat
1. Manually palpate the urinary bladder, immobilizing it with your fingers against the ventral or lateral abdomen.
2. Aseptically introduce a 1-inch, 22-gauge needle in a cat or a 2-inch, 22-gauge needle in the dog through the midline abdominal wall.
3. Extract the urine, noting the volume.
4. Infuse positive-contrast media or air so that there is minimal bladder distention.
5. Remove the needle.
6. Take lateral and ventrodorsal or oblique radiographs.

Comments and Tips
- There will likely be minimal leakage into the peritoneal cavity.
- To minimize possible leakage, do not apply any bladder compression after injection.

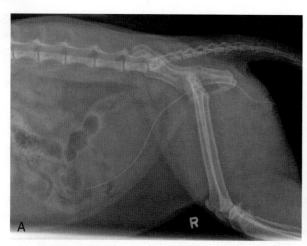

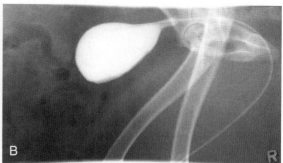

FIG. 23.17 A, Catheter injected with iodine before a cystogram. **B,** Lateral positive-contrast cystogram. (Courtesy Tara Wochesen, Ontario Veterinary College, Veterinary Teaching Hospital, Diagnostic Imaging at the University of Guelph.)

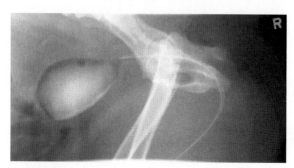

FIG. 23.18 Double-contrast cystogram. Note the bubble of air at the tip of the urinary catheter. (Courtesy Tara Wochesen, Ontario Veterinary College, Veterinary Teaching Hospital, Diagnostic Imaging at the University of Guelph.)

Excretory Urography[4–7]

Excretory urography is primarily used to determine the size, shape, location, and integrity of the kidneys, as well as the size, shape, and appearance of the collecting systems (Box 23.6). Although excretory urography is not a quantitative measurement of renal function, it can be used to assess the relative function of the kidneys and, indirectly, the pathophysical mechanism of renal failure.[6] The principle of the study is that sterile, water-soluble, iodinated contrast medium is injected intravenously, where it circulates; then the kidney concentrates and excretes the iodine, demonstrating the kidneys, ureters, and urinary bladder. The study was formerly called an *intravenous pyelogram (IVP)* or an *intravenous urogram (IVU)*. Ultrasound images the anatomy without using contrast media.

Further Urinary Tract Contrast Procedures

Box 23.7 includes further urinary tract contrast procedures.

Complete Urinary Tract Examination

Box 23.8 gives a summary of a complete urinary tract examination.

✎ TECHNICIAN NOTES

Some suggestions for minimizing reactions to contrast media injections are as follows[1]:

- Before the injection, check that the solution is clear and colorless.
- Check the expiration date, and discard outdated contrast material.
- Keep the contrast medium out of direct light for storage.
- There are no preservatives, so immediately use the bottle once it is opened, and discard the remainder.
- Keep the agent close to body temperature. The warmed solution decreases the viscosity for easier injection and reduces the potential for cardiovascular collapse.
- Use the minimum effective dose.
- To prevent incompatibility, do not administer other medications in the same syringe or IV administration set.
- Ensure patency of the catheter before the injection.
- If a contrast medium needs to be injected into a line, use normal saline (NS), dextrose and water (D/W), or lactated Ringer's solution (R/L). Potassium chloride (KCl) added to the IV is the *only* compatible medication. However, fluids dilute the concentration, lessening the contrast noted on an image.
- If a reaction occurs, stop injecting immediately and leave the catheter in the vein.
- Monitor carefully throughout.

✎ TECHNICIAN NOTES

- Properly prepare the patient.
- Obtain survey radiographs.
- Give the correct dose.
- Follow proper procedure; set the correct technical factors.
- Properly center, and include peripheral borders and position accurately.
- Monitor, monitor, monitor.

Normal Radiographic Anatomy of the Urinary Tract

Review the anatomy of the kidneys, bladder, urethra, and prostate found in Chapter 16 and Appendix C on the Evolve website.

Excretory urograms allow further quantitative measurements of the kidney and proximal ureters. The cortex is more radiopaque than the medulla in the early nephrogram phase. Generally the pyelogram is more radiopaque than the nephrogram. The normal nephrogram is most radiopaque within 10 to 30 seconds after administration of a bolus injection of contrast medium.[6] The pyelogram should be consistently opaque.

The ureter width varies because of peristalsis. The normal bladder wall is about 1 mm thick, regardless of the amount of distention.[6]

Prostate enlargement can be viewed on a survey radiograph as a soft tissue mass in the caudal abdomen. The displacement of the bladder due to prostatomegaly is more obvious with positive-contrast media.

BOX 23.6	Excretory Urography[5,6,12]

Indications for Excretory Urography

- Specific indications include abnormal urine or urination, suspected renal or urethral calculi, dysuria, pyuria, or intraabdominal mass that may involve or displace the kidney.
- Excretory urography can be used in both azotemic and nonazotemic patients provided there is adequate hydration.

Precautions

- Avoid the study if anuria, severe dehydration, severe uremia, or urethral obstruction is present.
- A temporary decrease in renal function may occur after excretory urography.
- Dehydration can result in kidney damage, so a dehydrated patient should be rehydrated before the procedure.
- Abdominal compression may have to be modified because of precluded conditions.
- Although they are rare, systemic reactions have occurred.
  - Kidney function parameters such as blood urea nitrogen (BUN) and serum creatinine levels should be checked before the start of the procedure.
  - It is important that the patient's hydration status be determined and corrected before administration of the agent.
- Even though the incidence of reaction to contrast media is low, especially with the use of low-osmolar, nonionic contrast media, it is imperative to be prepared and not to become complacent.
  - Reactions can occur quickly and without warning.
  - Most severe acute reactions occur within the first 1-5 minutes after administration.
  - Signs can range from mild to fatal.
  - The most common signs tend to be vomiting, defecation, urination, urticaria, tachycardia, and hypotension with or without collapse.
  - Most reactions can be reversed with immediate and proper intervention.
  - Vital signs should be monitored before, during, and after the procedure to observe for adverse reactions.
  - An emergency resuscitation kit should be on hand before the injection.
- Proper technique should be used to minimize iatrogenesis that may be caused by placement of the catheter.

Contrast Media and Dosage

- Water-soluble organic iodide, 600-700 mg/kg up to 880 mg/kg body weight.[5,6]
- A maximum dose of 90 mL in dogs and 15 mL in cats is suggested.
- A concentration of 300-400 mg iodine per mL is the suggested dilution if uremia is present.[5]
- Nonionic highly recommended: iopamidol (Isovue), iohexol (Omnipaque), or iodixanol (Visipaque).

Equipment/Supplies

- Indwelling intravenous catheter, syringe, and system for abdominal compression.
- Urethral catheter if continuing the study.
- Emergency resuscitation kit and oxygen.
- Markers to identify exposure time.

Patient Preparation

- No food for 24 hours before the study; water ad libitum.
- Perform a cleansing enema the previous evening if possible or at least 2 hours before (best if 4 hours to minimize gas artifacts).
- If urine samples are required for examination, they should be collected before infusion of the medium.
  - Contrast agents increase specific gravity, cause a false-positive increase in urinary protein as detected by sulfosalicylic acid, and may inhibit bacterial growth.
- Assess patient hydration, and proceed only if normal.
- Remove the urine so the contrast medium will not be diluted.
- Have image receptors, settings, markers, timers, protective gear, etc., ready, so that upon administration of the contrast agent, the image can be taken immediately.
- Position an indwelling catheter.
- Proper patient preparation is essential to ensure quality images.

Measure, Center, and Include

- Remember that for the full abdomen you are generally:
  - Measuring at the thickest part (liver), at the TL junction.
  - Center over caudal aspect of 13th rib at level of L2-L3 or over umbilicus for the canine and two to three finger widths caudal to 13th rib for the feline.
  - Include about an inch cranial to xiphoid and caudally to the acetabulum.

Continued

BOX 23.6 | Excretory Urography[5,6,12]—cont'd

- The cranial pole of the right kidney of a dog is generally found at T13.
- Place time markers at the cranial aspect for VD views and at the ventral cranial abdomen for lateral views.

Procedure for Excretory Urography

1. The patient is best sedated or anesthetized to minimize discomfort.
2. Obtain survey radiographs.
3. Place the patient in ventrodorsal recumbency with a patent intravenous indwelling catheter.
4. Inject the calculated warmed solution quickly as a bolus—within 2 minutes.
5. Flush the catheter with heparinized saline after the solution is administered.
6. Sequence the radiographs as follows after injection (Fig. 23.19):
   a. Immediately—within 5-20 seconds: ventrodorsal (arteriogram and nephrogram).
   b. 5 minutes: ventrodorsal and right lateral (pyelogram phase).
   c. If there is evidence of contrast agent within both kidneys, compression may be applied.
   d. 15- 20 minutes: ventrodorsal (both collecting systems should be filled with contrast medium (view ureters and urinary bladder).
   e. If compression has been applied, remove the compression band.
   f. 30-40 minutes or until a diagnosis is reached: right lateral and ventrodorsal oblique to view the bladder (optional if retrograde cystography is contraindicated).
   g. Further contrast study of the bladder can be completed:
      1. Positive-contrast retrograde cystography: Infuse positive-contrast medium solution retrogradely via the urethral catheter. The amount would be determined by pressure and what is noted on the previous radiographic image.
      2. Double-contrast retrograde cystography can be completed by infusing negative-contrast medium via the urethral catheter.

Comments and Tips

- For diagnostic reasons it is best if the bolus is administered fairly quickly, but the patient may be nauseous and may vomit if it is given too rapidly.
- Right lateral positioning is suggested as there is greater longitudinal separation of the right and left kidneys.
- For better visualization of the ureters, an oblique can be obtained after 5 minutes.
- Compression over the bladder can be applied for better visualization of the renal collecting system by delaying the drainage of the contrast media. If the urinary bladder is compressed, the intraluminal pressure increases and prevents drainage through the ureters.

- Compression can be applied by placing a flat radiolucent sponge on the central abdomen and securing it with elastic bandage. Commercially available compression devices can also be used.
- The agent can be administered more slowly and the sequence delayed for ureter examination.
- No abdominal compression should be used if diagnosing ectopic ureters so that a negative contrast cystogram can be performed.
- IV fluids should be stopped during the sequence because fluids reduce the concentration of the iodine and subsequent image on the radiograph.
- If the kidneys are highly compromised, contrast media may be noted in the liver.
- Various image sequences are listed in the literature, but the one described here probably provides the most diagnostic information.[6]
- The excretory urogram consists of the vascular (arteriogram), nephrogram, pyelogram, ureteral and drainage:
  - During the vascular phase, which is seen with rapid bolus infusion, the aorta and renal arteries are seen.
  - Opacification of the functional renal parenchyma (nephrons) occurs almost immediately and is known as the nephrographic phase.
    - The vascular supply and perfusion of the kidney are noted, helping differentiate the cortex from the medulla.
    - Absence in both kidneys may be due to disease or insufficient contrast media.
  - The pyelographic phase shows the renal pelvis, pelvic recesses, and ureters.
    - The renal collecting channels extend into the medulla from the pelvis of the kidneys.
    - A compression band slows the drainage from the pyelogram.
  - The ureteral and drainage phases occur when the agent is in the ureter and bladder.
- Proper distention of the urinary bladder cannot be achieved solely with an excretory urogram study.
  - Retrograde cystography is required. However, in traumatized female cats, it may be difficult to position a urethral catheter.
- The status of patient hydration, dosage rate, and renal function all affect the concentration, excretion, and opacification of the positive-contrast medium.
- Opaque material in the intestinal lumen, intestinal gas over the urinary bladder or urethra, and nipples can be mistaken for uroliths or filling defects.
  - Gas bubbles in the bladder or urethra introduced by urinary catheterization may appear as mineralized lesions in the tissues of the bladder wall.
- Additional views can be decided on the basis of individual findings.

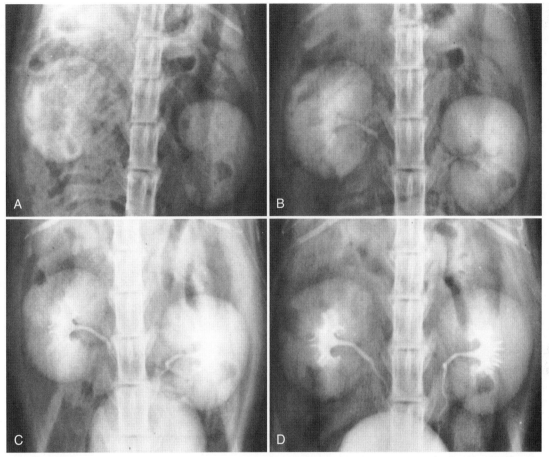

FIG. 23.19 Ventrodorsal views of a normal cat after intravenous administration of 400 mg iodine per pound of body weight in the form of sodium iothalamate. **A,** 10 seconds after injection; **B,** 5 minutes; **C,** 20 minutes; **D,** 40 minutes. (From Thrall DE. *Textbook of Veterinary Diagnostic Radiology*, 5th ed. St. Louis: Elsevier; 2007.)

BOX 23.7	Further Urinary Tract Contrast Procedures

Urethrography[4-7]

Overview

- Urethrography consists of filling the urethra with contrast medium for evaluation (Fig. 23.20).
- Can be accomplished in either a retrograde manner with a positive-, negative-, or double-contrast medium or by applying compression on a positive-contrast–filled bladder to cause a voiding urethrogram.
- The actual technique varies with the sex and species of the patient.
- Often performed after completion of a retrograde cystogram merely by repositioning the catheter tip more caudally.
- Most often performed in male dogs for evaluation of the urethra and suspected prostatic disease. Only indirect evidence of prostatic disease is provided, however.
- In females a combination vaginourethrogram can be completed (Fig. 23.21).

Indications

- Urethrography is indicated to determine the abnormal passage of urine due to urethral trauma, stricture, obstruction, or other pathological disturbances.

Precautions

- If injury results upon catheterization, injected air may enter the venous system, leading to fatal venous air embolism.
- Compression for a voiding urethrogram is contraindicated if the bladder is diseased because of the greater possibility of rupture.

Contrast Media and Dosage

- Positive-contrast organic ionic or nonionic agent (diluted to 150-200 mg of iodine/mL):
  - Dogs: 10-15 mL volume.
  - Cats: 5-10 mL volume.

Continued

BOX 23.7 | Further Urinary Tract Contrast Procedures—cont'd

Equipment/Supplies
- Sterile catheter with inflatable bulb if possible (Foley, Swan-Ganz).
- Skin prep solution, gauze, sterile gloves, sterile lubricating jelly.
- Catheter adapter/three-way stopcock.
- Large syringe.
- Sterile saline solution.
- 2% lidocaine jelly and lidocaine solution.
- Vaginal speculum or adapted otoscope for female dogs.

Measure and Center
- Measure and center at the crest of the ilium.

Patient Preparation
- Sedation is suggested, as the procedure may cause discomfort.
- Give a cleansing enema to remove fecal matter from the descending colon and rectum.
- Proper sterile technique is required. If the catheter was used for cystography, leave it aseptically inserted.
- If urine samples are required for examination, they should be collected before infusion of contrast media.

Procedure for Retrograde Positive-Contrast Urethrography
1. If not previously imaged, take ventrodorsal and lateral survey radiographs of the full urinary tract.
2. If the catheter is not yet inserted, fill the lumen of the catheter with contrast medium.
3. Insert the lubricated tip about 1-3 cm into the urethral orifice, and inflate the balloon.
   a. For prostatic urethra advance catheter to the level of ischial arch.[5]
4. Depending on the size of the patient, inject the warmed contrast medium until you feel back-pressure.
5. Take lateral radiographs toward the end of the infusion, repeating the administration if needed.
   a. Pull pelvic limbs cranially for a flexed lateral in males for a better view of the urethra (see Fig. 16.8).
6. A ventrodorsal oblique radiograph may be helpful.
7. Remove the catheter.

Comments and Tips
- If the catheter does not have a cuff, use a larger catheter to limit leakage of the contrast medium. Place a towel to absorb leaking contrast agent.
- Avoid using a stiff catheter to minimize iatrogenesis.
- Avoid the use of sterile lubricating jelly with a positive-contrast agent to prevent filling defects and false-positive diagnosis.
- Minimize the length of time the catheter balloon is inflated to avoid mild reversible inflammatory reaction.
- If the urinary bladder is fully distended with urine, contrast medium, or sterile saline during urethrography, there may be better distention of the urethra, especially the prostatic urethra.
- Vesicoureteral reflux and urethroprostatic reflux occur frequently in mature healthy dogs undergoing maximum distention urethrocystography.
- Left lateral recumbency is suggested when gas is being put in the bladder because the position will help the patient recover if an air embolus develops. Some radiographers prefer the typical right lateral position because it helps decrease renal overlap on images. If you suspect that an air embolus has developed during the procedure, immediately deflate the bladder and place the patient in left lateral recumbency.

Antegrade or Voiding Urethrogram
Procedure for Antegrade or Voiding Urethrogram
Because it is harder to catheterize female dogs and cats, the antegrade or voiding urethrogram is easier to complete than the retrograde study.
1. Apply gentle pressure on the positive-contrast–filled, distended bladder with a paddle or wooden spoon. Place a towel under the patient to absorb any leakage.
2. Take a lateral radiograph when urine is noted at the urethral orifice.

Vaginocystourethrography[6]
Procedure for Vaginocystourethrography
Vaginocystourethrography is another method of evaluating the urethra in female dogs.
1. If not previously imaged, take ventrodorsal and lateral survey radiographs of the full urinary tract.
2. Patients should be given general anesthesia.
3. If the catheter is not yet inserted, fill the lumen of the catheter with contrast medium (estimated dose- dogs 10-30 mL and cats 5-10 mL)[5]
4. Insert the lubricated tip into the vestibule and inflate the balloon to occlude outflow. The tip of the catheter distal to the balloon should be as short as possible to prevent it from entering the vagina.
5. It may be necessary to clamp the vulvar lips tightly to prevent reflux.
6. Inject amount of positive-contrast media for the size of the patient. The vagina will fill preferentially.
7. Infuse so the contrast medium will reflux into the urethra and bladder. Overdistention may result in expulsion of the contrast medium.[6]
8. Take lateral radiographs (optional VD and VD oblique) at the end of the infusion. The catheter can be pulled out at the same time.

Note: to avoid air bubbles that may be mistaken for calculi, prefill the catheter.

| BOX 23.8 | Summary of Complete Urinary Tract Examination |

Preparation

- No food for 12-24 hours. Give water ad libitum.
- Withhold water at least 1-2 hours or as required before sedation or anesthesia.
- Give an enema at least 4 hours before to lessen the chance of gas artifacts.
- Assess patient hydration and proceed only if normal.
- Have plates, settings, markers, protective apparel, etc., ready.
- Sedate patient and obtain survey radiograph—right lateral and ventrodorsal (VD)
- Aseptically place intravenous (IV) catheter in vein and urethral catheter in bladder.
- Place a three-way stopcock valve on the urethral catheter.
- Remove any urine from the bladder.
- Place the patient in dorsal recumbency.

Excretory Urography/Double-Contrast Cystogram/Urethrogram

- Inject nonionic iodinated contrast medium as a bolus within 2 minutes. Note maximum limits.

- Flush catheter with heparinized saline after the solution is administered.
- Take VD radiograph within 20-40 seconds of completing injection (vascular and nephrogram).
- Distend bladder with negative contrast media at about 1-2 mL/kg to keep iodine in kidney.
- Take VD and right lateral radiographs of the kidneys 5 minutes after IV injection (pyelogram).
- Gently palpate the bladder and determine whether more negative-contrast agent should be administered.
- At 20 minutes after IV injection, obtain VD, lateral, and oblique radiographs (optional) of kidneys, ureters, bladder (drainage and cystogram).
- Inject iodinated medium (5-15 mL) into the urethra as you withdraw the catheter.
- Take lateral radiograph as soon as you see contrast agent leaking from the external orifice of the urethra.

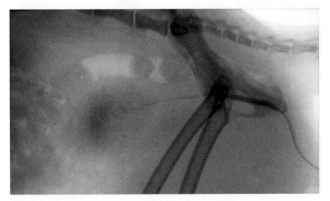

FIG. 23.20 Urethrogram with fluoroscopy of a dog positioned in right lateral recumbency. Iodine has been injected retrograde via a catheter. Some of the iodine has dispersed in the bladder. (Courtesy Tara Wochesen, Ontario Veterinary College, Veterinary Teaching Hospital, Diagnostic Imaging at the University of Guelph.)

FIG. 23.21 Fluoroscopy of a vaginogram iodine study with the patient positioned in lateral recumbency. (Courtesy Tara Wochesen, Ontario Veterinary College, Veterinary Teaching Hospital, Diagnostic Imaging at the University of Guelph.)

Additional Techniques

Myelography[4,6]

Myelography (Fig. 23.22 and Box 23.9) is the placement of radiopaque contrast agent into the subarachnoid space in either the cerebellomedullary cistern or the lumbar region for evaluation of the spinal cord. Computerized tomography (CT) and MRI are replacing the use of myelography for spinal evaluation in many practices because they are quicker and noninvasive.

Further Contrast Studies

Box 23.10 gives a brief overview of additional contrast radiography techniques, many of which have been replaced by ultrasound or other modalities. See other sources for more complete information.

Contrast Agents Used for Other Modalities

Ultrasound

Many substances may act as contrast agents in ultrasonography. Orally ingested fluid may expel gas from the stomach and create an acoustic window to the pancreas. Echo-free fluids such as water and saline may distend body cavities to improve visualization of the luminal walls. Contrast media for intravenous use have been limited to encapsulated microbubbles, which may produce up to a 25-dB increase in echo strength. They are generally used in Doppler ultrasonography of the heart. See Chapter 10 for ultrasound techniques.

Computerized Tomography

Generally, the nonionic contrast agents used in radiographic contrast studies are used in CT. See Chapter 12 for information on computerized tomography.

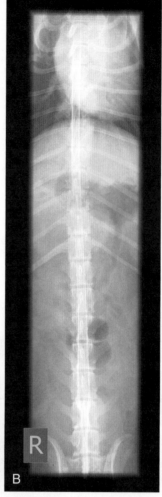

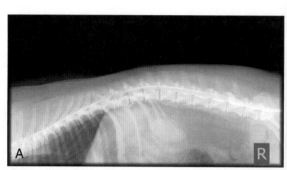

FIG. 23.22 A, Lateral projection during myelography study. **B,** Ventrodorsal view during a myelography study. (Courtesy of Carolyn Bennet, Ontario Veterinary College, Veterinary Teaching Hospital, Diagnostic Imaging at the University of Guelph.)

BOX 23.9 | Myelography

Indications

- Myelography helps localize and identify the cause of suspected transverse spinal myelopathy, such as the size of the lesion or the extent of cord compression.
- The location helps determine prognosis and course of treatment.
- Specific indications for myelography include paresis, paralysis, proprioceptive or sensory deficit, and spinal pain thought to be due to a transverse myelopathy.

Precautions

- General anesthesia is required; any contraindications need to be evaluated.
- The cerebrospinal fluid (CSF) should be examined to check that there is no systemic or local infection such as myelitis or meningitis.
- The needle must be aseptically placed.
- The anesthetic regimen should not include a phenothiazine derivative, which might lower the seizure threshold.
- Corticosteroids should not be administered intrathecally with the contrast agent.
- The patient should be adequately hydrated to help minimize side effects and complications due to delayed

elimination of contrast medium from the subarachnoid space.
- Incorrect procedure can cause trauma and have fatal consequences.
- Myelography may also cause intensification of preexisting neurological signs.

Contrast Media and Dosage

- Organic nonionic positive-contrast iodine: iopamidol (Isovue), 200-300 mg/mL, or iohexol (Omnipaque), 240 mg/mL.
- Dosage for the dog[4,13]:
  - Cisternal injection: cervical spine: 0.3 mL/kg; TL spine: 0.45 mL/kg.
  - Lumbar injection: cervical spine: 0.45 mL/kg; TL spine: 0.3 mL/kg.

Equipment/Supplies

- Clippers, scrub solutions, drape, sterile gloves.
- Dog: 20-gauge spinal needle with a flat bevel, 2-4 inches in length; two 10-mL syringes.
- Cat: 22-gauge spinal needle with a flat bevel, 1½ inches in length; two 5-mL syringes.

BOX 23.9	Myelography—cont'd

- Two 10 mL syringes for the dog and two 5 mL syringes for the cat. 18-gauge 1-inch needle, 3-mL syringe to collect cerebrospinal fluid.
- CSF collection tube, extension set, 0.22-μ nucleopore (millipore) filter.

Patient Preparation
- Use general anesthetic without a phenothiazine derivative.
- Shave the hair caudal to the skull (for cisternal) or over the lumbar spine (lumbar), and complete three scrubs.

General Procedure
For actual positioning of the needle, please consult more complete references. The veterinarian will usually perform the injection and administer the agent.

1. After obtaining the survey radiographs of the appropriate areas and anesthetizing the patient, aseptically prepare the region by shaving a 4-inch (10-cm) square; complete a surgical scrub and drape as follows.
2. Position the patient in perfect lateral recumbency with the aid of sandbags or foam sponges. See Chapter 20 for specific positioning.
3. Withdraw CSF in a volume that is at least equal to the volume of contrast agent to be injected.
4. Slowly inject the contrast medium.
5. Rotate the patient to ensure equal mixing of contrast agent and CSF.
6. Keeping the patient under general anesthesia for about an hour after injection lessens the frequency of postmyelography convulsions.
   a. Keep the head raised during recovery to prevent contrast medium from flowing into the ventricles of the brain, thereby increasing the pressure and the risk of convulsions.

Further Specifics for Cervical Myelography
1. Obtain surveys, shave, scrub, and place drape caudal to external occipital protuberance.
2. Position so that the head is in maximum ventral flexion (chin touching the sternum) with the aid of sandbags or foam pads and the midline of the head and neck is parallel to the table. The table can be tilted at 10 degrees with the patient's head at the raised end.
3. With the stylet in place, insert the needle into the cerebellomedullary cistern through the atlantooccipital space.
4. After withdrawing the CSF, inject the contrast medium over 3-4 minutes, and remove the needle.
5. Rotate the patient.
6. Keep the head elevated for a few minutes to allow contrast medium to flow caudally. The head may also need to be massaged.
7. A lateral radiograph can confirm the location of the contrast volumes. Take lateral views beginning at the site of injection and move caudally.
8. When contrast medium has reached the main area of interest, complete further lateral, ventrodorsal, and oblique radiographs for accurate identification and location of the lesion.

Further Specifics for Lumbar Myelography
1. Obtain surveys, shave, scrub, and place drape over L5-L6.

2. Position the patient flexing the pelvic limbs forward so the feet are along the abdomen. Sandbag in place.
3. With the stylet in place, insert the needle into the subarachnoid space.
4. Collect the CSF and slowly inject agent over 5 minutes. Keep the capped needle in place. This prevents the contrast from leaking into the needle tract and the epidural space
5. Rotate the patient.
6. Upon completion of the lateral view, remove the needle and immediately take the ventrodorsal view.[3]

Comments and Tips
- There must be no patient movement during the placement of the spinal needle and injection.
- The patient can remain in sternal recumbency for either injection. This position makes it more difficult to determine the depth of the needle, which is better evaluated and radiographed in the lateral position.
- Cautions for positioning of the needle for the cerebellomedullary cistern through the atlantooccipital space:
  - Incorrect lateral positioning would puncture the vertebral sinus and cause bleeding.
  - Incorrect cranial positioning may put the tip in the hind brain, causing respiratory collapse and death.
  - Any movement during positioning may lacerate the spinal cord or medulla.
- If the needle position is accurate for the cervical injection, the most common problem is that the contrast medium does not flow caudally to fully visualize the lesion:
  - The contrast medium flows rostrally into the ventricular system when resistance to caudal flow is met, so only the cranial margin of a compressive lesion may be identified.
  - Positioning the head up during the injection or after removal of the spinal needle and massaging the neck may assist in the flow.
  - Cervical myelography is not likely diagnostic if there is severe thoracolumbar cord swelling.
- There is less danger in incorrect positioning of the needle for lumbar myelography but keep in mind the following:
  - Lateral placement punctures the venous sinuses, creating a bloody tap and compromising the interpretation of the CSF.
  - The most common problem with lumbar punctures is the injection of the contrast agent into the epidural space and/or into the venous sinuses.
  - Extradural passage of contrast agent decreases the amount available in the subarachnoid space.
- If there is a bloody tap, do not inject the contrast agent, because the mixture of blood and contrast agent is highly irritative in the subarachnoid space.
- If postmyelography convulsions occur, intravenous diazepam in therapeutic doses is recommended. If this is not effective, intravenous barbiturates are suggested.
- Keep in mind the suggestions for minimizing reactions to contrast media injections as described in the Technician Notes box for excretory urography.

BOX 23.10	Additional Contrast Radiography Techniques		
STUDY	**AGENT(S) USED**	**INDICATION/PROCEDURE**	**COMMENTS**
Angiocardiography—nonselective (selective study is direct injection into the right ventricle)	Water-soluble organic iodide.	Inject into the cephalic or jugular vein to obtain information on cardiac abnormalities such as occlusion of a particular blood vessel, to demonstrate pathological lesions of the vascular system, or to provide evidence of a tumor noted on the survey. Use when echocardiography is unavailable.	Sedation or anesthesia usually required. Fluoroscopy or a method of rapidly exposing multiple images is recommended because a series of radiographs is to be taken every second.
Arthrography	Water-soluble organic iodide—nonionic low-osmolar agent. Pneumoarthrogram can be completed with carbon dioxide or nitrous oxide, which is preferred to air which could cause an air embolism. Carbon dioxide is resorbed much more quickly than other gases.	Injection into the synovial fluid to contrast the articular surfaces and joint capsule. An arthrogram can be used to evaluate a ruptured joint capsule, the presence of a cartilaginous flap, meniscal injuries, or the necessity for surgery.	Dilute with sterile saline to a concentration of 20%-40%. General anesthesia and a surgically prepared 8 cm × 8 cm area are required. Contraindicated if there is infection of surrounding soft tissues.
Bronchography	Nonionic water-soluble iodine.	Tracheobronchial lesions that cause coughing or dyspnea.	CT and MRI have displaced this procedure.
Celiography—positive-contrast	Water-soluble organic iodide.	Evaluates the abdominal cavity and the integrity of the diaphragm often to determine a diaphragmatic hernia.	Surgical preparation of the site just caudal to the umbilicus.
Fistulography	Water-soluble organic iodide (nonionic preferred) or negative contrast media.	Evaluates the extent of fistulous tracts, sinus cavities, or draining wounds. Will detect radiolucent foreign bodies. Infuse into the fistulous tract with a syringe and flexible catheter, preferably one with a balloon tip.	Infection in the area may disseminate into the site. Often the site of the wound is distant from the site of drainage.
Pneumoperitoneography, peritoneography, and herniography. (These are generally replaced by CT, MRI, or ultrasound.)	Negative contrast media with carbon dioxide and nitrous oxide are preferred gases because of their more rapid absorption in the body. Room air also has an increased incidence of air embolism.	Evaluates the abdominal cavity and integrity of the diaphragm. Often used to determine a diaphragmatic hernia. A horizontal beam should be used. The gas does not need to be removed.	Sedation is usually required. Surgical preparation caudal to the umbilicus is required. Use a stylet and syringe. Fasting and a full bladder are suggested.

Magnetic Resonance Imaging

In cases in which it is difficult to differentiate between two types of tissue on MRI, the solution is to add a contrast agent to one of them. An MRI contrast agent works by affecting the time it takes for the hydrogen atoms to return to their original energy state. See Chapter 13 for MRI information.

The contrast agent increases the difference in the signal intensity from the two types of tissue, thus increasing the degree of contrast on the image. The contrast medium becomes evenly distributed in the blood and is then excreted by the kidneys.

Most MRI contrast media contain the heavy-metal gadolinium encapsulated in a chelate that makes it less toxic.

Sometimes the gadolinium is given midway through the MRI session by injection into a vein to highlight areas of a tumor or inflammation. All gadolinium chelates are administered intravenously. Each injection of gadolinium is followed by a saline flush. The rate of injection should be slower than 10 mL per minute.

Some gadolinium products in common use today are as follows (see Fig. 23.23A):
- Gadopentetate dimeglumine (Magnevist)
- Gadoteridol injection (ProHance)
- Gadodiamide injection (Omniscan)
- Gadobutrol (Gadavist)

Positron Emission Tomography and Nuclear Medicine Imaging Agents

Nuclear imaging (or scintigraphy) requires use of radioactive contrast agents (called *radiopharmaceuticals*) to obtain images (Fig. 23.23B). Some agents used for positron emission tomography (PET) provide information about tissue metabolism or some other specific molecular activity. The most commonly used agent in veterinary medicine is technetium 99mTc, which is used to radiolabel many different common radiopharmaceuticals. It is used most often in bone and heart scans. See Chapter 14 for further information.

Summary

Box 23.11 provides an overview of the contrast studies explained in this chapter.

Fig. 23.24 is a mystery radiograph. Review it and answer the question presented with it.

Image Gallery

Figs. 23.25 to 23.30 provide additional images of contrast studies.

BOX 23.11 Quick Review of Gastrointestinal, Urinary, and Spinal Contrast Studies

Esophagus Contrast Study:
1. Prepare the patient, including survey radiographs.
2. Administer the barium, and immediately expose radiographs with the patient in lateral position.
3. Administer more barium, and take further positions as required.

LGI Contrast Study
1. Prepare the patient, including fasting, enema, sedation, and survey radiographs.
2. Make sure everything is ready.
3. Administer the barium.
4. Place the patient in position and follow the required sequence for times and positioning for proper completion of a positive-contrast LGI.
5. Follow up with a negative-contrast study if required.

Retrograde Cystography
1. Prepare the patient, including fasting, enema, emptying of the bladder, insertion of the urinary catheter, survey radiographs, and sedation/anesthesia. Follow proper aseptic technique.
2. Have everything ready before administering the contrast media.
3. Administer the required solution—warmed positive-contrast water-soluble organic iodide and/or negative-contrast medium.
4. Obtain the required radiographs shortly after administration.
5. If required, follow up with the opposite-contrast media for the bladder or urethra.
6. Remove contrast medium; insert antibiotic if required; remove the catheter, and recover the patient.

Retrograde Urethrography and Vaginocystourethrography
1. Prepare the patient, including fasting, enema, emptying of the bladder, insertion of the urinary catheter, survey radiographs, and sedation/anesthesia. Follow proper aseptic technique.
2. Have everything ready before administering the contrast medium.
3. Administer the warmed positive-contrast water-soluble organic iodide via the catheter.
4. Obtain the required radiographs shortly after administration.
5. Remove the contrast medium; insert antibiotic if required; remove the catheter; and recover the patient.

UGI Study
1. Prepare the patient, including fasting, an enema, survey radiographs.
2. Make sure everything is ready so the exposure can be made immediately.
3. Administer the barium antegrade.
4. Place the patient in position, and follow the required sequence for times and positioning for proper completion of positive-contrast UGI study.
5. Follow up with a negative-contrast study if required.

Use of BIPS
1. Prepare the patient, including fasting or feeding as required and survey radiographs.
2. Administer the capsules.
3. Expose lateral and VD views at the suggested time, depending on the condition. Repeat radiographs if required.
4. Follow up with barium study or negative-contrast study if required.

Excretory Urography
1. Prepare the patient, including fasting, enema, emptying of the bladder, insertion of IV line and urinary catheters, survey radiographs, and sedation/anesthesia. Follow proper aseptic technique.
2. Have everything ready so exposures can be made immediately after administration of contrast medium.
3. Administer the warmed contrast water-soluble organic iodide IV as a quick bolus.
4. Expose the required radiographs in the correct time sequence.
5. Apply compression if required, and continue the sequence of exposure.
6. Follow up with a positive or negative retrograde contrast medium if required for the bladder or urethra.
7. Remove the contrast medium, insert an antibiotic if required, remove the catheter, and recover the patient.

Myelography
1. Prepare the patient, including fasting, enema (if required), survey radiographs, general anesthesia, and shaving and scrubbing of the site. Follow proper aseptic technique.
2. Have everything ready.
3. Place the needle; remove CSF, and slowly inject warmed organic nonionic positive-contrast iodine.
4. Obtain the required lateral, VD, and oblique radiographs.
5. Recover the patient when appropriate.

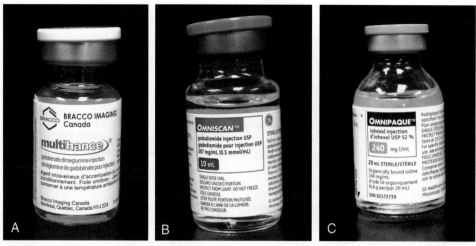

FIG. 23.23 MRI contrast agents. **A,** Gadobenate dimeglumine (MultiHance). **B,** Gadodiamide (Omniscan). **C,** Omnipaque, a nonionic contrast agent used for radiography and CT studies.

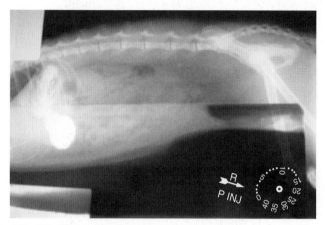

FIG. 23.24 Mystery radiograph. Why is there a difference in density on the lower portion of the radiograph?

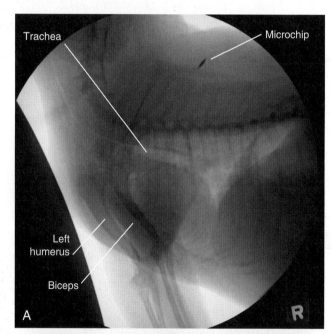

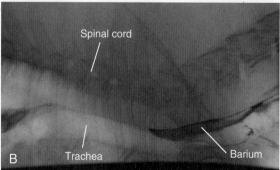

FIG. 23.25 A, Fluoroscopy in right lateral recumbency without any contrast study. Note that the trachea is white and the bones are dark. **B,** Fluoroscopy of the esophagus in right lateral recumbency with barium. (Courtesy Tara Wochesen, Ontario Veterinary College, Veterinary Teaching Hospital, Diagnostic Imaging at the University of Guelph.)

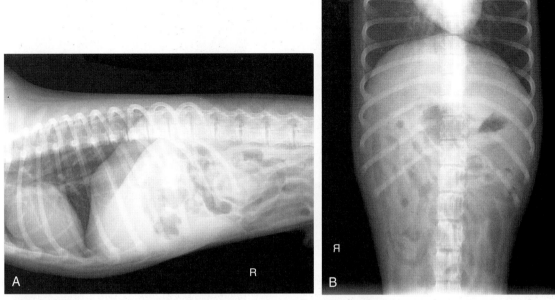

FIG. 23.26 A, Right lateral survey. **B,** Ventrodorsal survey radiograph. (Courtesy Tara Wochesen, Ontario Veterinary College, Veterinary Teaching Hospital, Diagnostic Imaging at the University of Guelph.)

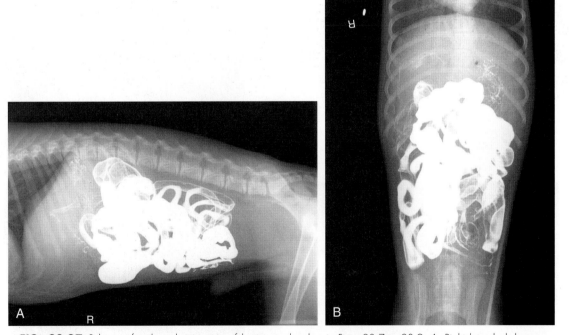

FIG. 23.27 3 hours after the administration of barium to the dog in Figs. 23.7 to 23.9. **A,** Right lateral abdomen. **B,** Ventrodorsal abdomen. (Courtesy Tara Wochesen, Ontario Veterinary College, Veterinary Teaching Hospital, Diagnostic Imaging at the University of Guelph.)

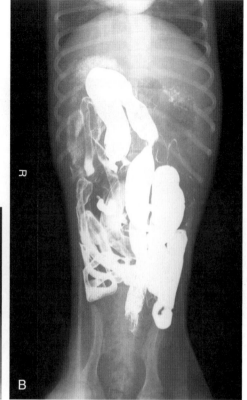

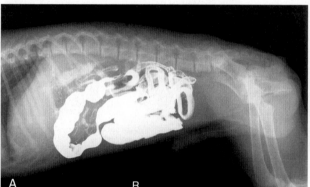

FIG. 23.28 4 hours after the administration of barium to the dog in Figs. 23.7 to 23.9. **A,** Right lateral abdomen. **B,** Ventrodorsal abdomen. (Courtesy Tara Wochesen, Ontario Veterinary College, Veterinary Teaching Hospital, Diagnostic Imaging at the University of Guelph.)

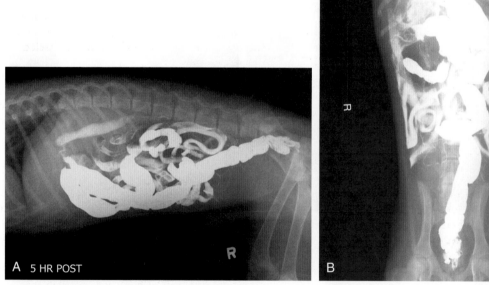

FIG. 23.29 5 hours after the administration of barium to the dog in Figs. 23.7 to 23.9. **A,** Right lateral abdomen. **B,** Ventrodorsal abdomen. (Courtesy Tara Wochesen, Ontario Veterinary College, Veterinary Teaching Hospital, Diagnostic Imaging at the University of Guelph.)

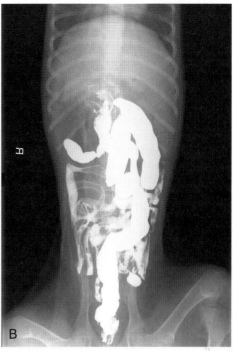

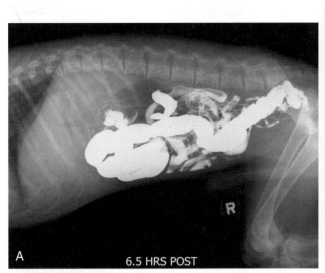

FIG. 23.30 6.5 after the administration of barium to the dog in Figs. 23.7 to 23.9. **A,** Right lateral abdomen. **B,** Ventrodorsal abdomen. (Courtesy Tara Wochesen, Ontario Veterinary College, Veterinary Teaching Hospital, Diagnostic Imaging at the University of Guelph.)

✳ KEY POINTS

1. Contrast medium enhances the surrounding tissue or organ to make it more visible radiographically.
2. Positive-contrast medium has a greater atomic number than the elements of soft tissue and bone, and it is denser. Thus agents such as barium (atomic number 56) attenuate the x-rays to a greater degree, absorb more x-rays, and create a whiter image on the radiograph than bone or tissues.
3. Negative-contrast media have lower atomic numbers and are less dense than soft tissue, so the x-rays will not be attenuated. X-rays pass through more easily, causing a black image to appear on the radiograph. Carbon dioxide and nitrous oxide are the negative-contrast agents of choice because according to the literature, room air can create air emboli.
4. Double-contrast studies utilize both positive- and negative-contrast agents. Depending on the study, the negative-contrast medium is often administered first and the positive-contrast agent second.
5. A contrast study is generally more effective for determining the change in morphology than for determining the function of an organ.
6. There is a risk involved in any contrast study. The benefits and contraindications need to be weighed by the veterinarian.
7. Various dilutions of barium sulfate suspension are the most commonly used positive-contrast agent for GI studies.
8. Barium should not be used if there is a suspected perforation, because barium is physiologically inert. It resists dilution in the peritoneal cavity and is completely insoluble. If it were leaked into the peritoneal cavity, a granuloma or adhesions may occur. Barium should never be injected intravenously.
9. Water-soluble organic iodides can be used if there is suspected intestinal perforation. They have a rapid transit time, are readily absorbed from the peritoneal cavity across the mucosa, and are excreted by the kidney.
10. Water-soluble organic ionic iodine is hypertonic and can cause electrolyte imbalance, dehydration, nausea, vomiting, decreased blood pressure, and other physiological problems.
11. Water-soluble organic nonionic iodine with a dimer chemical structure is almost isotonic to blood and cerebral fluid and has fewer side effects than ionic iodine.
12. Patient and other preparation are essential for the full benefit of the contrast study to be obtained.

Continued

✳ KEY POINTS—cont'd

Depending on the study, this could include fasting, enema administration, and/or sedation. Make sure that the correct concentration in sufficient amount is given and that enough radiographs are made at the appropriate times. Have image receptors, markers, timers, protective apparel, etc., ready before the administration of the contrast agent.

13. Survey radiographs before the administration of the contrast agent are essential for ensuring that the correct exposure is made, that patient preparation is adequate, and that the contrast study still needs to be completed.

14. The actual procedure and radiographs taken are dictated by the clinical signs in the patient and by the veterinarian's assessment. Only one area may need to be evaluated, or a full-system contrast study may be required.

15. Ultrasound and other imaging modalities, when available, have replaced contrast radiography for many evaluations.

16. The nonionic contrast agents used for radiography are generally used for CT. Gadolinium can be used for MRI, and radiopharmaceuticals are used for PET or nuclear medicine imaging.

REVIEW QUESTIONS

1. A contrast agent solution is completely insoluble, radiopaque, and physiologically inert. This would be in reference to:
   a. Barium
   b. Iodine
   c. Air
   d. BIPS

2. To increase the viscosity of organic nonionic dimer solutions, it is best to:
   a. Chill the solution
   b. Warm the solution
   c. Keep the solution at room temperature
   d. Add saline to the solution

3. To increase the transit time of barium for a UGI study, it is best to:
   a. Chill the solution
   b. Warm the solution
   c. Keep the solution at room temperature
   d. Add saline to the solution

4. Vomiting, defecation, urination, urticaria, tachycardia, and hypotension with or without collapse are more likely to occur when administrating a/an:
   a. Nonionic monomer contrast agent
   b. Nonionic dimer contrast agent
   c. Ionic monomer contrast agent
   d. Ionic dimer contrast agent

5. Urinary samples are best collected_____ administration of the contrast agents because:
   a. after; bacterial growth is not inhibited by contrast media
   b. after; there will not be a false positive in urinary protein
   c. before; bacterial growth is inhibited by contrast media
   d. either before or after; there will be no change in either urinary protein or bacterial growth

6. A nonionic dimer, iodine-based contrast agent is almost isotonic because:
   a. The ionizing carboxyl group is replaced with a group that does not dissociate
   b. The cations separate when injected into the blood or given orally
   c. There are three iodine atoms to every two particles in solution
   d. It has a low viscosity

7. A hypertonic contrast agent is likely to cause:
   a. Water to move from the vessels into the extravascular tissues and red blood cells
   b. Minimal side effects as the plasma and the agent are almost the same osmolality
   c. Crenation, vasodilation, and decreased blood pressure
   d. Elimination to take place through the liver and not the kidney

8. You have just administered barium via gastric gavage to a cat. For a full study, it is best to take the radiographs:
   a. At 15, 30, 60, and 90 minutes and then hourly until completed
   b. Immediately; at 5, 10, 20, and 60 minutes; and then hourly
   c. Immediately; at 15, 30, 60, and 90 minutes; and then hourly until completed
   d. Immediately; at 30, 60, and 90 minutes; and then hourly until completed

9. You are looking at a radiograph of a terrier in right lateral recumbency. Barium has just reached the cecum. The time of the radiograph, assuming average filling, is probably:
   a. 15 minutes
   b. 30 minutes
   c. 1 hour
   d. 2 hours

10. Five small BIPS and two large BIPS are still remaining in the stomach of a Doberman. In the large intestine there are 15 small BIPS and 3 large BIPS. The rest of the BIPS are all accounted for in the small intestine. The orocolic transit time for the large BIPS is:
    a. 20%
    b. 30%
    c. 50%
    d. 70%

11. The primary function of the large barium-impregnated polyethylene spheres is to:
    a. Determine extramural, mural, or intramural lesions
    b. Mimic the passage of food and calculate transit times
    c. Detect gastrointestinal tract obstructions
    d. Visualize the mucosal irregularities of the large intestine

12. A retrograde double-contrast cystogram is to be performed. The patient is best fasted:
    a. 12 to 24 hours
    b. 4 to 12 hours
    c. 1 to 4 hours
    d. not at all as fasting is not needed for this study

13. An esophagogram is to be completed. An enema should be given:
    a. 1 to 4 hours
    b. 4 to 12 hours
    c. 12 to 24 hours
    d. Not at all as an enema is not needed for this study

14. The best radiograph contrast procedure to assess the urinary bladder mucosa is:
    a. Excretory urography
    b. Double-contrast cystography
    c. Positive-contrast cystography
    d. Negative-contrast cystography (pneumocystogram)

15. The nephrogram phase of an excretory urogram shows the:
    a. Vascular supply and perfusion of the kidneys and should be taken immediately
    b. Vascular supply and perfusion of the kidneys and should be taken at 5 minutes
    c. Renal collection system and should be taken immediately
    d. Renal collection system and should be taken at 5 minutes

16. The most appropriate contrast medium for a positive-contrast cystography in dogs is:
    a. Barium sulfate paste
    b. Barium sulfate solution
    c. Air
    d. Iodinated water-soluble liquid

17. You are going to perform a positive-contrast retrograde cystography on a 35-kg male retriever. If the total dose is 240 mL of a 10% diluted meglumine diatrizoate (Hypaque M), how much diluent will you add if the original Hypaque M solution is 60%?
    a. 40 mL
    b. 160 mL
    c. 200 mL
    d. 280 mL

18. When radiographing for a double-contrast cystogram of a large dog, the central ray should be at:
    a. The umbilicus
    b. L2 or L3
    c. The caudal portion of the wings of the ilia
    d. The cranial portion of the wings of the ilia

19. The peripheral borders for a double-contrast cystogram for a large dog will likely be:
    a. T13 to the caudal portion of the ischium
    b. T8 to the caudal portion of the ischium
    c. L2 to the cranial portion of the ischium
    d. L2 to the caudal portion of the ischium

20. For a double-contrast cystogram of a male retriever, it is best to obtain right lateral:
    a. left lateral, VD (optional), and DV
    b. left lateral, and oblique (VD optional)
    c. and VD
    d. VD, and oblique (optional)

Answers to Review Questions can be found on the Evolve website.

References

1. Kelly EA. Ontario Association of Medical Radiation Technologists (OAMRT): Intravenous contrast injection for medical radiation technologists & related allied health professionals, revised November 2010. File No: 4010-4036. Ontario Association of Medical Radiation Technologists.
2. American Society of Health-System Pharmacists. Quick guide to contrast media, 2010. http://www.ashp.org/Import/PRACTICE ANDPOLICY/PracticeResourceCenters/ContrastMedia/QuickGuide toContrastMedia.aspx.
3. Han C, Hurd C. *Practical Diagnostic Imaging for the Veterinary Technician*. 3rd ed. St. Louis: Mosby; 2005.
4. Morgan JP. *Techniques of Veterinary Radiography*. Ames, IA: Iowa State University Press; 1993.
5. Muhlbauer MC, Kneller SK. *Radiography of the Dog and Cat: Guide to Making and Interpreting Radiographs*. Oxford: Wiley-Blackwell; 2013. Ch 3.
6. Thrall DE. *Textbook of Veterinary Diagnostic Radiology*. 6th ed. St. Louis: Elsevier; 2013. Ch. 27, 39.
7. Rendano V. UGI-stomach-ohiostate.htm/Veterinary Radiography. In: *Proceedings of the Ontario Association of Veterinary Technician Conference*. Toronto: February 2005.
8. Lester NV, Roberts GD, Newell SM, et al. Assessment of barium impregnated polyethylene spheres (BIPS) as a measure of solid-phase gastric emptying in normal dogs—comparison to scintigraphy. *Vet Radiol Ultrasound*. 1999;40:465-471.
9. Goggin JM, Hoskinson JJ, Kirk CA, et al. Comparison of gastric emptying times in healthy cats simultaneously evaluated with radiopaque markers and nuclear scintigraphy. *Vet Radiol Ultrasound*. 1999;40:89-95.

10. Wyse CA, McLellan J, Dickie AM, et al. A review of methods for assessment of the rate of gastric emptying in the dog and cat: 1898-2002. *J Vet Intern Med*. 2003;17:609-621.

11. Medical ID Systems, Inc. BIPS Manual. Published 2008. http://www.medid.com/manual_bipers.pdf.

12. Bennet C. Ontario Veterinary College, University of Guelph, March 2016.

13. Ayers S. *Small Animal Radiographic Techniques and Positioning*. Oxford: Wiley-Blackwell; 2013.

Bibliography

American College of Radiology Imaging Network. About imaging exams and agents. Published 2011. http://www.acrin.org/PATIENTS/ABOUTIMAGINGEXAMSANDAGENTS/ABOUTIMAGINGAGENTSORTRACERS.aspx.

Carrig CB. The use of compression in abdominal radiography of the dog and cat. *Vet Radiol*. 1976;17:178-181.

Colville T, Bassert J. *Clinical Anatomy and Physiology for Veterinary Technicians*. 3rd ed. St. Louis: Mosby; 2016.

Done SH, Goody PC, Stickland NC, et al. *Color Atlas of Veterinary Anatomy, the Dog and Cat*. London: Mosby; 2009.

Douglas SW. *Principles of Veterinary Radiography*. London: Bailliere Tindall; 1980.

Dyce KM, Sack WO, Wensing CJG. *Textbook of Veterinary Anatomy*. 4th ed. St. Louis: Saunders; 2010.

Evans H, de Lahunta A. *Guide to the Dissection of the Dog*. 8th ed. St. Louis: Saunders; 2017.

Lester NV, Roberts GD, Newell SM, et al. Assessment of barium impregnated spheres (BIPS) as a measure of solid-phase gastric emptying in normal dogs-comparison to scintigraphy. *Vet Radiol Ultrasound*. 1999;40:465-471.

Owens JM, Biery DN. *Radiographic Interpretation for the Small Animal Clinician*. 2nd ed. Baltimore: Williams & Wilkins; 1999.

Sirois M, Anthony E, Mauragis D. *Handbook of Radiographic Positioning for Veterinary Technicians*. Clifton Park, NY: Delmar Cengage Learning; 2010.

Solomon R. Role of osmolality in the incidence of contrast induced nephropathy: a systemic review of angiographic contrast media in high risk patients. *Kidney Int*. 2005;68:2257.

Tighe M, Brown M. *Mosby's Comprehensive Review for Veterinary Technicians*. 4th ed. St. Louis: Elsevier; 2015.

CHAPTER 24

Equine and Large Animal Radiography*

Marg Brown, RVT, BEd Ad Ed

The essential joy of being with horses is that it brings us in contact with the rare elements of grace, beauty, spirit, and fire.
—Sharon Ralls Lemons, Author and equestrian

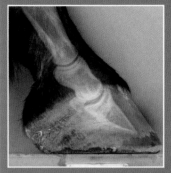

(Courtesy EponaTech LLC, Paso Robles, California.)

OUTLINE

---

*Special thanks to Shannon T. Brownrigg, RVT, who co-wrote this chapter for the previous edition.

LEARNING OBJECTIVES

When you have finished this chapter, you will be able to:

1. Understand the terminology used in equine and large-animal radiography.
2. Identify skeletal anatomy.
3. Produce a diagnostic radiograph for common radiographic procedures of the equine/large-animal patient, using proper safety and positioning techniques.

4. Identify the less common views.
5. Identify normal equine and large-animal anatomy found on a radiograph.

KEY TERMS

Key terms are defined in the Glossary on the Evolve website.

Caudoproximal-craniodistal
  (CdPr-CrDi)
Cranioproximal-caudodistal
  (CrPr-CdDi)
Crena
Dorsolateral-palmaromedial
  oblique (DLPMO)
Dorsolateral-ventrolateral
  oblique (DLVLO)

Dorsomedial-palmarolateral
  oblique (DMPLO)
Dorsoproximal-dorsodistal
  oblique (DPr-DDi)
Dorsoproximal-palmarodistal
  (DPr-PaDi)
Flexor view
High coronary view
Lateromedial (LaM)

Midsagittal plane
Occlusal
Palmaroproximal-
  palmarodistal oblique
  (PaPr-PaDi)
Plantaroproximal-
  plantarodistal (PlPr-PlDi)
Positional terminology
Skyline

Sulcus
Tangential
Ungular or collateral
  cartilages
Upright pedal route
Ventrolateral-dorsolateral
  oblique
Weight bearing

TECHNICAL NOTE: To preserve space, the radiographs presented in this chapter do not show collimation. For safety, always collimate so that the beam is limited to within the image receptor edges. In film radiography, you should see a clear border of collimation (frame) on every radiograph. In some jurisdictions, evidence of collimation is required by law.

Imaging large animals requires good planning, good teamwork, lots of patience, and being prepared to expect the unexpected. The common principles of radiography that apply to small animals also apply to large animals, with the major differences being due to patient size and posture, which necessitate special consideration for areas of patient restraint, equipment, preparation, radiation safety, and positioning devices. Safety of personnel and patient is critical.

Compare the large-animal anatomy with human and small-animal anatomy (Fig. 24.1). The technical terms are similar but common terms differ.

Special Considerations

Restraint and Patient Preparation

Large animals in the standing position are minimally restrained, which is a concern for both human and machine safety. Large animals can easily become startled when confronted with unfamiliar objects, so it is important to minimize sudden movements and loud noises. Keep the behavior of the particular patient in mind, and modify your restraint to take advantage of that behavior, being aware that any sights or sounds such as uncoiling electrical cords or moving positioning devices can startle a typically quiet horse.

Ensure there is a solid ground surface that is level, clean, and nonslippery. The area should be quiet, free of obstacles, and large enough for personnel to move around the horse safely. Sedation may calm the patient and curtail startling that can cause movement blur on the image. Depending on the patient, consider various strategies such as raising the opposite limb, using a twitch, offering food, or using stocks.

A competent handler is essential if the horse is being difficult or sedation is not an option.

Movement artifacts, poor positioning of the patient or the x-ray beam, and inadequate exposure are the most common reasons that images must be repeated. Among other inconveniences, any repetition means further radiation dose for the restrainer or the patient. To help minimize repeat radiographs, take the time to make sure that the patient is properly positioned, the image receptor is properly placed, and the central ray is directed correctly.

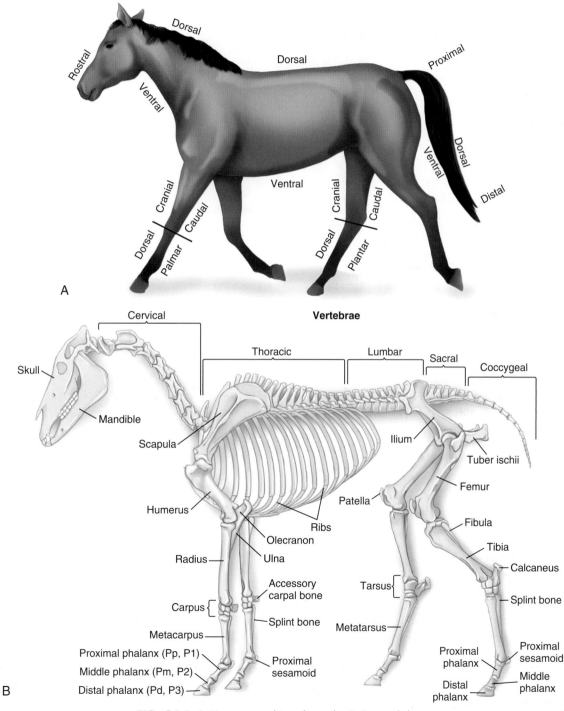

FIG. 24.1 A, Key terms used in radiography. B, Equine skeleton.   *Continued*

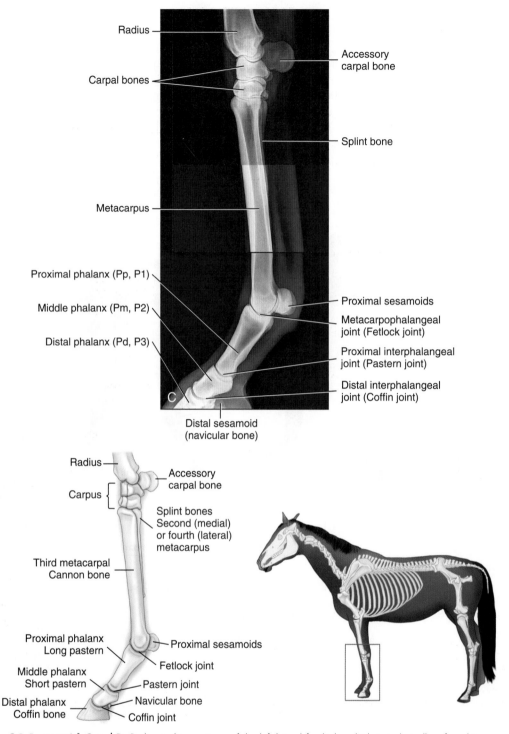

FIG. 24.1, cont'd C and D, Radiographic anatomy of the left lateral forelimb, which is technically referred to as a lateromedial view.

Proper patient preparation is essential to obtain high-quality radiographs and to minimize radiation exposure. The hair coat should be dry, brushed, and cleared of dirt or other debris. If the foot is being radiographed, it is important to prevent overlying shadows superimposed on the field of view. This is especially true of dorsopalmar/dorsoplantar and oblique views. Remove the shoe and trim back any overgrown portions of the foot. Pick and thoroughly clean the sole and clefts, and then pack the sulci adjacent to and in the center of the frog with a substance of similar radiographic opacity, such as Play-Doh, methylcellulose, or softened soap, to eliminate gas shadows due to the grooves of the frog (Fig. 24.2).

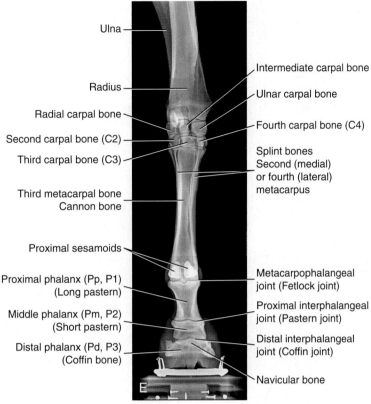

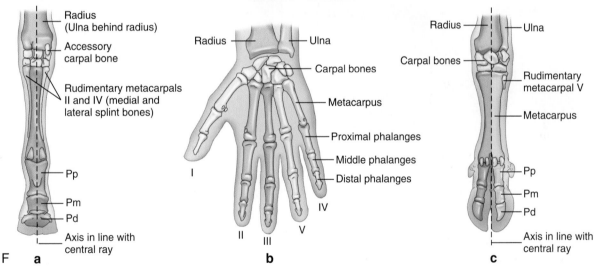

FIG. 24.1, cont'd E, Radiographic anatomy of the DP or dorsopalmar (dorsoproximal-palmarodistal) of left forelimb. F, Comparison of the palmar views of the (a) horse's limb, (b) human hand, and (c) ruminant's limb. (C and E courtesy Vetel Diagnostics, San Luis Obispo, California, and Seth Wallack, DVM, DACVR, AAVR, Director and CEO of Veterinary Imaging Centre of San Diego.)

Double-check that you have all proper equipment and supplies with you, including foot blocks, as well as protective equipment and devices for all personnel to be as far from the primary beam as possible. If film cassettes are used and radiographs are being taken off site, make sure to take enough cassettes and film to the facility to allow for "repeats" and unexpected views. For digital radiography make sure that all required equipment such as spare cords, hand switches, or required batteries is on hand.

🖊 TECHNICIAN NOTES

Debris such as shavings, mud, sand, small stones, and manure may cause radiographic artifacts. Sweep the area you are working in to keep the packing clean and minimize artifacts. Visually inspect and clean the legs and hooves well before taking images of the area. Depending on the size of the foot, try brown paper bags, craft paper, sandwich bags, plastic wrap, paper towel, or dry gauze to keep the packing material from picking up particles.

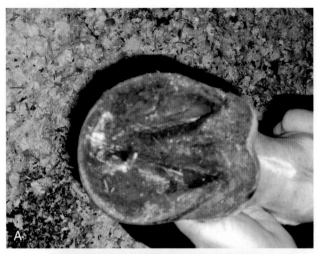

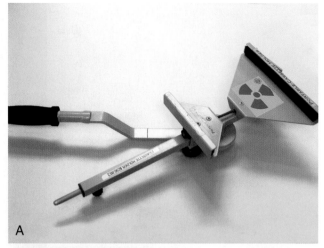

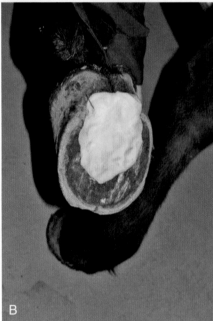

FIG. 24.2 For diagnostic radiographs of the distal foot, the shoe should be removed and the sole cleaned (**A**), then packed with a radiolucent material (**B**). (**A** courtesy Shannon Brownrigg.)

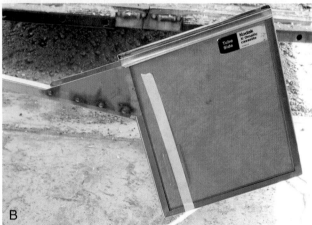

FIG. 24.3 A and B, Commercial cassette holders used for equine positioning.

Radiation Safety and Positioning Devices

All of the radiation safety principles applied to small animals equally apply to large animals. When working with large animals, concern for physical safety often supersedes radiation safety. Thus it is essential to constantly keep the three tenets of radiation safety in mind (shielding, distance, and time).

Portable machines can be particularly dangerous with regard to radiation exposure as they can be aimed in any direction and they use longer exposure times than stationary units to produce diagnostic images due to limited machine power. It is critical for all individuals who will be in the path of the beam, near the beam, or holding the portable x-ray unit to have appropriate and proper fitting protective lead attire, thyroid collars, and a monitoring badge (see Chapter 3).

All personal protective equipment (PPE) must undergo a routine maintenance schedule to evaluate weaknesses and breakage (see Chapters 3 and 9). Proper storage of PPE is important; avoid folding gowns and gloves.

The most significant safety action is to increase one's distance from the primary beam through the use of a cassette holder (Fig. 24.3) and the use of a tripod to hold the x-ray unit if space and circumstances allow. Because the construction of x-ray machines does not allow the primary beam to be centered less than about 10 cm (4 inches) from the ground, a positioning block is needed to raise the affected foot (Fig. 24.4) for most views of the foot and pastern.

Always collimate. The primary beam should only include the area of interest so that all margins of the primary beam are visible on the processed film. In digital imaging the algorithm depends on proper collimation. Stand out of direct or bright light to see the collimator guide-light. Because the horizontal beam is standard, always be conscious of where the beam is directed and where individuals are standing; a cassette holder should be used when possible. To help decrease exposure time, use a fast combination of film and screen if using this system.

The source-image distance (SID) is generally less for large animals, with the common SID being 26 to 30 inches

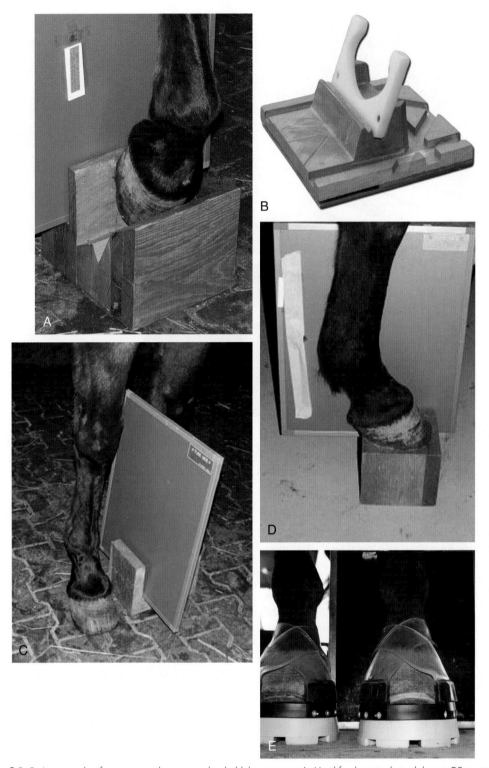

FIG. 24.4 An example of positioning devices used to hold the cassette. **A,** Used for the upright pedal route DP positions. **B,** Redden Navicular x-ray block. **C,** Ideal for lateral views of the metacarpus. **D,** Use for the lateral phalanx and sesamoids. The block can be rotated for a DP weight-bearing view so the beam is parallel to the ground. **E,** EZ Blox-Strap on X-ray blocks. *Continued*

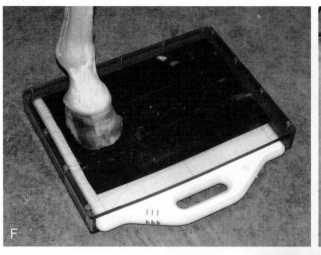

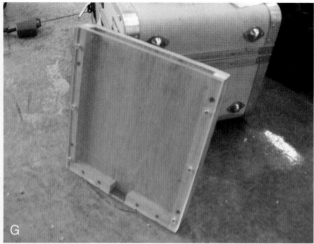

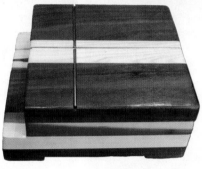

FIG. 24.4, cont'd F, Use of a radiolucent cassette tunnel for the digital plate. G, Homemade cassette tunnel for film cassette. H, Redden offset lateral and DP x-ray positioning block. (B and H courtesy NANRIC, www.nanric.com; E courtesy Equine Digit Support System, Inc., www.ezxrayblox.com.)

(66 cm-76.2 cm), compared with 40 inches (100 cm) in radiography of small animals. Always use the retractable tape measure to determine the proper SID based on the technique chart. Do not guess! Some units have two small laser pointers at precise angles that merge at the correct distance when the collimator light is on. A shorter SID also helps decrease the exposure time. If the SID changes from what is suggested on the technique chart, keep this formula in mind to change the mAs:

$$\text{Old mAs} \times \frac{(\text{New SID})^2}{(\text{Old SID})^2} = \text{New mAs}$$

Review Chapters 5 and 6 if you need to adjust the image technique.

A cassette tunnel is also useful for digit radiographs to protect the image receptor for dorsopalmar/dorsoplantar and oblique views of the foot. A cassette tunnel can be purchased or can be manufactured out of radiolucent wood (avoid use of nails) or hard plastic durable enough to withstand the weight of the horse. If using a cassette tunnel, make sure it is strong enough to support the weight of the horse and is translucent to minimize artifacts on the film (Fig. 24.4F and G). To minimize a slippery surface, cover with duct tape or use a mouse pad or section of yoga mat between the hoof and tunnel.

If using a foot block, have it high enough so that the beam can be directed in a horizontal plane on the area of interest. Ideally, the block should have a slot to support the cassette close to the limb to minimize distortion (Fig. 24.4D). If only the lateromedial view of the digit is needed, then shoe removal, sole cleaning, and foot trimming are not essential. For equal weight-bearing, both front feet should be on a foot block. If only the affected foot is placed on the block, improper pressure of the distal limb joints may affect the accuracy of the diagnosis.

The opposite limb may need to be lifted to ensure full weight-bearing and to prevent motion if equal weight-bearing is not required.

Keep the image receptor as close and parallel to the limb as possible to minimize object-film distance (OFD) and distortion. The suggested angle with the ground may change depending on the limb confirmation of the patient. The central ray should always be perpendicular to the limb axis being radiographed.

> **✐ TECHNICIAN NOTES**
>
> *ALWAYS* keep the three principles of radiation safety in mind—time, distance, and shielding—when imaging large animals. Also remember to collimate, collimate, collimate.

Equipment

Of the three types of x-ray machines available—portable, mobile, and ceiling mounted—the portable unit is the most practical for those in ambulatory practices. Portable units are small and can be set up wherever there is a power supply.

Ensure there is an adequate power supply, as line voltage may vary, causing inconsistency in the exposures. These units are generally adequate for radiography of the equine distal limbs, skull, and cranial cervical vertebrae. Keep cords well away from feet to prevent tangling or damage from being stepped on. Position the horse so the cords can reach both the left and right sides. Although the portable equipment is built to withstand a certain amount of rough handling, transportation and frequent movement of radiographic equipment increase the opportunity for damage to x-ray equipment. Units should never be left in the vehicle overnight during below-freezing temperatures unless a sufficient warm-up time is taken into consideration before the first exposure.

Depending on the type of unit, the kilovoltage (kV) and milliampere (mA) are generally preset, giving power anywhere from 40 to 120 kV and 15 to 100 mA. Time is usually the variable control, providing values of 0.3 to generally 50 milliampere-seconds (mAs). Newer units have variable kV and mAs. The digital displays allow adjustments of 1- to 5-kV increments. Because of the relatively low mA capacity, movement is a concern. Mobile units can be wheeled from room to room in the same premises, but are generally too cumbersome to be easily moved and transported. The kV and mA capacity is higher, allowing for shorter exposure times and less chance of motion artifacts than with the portable units.

Veterinary specialty referral practices commonly use large units permanently mounted on a set of ceiling rails to allow horizontal and vertical movement. These high-capacity units have the greatest output range (between 800 and 1000 mA), capable of obtaining high-quality radiographs of regions such as the thorax, pelvis, and thoracolumbar vertebrae. It may be difficult to obtain parallel views of the feet because the unit may not reach the ground close enough to prevent obliquity. A supplementary portable unit is often used in these situations.

Exposure factors vary for each machine, so contact the generator manufacturer for a technique chart that can be used as a starting point. See Chapters 5 and 8 for suggested equine charts.

Regular maintenance and calibration of all x-ray units are essential to the consistent production of quality radiographs and maintenance of a safe working environment. Inspections should be implemented as per local regulations.

See Chapter 8 for further information on digital equipment.

> ### ✐ TECHNICIAN NOTES
>
> Electrical power may vary in different barn settings. Power may not have the consistency (brownouts) to produce quality radiographs. Have suitable and safety-approved extension cord(s) for exterior use as part of your equipment list. Proper-length cords are best (the shorter the better).

Equine Radiography

Radiographic Interpretation and Diagnosis

You should have an understanding of the normal equine anatomy. Use a systematic approach, making sure to view the whole image. Review the radiography checklist found in Chapter 15.

The purpose of most radiographs taken in equine practice is to evaluate the bones of the skeleton; thus any response of the bone to insult or disease is relevant. Any changes such as sclerosis (causing more of a radiopaque image) or demineralization (radiolucent appearance) may not be visible on the radiograph, as a change of at least 30% in the bone mineral matrix is required before radiographic changes are evident.[1]

Consideration may need to be given to additional imaging for accurate diagnosis and prognosis. This would include ultrasonography as well as cross-sectional imaging modalities such as computerized tomography (CT), magnetic resonance imaging (MRI), scintigraphy, and further diagnostic testing. CT and MRI show the most detail in all structures, indicating actual soft tissue and cartilage within the foot. Modalities such as nuclear scintigraphy and thermography show problem areas to the bone and soft tissue, such as ligaments, tendons, and articular cartilage that are poorly imaged on radiographs (see Fig. 24.64).

Prepurchase Examinations

Equine clients often request a prepurchase examination of a horse before buying a competitive or breeding prospect. This examination is done to reduce the buyer's risk and assess the current health and athletic soundness of the horse. The examination is not a guarantee of the health or soundness of the horse, but an interpretation of the ability of the horse to meet the intended purpose of the procurer. Depending on the level of expected performance or value of the purchase, this examination may include extensive radiographs.

It is critical for all parties to identify any potential conflict of interest that may exist. The veterinarian requested to perform such an examination must clearly identify his or her relationship with, or prior knowledge of, the horse to be purchased and its owners or trainers. It is recommended to have a legal agreement prepared and signed that clearly identifies any relationship or knowledge to protect the interest of the performing veterinarian.

> ### ✐ TECHNICIAN NOTES
>
> Unless otherwise indicated, when the limb is described in this chapter, the forelimb terminology is used, but it is understood that the same principles apply to the hind limb.

Labeling and Terminology

For proper diagnosis and legal requirements, correct labeling is mandatory. As with radiography of small animals, permanent identification of the patient and owner (or purchaser for a prepurchase examination) is required. The specific limb being radiographed should also be identified, as well as the actual position. This includes indicating forelimbs and hind limbs, especially distal to the carpus/tarsus.

As in small-animal radiography, the proximal end of the extremity is at the top of the viewer for DP/PD/CrCd/CdCr views. For the lateral or oblique radiographs, the proximal end points up, and the cranial or dorsal aspect of the limb is to your left.

Conventionally, limb markers should be placed dorsally or laterally. Place directional markers (right/left, front/rear) on the lateral aspect of the limb for DP(CrCd) and oblique views and at the dorsal/cranial aspect for lateromedial views. Use Velcro tabs or duct tape to affix to plate. If there is a swelling on the limb, a marker such as a BB pellet taped on the skin might be useful. If using a digital plate, take images in the order of DP, DLPMO, DMPLO, and LM to move the markers only once.

Because equine skeletal structures are large and complex, multiple views are required. In small animals, generally two views perpendicular to each other are taken. Horses generally require a minimum of four views for most positions, and six for many joints.

Refer to Chapter 15 for a review of some of the basic terminology.

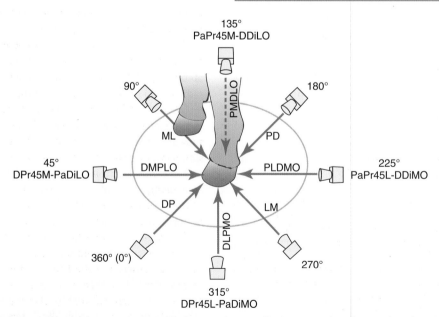

FIG. 24.5 Terminology of the equine proximal limb views. *Inner circle:* Common terminology and angles. *Outer circle:* Proper directional terms for the oblique views taken at the level of the metacarpus. *P* and *Pa,* palmar; *D,* dorsal; *Pr,* proximal; *Di,* distal; *M,* medial; *L,* lateral; *O,* oblique.

Dorsolateral-Palmaromedial Oblique (DLPMO)

For the dorsolateral-palmaromedial oblique (DLPMO) view (Fig. 24.6B), the central ray faces the dorsal part of the limb aimed 45 degrees laterally from the midline. The image receptor is on the palmaromedial aspect of the limb so that it is perpendicular to the beam. Remember "point of entry to point of exit"; the beam travels from dorsolateral to palmaromedial. The film marker is placed along the lateral aspect of the image receptor. So that there is no confusion as to what angle should be used, the proper description for this 45-degree DLPMO view is dorsoproximal 45-degree lateral palmarodisto-medial oblique (DPr45L-PaDiMO).

What is actually being highlighted on this DLPMO projection (Fig. 24.6B) is the portion that is not against the film—specifically the lateral sesamoid in Fig. 24.6B. Note that because this is taken at an oblique angle, the image of the medial proximal sesamoid is obstructed by the distal metacarpus (see Technician Notes). Thus an oblique projection allows the portion of the bone farther from the film to be in profile. The radiograph is like a shadow: the way the beam is directed, the body part on the film is superimposed in the oblique, and the opposite edges are highlighted.

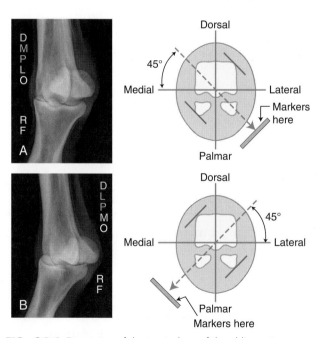

FIG. 24.6 Description of the terminology of the oblique views on a fetlock radiograph. The dotted lines are the direction of the beam and the red lines are the surfaces of the limbs being imaged. **A,** DMPLO or dorsoproximal 45-degree medial–palmarodistolateral oblique (DPr45M-PaDiLO). Following the rule and taking the middle two and outer two letters, you are looking at the dorsolateral and palmaromedial surfaces of the limb/medial sesamoid. **B,** DLPMO or dorsoproximal 45-degree lateral–palmarodistomedial oblique (DPr45L-PaDiMO). Following the rule and taking the middle two and outer two letters, you are looking at the dorsomedial and palmarolateral surfaces of the limb/lateral sesamoid. (Courtesy Carolyn Bennet, Ontario Veterinary College, Veterinary Teaching Hospital, Diagnostic Imaging at University of Guelph, Ontario.)

The view is correctly described first from where the beam enters on the limb and then where it exits. Using point of entry to point of exit the DLPMO is technically termed a *medial oblique* because the beam enters off the midline on the lateral aspect and exits on the medial aspect. The medial aspect is against the film. However, because the lateral portion of the bone is in profile in a DLPMO, practicing veterinarians may refer to the position as a *lateral oblique.*

Dorsomedial-Palmarolateral Oblique (DMPLO)

The same principle applies to the dorsomedial-palmarolateral oblique (DMPLO) (Fig. 24.6A), but this time the central ray is aimed at the dorsal part of the limb 45 degrees medially to the midline. The image receptor is on the palmarolateral aspect of the limb and is perpendicular to the beam. The beam travels from dorsomedial (point of entry) to palmarolateral (point of exit). The film marker is placed along the lateral aspect of the image receptor, appearing to be on the dorsal part of the limb in the radiograph. So that there is no confusion as to what angle should be used, the proper description for this 45-degree DMPLO is dorsoproximal 45-degree medial–palmarodistolateral oblique (DPr45M-PaDiLO).

Taking the two middle and two outer letters once the "O" is removed tells us that the dorsolateral and mediopalmar surfaces (*red lines* on Fig. 24.6A) will be highlighted. The medial proximal sesamoid is in profile.

Remember the view is correctly described first from where the beam enters on the limb and then where it exits. Using point of entry to point of exit, the DMPLO is technically termed a lateral oblique since the beam enters off the midline on the medial aspect and exits on the lateral aspect. The lateral aspect is against the film. However, because the medial portion of the bone is in profile in a DMPLO, practicing veterinarians may refer to the position as a *medial oblique.*

In practice, you may hear common terms that are used in place of the correct anatomical terms (Table 24.1) or different modes of describing the beam. Anterior posterior (AP), a human term, is still sometimes used in practice; however, the correct nomenclature is *dorsopalmar* or *dorsoplantar (DP).* Common terms are listed here for the purpose of further understanding but are not necessarily the proper nomenclature.

TABLE 24.1	Comparative Terminology of the Human and Equine Limbs		
ANATOMICAL TERM	**FURTHER TERM/ABBREVIATION**	**COMMON LAY TERM**	**HUMAN EQUIVALENT**
Distal phalanx (Pd)	Third phalanx (P3)	Coffin or pedal bone	Distal phalanx (finger tip)
Distal interphalangeal joint		Coffin joint	Distal interphalangeal joint
Distal sesamoid		Navicular bone	
Middle phalanx (Pm)	Second phalanx (P2)	Short pastern	Middle phalanx
Middle interphalangeal joint		Pastern joint	Middle interphalangeal joint
Proximal phalanx (Pp)	First phalanx (P1)	Long pastern	Proximal phalanx
Proximal sesamoid bones		Fetlock	
Metacarpal interphalangeal joint		Fetlock joint	Metacarpal interphalangeal joint—knuckle
Metacarpus/metatarsus	Third metacarpal/metatarsal bone (M3)	Cannon bone	Metacarpus /Metatarsus
	Second metacarpal bone/ metatarsal bone (M2)	Short splint bone	
	Fourth metacarpal bone/metatarsal bone (M4)	Long splint bone	
Carpometacarpal/ carpometatarsal joint		Knee joint/hock joint	Wrist joint/ankle joint
Carpus/tarsus		Knee/hock	Wrist/ankle
Brachioantebrachial/ femorotibial joints	Elbow/stifle	Elbow/stifle	Elbow/knee
Shoulder/pelvis		Shoulder/hip	Shoulder/pelvis

Data from Butler JA, Coles CM, Dyson SJ, et al: *Clinical Radiology of the Horse*, Osney Mead, Oxford, 1993, Blackwell Science Ltd; Morgan JP: *Techniques of Veterinary Radiography*, Ames, IA, 1993, Iowa State University Press; Thrall DE: *Textbook of Veterinary Diagnostic Radiology*, St Louis, 2007, Saunders; Weaver M, Barakzai S: *Handbook of Equine Radiography*, London, 2010, Saunders.

TECHNICIAN NOTES

To demonstrate that the opposite projections will be in profile, tape two different objects, such as a pen and pencil, to an empty paper towel roll. Label four sides dorsal, palmar, lateral, and medial, and place a piece of paper behind your "limb." Use your finger as the x-ray beam and try the oblique views. Notice that the opposite protrusion is in profile. Using a flashlight may also help you visualize the projections better. The radiograph is like a shadow with the way the beam is directed—the part on the film is superimposed, but the opposite edges are highlighted.

TECHNICIAN NOTES

A human middle finger is equivalent to the front foot of the horse, whereas the hind foot is a human's middle toe (Fig. 24.7). Imagine standing on your middle toes all day. It is no wonder the foot is the most frequently imaged for equine lameness issues.

Equine Radiographic Positioning

Table 24.2 lists the views that are used in equine limb examination.

TECHNICIAN NOTES

Keep the principles of good radiographic imaging in mind every time. The body part should be close to and parallel to the image receptor, and the central ray is perpendicular to both. Think radiation safety for each exposure.

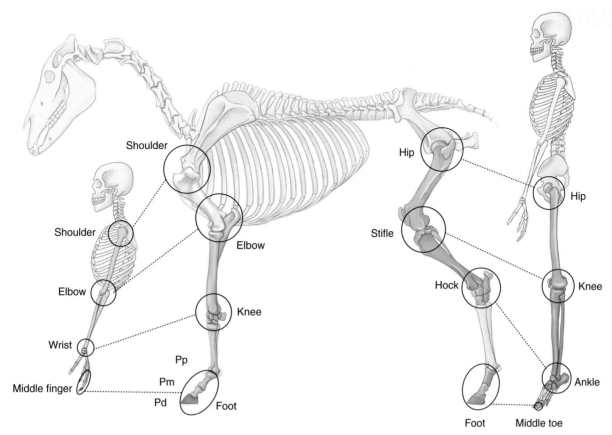

FIG. 24.7 Comparison of human and equine skeletal structures.

TABLE 24.2	Views of the Equine Limb Examination	
STRUCTURES EVALUATED/ COMMENTS	**VIEWS/COMMENTS**[a]	**COMMON TERMINOLOGY**
P3	Dorsal 65-degree proximal–palmarodistal oblique (D65Pr-PaDiO); beam angled to ground, high coronary or upright pedal routes.	Dorsopalmar (DP)
	Dorsoproximal-palmarodistal (DPr-PaDi) with horizontal beam	
	Lateromedial (LM) with foot on block (optional).	Lateral (L)
	Oblique views especially if a P3 fracture is suspected:	
	(1) Dorsal 65-degree proximal, 45-degree lateral–palmarodistomedial oblique (D65Pr-45L–PaDiMO)	(1) DLPMO
	(2) Dorsal 65-degree proximal, 45-degree medial–palmarodistolateral oblique (D65Pr-45M-PaDiLO)	(2) DMPLO
Distal interphalangeal joint	Dorsal 65-degree proximal–palmarodistal oblique (D65Pr-PaDiO) high coronary route with beam angled to ground	Dorsopalmar (DP)
	Lateromedial (LM) with foot on block to include solar margin of P3 and soft tissues of sole on the radiograph	Lateral (L)
Optional views	Oblique views	
	(1) Dorsal 65-degree proximal, 45-degree lateral–palmarodistomedial oblique (D65Pr-45L–PaDiMO)	(1) DLPMO
	(2) Dorsal 65-degree proximal, 45-degree medial–palmarodistolateral oblique (D65Pr-45M-PaDiLO)	(2) DMPLO

Continued

TABLE 24.2 Views of the Equine Limb Examination—cont'd

STRUCTURES EVALUATED/ COMMENTS	VIEWS/COMMENTS[a]	COMMON TERMINOLOGY
Navicular	Lateromedial (LM)	Lateral (L)
	Dorsoproximal-palmarodistal oblique (DPr-PaDiO):	Dorsopalmar (DP)
	(1) High coronary stand-on route:	
	45 degrees: projects proximal border and extremities (D45Pr-PaDiO)	
	65 degrees: projects both borders and extremities (D65Pr-PaDiO)	
	OR	
	(2) Upright pedal route (on a block):	Dorsopalmar (DP)
	D90Pr-PaDiO Projects proximal border and extremities	
	D80Pr-PaDiO: Projects both borders and extremities	
	Palmaroproximal-palmarodistal oblique view (PaPr-PaDiO):	Flexor or skyline
	D65Pr45L-PaDiMO	DLPMO
	D65Pr45M-PaDiLO	DMPLO
Pastern P1, proximal interphalangeal joint, P2	Lateromedial (LM)	Lateral (L)
	Dorsoproximal-palmarodistal oblique (D30-45Pr-PaDiO)	Dorsopalmar (DP)
	Dorsal 35-degree proximal, 35-degree lateral–palmarodistomedial oblique (D35Pr-35L-PaDiMO)	DLPMO
	Dorsal 35-degree proximal, 35-degree medial–palmarodistolateral oblique (D35Pr-35M-PaDiLO)	DMPLO
Metacarpophalangeal/ metatarsophalangeal joint/proximal sesamoid bones (fetlock)	Dorsal 10-degree proximal–palmarodistal oblique (D10Pr-PaDiO)	Dorsopalmar (DP)
	Lateromedial (LM) extended	Lateral (L)
	Lateromedial (LM) flexed	Flexed lateral (L)
	Dorsoproximal 45-degree lateral–palmarodistomedial oblique (DPr45L-PaDiMO)	DLPMO
	Dorsoproximal 45-degree medial–palmarodistolateral oblique (DPr45M-PaDiLO)	DMPLO
Optional views	Palmaroproximal-palmarodistal oblique view (PaPr-PaDiO)	Flexor/skyline/ caudal tangential
	Dorsoproximal-dorsodistal oblique (DPr-DDiO)	Extensor surface/ skyline
Metacarpal/ metatarsal cannon bone (M3)	Dorsoproximal-palmarodistal (DPr-PaDi)	Dorsopalmar (DP)
	Lateromedial (LM)	Lateral (L)
Lateral splint bone (M4)	Dorsoproximal 45-degree lateral–palmarodistomedial oblique (DPr45L-PaDiMO)	DLPMO
Medial splint bone (M2)	Dorsoproximal 45-degree medial–palmarodistolateral oblique (DPr45M-PaDiLO)	DMPLO
Carpus	Dorsoproximal-palmarodistal (DPr-PaDi)	Dorsopalmar (DP)
	Lateromedial extended (LM)	Lateral (L)
	Lateromedial flexed (LM)	Flexed lateral (L)
	Dorsoproximal 45-degree lateral–palmarodistomedial oblique (DPr45L-PaDiMO)	DLPMO
	Dorsoproximal 45-degree medial–palmarodistolateral oblique (DPr45M-PaDiLO)	DMPLO
Optional views	Dorsoproximal-dorsodistal oblique flexed (DPr-DDiO)	Skyline

TABLE 24.2	Views of the Equine Limb Examination—cont'd	
STRUCTURES EVALUATED/ COMMENTS	**VIEWS/COMMENTS[a]**	**COMMON TERMINOLOGY**
Tarsus	Dorsoproximal-plantarodistal (DPr-PlDi) Lateromedial (LM) extended Lateromedial flexed (LM) Dorsoproximal 45-degree lateral–plantarodistomedial oblique (DPr45L-PlDiMO) Dorsoproximal 45-degree medial–plantarodistolateral oblique (DPr45M-PlDiLO)	Dorsoplantar (DP) Lateral (L) Flexed lateral (L) DLPMO DMPLO
Tuber calcaneus	Flexed plantaroproximal-plantarodistal (PlPr-PlDi)	Skyline
Radius	Cranioproximal-caudodistal (CrPr-CdDi) Lateromedial (LM)	Craniocaudal (CrCd) Lateral (L)
Optional views	Caudoproximal-craniodistal (CdPr-CrDi) Cranioproximolateral-caudodistomedial oblique (CrPrL-CdDiMO) Cranioproximomedial-caudodistolateral oblique (CrPrM-CdDiLO)	Caudocranial (CdCr) CrLCdMO CrMCdLO
Elbow joint	Cranioproximal-caudodistal (CrPr-CdDi)—standing Mediolateral standing (ML)	Craniocaudal (CrCd) Lateral (L)
Optional views	Cranioproximal-craniodistal oblique (CrPr-CrDiO) of olecranon Lateromedial (LM) Mediolateral through the thoracic cavity Cranioproximal-caudodistal (CrPr-CdDi)—recumbent Mediolateral (recumbent) (ML) Craniomedial-caudolateral oblique	Skyline or flexor Lateral (L) Mediolateral (ML) Craniocaudal (CrCd) Lateral (L) CrMCdLO
Shoulder	Mediolateral (ML)	Lateral (L)
Optional views	Cranioproximal 45-degree medial–caudodistolateral oblique (CrPr45M-CaDiLO) Cranioproximal 45-degree lateral–caudodistomedial oblique (CrPr45L-CaDiMO)	CrMCdLO CrLCdMO
Stifle	Lateromedial (LM) Caudoproximal-craniodistal (CdPr-CrDi)	Lateral (L) Caudocranial (CdCr)
Lateral trochlear ridge and medial femoral condyle (stifle)	Caudoproximal 60-degree lateral–craniodistomedial oblique (Cd60L-CrMO)	CdLCrMO
Optional stifle	Cranioproximal-caudodistal (CrPr-CdDi) Cranioproximal-craniodistal oblique(CrPr-CrDiO) Lateromedial flexed (LM)	Craniocaudal (CrCd) Skyline patella Flexed lateral (L)

[a]*Palmar* is used in this chart and chapter with the understanding that *plantar* can be substituted when referring to the hind limb.
Data from Weaver M, Barakzai S: *Handbook of equine radiography,* London, 2010, Saunders Elsevier; Morgan JP: *Techniques of veterinary radiography.* Ames, IA, 1993, Iowa State University Press; Butler JA, Coles CM, Dyson SJ, et al: *Clinical radiology of the horse,* Osney Mead, Oxford, 2008, Wiley-Blackwell; Thrall DE: *Textbook of veterinary diagnostic radiology,* ed 6, St. Louis, 2013, Elsevier.

The Digit (Foot)

The distal phalanx and the navicular bone comprise the digit or foot. Common indications for imaging the equine foot include localized lameness by clinical examination (pain on pressure from foot testers, increased digital pulses, etc.) or by diagnostic analgesia, laminitis, penetrating wounds, or as required for a prepurchase examination.[1]

Dorsopalmar (DP): Dorsoproximal-Palmarodistal View of the Digit

The three following views can be taken for the dorsoproximal-palmarodistal (DPr-PaDi) views of the foot. The terminology changes slightly depending on the actual positioning. Because the foot or the beam is at an angle to the ground, the high coronary and upright pedal routes are technically termed *DPr-PaDiO views.* Note that there is no lateral or medial distinction, so do not get confused.

High coronary view: Dorsal 65-degree proximal–palmarodistal oblique (D65Pr-PaDiO).

- The beam is angled to the ground 65 degrees dorsoproximal (stand-on route) (see Fig. 24.8).
- The foot is on top of the cassette tunnel, which is placed on the ground.
- The foot is placed near the center and the toe close to the front edge of the tunnel.
- This view tends to be most common

Upright pedal route: Dorsoproximal-palmarodistal oblique (DPr-PaDiO).

- The beam is horizontal and parallel to the ground with the toe pointed down (Fig. 24.9).
- Point the toe of the foot downward so it is resting on a block, or use a navicular block.
- The sole is perpendicular to the ground, and the dorsal hoof wall is 65 degrees to the horizontal for the coffin bone.
- A positioning block with a slot (see Fig. 24.4A) or the Redden Navicular Block (Fig. 24.4B) can be used so that the hoof angle is 65 degrees.

Position 3: True dorsopalmar view (Fig. 24.10).

- The beam is horizontal and parallel to the ground, with the foot being weight-bearing.
- The foot is placed on the foot block to raise it to the level of the x-ray tube.

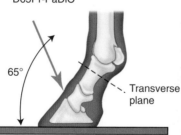

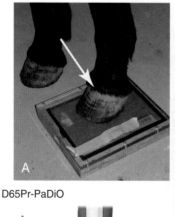

D65Pr-PaDiO

65°

Transverse plane

Supporting surface

B

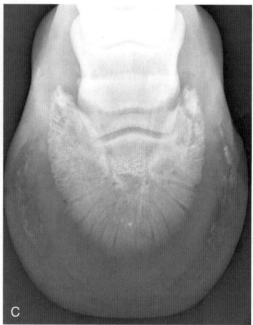

C

FIG. 24.8 A, Positioning for the dorsoproximal (DP) view of the digit using a tunnel cassette for the high coronary stand-on view angled 65 degrees to the ground. The foot is best placed closer to the front of the cassette so that the foot shadow and thus relevant structures are included. **B,** Dorsoproximal-palmarodistal oblique (D65Pr-PaDiO) view of the equine distal phalanx and distal sesamoid bone (navicular) made at 65 degrees proximal to the supporting surface. This is often referred to as a DP, high coronary view. **C,** Radiograph of the dorsoproximal distal phalanx with the high coronary view route. (**C** courtesy Carolyn Bennet, Ontario Veterinary College, Veterinary Teaching Hospital, Diagnostic Imaging at University of Guelph, Ontario.)

Dorsopalmar (DP): Dorsoproximal-Palmarodistal View of the Digit—cont'd

- The image receptor is positioned vertically for the true DP and directly caudal to the foot on the ground or in the cassette holder groove.

For all 3 positions:
Central Ray: On the *midsagittal plane* (MSP) of the pedal bone (dorsal foot wall) 2 cm above the dorsal coronary band.
Include: The full digit—foot wall, pedal bone, superimposed navicular bone, middle phalanx (P2), and the distal part of the proximal phalanx (P1).
Collimate: To include area of interest, ensuring that labels are included and borders are visible.

Comments

- Aim the central ray at right angles to the correctly trimmed foot wall.
- When the beam is at an angle to the ground or to the limb, the view is technically called a *DP oblique* (note there is no mention of medial or lateral so the beam is on the MSP).
- Lift the opposite limb for restraint for the high coronary view.

- Proper full preparation of the sole is essential.
- Wings of the coffin bone and distal sesamoids should be equidistant.
- Increase the mAs to view the navicular bone, and decrease the mAs for the solar margin.
- The purpose of the high coronary study is to note the number, size, and character of the vascular channels. The *crena,* which is the large notch in the solar border; the palmar processes, or wings formed by the solar border; and the *ungular or collateral cartilages* are all noted.[2] This is the preferred view for the interphalangeal joint.
- The upright pedal route better shows the extensor process, conformation, quality of hoof care, and relationship of foot to the surface and is preferred for the bones.[1,2]
- The true DP with the foot weight-bearing on a block and the beam parallel to the ground is slightly more limited than the high coronary view, but does assess lateromedial foot imbalance, some distal phalanx fractures, and ossification of the collateral cartilages of P3.[1,2]
- These views also apply to the hind limb, with the term *plantar* being substituted for *palmar.*

✎ TECHNICIAN NOTES

The high coronary stand-on route literally means stand on the cassette tunnel. The upright pedal route has the pedal bone (digit) pointing downward, sole flat on the cassette and both perpendicular to the ground. In both of these cases the beam or the area of interest is at an angle to the ground.

✎ TECHNICIAN NOTES

Do not get confused when you see the dorsoproximal-palmarodistal oblique view for the lower limb. This is called oblique because the central ray that is focused on the midsagittal plane is angled to the ground due to hoof conformation. There is no lateral or medial designation in these DP views, and the angle degree to the ground is placed right after the dorsal designation. The beam is always perpendicular to the area of interest.

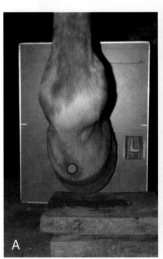
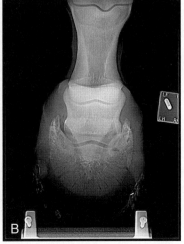

FIG. 24.9 A, Positioning for the dorsoproximal (DP) digit and the navicular bone using the upright pedal position. The beam is horizontal and parallel to the ground. Referred to as the dorsal 65-degree proximal–palmarodistal oblique (D65Pr-PaDiO). **B,** Radiograph of the dorsoproximal distal phalanx with the upright pedal position. (**A** courtesy Shannon Brownrigg; **B** courtesy Stacey Thompson, BSc, RVT, McKee-Pownall Equine Services.)

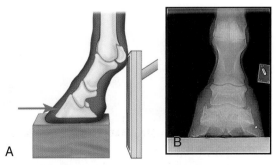

FIG. 24.10 A, Positioning of the foot on a foot block to obtain a weight-bearing DP view of the digit. **B,** Radiograph of the true dorsopalmar view with the foot on a block. (Courtesy Stacey Thompson, BSc, RVT, McKee-Pownall Equine Services.)

Lateral: Lateromedial View of the Digit

The lateromedial view of the distal phalanx is used for all of the bones and joints of the foot.

Patient: Is weight-bearing in a natural position.

Place the Foot: On a block and the image receptor on the medial side of the leg in the positional slot of a block (Fig. 24.11).

Central Ray: 90 degrees to the midsagittal plane of the foot wall, just below the coronary band so that the bulbs of the heel are visually superimposed.

Beam: Should be parallel to the ground, midway between the dorsal foot wall and the bulbs of the heel.

Include: The entire foot—whole foot wall, distal phalanx (P3), middle phalanx (P2), distal portion of P1, navicular bone, and distal interphalangeal and proximal interphalangeal joints.

Collimate: To include area of interest, ensuring that labels are included and borders are visible.

Comments

- The bulbs of the heel should be superimposed and in a straight line with the central ray.

- Care must be taken when assessing the foot pattern axis, which may be altered if the horse is not fully weight-bearing on a level surface.[3]
- Aim for a square stance unless the horse is painful or almost non–weight-bearing in which the affected foot can be pulled forward.
- Wings of the coffin bone and distal sesamoids should be superimposed when viewing the radiograph.
- Consider taping radiodense wire or a line of barium paste placed on the dorsal wall of the hoof, beginning at the coronet band and working down, to make it easier to visualize if there has been any rotation or sinking of P3 in laminitis. If using barium, always complete the other views before the barium is applied.
- For this view of the distal phalanx, the purpose is to see the relationship between the dorsal foot wall and the dorsal border of the distal phalanx. The palmar processes may appear to be irregular with separate bony fragments. They are normally separated from the distal phalanx cartilages by a prominent parietal *sulcus*.[2]
- This view also applies to the hind limb, with the term *plantar* being substituted for *palmar*.

TECHNICIAN NOTES

Minimizing obliquity is a concern for the lateral view, so it is important to make sure that the floor is level and the central ray is lined up so that the bulbs of the heel are superimposed.

TECHNICIAN NOTES

The same principles apply to the hind limb. Substitute the term *plantar* for *palmar*.

TECHNICIAN NOTES

A common cause of nondiagnostic radiographs of the foot is lack of preparation. Artifacts need to be eliminated—remove the shoe; remove dirt, debris, and excess horny tissue; and pack the sulcus to eliminate air artifacts.

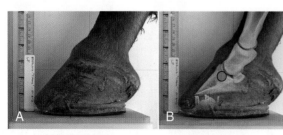

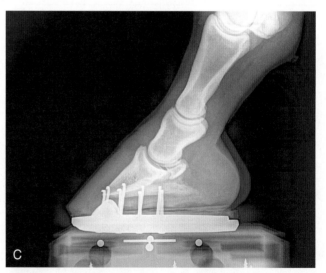

FIG. 24.11 A, Positioning for the lateromedial view of the distal phalanx. **B,** Radiographic anatomy of the lateromedial left equine distal phalanx. **C,** Radiograph of the lateromedial left equine distal phalanx of the above patient with the shoe in place. The shoe needs to be removed for other views of the digit. (**C** courtesy Vetel Diagnostics, San Luis Obispo, California; and Seth Wallach, DVM, DACVR, AAVR, Director and CEO of Veterinary Imaging Centre of San Diego.)

Oblique Views of the Digit

Oblique views of the distal phalanx and navicular bone are as follows:

DLPMO: Dorsal 65-degree proximal, 45-degree lateral–palmarodistomedial oblique (D65Pr45L-PaDiMO). The medial oblique aspect of the limb is against the film. The DLPMO view allows visualization of the lateral wing of the coffin bone. See Fig. 24.6B and Fig. 24.12.

DMPLO: Dorsal 65-degree proximal, 45-degree medial–palmarodistolateral oblique (D65Pr45M-PaDiLO). The lateral oblique aspect is against the film. The DMPLO view allows visualization of the medial wing of the coffin bone. See Fig. 24.6A and Fig. 24.13.

Patient: Is weight-bearing.

Foot: Is placed on the tunnel cassette with the foot off-center, slightly toward the side to be studied. The angle to be projected is closer to the edge of the image receptor.

Beam: Angled 65 degrees on the dorsal surface downward on the DP line just below the coronary band and 45 degrees either lateral or medial to the midsagittal plane.

Central Ray: Just distal to the coronary band, half the distance between the dorsal wall and the heels.

Collimate: To include area of interest, ensuring that labels are included and borders are visible.

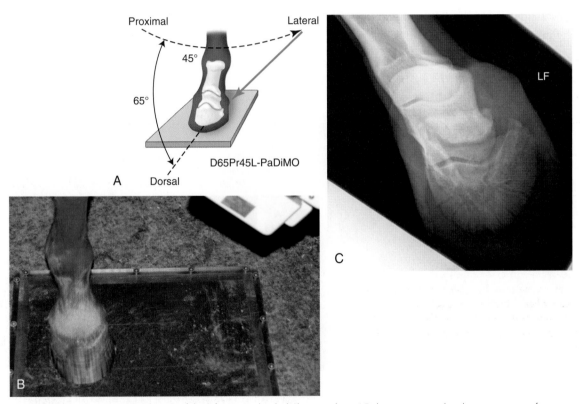

FIG. 24.12 A, A DLPMO view of the left equine distal phalanx made at 65 degrees proximal to the supporting surface and 45 degrees lateral to the dorsopalmar line or the midsagittal plane. The blue arrow indicates the side the beam is directed from. Specifically, this projection would be termed D65Pr45L-PaDiMO. **B,** Positioning for the DLPMO radiograph of the left front distal phalanx to view the lateral wing of the coffin bone. The beam is 65 degrees to the ground and 45 degrees lateral to the midsagittal plane. The foot is best placed closer to the side of the cassette facing the tube head to allow the full foot shadow to appear on the image. **C,** Radiograph of the DLPMO position of the digit as described in *A* and *B*. (**B** courtesy Dr. Usha Knabe, Knabe Equine Veterinary Services, Orangeville, Ontario; **C** courtesy Carolyn Bennet, Ontario Veterinary College, Veterinary Teaching Hospital, Diagnostic Imaging at University of Guelph, Ontario.)

Continued

Oblique Views of the Digit—cont'd

Comments

- Keep the beam perpendicular to the foot axis; this is normally about 65 degrees to the ground (D65Pr).
- Ensure that the foot is clean, the sole picked, and shoes have been removed.
- The oblique views help detect nondisplaced fractures in the quarters of the solar border and in the plantar or palmar processes of the distal phalanx.
- The DLPMO view visualizes the lateral wing of the coffin bone, which appears larger due to increased OFD. Because there is no superimposition, the lateral wing of the coffin bone appears grayer.
- The DMPLO view visualizes the medial wing of the coffin bone, which appears larger due to increased OFD. Because there is no superimposition, the medial wing of the coffin bone appears grayer.
- This positioning also applies to the hind limb, with the term *plantar* being substituted for *palmar*.

> ### ✎ TECHNICIAN NOTES
>
> As with small-animal imaging, plan so you minimize retakes. Your mental checklist includes but is not limited to the following: machine ready and settings correct, correct SID, PPE donned, use of a cassette holder or positioning device if possible, proper location of markers, patient properly prepared and restrained, correct body part and view, properly centered and borders included, and correct angle of the central ray so it is perpendicular to the body part and the image receptor.

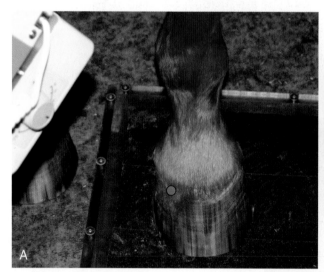 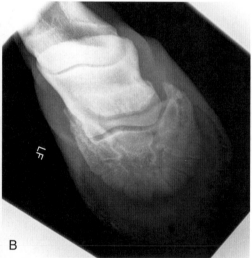

FIG. 24.13 A, Positioning for the DMPLO [D65Pr45M-PaDiLO] view of the left front distal phalanx. The beam is 65 degrees to the ground and 45 degrees medial to the midsagittal plane. Note placement of foot to ensure the full image will be shown. **B,** DMPLO radiograph of the distal phalanx to view the medial wing of the coffin bone. (**A** courtesy Dr. Usha Knabe, Knabe Equine Veterinary Services, Orangeville, Ontario; **B** courtesy Carolyn Bennet, Ontario Veterinary College, Veterinary Teaching Hospital, Diagnostic Imaging at University of Guelph, Ontario.)

Navicular Bone (Distal Sesamoid)

Lateral: Lateromedial View of the Navicular Bone

Positioning, Central Ray, and Collimation

Positioning, central ray, and collimation instructions are the same as those for the lateromedial view of the distal phalanx (Fig. 24.14).

Comments

- This view assists in evaluating the changes in the shape of the bone that are often associated with chronic degenerative changes of navicular disease.[1,2]
- If only a lateral view is required, the shoe does not have to be removed; only cleaning and brushing of the wall are required.

- This view gives a foreshortened projection along the axis of the bone. Both borders and both surfaces will be projected in profile.

✎ **TECHNICIAN NOTES**

If a radiodense wire is taped or barium paste is applied on the midsagittal plane of the dorsal hoof wall, it is easier to see the hoof wall axis on an image.

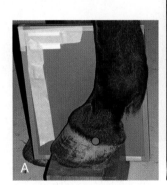
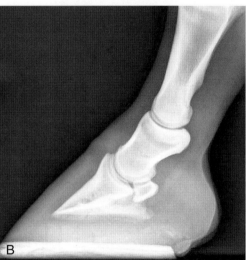

FIG. 24.14 **A,** Positioning for the lateromedial view of the navicular bone standing on a block. **B,** Lateromedial radiograph of the navicular bone. (**B** courtesy Carolyn Bennet, Ontario Veterinary College, Veterinary Teaching Hospital, Diagnostic Imaging at University of Guelph, Ontario.)

Dorsopalmar (DP): Dorsoproximal-Palmarodistal Oblique Views of the Navicular Bone

High Coronary Stand-on Routes
Dorsal 65-Degree Proximal–Palmarodistal Oblique (D65Pr-PaDiO) of the Navicular Bone

The D65Pr-PaDiO view projects both borders and extremities of the navicular, and the distal border can be seen through the distal and palmar (plantar) portions of the middle phalanx (Fig. 24.15).

Patient: Is weight-bearing.

Foot: Placed on the cassette tunnel, which is flat on the ground. Position the foot near the center and the toe close to the front edge of the tunnel.

Beam: 65 degrees with the ground and at 110 degrees with the hoof wall.

Central Ray: On the midsagittal plane just distal to the coronary band centered between the bulbs of the heel, which are level.

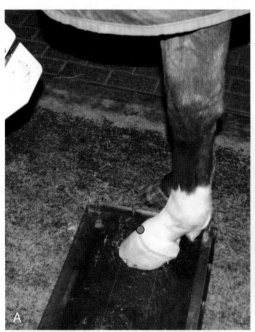 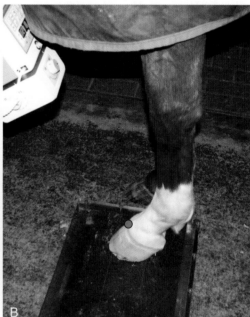

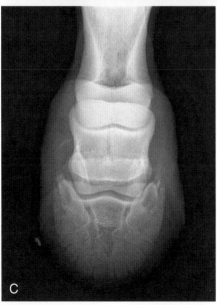

FIG. 24.15 A, Positioning for the dorsoproximal (DP) view of the navicular with the high coronary view angled 45 degrees to the ground (dorsal 45-degree proximal–palmarodistomedial oblique). B, Positioning for the dorsoproximal (DP) view of the navicular with the high coronary view angled 65 degrees to the ground. C, Radiograph of the DP (D60-65Pr-PaDiO)-high coronary navicular position. Note the air artifact along the clefts of the frog due to improper packing of the sole. (A and B courtesy Dr. Usha Knabe, Knabe Equine Veterinary Services, Orangeville, Ontario.)

Dorsopalmar (DP): Dorsoproximal-Palmarodistal Oblique Views of the Navicular Bone—cont'd

Include: All of P3, the navicular, and P2.

Collimate: To include area of interest, ensuring that labels are included and borders are visible.

Dorsal 45-Degree Proximal–Palmarodistal Oblique (D45Pr-PaDiO) of the Navicular Bone

The D45Pr-PaDiO view projects the proximal border and extremities.

Patient: Is weight-bearing.

Foot: Placed on the cassette tunnel, which is flat on the ground. Position the foot near the center and the toe close to the front edge of the tunnel.

Beam: 45 degrees with the ground and 90 degrees with the foot wall.

Central Ray: On the midsagittal plane above the coronary band, centered between the bulbs of the heel.

Include: All of P3, navicular, and P2.

Collimate: To include area of interest, ensuring that labels are included and borders are visible.

> ### ✎ TECHNICIAN NOTES
>
> The 45-degree high coronary stand-on and the 90-degree upright pedal routes show the undistorted proximal navicular border.
>
> The 65-degree high coronary stand-on and the 80-degree upright pedal routes show both the distal and proximal borders.

Upright Pedal Route of the Navicular Bone

Place the foot with the toe tipped so that the dorsal wall is positioned 80 degrees or 90 degrees from the horizontal for the navicular bone (Fig. 24.16).[3]

Dorsal 90-Degree Proximal-Palmarodistal Oblique (D90Pr-PaDiO) of the Navicular Bone

The D90Pr-PaDiO view projects the proximal border and extremities (equivalent to 45-degree high coronary view).

Foot: Placed on a block with the toe pointing downward, the sole perpendicular to the ground, and the dorsal foot wall about 90 degrees to the horizontal.

Use of Special Navicular Block: Place the foot in the slot closest to the front of the block or the 45-degree slot.

Beam: Horizontal to the ground.

Central Ray: Midsagittal plane just distal to the coronary band, centered between the bulbs of the heel.

Include: All of P3, navicular, and P2.

Collimate: To include area of interest, ensuring that labels are included and borders are visible.

> ### ✎ TECHNICIAN NOTES
>
> Be consistent when viewing a series of radiographs from the same patient so that the images are oriented in the same direction.

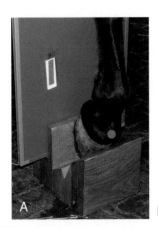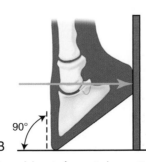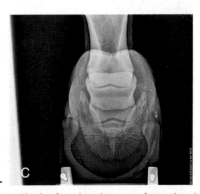

FIG. 24.16 A, An alternate upright pedal route for navicular positioning. The hoof is placed in one of two slots that change the angle at which the central ray strikes the navicular, giving both 80-degree and 90-degree DP views. This block was custom made but commercial 45 and 65 degree navicular blocks can be purchased. B, Positioning for the upright pedal route of the navicular with the foot tipped so that the dorsal wall is positioned 90 degrees from the horizontal to show the proximal border and extremities of the distal sesamoid. The arrow indicates the horizontally directed central ray. C, Radiograph of the DP equine upright pedal route for the navicular with the dorsal wall positioned 80 degrees. (C courtesy Vetel Diagnostics, San Luis Obispo, California; and Seth Wallach, DVM, DACVR, AAVR, Director and CEO of Veterinary Imaging Centre of San Diego.)

Continued

Dorsopalmar (DP): Dorsoproximal-Palmarodistal Oblique Views of the Navicular Bone—cont'd

Dorsal 80-Degree Proximal–Palmarodistal (D80Pr-PaDiO) of the Navicular Bone

The D80Pr-PaDiO view projects both the proximal and distal borders and the extremities (equivalent to 65-degree high coronary view).

Foot: Placed on a block with the toe pointing downward, the sole perpendicular to the ground, and the dorsal foot wall about 80 degrees with the ground.

Use of a Special Navicular Block: Place the toe in the position closest to the image receptor or the 65-degree slot (Fig. 24.16).

Beam: Horizontal and parallel to the ground.

Central Ray: On the midsagittal plane 2 cm proximal to the coronary band between the bulbs of the heel.

Include: All of P3, the navicular, and P2.

Collimate: To include the area of interest, ensuring that labels are included and borders are visible.

Comments

- Important: The foot needs to be properly trimmed and the sole cleaned for the DP views.
- The frog should be packed to eliminate air artifact.
- Proper angulation of the central ray is important for the high coronary views. The high coronary view requires less restraint but involves more geometric distortion because the beam is not perpendicular to the image receptor.
- A Redden Navicular x-ray block (Fig. 24.4B) can also be used, which utilizes a 65-degree DP. The central ray is directed horizontally.
- Collimate the beam for better image quality to decrease scatter radiation.
- A lead shield (navicular mask) can be cut so that only the area of interest is exposed. This shield, along with placement of a lead sheet under the cassette tunnel for the high coronary stand-on route or behind the image receptor for the upright pedal route, minimizes scatter radiation and fogging from reaching the image.
- These views also apply to the hind limb, with the term *plantar* being substituted for *palmar*.

✎ TECHNICIAN NOTES

When using the cassette tunnel, keep in mind how the "shadow" or image will project onto the receptor. If the affected limb is not properly positioned on the image receptor for the oblique or DP views, the area of interest may be projected beyond the detector.

Flexor/Caudal Tangential/Skyline (Palmaroproximal-Palmarodistal Oblique) View of the Navicular Bone

Image Receptor: Placed directly under the foot slightly toward the back of the tunnel to project the image slightly forward.

Position: The affected navicular bone more caudally than the contralateral foot.

Extend: The fetlock, causing the middle phalanx to be vertical and isolating the navicular bone (Fig. 24.17).

Central Ray: On the midpoint between the bulbs of the heel at the distal-palmar (or distal-plantar) fetlock. The central ray must be angled tangentially in the same plane as the flexor cortex.

Beam: Along the palmar or plantar surface on the midsagittal plane at about 65 degrees with the ground.

Collimate: To include area of interest, ensuring that labels are included and borders are visible.

Comments

- This view shows the flexor surface, palmar cortex, and medulla of the navicular bones.[3]
- Decrease the SID to 20 inches and adjust the exposure factors accordingly.

- Full patient preparation is required.
- Take advantage of any nerve blocks, and perform the study before the anesthetic wears off, if possible.
- Keep a small field of exposure to minimize scatter radiation.
- Extending the affected foot caudally to the opposite limb and leaning the limb and fetlock slightly forward keeps the fetlock out of the field of view.
- This view also applies to the hind limb. For radiographing the rear feet, it is physically safer for the machine and restrainer if the hind limbs are kept in a normal position.

> **✎ TECHNICIAN NOTES**
>
> Common problems for imaging the skyline of the navicular bone of the front limb include not extending the foot far enough forward, improper foot preparation (cleaning and packing), and not angling the central ray proximally enough.

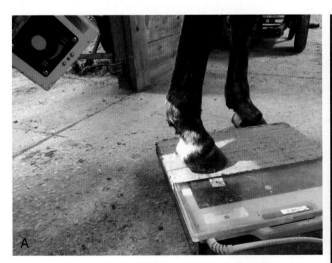

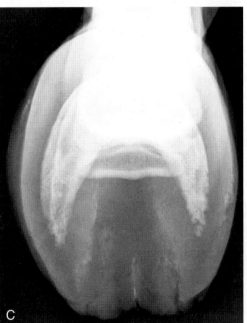

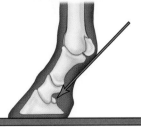
B Cassette

FIG. 24.17 **A,** Positioning for the palmaroproximal-palmarodistal oblique (flexor/caudal tangential/skyline) view of the navicular bone. **B,** Anatomy of the skyline view of the navicular bone. This view highlights the flexor surface of the navicular bone and allows the distinction between the cortex and medulla to be visualized. **C,** Radiograph of the palmaroproximal skyline of the navicular bone. (**A** courtesy Stacey Thompson, BSc, RVT, McKee-Pownall Equine Services; **C** courtesy Carolyn Bennet, Ontario Veterinary College, Veterinary Teaching Hospital, Diagnostic Imaging at University of Guelph, Ontario.)

Oblique Views of the Navicular Bone

Oblique views of the navicular bone are as follows:

DLPMO: Dorsal 65-degree proximal, 45-degree lateral–palmarodistomedial oblique (D65Pr45L-PaDiMO)

DMPLO: Dorsal 65-degree proximal, 45-degree medial–palmarodistolateral oblique (D65Pr45M-PaDiLO)

The oblique views do not superimpose the wings, so fractures are more easily diagnosed.

Positioning, Central Ray, and Collimation

Positioning, central ray, and collimation instructions are the same as those for the oblique views of the distal phalanx (see Fig. 24.12).

The Pastern

Middle and Proximal Phalanx, Proximal Interphalangeal Joint (Pastern)

The main indications for radiography of the middle and proximal phalanx and proximal interphalangeal joint are lameness localized with clinical examination or diagnostic analgesia and penetrating wounds. Specific views of this area are best obtained with the horse bearing weight squarely on all four limbs.

Lateral: Lateromedial View of the Pastern

The lateromedial view of the pastern provides information on the integrity of the foot axis and the bones and joints in the digit.

Patient: Is weight-bearing.

Foot: Placed on a block.

Image Receptor: Placed on medial side of leg, perpendicular to the ground (Fig. 24.18).

Central Ray: On proximal pastern joint (interphalangeal joint) or the joint of interest.

Beam: Is parallel to the ground, 90 degrees to the midsagittal plane.

Include: P2, the proximal interphalangeal joint, P1, and the interphalangeal-metacarpal joint.

Collimate: To include the area of interest, ensuring that labels are included and borders are visible.

Comments

- Look at the foot from the front to see whether there is angulation of the digit.
- If there is a conformation problem, the angle of the beam may need to be adjusted.
- This view also applies to the hind limb, with the term *plantar* being substituted for *palmar*.

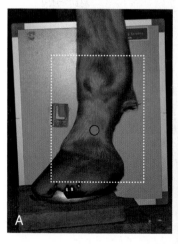
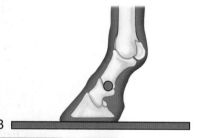
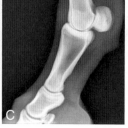

FIG. 24.18 **A**, Positioning for the lateromedial view of the middle and proximal phalanx and proximal interphalangeal joint (pastern). **B**, Radiographic anatomy of the middle and proximal phalanx and proximal interphalangeal joint (pastern). **C**, Radiograph of lateromedial middle and proximal phalanx and proximal interphalangeal joint (pastern). (**A** courtesy Shannon Brownrigg; **C** courtesy Carolyn Bennet, Ontario Veterinary College, Veterinary Teaching Hospital, Diagnostic Imaging at University of Guelph, Ontario.)

> ✎ **TECHNICIAN NOTES**
>
> The technique is similar for imaging the lateral views of the lower limbs. What differs is the centering and what is included.

Dorsopalmar (DP): Dorsoproximal-Palmarodistal Oblique (D30-45Pr-PaDiO) View of the Pastern

The dorsopalmar (D30-45Pr-PaDiO) view of the pastern is a standard view to evaluate the causes of forelimb and hind limb lameness. Additional views of the opposite limb are indicated in patients less than 9 months of age. Comparison studies permit evaluation of physeal closure.[2]

Patient: Is weight-bearing. Clean the hair coat.

Image Receptor: Placed caudal to the limb (palmar or plantar), keeping it parallel to the phalanges (Fig. 24.19).

Beam: On the midsagittal plane perpendicular to the foot axis.

Central Ray: About 30-degree to 45-degree angle with the ground but always perpendicular to the foot axis.

Include: P2, the proximal interphalangeal joint, P1, and the interphalangeal-metacarpal joint.

Collimate: To include the area of interest, ensuring that labels are included and borders are visible.

Comments

- The joint space appears narrowed on one side if the horse is not standing straight. Elevate the opposite forefoot to ensure that the horse is bearing full weight.
- This view also applies to the hind limb, with the term *plantar* being substituted for *palmar*.

✎ **TECHNICIAN NOTES**

Because of the foot conformation, the central ray is angled to the ground but perpendicular to the hoof wall. Thus the DP views of the foot taken with an angled beam with the ground are correctly referred to as *dorsoproximal-palmarodistal oblique views* (e.g., D30-45Pr-PaDiO means that the beam is angled 30-45 degrees to the ground). Note the angle is between the dorsal (D) and proximal (Pr) designations, indicating beam direction from the front of the limb. There is no lateral or medial designation.

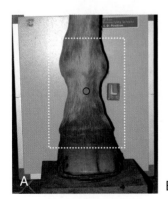
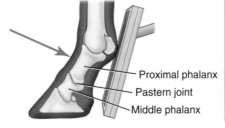
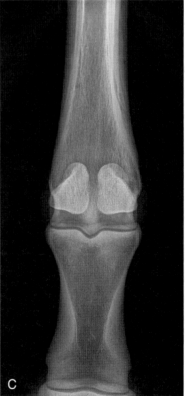

FIG. 24.19 **A,** Positioning for the dorsopalmar/dorsoplantar view of the middle and proximal phalanx and proximal interphalangeal joint (pastern). **B,** Radiographic anatomy of the dorsal aspect of the middle and proximal phalanx and proximal interphalangeal joint (pastern). **C,** Radiograph of the dorsopalmar/dorsoplantar view of the middle and proximal phalanx and proximal interphalangeal joint (pastern). (**A** courtesy Shannon Brownrigg; **C** courtesy Carolyn Bennet, Ontario Veterinary College, Veterinary Teaching Hospital, Diagnostic Imaging at University of Guelph, Ontario.)

Oblique Views of the Pastern

Oblique views of the pastern are as follows (Fig. 24.20):

DLPMO: Dorsal 35-degree proximal, 35-degree lateral–palmarodistomedial oblique (D35Pr35L-PaDiMO).
DMPLO: Dorsal 35-degree proximal, 35-degree medial–palmarodistolateral oblique (D35Pr35M-PaDiLO).

Patient: Is weight-bearing.
Foot: Placed on a block.
Image Receptor: Placed perpendicular to the ground against the lateral side of the limb for the DMPLO view and against the medial side for the DLPMO.
Limb: Can be positioned as for a DP view, with the image receptor directly caudal to the limb, if a cassette slot is used, but there will be distortion of the limb.

Central Ray: On the proximal interphalangeal joint or the area of interest.
Beam: At a 35-degree angle with the ground and perpendicular to the foot axis.
X-ray Tube: Rotated as follows:
  • To a 35-degree angle from the midsagittal plane toward the lateral side for the DLPMO view.
  • To a 35-degree angle from the midsagittal plane toward the medial part of the limb for the DMPLO view.
Include: P2, the proximal interphalangeal joint, P1, and the interphalangeal-metacarpal joint.
Collimate: To include the area of interest, ensuring that labels are included and borders are visible.

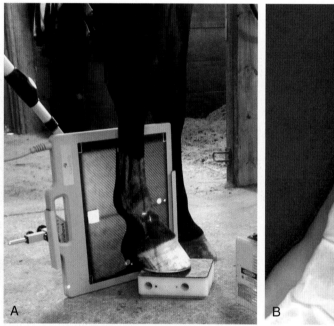 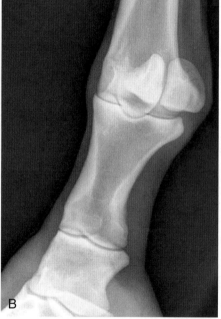

FIG. 24.20 A, Positioning for the DLPMO view of the right front pastern. B, Radiograph of the DLPMO view of the pastern.

Oblique Views of the Pastern—cont'd

Comments

- Note that the beam is at an oblique angle both to the ground (D35Pr) and to the midsagittal plane (35L or 35M).
- These oblique views detect areas of new bone production that are located medially and laterally from the palmar/plantar and dorsal borders of the phalanges, as well as indicating new bone formation around the joints.[3]
- Chip fractures of the phalanges are best visualized on oblique views.[3]
- Dorsoproximal-palmarodistal oblique views made by aligning the beam at right angles to the dorsal surface of the pastern and the parallel image receptor result in less distortion, specifically for assessment of the middle phalanx or proximal interphalangeal joint.[3]

- Using a wood block with a 35-degree groove (to hold the image receptor) eliminates the need for a person to hold the plate.
- This view also applies to the hind limb, with the term *plantar* being substituted for *palmar*.

> ✎ **TECHNICIAN NOTES**
>
> Remember that for DLPMO/DMPLO views, the last letter before the O (oblique) tells us which side is against the film, so the beam has to come from the opposite side. To tell which bones will be in profile, after the "O" is dropped, take the middle two and outer two letters. Thus for a DLPMO view, you can see the lateral sesamoid (which is grayer and more magnified), so it is the dorsomedial and lateropalmar surfaces that are highlighted.

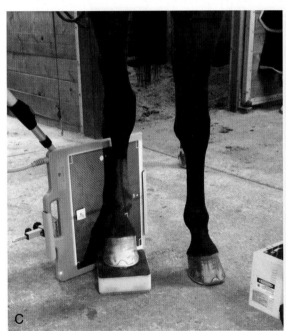
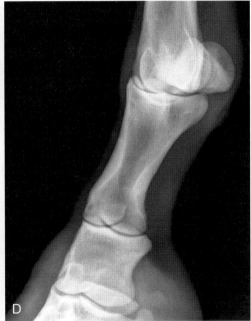

FIG. 24.20, cont'd C, Positioning of the DLPMO view of the right front pastern. D, Radiograph of the DMPLO view of the pastern. (A and C courtesy Stacey Thompson, BSc, RVT, McKee-Pownall Equine Services; B and D courtesy Carolyn Bennet, Ontario Veterinary College, Veterinary Teaching Hospital, Diagnostic Imaging at University of Guelph, Ontario.)

Metacarpophalangeal/Metatarsophalangeal Joint/Proximal Sesamoid Bones (Fetlock)

Dorsopalmar (DP): Dorsal 10-Degree Proximal–Palmarodistal Oblique (D10Pr-PaDiO) View of the Fetlock

Patient: Is weight-bearing. Ensure that hair is free of all debris.

Foot: Placed on the ground or on a block.

Image Receptor: Caudal to the limb (palmar or plantar position) (Fig. 24.21).

Central Ray: Perpendicular to the foot axis and approximately 10- to 20-degree angle with the ground.

Beam: On the midsagittal plane of the fetlock joint parallel to the pastern.

Include: P1, the fetlock, and one-third of the cannon bone.

Collimate: To include the area of interest, ensuring that labels are included and borders are visible.

Comments

- Superimposition of the proximal sesamoid bones over the joint space can be avoided by angling the image receptor and central ray with the ground proximodistally 10 degrees for the dorsopalmar view and 15 degrees for the dorsoplantar view.[3]
- This view provides visibility of the fetlock joint and the proximal sesamoid bones.
- Additional views of the opposite limb are indicated in patients less than 12 months of age.[2]
- This view also applies to the hind limb, with the term *plantar* being substituted for *palmar*.

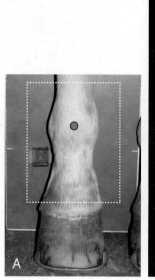
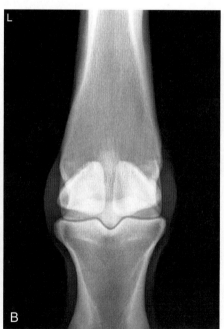

FIG. 24.21 **A,** Positioning for the dorsopalmar view of the metacarpophalangeal/metatarsophalangeal joint/proximal sesamoid bones (fetlock). **B,** Radiograph of dorsopalmar view of the metacarpophalangeal joint/proximal sesamoid bones (fetlock). (**A** courtesy Shannon Brownrigg; **B** courtesy Carolyn Bennet, Ontario Veterinary College, Veterinary Teaching Hospital, Diagnostic Imaging at University of Guelph, Ontario.)

Lateral: Lateromedial (LM) Extended View of the Fetlock

Patient: Is weight-bearing. Clean the hair coat (Fig. 24.22).

Foot: Placed on the ground or a block.

Image Receptor: Against medial aspect of limb and perpendicular to the ground.

Central Ray: Medial aspect of the fetlock.

Beam: Parallel to the ground and directed 90 degrees from the midsagittal plane.

Include: P1, the fetlock, and a third of the cannon bone.

Collimate: To include the area of interest, ensuring that labels are included and borders are visible.

Comments

- Aligning the beam parallel to a line tangential to the bulbs of the heel results in a true lateromedial view. Palpation of the medial and lateral epicondyles of the third metacarpal bone may be helpful.[3]
- If there is not a good image of the joint space, the horse may need to be repositioned.
- This view contains the fetlock joint and a portion of the bones proximal and distal. A true lateromedial view displays the metacarpal condyles and superimposed sesamoids, with a visible joint space.[4]
- This view also applies to the hind limb, with the term *plantar* being substituted for *palmar*.

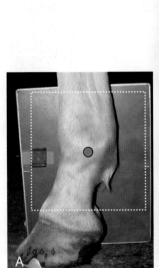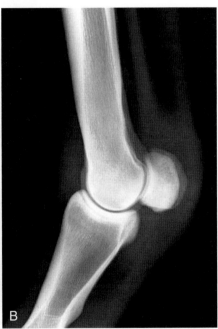

FIG. 24.22 A, Positioning for the lateromedial view of the metacarpophalangeal/metatarsophalangeal joint/proximal sesamoid bones (fetlock). **B,** Radiograph of the lateromedial view of the metacarpophalangeal proximal sesamoid bones (fetlock). (**A** courtesy Shannon Brownrigg; **B** courtesy Carolyn Bennet, Ontario Veterinary College, Veterinary Teaching Hospital, Diagnostic Imaging at University of Guelph, Ontario.)

Lateral: Lateromedial Flexed (LM) View of the Fetlock

Foot: Supported off the ground. Completely flex the fetlock, avoiding any obliquity by pointing the midsagittal ridge at the ground (Fig. 24.23). Do not abduct the foot laterally.

Central Ray: At the medial aspect of the fetlock joint.

Beam: Parallel to the ground and directed 90 degrees from the midsagittal plane.

Include: P1, the fetlock, and the proximal cannon bone.

Collimate: To include the area of interest, ensuring that labels are included and borders are visible.

Comments

- The flexed lateromedial view allows for greater visualization of the spatial area of the metacarpophalangeal joint. The distal articular surface of metacarpal/tarsal bone is shown.
- This view also applies to the hind limb, with the term *plantar* being substituted for *palmar*.

⬙ TECHNICIAN NOTES

Ensure that the restrainer is not within the beam direction and is wearing proper PPE. Collimate.

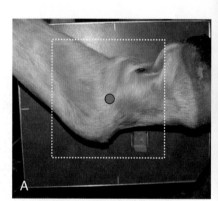
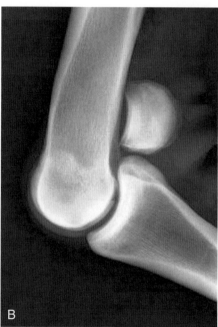

FIG. 24.23 A, Positioning for the lateromedial flexied view of the metacarpophalangeal joint/proximal sesamoid bones or fetlock. **B,** Radiograph of the lateral flexed view of the fetlock. (**A** courtesy Shannon Brownrigg; **B** courtesy Carolyn Bennet, Ontario Veterinary College, Veterinary Teaching Hospital, Diagnostic Imaging at University of Guelph, Ontario.)

Oblique Views of the Fetlock

Oblique views of the fetlock are as follows:

DLPMO: Dorsoproximal 45-degree lateral–palmarodistomedial oblique (DPr45L-PaDiMO) (Fig. 24.24A-B).
DMPLO: Dorsoproximal 45-degree medial–palmarodistolateral oblique (DPr45M-PaDiLO)

The DLPMO view is used to view the lateral sesamoid (see Fig. 24.6B and Fig. 24.24A-B), and the DMPLO to view the medial sesamoid (see Fig. 24.6A and Fig. 24.24C-D).

Patient: Is weight-bearing.
Foot: Placed normally under the body.
Beam: Parallel to the ground at the middle of the joint.
Central Ray: Angled 30 degrees to 45 degrees from the midsagittal plane in the medial or lateral direction.

Collimate: To include area of interest, ensuring that labels are included and borders are visible.

Comments
- The oblique views of the fetlock allow visualization of the medial and lateral sesamoid bones on the palmar/plantar aspect of the limb.
- Depending on the personal preference of the veterinarian, the receptor can be angled slightly and the central ray is tipped to match to elevate the sesamoids away from the joint space for better visualization.
- This view also applies to the hind limb, with the term *plantar* being substituted for *palmar*.

> ✐ **TECHNICIAN NOTES**
>
> The precise position of the central ray may vary depending on the patient conformation. It is important to be perpendicular to the area of interest and the image receptor.

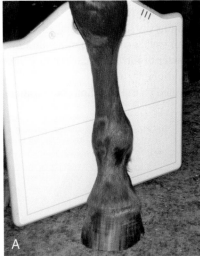

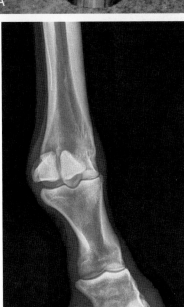

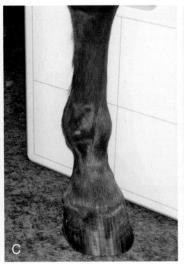

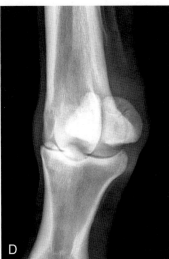

FIG. 24.24 **A,** Positioning for the DLPMO view of the left fetlock. Proper description of the view is dorsoproximal 45-degree lateral–palmarodistomedial oblique (DPr45L-PaDiMO). **B,** DLPMO view of the proximal sesamoids or fetlock joint. **C,** Positioning for the DMPLO view of the left front proximal sesamoids or fetlock joint. **D,** Radiograph of the DMPLO (DPr45M-PaDiLO) view of the proximal sesamoids or fetlock joint. (A courtesy Dr. Usha Knabe, Knabe Equine Veterinary Services, Orangeville, Ontario; B and D courtesy Carolyn Bennet, Ontario Veterinary College, Veterinary Teaching Hospital, Diagnostic Imaging at University of Guelph, Ontario.)

Flexor/Skyline/Caudal Tangential (Palmaroproximal-Palmarodistal Oblique [PaPr-PaDiO]) View of the Fetlock (Optional View)

Patient: Is weight-bearing.

Foot: Placed as far back under (or behind for the hind foot) the horse as possible.

Image Receptor: Positioned in the tunnel with the foot centered on the tunnel.

Central Ray: In between the proximal sesamoid bones.[1,2]

Beam: Should be perpendicular to the ground caudal to the front limb.

Collimate: To include the area of interest, ensuring that labels are included and borders are visible.

Comments

- SID is decreased because there is minimal space caudal to the front limb when the x-ray tube is placed under the horse.
- This view allows visualization of the axial surface and abaxial recess of the proximal sesamoid bone.[1,2]
- This study can also be made using an oblique view with the tube shifted either medially or laterally.
- This view also applies to the hind limb, with the term *plantar* being substituted for *palmar*.

Extensor Surface/Skyline (Dorsoproximal-Dorsodistal [DPr-DDi]) View of the Fetlock (Optional View)

Fetlock Joint: Fully flexed and leg is positioned forward.

Image Receptor: Positioned against the dorsal surface of the proximal phalanx and parallel to the ground (Fig. 24.25).

Central Ray: On the dorsodistal end of the third metacarpal (tarsal) bone.

Beam: Positioned directly above the distal end of the third metacarpal (tarsal) bone almost perpendicular to the ground.

Collimate: To include the area of interest, ensuring that labels are included and borders are visible.

Comments

- The SID is decreased to 50 cm (20 inches).
- This study evaluates lesions dorsal to the distal end of the third metacarpal bone, as well as soft tissue mineralization. It also detects the character of intraarticular fracture lines of the distal metacarpal bone.[1,2]
- This study can be performed on the hind limb, but positioning is more difficult.

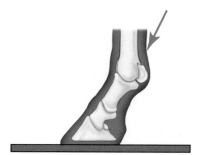

FIG. 24.25 Flexor (skyline/caudal tangential) view of the fetlock. The proper term is palmaroproximal-palmarodistal oblique (PaPr-PaDiO).

Metacarpus/Metatarsus (Cannon Bone, MII, and MIV)

Dorsopalmar (DP): Dorsoproximal-Palmarodistal (DPr-PaDi) View of the Metacarpus (Mc)/Metatarsus (Mt)

Patient: In natural weight-bearing position.

Image Receptor: Caudal to the palmar or plantar aspect of the limb and perpendicular to the ground (Fig. 24.26).

Central Ray: On the midsagittal plane of the third metacarpus/third metatarsus (cannon bone).

Beam: Is parallel to the ground and perpendicular to the limb and image receptor.

Include: Cannon bone, fetlock, and carpal/tarsal joints.

Collimate: To include the area of interest, ensuring that labels are included and borders are visible.

Comments

- Larger image receptors are recommended for this area.
- This view may include both joints (distal and proximal to metacarpus). If the image receptor is not large enough, include one joint to provide orientation. Distortion is possible because of the length of the area.
- This view also applies to the hind limb, with the term *plantar* being substituted for *palmar*.

> ✎ **TECHNICIAN NOTES**
>
> When taking radiographs, mark the center of the area to be examined with a radiolucent indicator such as tape. This maneuver may minimize repeat radiographs due to inaccurate centering and also gives a reference point if the position is to be repeated.

> ✎ **TECHNICIAN NOTES**
>
> Because the central ray is parallel to the ground and not angled, there is no oblique (O) to the DP views proximal to and including the metacarpus/metatarsus.

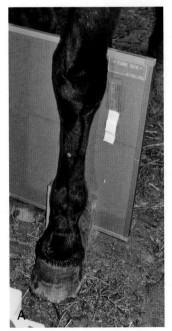
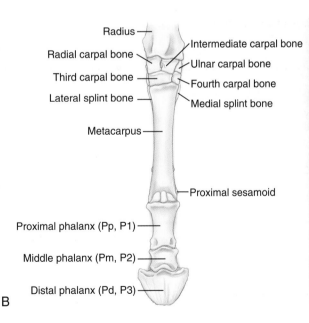
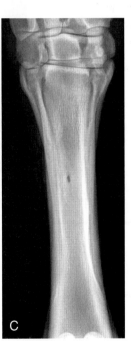

Radius
Radial carpal bone
Third carpal bone
Lateral splint bone
Intermediate carpal bone
Ulnar carpal bone
Fourth carpal bone
Medial splint bone
Metacarpus
Proximal sesamoid
Proximal phalanx (Pp, P1)
Middle phalanx (Pm, P2)
Distal phalanx (Pd, P3)

FIG. 24.26 A, Positioning of the dorsopalmar or DP of the third metacarpals (cannon bone), M2, and M4 (splint bones). Proper description of the view is dorsoproximal-palmarodistal (DPr-PDi). **B,** Anatomy of the third metacarpus (cannon bone), M2, and M4 (splint bones). **C,** Radiograph of the dorsopalmar view of the third metacarpus (cannon bone), M2, and M4 (splint bones). (**C** courtesy Carolyn Bennet, Ontario Veterinary College, Veterinary Teaching Hospital, Diagnostic Imaging at University of Guelph, Ontario.)

Lateral: Lateromedial (LM) View of the Metacarpus (Mc)/Metatarsus (Mt)

Patient: In natural weight-bearing position.

Image Receptor: Against the medial aspect of the cannon bone (Fig. 24.27).

Central Ray: On the midshaft of the cannon bone (MIII).

Beam: Is parallel to the ground and angled 90 degrees from the midsagittal plane.

Include: From the carpus/tarsus to the fetlock.

Collimate: To include the area of interest, ensuring that labels are included and borders are visible.

Comments

- The image receptor must be large enough to include at least one joint to provide orientation.
- This view also applies to the hind limb, with the term *plantar* being substituted for *palmar*.

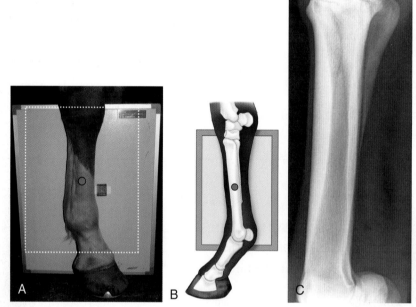

FIG. 24.27 A, Positioning for the lateral extended (lateromedial) view of the third metacarpus (cannon bone), M2, and M4 (splint bones). **B,** Anatomy of the lateral extended (lateromedial) view of the third metacarpus (cannon bone), M2, and M4 (splint bones). **C,** Radiograph of the lateral extended (lateromedial) of the third metacarpus (cannon bone), M2, and M4 (splint bones). (**A** courtesy Shannon Brownrigg; **B** courtesy Carolyn Bennet, Ontario Veterinary College, Veterinary Teaching Hospital, Diagnostic Imaging at University of Guelph, Ontario.)

Oblique Views of the Splint Bones

Oblique views of the metacarpus/metatarsus to view the splint bones are as follows:

DLPMO: Dorsoproximal 45-degree lateral–palmarodistomedial oblique (DPr45L-PaDiMO)
DMPLO: Dorsoproximal 45-degree medial–palmarodistolateral oblique DPr45M-PaDiLO

The DLPMO view is used to evaluate the lateral splint bone (M4), and the DMPLO to evaluate the medial splint bone (M2).

Patient: In natural weight-bearing position.
Image Receptor: Is placed on the lateral or medial aspect of the limbs, against the plantar or palmar surface (Fig. 24.28).
Beam: Is centered on the midshaft of the cannon bone parallel to the ground as follows:

DLPMO view: **Central ray:** directed 35 degrees to 45 degrees laterally from the midsagittal plane. The image receptor is against the medial plane of the metacarpus.
DMPLO view: **Central ray:** directed 35 degrees to 45 degrees medially from the midsagittal plane. The image receptor is against the lateral plane of the metacarpus.
Collimate: To include the area of interest, ensuring that labels are included and borders are visible.

Comments
- This view also applies to the hind limb, with the term *plantar* being substituted for *palmar*.
- The oblique views provide an unobstructed view of the splint bones (second and fourth metacarpus/metatarsus).

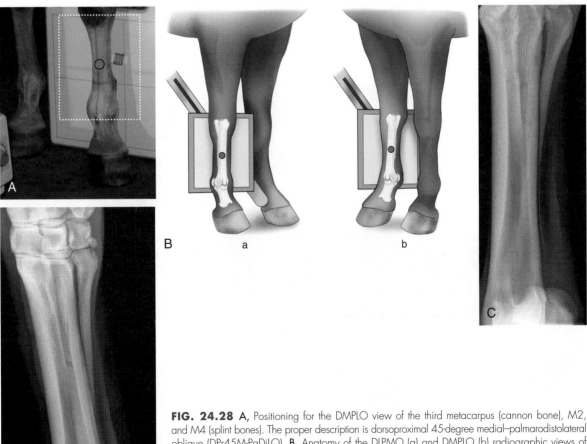

FIG. 24.28 A, Positioning for the DMPLO view of the third metacarpus (cannon bone), M2, and M4 (splint bones). The proper description is dorsoproximal 45-degree medial–palmarodistolateral oblique (DPr45M-PaDiLO). **B,** Anatomy of the DLPMO (a) and DMPLO (b) radiographic views of the third metacarpus (cannon bone), M2, and M4 (splint bones). **C,** Radiograph of the DLPMO view of the third metacarpus (cannon bone), M2, and M4 (splint bones), to show the lateral splint bone or M4. **D,** DMPLO radiograph to show the medial splint bone or M2. (**A** courtesy Dr. Usha Knabe, Knabe Equine Veterinary Services, Orangeville, Ontario; **C** and **D** courtesy Carolyn Bennet, Ontario Veterinary College, Veterinary Teaching Hospital, Diagnostic Imaging at University of Guelph, Ontario.)

Carpus

The carpus consists of three principal joints with articulation between adjacent bones in each row of carpal bones. This causes overlying images, which may confuse interpretation.

Consequently, it is recommended to obtain a minimum of five standard views.[3]

Dorsopalmar (DP): Dorsoproximal-Palmarodistal (DPr-PaDi) View of the Carpus

Patient: In natural weight-bearing position.

Image Receptor: Placed vertically on the palmar aspect of the limb and perpendicular to the beam and ground (Fig. 24.29).

Opposite Limb: May have to be elevated.

Central Ray: To the middle of the carpus at a true DP plane, centering on an imaginary line from the middle of the foot wall to the radius.

Beam: Is parallel to the ground and perpendicular to the carpus and image receptor.

Include: The entire carpus and a portion of each of the metacarpal bones and radius/ulna.

Collimate: To include the area of interest, ensuring that labels are included and borders are visible.

Comments

- To see whether there is closure of the distal radial physis in young horses, the other limb may be required for comparison.
- The orientation of the central ray is perpendicular to the limb in question, not to the body of the horse.
- On the radiograph, the intercarpal space between the radial and intermediate carpal bones should be visible with no superimposition.

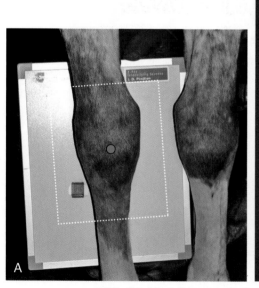
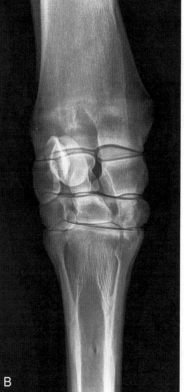
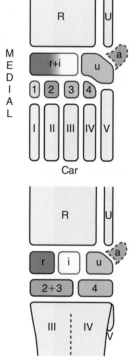
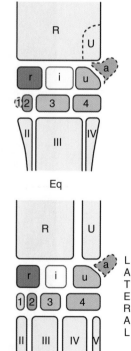

FIG. 24.29 A, Positioning for the DP (dorsoproximal-palmarodistal) (DPr-PaDi) view of the carpus. **B,** Radiograph of the DP (dorsoproximal-palmarodistal) (DPr-PaDi) view of the carpus. **C,** Schematic diagrams of the bones of the carpal skeleton in carnivore *(Car),* horse *(Eq),* cattle *(Bo),* and pig *(Su).* **(A** courtesy Shannon Brownrigg; **B** courtesy Carolyn Bennet, Ontario Veterinary College, Veterinary Teaching Hospital, Diagnostic Imaging at University of Guelph, Ontario.)

Lateral: Lateromedial (LM) Extended View of the Carpus

Patient: In natural weight-bearing position.

Image Receptor: Placed vertically at the medial aspect of the limb (Fig. 24.30).

Central Ray: Angled 90 degrees from the dorsal midline.

Beam: Parallel to the ground and perpendicular to the carpus and image receptor.

Include: Entire carpus.

Collimate: To include the area of interest, ensuring that labels are included and borders are visible.

Comments

- A true LM view displays all carpal bones superimposed over one another, allowing for a clear view of the dorsal surfaces. A small portion of the distal and proximal bones, along with a full view of the carpus, should be visible. The carpus is a very complex joint. Multiple views may be required.
- Consideration must be given to mature versus immature development.

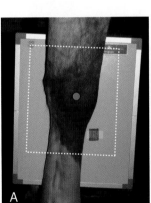 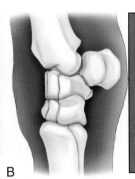 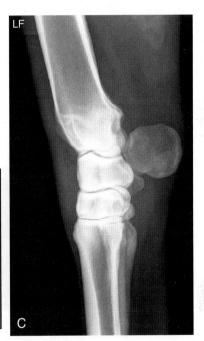

FIG. 24.30 A, Positioning for the lateromedial view of the carpus. **B,** Anatomy of the lateromedial view of the carpus. **C,** Radiograph of the lateromedial view of the carpus. (**A** courtesy Shannon Brownrigg; **C** courtesy Carolyn Bennet, Ontario Veterinary College, Veterinary Teaching Hospital, Diagnostic Imaging at University of Guelph, Ontario.)

Lateral: Lateromedial (LM) Flexed View of the Carpus

Limb of Interest: Elevated and carpus flexed to approximately three-quarters of full flexion. Support the foot at the level of the carpus of the opposite limb so the carpus is slightly dorsal to the limb. Keep the carpus under the body, and prevent abduction (Fig. 24.31).

Image Receptor: Vertically against the medial aspect of the carpus.

Central Ray: Over the lateral aspect of the limb in the middle of the carpus.

Beam: Parallel to the ground, 90 degrees from the midsagittal plane, and perpendicular to the image receptor.

Include: Entire carpus.

Collimate: To include the area of interest, ensuring that labels are included and borders are visible.

Comments

- The flexed lateromedial view displaces the patella distally to better visualize the proximal femoral trochlear ridges, medial femoral condyle proximal tibia, and apex of the patella.

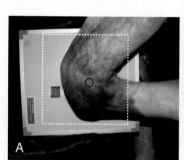 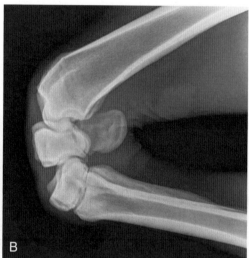

FIG. 24.31 **A,** Positioning for lateromedial flexed view of the carpus. **B,** Radiograph of the lateromedial flexed view of the carpus. (**A** courtesy Shannon Brownrigg; **B** courtesy Carolyn Bennet, Ontario Veterinary College, Veterinary Teaching Hospital, Diagnostic Imaging at University of Guelph, Ontario.)

Oblique Views of the Carpus

Oblique views of the carpus are as follows:

DLPMO: Dorsoproximal 45-degree lateral–palmarodistomedial oblique (DPr45L-PaDiMO)
DMPLO: Dorsoproximal 45-degree medial–palmarodistolateral oblique (DPr45M-PaDiLO)

Patient: In natural weight-bearing position.
Image Receptor: Is placed vertically against the palmarolateral or the palmaromedial side, depending on the projection (Fig. 24.32).
X-ray Tube: In front of the limb and perpendicular to the image receptor.
Central Ray: On middle of the carpus.

Include: Entire carpus and a portion of the metacarpal bones and radius if possible.
Beam: Is parallel to the ground and perpendicular to the image receptor.
 DMPLO view: Position the central ray medially 45 degrees to 60 degrees from the dorsal midline (with the image receptor against the palmarolateral aspect).
 DLPMO view: Position the central ray laterally 45 degrees to 60 degrees from the dorsal midline (with the image receptor against the palmaromedial aspect).
Include: The dome of the carpus.
Collimate: To include the area of interest, ensuring that labels are included and borders are visible.

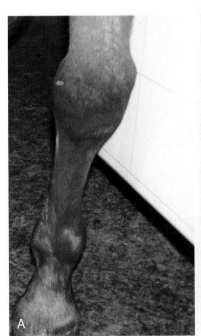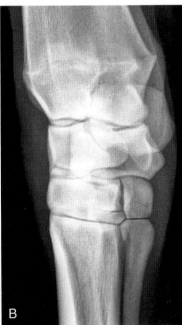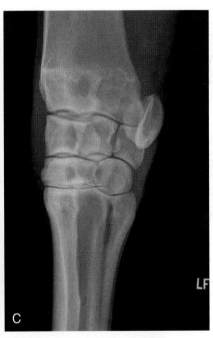

FIG. 24.32 A, Positioning for the DMPLO view of the carpus. The proper description is the dorsoproximal 45-degee medial–palmarodistolateral oblique (DPr45M-PaDiLO). Place the limb as close as possible to the image receptor. **B,** Radiograph of the DMPLO view of the carpus. **C,** Radiograph of the DLPMO view of the carpus. (A courtesy Dr. Usha Knabe, Knabe Equine Veterinary Services, Orangeville, Ontario; B and C courtesy Carolyn Bennet, Ontario Veterinary College, Veterinary Teaching Hospital, Diagnostic Imaging at University of Guelph, Ontario.)

Skyline: Flexed Dorsoproximal–Dorsodistal Oblique (DPr-DDiO) Views of the Distal Radius, Proximal Row of Carpal Bone, and the Distal Carpal Row[1]

Limb: Elevated and carpus flexed so the metacarpals are horizontal and parallel to the ground for all the views.

Image Receptor: Placed firmly against the dorsal surface of the proximal metacarpus, parallel to the ground (Fig. 24.33).

Central Ray: Aimed toward the midsagittal plane of the dorsal surface of the carpus. The exact location and angle of the beam to the image receptor vary, depending on the row of carpal bones being imaged, is as follows:

Flexed D65Pr-DDi-skyline view of the dorsodistal radius:
* The radius is vertical to the ground at the level of the opposite carpus.
* The central ray is angled 65 degrees to the image receptor.

Flexed D45Pr-DDi-skyline view of the dorsal aspect of the proximal row of the carpal bones:
* The radius is angled at 45 degrees with the ground and slightly cranially so the flexed carpus is slightly in front of the opposite carpus.

* The central ray is angled to 45 degrees to the cassette.

Flexed D30Pr-DDi-skyline view of the dorsal aspect of the distal carpal row:
* The carpus is maximally flexed so that the radius is angled 60 degrees to the ground.
* The flexed carpus is positioned cranial and proximal the opposite carpus.
* The central ray is angled 30 degrees with the image receptor.

Include: Carpus.

Collimate: To include the area of interest, ensuring that labels are included and borders are visible.

Comments
* There will be distortion if the image receptor is not perpendicular to the carpal bones.
* Avoid the tendency to abduct the flexed carpus.

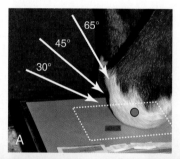

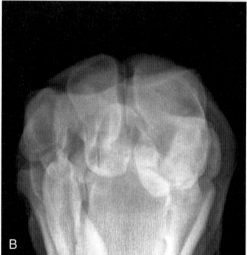

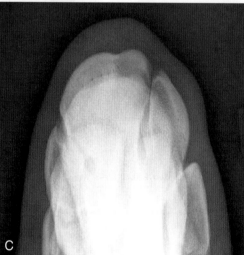

FIG. 24.33 **A,** Positioning for the skyline view of the carpus or the dorsoproximal–dorsodistal oblique flexed views (DPr-DDiO). **B,** Radiograph of a 60-degree, dorsoproximal-dorsodistal oblique flexed (skyline) view (D60Pr-DDiO) of the distal row of carpal bones. **C,** Radiograph of the distal row of carpal bones with a 30-degree angle. (**A** courtesy Dr. Usha Knabe, Knabe Equine Veterinary Services, Orangeville, Ontario; **B** and **C** courtesy Carolyn Bennet, Ontario Veterinary College, Veterinary Teaching Hospital, Diagnostic Imaging at University of Guelph, Ontario.)

Radius/Ulna

Craniocaudal (CrCd): Cranioproximal-Caudodistal (CrPr-CdDi) View of the Radius/Ulna

Patient: In natural weight-bearing position.

Image Receptor: Is on the caudal aspect of the limb and perpendicular to the ground (Fig. 24.34).

Central Ray: Cranioproximally on the midsagittal plane of the radius/ulna at the point of injury or the location of pain or swelling.

Beam: Is directed slightly downward so it is perpendicular to the limb and image receptor.

Include: At least one joint for orientation.

Collimate: To include the area of interest, ensuring that labels are included and borders are visible.

Comments

- Studies made of the area generally require a long image receptor. It is difficult to include the entire bone on a single radiograph.
- A cassette holder should be utilized to decrease radiation exposure to personnel.
- If the affected limb is uppermost in a recumbent patient, either a craniocaudal or caudocranial view is possible.

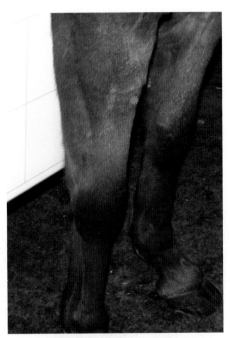

FIG. 24.34 Positioning for the craniocaudal (CrCd) (cranioproximal-caudodistal) view of the radius and ulna. (Courtesy Dr. Usha Knabe, Knabe Equine Veterinary Services, Orangeville, Ontario.)

Lateral: Lateromedial (LM) View of the Radius/Ulna

Patient: In natural weight-bearing position.

Image Receptor: Is against the medial aspect of the radius/ulna (Fig. 24.35).

Beam: Is parallel to the ground and angled 90 degrees from the midsagittal plane.

Center: On the radius/ulna at the point of injury or pain.

Include: At least one joint to provide orientation.

Collimate: To include the area of interest, ensuring that labels are included and borders are visible.

Comments

- If the affected limb can be pulled forward to position the plate laterally, the beam can be directed in a medial-to-lateral direction, though this is more difficult and not common.

Optional Views

- Oblique views can be taken as required following the principles of positioning and beam direction.

- Views of the opposite limb are suggested in horses with open physes.

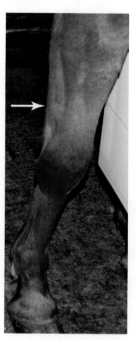

FIG. 24.35 Positioning for the lateral view of the radius and ulna. (Courtesy Dr. Usha Knabe, Knabe Equine Veterinary Services, Orangeville, Ontario.)

Elbow (Brachioantebrachial Joint)

The elbow joint is difficult to radiograph while the animal is in a standing position because of its proximity to the ventral body wall. The use of general anesthesia is preferred if possible.

Because of the increased thickness of the limb, higher-capacity x-ray equipment is required.

Craniocaudal (CrCd): Cranioproximal-Caudodistal (CrPr-CdDi) View of the Elbow

Patient: In standing position, extend the limb as far cranial as possible. If the patient is anesthetized and in lateral recumbency, abduct the limb and extend it away from the body wall.

Foot: Elevated off the ground.

Image Receptor: Placed against the radius/ulna, pushing medially against the ventrolateral thorax caudal to the olecranon (Fig. 24.36).

Central Ray: In a cranioproximal-caudodistal direction through the cranial aspect of the joint.

Beam: Perpendicular to the image receptor and the limb.

Include: The olecranon and a portion of the radius and ulna.

Collimate: To include the area of interest, ensuring that labels are included and borders are visible.

Comments

- Because of its proximity to the ventral body wall, this joint is difficult to radiograph.
- It may be beneficial to have a different person flexing the tarsus than supporting the receptor plate, but ensure all wear PPE.
- This view shows the humeroradial joint space and medial and lateral aspects of the humerus and radius.
- Lifting the foot off the ground partially separates the elbow from the chest wall.
- If the patient is weight-bearing, the central ray will be more horizontal to the ground. Place the image receptor with the long edge pressed firmly against the ventrolateral thorax at the caudal aspect of the elbow. Extend the lower inner corner ventral to the thorax to include the distal humerus.

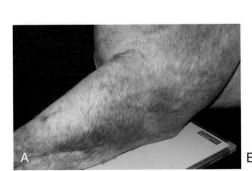
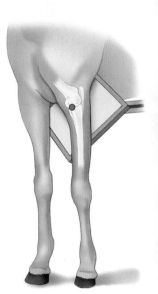
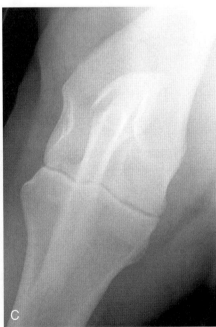

FIG. 24.36 A, Positioning for the craniocaudal view of the elbow (brachioantebrachial joint). **B,** Anatomy of the craniocaudal view of the elbow. **C,** Radiograph of the craniocaudal view of the elbow. (**C** courtesy Carolyn Bennet, Ontario Veterinary College, Veterinary Teaching Hospital, Diagnostic Imaging at University of Guelph, Ontario.)

Lateral: Mediolateral (ML) View of the Elbow

With the patient standing, the mediolateral view is the easiest positioning for the elbow and is often suitable for a portable x-ray unit.

Affected Limb: Pulled cranially as far as possible.

Limb: Is elevated and manually pulled forward so the radius is parallel to the ground.

Image Receptor: Firmly placed against the lateral aspect of the limb, with the elbow joint centered to the image receptor. The image receptor must remain perpendicular to the ground (Fig. 24.37A).

Central Ray: On the elbow joint.

Beam: Parallel to the ground, toward the medial side of the elbow joint just cranial to the opposite forelimb.

Include: The entire joint in collimation.

Collimate: To include the area of interest, ensuring that labels are included and borders are visible.

Comments

- Forward extension is required for an adequate projection.
- It may be beneficial to have a different person flexing the tarsus than supporting the receptor plate, but ensure all wear PPE.
- If the limb cannot be extended, the patient may need to be bearing weight on the limb and a lateromedial view obtained with the image receptor positioned against the medial aspect (see Fig. 24.37C). The distal humerus or olecranon is not as well visualized with this position.
- A recumbent study is best with the patient in lateral recumbency.

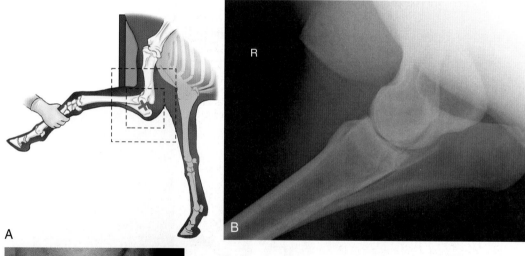

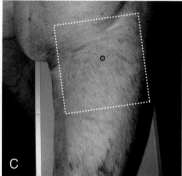

FIG. 24.37 A, Positioning for the mediolateral view of the elbow. **B,** Radiograph of the mediolateral view of the elbow. **C,** Lateromedial view of the elbow. (**B** courtesy Carolyn Bennet, Ontario Veterinary College, Veterinary Teaching Hospital, Diagnostic Imaging at University of Guelph, Ontario; **C** courtesy Shannon Brownrigg.)

Shoulder

To attain quality projections of the shoulder joint, the use of general anesthesia and placement of the patient in lateral recumbency are recommended. The standing position may be possible if the patient tolerates manipulation. The easiest and maybe only view of the shoulder that can be obtained is the mediolateral.

Lateral: Mediolateral (ML) View of the Shoulder

Affected Limb: Elevated forward and pulled cranially with the radius parallel to the ground. Superimpose the humeral head over the soft tissue of the neck.

Image Receptor: Firmly placed against the lateral aspect of the shoulder joint (Fig. 24.38).

X-ray Tube: On the opposite side of the patient.

Beam: Parallel to the ground and perpendicular to the image receptor, centered on the joint.

Central Ray: On the scapulohumeral joint, palpate the distal aspect of the spine of the scapula of the opposite limb and aim cranial and proximal 10 cm (4 inches).[1]

Include: The proximal humerus and distal spine of the scapula.

Collimate: To include the area of interest, ensuring that labels are included and borders are visible.

Comments

- If injury to the supraglenoid process is suspected, direct the central ray more dorsocaudally.
- If there is injury to the tubercles, direct the central ray more ventrocaudally.[2]

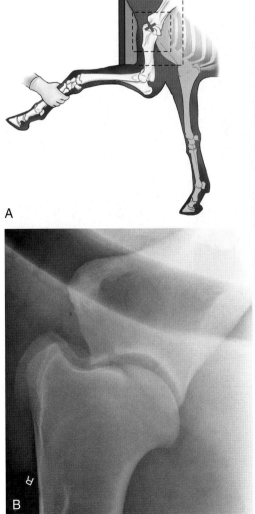

A

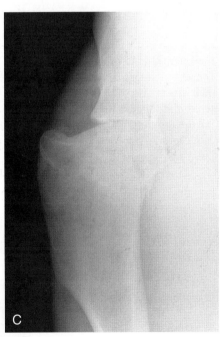

C

FIG. 24.38 A, Positioning for the mediolateral view of the shoulder joint. B, Radiograph of the mediolateral view of the equine shoulder joint. C, Radiograph of the CrPr45M-CaDiLO of the shoulder joint. (B and C courtesy Carolyn Bennet, Ontario Veterinary College, Veterinary Teaching Hospital, Diagnostic Imaging at University of Guelph, Ontario.)

Oblique View of the Shoulder

CrMCdLO[1]: Cranioproximal 45-degree medial–caudodistolateral oblique (CrPr45M-CaDiLO) (Fig. 24.38C)

Patient: Standing with the affected limb in a normal position slightly cranial to the opposite limb. An assistant should pull the distal aspect of the affected limb cranially as far as possible.

Image Receptor: Placed cranial and lateral to the affected shoulder joint against the pectoral muscle mass.

Beam: Parallel to the ground directed craniomedial to caudolateral aimed at the shoulder joint.

Include: The proximal humerus and distal spine of the scapula.

Collimate: To include the area of interest, ensuring that labels are included and borders are visible.

Comments

- Because the central ray hits the image receptor at an angle, there is distortion of the underlying bones.
- It is difficult to adequately evaluate the shoulder joint space with this view.
- These views are used to evaluate an area of suspected injury at the point of the shoulder, such as tubercles.

Pelvic Limb Proximal to and Including the Tarsus

Tarsus

Dorsoplantar (DP): Dorsoproximal-Plantarodistal (DPr-PlDi) View of the Tarsus

Patient: In natural weight-bearing position for the affected limb; opposite limb may have to be elevated.

Image Receptor: The vertical image receptor is caudal to the limb on the plantar aspect (Fig. 24.39).

Central Ray: Centered mid-joint on the midsaggital plane.

Beam: Is parallel to the ground and perpendicular to the tarsus and image receptor.

Include: The entire tarsus, a portion of each of the metatarsal bones, and the medial and lateral malleoli of the tibia.

Collimate: To include the area of interest, ensuring that labels are included and borders are visible.

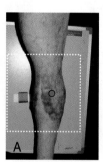

FIG. 24.39 A, Positioning for the DP (dorsoproximal-plantarodistal) (DPr-PlDi) view of the tarsus.

Dorsoplantar (DP): Dorsoproximal-Plantarodistal (DPr-PlDi) View of the Tarsus—cont'd

Comments

- This view demonstrates the tarsal joint and a portion of the bones proximal and distal to it.

- The primary beam is usually directed horizontally, but in some horses, it is best to direct the beam 5 degrees to 10 degrees proximodistally to visualize the joint more clearly.

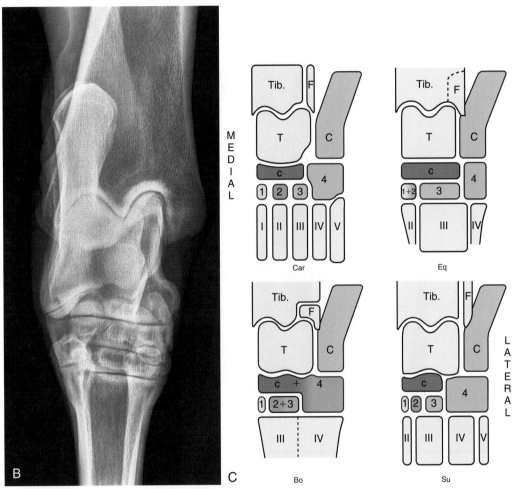

FIG. 24.39, cont'd B, Radiograph of the DP view of the tarsus. C, Schematic diagrams of the bones of the tarsal skeleton in carnivore (Car), horse (Eq), cattle Bo), and pig (Su). (A courtesy Shannon Brownrigg; B courtesy Carolyn Bennet, Ontario Veterinary College, Veterinary Teaching Hospital, Diagnostic Imaging at University of Guelph, Ontario.)

Lateral: Lateromedial (LM) Extended View of the Tarsus

Patient: In natural weight-bearing position. Keep the tarsus under the body, and prevent abduction (Fig. 24.40).

Image Receptor: Perpendicular to the ground against the medial aspect of the tarsus.

Central Ray: Over the lateral aspect of the limb in the middle of the tarsal joint.

Beam: Parallel to the ground and 90 degrees from the midsagittal plane.

Include: The entire tarsal joint and calcaneus.

Collimate: To include the area of interest, ensuring that labels are included and borders are visible.

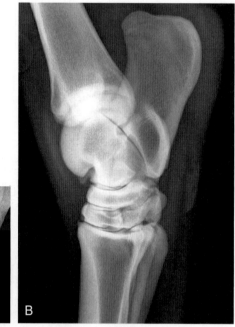
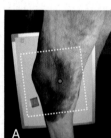

FIG. 24.40 A, Positioning for the lateromedial (LM) view of the tarsus. B, Radiograph of lateromedial (LM) view of the tarsus. (A courtesy Shannon Brownrigg; B courtesy Carolyn Bennet, Ontario Veterinary College, Veterinary Teaching Hospital, Diagnostic Imaging at University of Guelph, Ontario.)

Lateral: Lateromedial Flexed (LM) View of the Tarsus

Limb of Interest: Is elevated, and the tarsus as flexed as the horse will allow. Support the foot at the level of the tarsus of the opposite limb with the affected tarsus slightly dorsal to the limb. Keep the tarsus under the body, and prevent abduction (Fig. 24.41).

Image Receptor: Vertically placed against the medial aspect of the tarsus.

Central Ray: Perpendicular to the image receptor over the lateral aspect of the limb at the talus.

Beam: Parallel to the ground and angled 90 degrees from the midsagittal plane.

Include: Point of the hock, distal tibia, and proximal metatarsal bones.

Collimate: To include the area of interest, ensuring that labels are included and borders are visible.

Comments

- Care must be taken when flexing the tarsus to monitor the comfort level of the patient.
- It may be beneficial to have a different person flexing the tarsus than supporting the receptor plate. All must wear PPE.

✎ **TECHNICIAN NOTES**

If joint space is not properly visible on the radiograph, try repositioning the horse. Minor adjustments to their stance can greatly affect the ability to properly image the joint spaces.

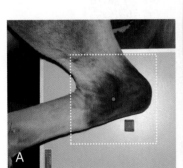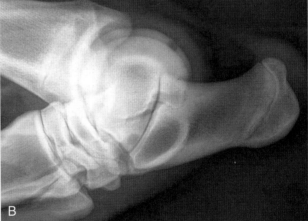

FIG. 24.41 A, Positioning for the lateromedial flexed view of the tarsus. **B,** Radiograph of the lateromedial flexed view of the tarsus. (**A** courtesy Shannon Brownrigg; **B** courtesy Carolyn Bennet, Ontario Veterinary College, Veterinary Teaching Hospital, Diagnostic Imaging at University of Guelph, Ontario.)

Oblique Views of the Tarsus

Oblique views of the tarsus are as follows:

DLPMO: Dorsoproximal 45-degree lateral–plantarodistomedial oblique (DPr45L-PlDiMO).
DMPLO: Dorsoproximal 45-degree medial–plantarodistolateral oblique (DPr45M-PlDiLO).

Patient: In natural weight-bearing position.
Image Receptor: Placed vertically against the plantaromedial or plantarolateral aspect of the tarsus (Fig. 24.42).
Central Ray: Directed horizontally to center on the central tarsal bone.
Beam: Parallel to the ground at 45 degrees laterally or medially to the MSP.
X-ray Tube: In front of the limb and perpendicular to the image receptor.

DLPMO view: Position the central ray laterally 45 degrees to 60 degrees from the dorsal midline (with the image receptor against the plantaromedial aspect).
DMPLO view: Position the central ray medially 45 degrees to 60 degrees from the dorsal midline (with the image receptor against the plantarolateral aspect).
Collimate: To include the area of interest, ensuring that labels are included and borders are visible.

Comments

- The actual position of the central ray in relation to the dorsal midline may vary depending on the conformation.
- There will be greater magnification with the DLPMO view due to increased OFD, which is caused by the angulation of the distal tibia.

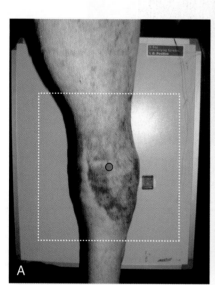
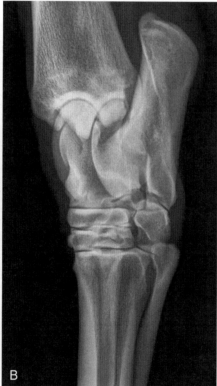
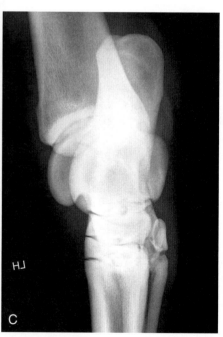

FIG. 24.42 **A,** The DLPMO of the tarsus. The accurate positioning term is dorsoproximal 45-degree lateral-plantarodistomedial oblique (DPr45L-PlDiMO). **B,** Radiograph of the DLPMO view of the tarsus. **C,** Radiograph of the DMPLO view of the tarsus. (**A** courtesy Shannon Brownrigg; **B** courtesy Carolyn Bennet, Ontario Veterinary College, Veterinary Teaching Hospital, Diagnostic Imaging at University of Guelph, Ontario.)

Skyline: Flexed Plantaroproximal-Plantarodistal (PlPr-PlDi) View of the Tuber Calcaneus and Sustentaculum Tali

Limb: Elevated and tarsus joint flexed so that the metatarsal bones are parallel with the ground and horizontal for all views.

Image Receptor: Placed horizontally and firmly against the plantar surface of the calcaneus, parallel to the ground (Fig. 24.43).

Central Ray: On the tuber calcaneus.

Beam: Directly above the tarsus, perpendicular to the ground, and aimed straight down, being as perpendicular to the image receptor as possible, with a slight cranial angulation, to avoid the thigh musculature.

Include: Only the calcaneus and sustentaculum tali.

Collimate: To include the area of interest, ensuring that labels are included and borders are visible.

Comments

- This skyline flexed view provides evaluation of the calcaneus and the sustentaculum tali from a proximal-to-distal direction without overlying bony shadows.[1,2]
- It may be beneficial to have a different person flexing the tarsus than supporting the receptor plate, but ensure all wear PPE.
- The use of a ceiling-mounted x-ray unit is preferred because of the height of the positioning of the tube head required.

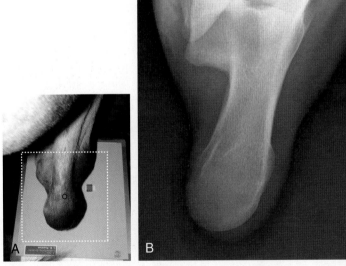

FIG. 24.43 A, Positioning of the tuber calcaneus for the skyline flexed or plantaroproximal-plantarodistal (PlPr-PlDi) view. B, Radiograph of the tuber calcaneus for the skyline flexed or plantaroproximal-plantarodistal (PlPr-PlDi) view. (A courtesy Shannon Brownrigg; B courtesy Carolyn Bennet, Ontario Veterinary College, Veterinary Teaching Hospital, Diagnostic Imaging at University of Guelph, Ontario.)

Tibia/Fibula

Caudocranial (CdCr): Caudioproximal-Cranioodistal (CdPr-CrDi) View of the Tibia/Fibula

Patient: In natural weight-bearing position.

Image Receptor: Cranial to the cranial aspect of the limb and parallel with the limb (Fig. 24.44).

Central Ray: On the midsagittal plane of the tibia/fibula at the point of injury or the location of pain or swelling.

Beam: Slightly directed downward so it is perpendicular to the limb and image receptor.

Include: At least one joint for orientation.

Collimate: To include the area of interest, ensuring that labels are included and borders are visible.

Comments

- Studies made of the area generally require a long image receptor. It is difficult to include the entire bone on a single radiograph.
- A cassette holder should be utilized to decrease both physical and radiation danger.
- The study can be made as the craniocaudal view, with the image receptor against the caudal aspect of the limb and the x-ray tube positioned cranially. However, there is increased OFD and concern with positioning safety.

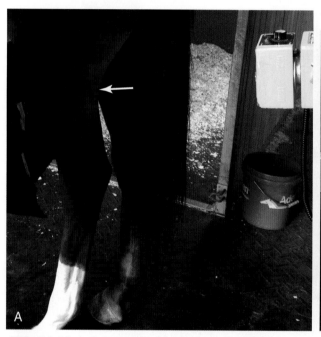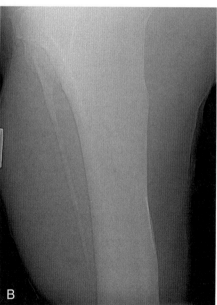

FIG. 24.44 **A,** Positioning for the CdCr view of the tibia/fibula. **B,** Radiograph of the CdCr view of the tibia/fibula. (Courtesy Stacey Thompson, BSc, RVT, McKee-Pownall Equine Services.)

Lateral: Lateromedial (LM) View of the Tibia/Fibula

Patient: In natural weight-bearing position.

Image Receptor: Against the medial aspect of the tibia/fibula (Fig. 24.45).

Central Ray: On the tibia/fibula at the point of injury or pain.

Beam: Parallel to the ground and angled 90 degrees from the midsagittal plane.

Include: The tibia/fibula and at least one joint to provide orientation.

Collimate: To include the area of interest, ensuring that labels are included and borders are visible.

Comments

- Studies made of the area generally require a long image receptor. It is difficult to include the entire bone on a single radiograph.
- A cassette holder should be utilized to decrease both physical and radiation danger.
- Oblique views can be taken but are not as common.

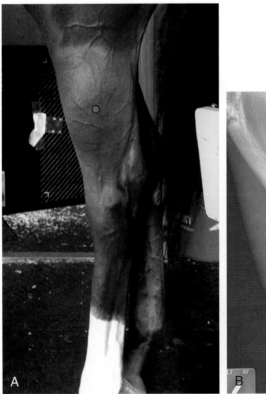
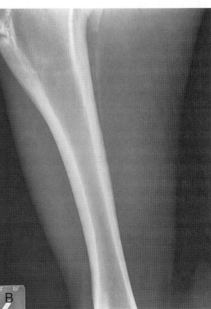

FIG. 24.45 A, Positioning for the lateromedial view of the tibia/fibula. **B,** Radiograph of the lateromedial view of the tibia/fibula. (Courtesy Stacey Thompson, BSc, RVT, McKee-Pownall Equine Services.)

Stifle (Femorotibial Joint)

Radiography of the femorotibial joint (stifle) is difficult because of the thickness of the surrounding tissue and the sensitive nature of this region. Because of the depth of the muscle in the femoral region, the caudocranial projection demonstrates little above the joint space. Radiographs of this region should be attempted only if the patient is cooperative. Safety is paramount in radiography of the hind region of the horse. Sedation or a twitch may be used; general anesthesia is also to be considered.

Lateral: Lateromedial (LM) View of the Stifle

Patient: In natural weight-bearing position.

Image Receptor: Angled and cautiously placed against the medial side of the stifle joint (Fig. 24.46A). Use gentle force to push the flat edge of the image receptor as far into the medial aspect of the stifle (flank) as possible. Most patients object to this image receptor placement.

Central Ray: 5 to 7 cm (2 inches) proximal to the tibial plateau between cranial and middle third of the stifle region.[5]

Beam: Is parallel to the floor, perpendicular to the image receptor, and 90 degrees laterally from the MSP.

Include: The entire patellae and proximal tibia.

Collimate: To the size of a large image receptor, ensuring that labels are included and borders are visible.

Comments

- If the limb being imaged is slightly caudal to the opposite limb, the space may open up on the medial side of the stifle for the receptor. Angle the receptor so it is aligned with the tibia.

- Great care must be taken because of the sensitivity of the patient in this region of the body. Gentle, calm movements are needed. All personnel involved must be prepared to respond to the patient at any moment.
- Gently touching the medial stifle region and the flank before inserting the image receptor may help with patient compliance.
- It is helpful to elevate the front limb to minimize motion.
- Sedation is highly recommended, especially if kicking seems likely.
- This view visualizes the articular surfaces of the femorotibial joints.
- To obtain a *flexed* view: Either lift the limb or rest the toe on the ground, creating a "dropped" stifle position.
  - The horse may prefer to rest the toe over a full weight-bearing position of the opposite limb.
  - It may be beneficial to have a different person flexing the tarsus than supporting the receptor plate, but ensure all wear PPE.

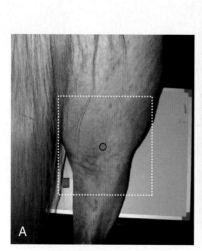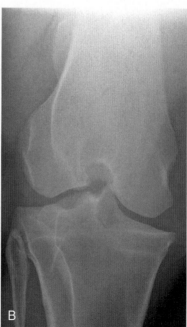

FIG. 24.46 A, Positioning for caudocranial (caudoproximal-craniodistal) view of the stifle. **B,** Radiograph of the caudocranial view of the stifle.

Caudocranial (CdCr): Caudoproximal-Craniodistal (CdPr-CrDi) View of the Stifle (Optional)

Patient: In natural weight-bearing position.

Image Receptor: Placed cranially to the stifle and tilted so that the long edge is snug against the body wall (Fig. 24.47). To increase the ease of image receptor placement, extend the hind limb caudally and angle the central ray 10 degrees to 20 degrees proximodistally[3] (downward).

X-ray Tube: Positioned caudally to the stifle joint.

Beam: Almost perpendicular to the image receptor.

Central Ray: Over the stifle joint approximately 10 cm (4 inches) distal to the patella angled 10 degrees to 15 degrees proximodistally so the ray exits at the proximal cranial tibia level.[1]

Include: The entire patellae and proximal tibia.

Collimate: To include the area of interest, ensuring that labels are included and borders are visible.

Comments

- This view is indicated to identify secondary bone growth within the joint space. The distal growth center of the femur closes at age 20 to 30 months. The apophyseal center of the tibial tuberosity joins the proximal tibial growth center at 9 to 12 months, and the combined growth centers join the tibial shaft at 20 to 30 months.[2]
- Personal preference may have the receptor tipped to the angle of the tibia or directly perpendicular to the ground as long as the angle is accounted for with the central ray.
- This view is potentially dangerous; have the receptor in position before moving in with the x-ray tube.
- This view helps detect changes indicative of secondary joint disease and evaluate the joint width.

> ### ✎ TECHNICIAN NOTES
>
> A firm touch is less irritating than a light touch for the patient. Introduce a gloved hand before introducing the image receptor. Be sure not to come in contact with the sheath of a male horse. Keep alert to any signs of agitation displayed by the patient.

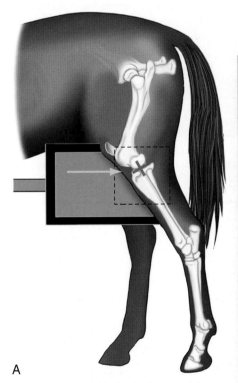
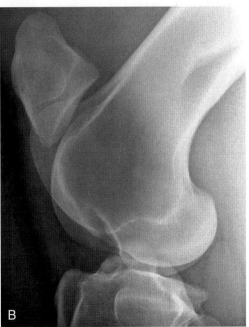

FIG. 24.47 A, Positioning for the lateromedial view of the stifle. Centering of the stifle is assisted if a piece of tape is placed at the proximal end of the tibia *(arrow).* **B,** Radiograph of the lateromedial view of the stifle. (**B** courtesy Carolyn Bennet, Ontario Veterinary College, Veterinary Teaching Hospital, Diagnostic Imaging at University of Guelph, Ontario.)

CdLCrMO: Caudoproximal 60-Degree Lateral–Craniodistomedial Oblique (CdPr60L-CrDiMO) View of the Stifle (Optional)

Patient: In natural weight-bearing position. (Fig. 24.48).

Image Receptor: Pushed as far into the flank as possible, resting it against the medial ridge of the trochlea.[2]

Central Ray: Approximately 10 cm (4 inches) on the caudal aspect of the limb at the level of the femorotibial joint[3] at a downward angle of 10 degrees.[1]

Beam: Directed horizontally, positioned caudally and laterally 60 degrees.[1]

Include: The entire patellae and proximal tibia.

Collimate: To include the area of interest, ensuring that labels are included and borders are visible.

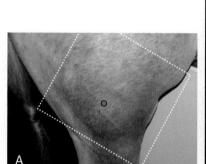
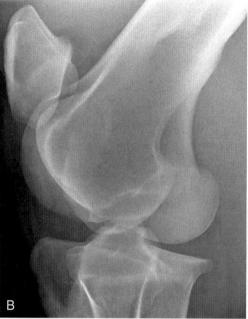

FIG. 24.48 **A,** Positioning of the caudolateral-craniomedial oblique view of the stifle. **B,** Radiograph of the caudolateral-craniomedial oblique view of the stifle. (**A** courtesy Shannon Brownrigg; **B** courtesy Carolyn Bennet, Ontario Veterinary College, Veterinary Teaching Hospital, Diagnostic Imaging at University of Guelph, Ontario.)

Skyline: Cranioproximal-Craniodistal Oblique (CrPr-CrDiO) View of the Stifle (Optional)

Patient: In natural weight-bearing position. Lift the distal hind limb, flex, and retract it caudally to place the tibia horizontally

Image Receptor: Positioned horizontal to the ground facing the stifle so the caudal part of the plate touches the tibial crest.

Beam: Position dorsally and angled down to the stifle (Fig. 24.49).

Central Ray: Downward distally and 10 degrees lateral to medial.

Include: Cranial patella.

Collimate: Tightly to include the area of interest, ensuring that labels are included and borders are visible.

Comments

- It may be beneficial to have a different person flexing the tarsus than supporting the receptor plate, but ensure all wear PPE.
- This view is used to access fractures of the patella. The medial and lateral trochlear ridges, as well as the intertrochlear groove of the femur, are visualized.[1]

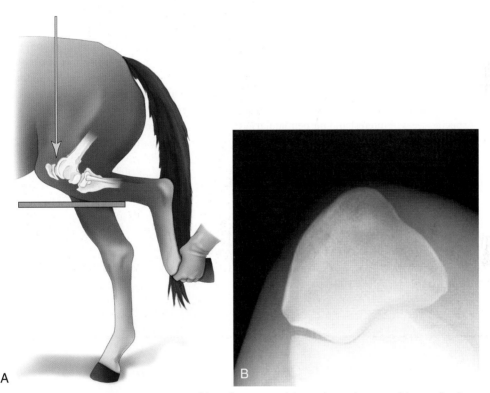

FIG. 24.49 **A,** Positioning for the skyline view of the stifle joint. **B,** Skyline radiographic view of the patella. (**B** courtesy Carolyn Bennet, Ontario Veterinary College, Veterinary Teaching Hospital, Diagnostic Imaging at University of Guelph, Ontario.)

Pelvis and Hip Joints

General anesthesia is required for the pelvic radiographic study of a large animal patient. Young foals (or calves) can be successfully radiographed in the field, whereas larger patients (horses or cows) must be radiographed in the hospital setting because of the specific high-powered radiographic equipment required, such as a mobile or ceiling-mounted unit, to provide proper output (high kV exposure). Views may be segmented to obtain a complete pelvic view (multiple images used for a single view). If using film, the use of a table with an embedded cassette tunnel is preferred to increase ease of positioning and cassette exchange. Due to the thickness of this region, the use of a grid is suggested.

Before administration of a general anesthetic, special consideration must be given to the anesthesia recovery process for patients with pelvic fractures or luxation. As a result, a pelvic radiographic study may be contraindicated.

Ventrodorsal (VD) View of the Pelvis

Patient: In dorsal recumbency with the hind limbs flexed in a "frog-leg" position (Fig. 24.50). Evacuation of the rectum may be required to minimize artifacts for an evaluation of the pelvic symphysis.

Image Receptor: Under the pelvis.

Limbs: Positioned about 20 degrees to 30 degrees above the surface, not touching the ground or table.

Beam: Directly vertical to the pelvis with the beam centered over the image receptor. Multiple views may be required, depending on the size of the patient.

Central Ray: Over specific areas of interest and perpendicular to the image receptor to minimize distortion.

Include: Entire pelvis if possible.

Collimate: Tightly to include the area of interest, ensuring that labels are included and borders are visible.

Comments

- It is important for both legs to be positioned at the same angle and flexion to maintain symmetry of the pelvic joints.
- If more than one projection is necessary, each centering point should be marked with a marker or tape. Marking the centering points allow adjustments to be made from the previously exposed site.
- For a thorough assessment, five to seven overlapping radiographs may be required.

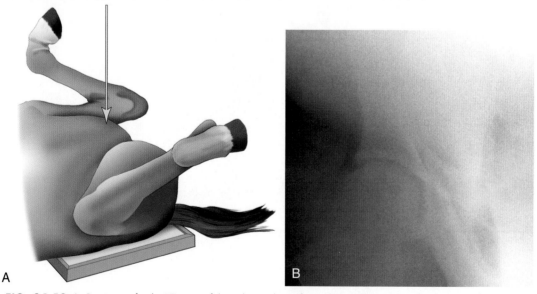

FIG. 24.50 **A,** Positioning for the VD view of the pelvis and coxofemerol joint. The arrow is the direction of the central ray. **B,** Radiograph of the acetabulum of an anesthetized patient in a ventrodorsal view. (**B** courtesy Carolyn Bennet, Ontario Veterinary College, Veterinary Teaching Hospital, Diagnostic Imaging at University of Guelph, Ontario.)

Ventrodorsal Oblique View of the Pelvis (for Each Hip)

Patient: Placed in a ventrodorsal position, with the hind limbs flexed (frog-leg), and pelvis then shifted 10 degrees to 20 degrees to elevate the unaffected side away from the tabletop. Rectal evacuation is not required for this position.

Image Receptor: Positioned under the patient.

Beam: Angled perpendicular to the image receptor.

Central Ray: Directly vertical to the hip joint and center laterally from the midline over the hip joint of interest.[2]

Include: The entire pelvis if possible.

Collimate: Tightly to include the area of interest, ensuring that labels are included and borders are visible.

Comments

- The oblique views are to isolate and evaluate the individual hip joint. Comparative radiographs are recommended.

- A specific angle is not critical, provided it is possible to repeat the same angle on the opposite side.
- X-ray positioning devices may be helpful to maintain and repeat the angle of the pelvis. Ensure that both the hind and front ends of the horse are rotated.
- Secure the patient to prevent injury and unexpected movement. The use of ropes is critical to secure the patient on the tabletop.
- Protective padding is recommended with the use of ropes to prevent tendon and ligament injuries.
- The use of a cassette tunnel is preferred for ease of changing image receptors.
- The proximal femur can also be radiographed if the beam is centered more laterally.

Head, Neck, Thorax, and Abdomen

Note that for all positions:

Image Receptor: Is placed against the side of the skull (see Fig. 24.52) closest to the area of interest (i.e., lesion).

X-ray Tube: Is positioned on the opposite lateral side.

Position: The patient in a natural standing posture.

Central Ray: On the area of interest and perpendicular to the image receptor.

Collimate: Tightly to include the area of interest, ensuring that labels are included and borders are visible.

See Table 24.3 for further specifics.

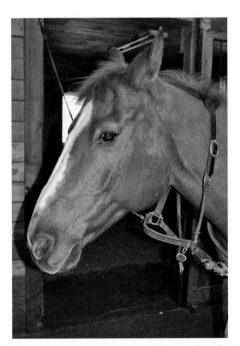

FIG. 24.51 Use of halter or lead shank to prevent artifacts for skull imaging.

Continued

Head, Neck, Thorax, and Abdomen—cont'd

TABLE 24.3	Imaging of the Equine Head, Neck, Thorax, and Abdomen				
BODY PART	**PROJECTION**	**IMAGE RECEPTOR PLACEMENT**	**X-RAY TUBE**	**CENTRAL RAY**	**FURTHER COMMENTS**
Skull	Lateral (Fig. 24.52)	Against the affected side.	Opposite lateral side.	From the opposite side on area of interest.	
Skull	Dorsoventral (DV) (Fig. 24.53)	Horizontal ramus against the ventral aspect of the mandible.	At the dorsal aspect.	Along the midline of dorsal skull on area of interest, perpendicular to the horizontal ramus of mandible.	Easier to note asymmetry. Will need increased exposure.
Maxillary sinuses, nasal passage	Oblique views: Dorso 45-degree lateral–ventrolateral oblique (D45L-VLO) (Fig. 24.54)	Ventral, against affected side. Plate is angled 45 degrees.	Dorsolateral above the head on the opposite unaffected side.	On third and fourth cheek teeth and 45 degrees from parallel plane directed downward.	Avoids superimposition of cheek teeth. Best views for maxillary sinuses, frontal sinuses, and both dental arcades. Bilateral recommended.
Incisor	D45L-VLO	Below affected jaw and laterally.	Above affected jaw and opposite lateral.	45-degree angle directed downward on area of interest.	
Upper dental arcade	D45L-VLO	Against affected side laterally.	Position laterally against unaffected side on the dorsal head.	Downward 45 degrees from horizontal on area of interest.	Can reverse so image receptor against unaffected side and beam aimed upward 45 degrees (V45L-DLO).
Lower dental arcade	D45L-VLO	Unaffected side ventrally.	Laterally to affected side of head dorsally.	Downward 45 degrees from horizontal on area of interest.	
Frontal region	D30L-VLO	Affected side slightly ventrally.	Opposite unaffected side slightly above head.	30 degrees centered on midline behind eye on the affected side.	Avoid inadvertent rostrocaudal angulation. Will need less exposure than if imaging teeth.
Teeth	V45L-DLO (Fig. 24.55)	Above affected jaw (dorsally) and laterally.	Below affected jaw (ventrally) and from opposite lateral.	45-degree angle directed upward.	Alternative view for oblique teeth. For upper dental arcade, the image receptor is placed against the unaffected side.
Teeth	Occlusal (Fig. 24.56)	In the mouth as far caudal as the patient will allow.	Maxillary: dorsal to head. Mandibular: ventral to head.	Maxillary: direct beam downward. Mandibular: direct beam upward at 60-80 degrees from vertical, depending on the conformation of incisors.	Difficult as patient not likely to cooperate without chemical restraint. Need lower exposure than for cheek teeth.

Head, Neck, Thorax, and Abdomen—cont'd

TABLE 24.3	Imaging of the Equine Head, Neck, Thorax, and Abdomen—cont'd				
BODY PART	**PROJECTION**	**IMAGE RECEPTOR PLACEMENT**	**X-RAY TUBE**	**CENTRAL RAY**	**FURTHER COMMENTS**
Guttural pouch/ larynx/ pharynx/ hyoid bones	Lateral (Fig. 24.57)	Lateral side of the caudal skull.	Horizontal beam opposite lateral side of the skull.	Caudal to vertical ramus of mandible (over guttural pouch region). At caudoventral angle of the mandible for the nasopharynx, larynx, and proximal trachea.	Portable unit may be used due to soft tissue density. Position as for routine skull views. Oblique views can be taken with 10- to 20-degree caudorostral angle.[1] Endoscopy is preferred for nasopharynx, larynx, and proximal trachea.
	Dorsoventral (DV)	Ventral: under the mandible.	Dorsal to the head.	Midline of the skull over the area of interest.	Sedation is highly recommended.
Cervical spine	Lateral (Fig. 24.58)	Side of the cervical region.	Opposite side of neck.	Centered on region of choice: C2 C4 C6	Because of the size of the patient, the cervical spine must be exposed in three views. The patient can be standing or recumbent.
Thoracic spine	Lateral (Fig. 24.59)	Side of the patient on area of interest.	Opposite side.	Area of interest perpendicular to the image receptor.	Often completed for the dorsal spinous processes (withers).
Thorax	Lateral (Fig. 24.60)	Affected side	Horizontal beam on opposite side.	See comments later for specifics: (1) Midcraniodorsal (2) Midcaudodorsal (3) Midcranioventral (4) Midcaudoventral	Patient standing. Portable unit not powerful enough.
Abdomen	Lateral (Fig. 24.61)	On side (most lesions on midline).	Opposite side.	Last rib for small horses: (1) Midcranioventral (2) Midabdominal (3) Midcaudodorsal	Multiple laterals required for larger patients.

Continued

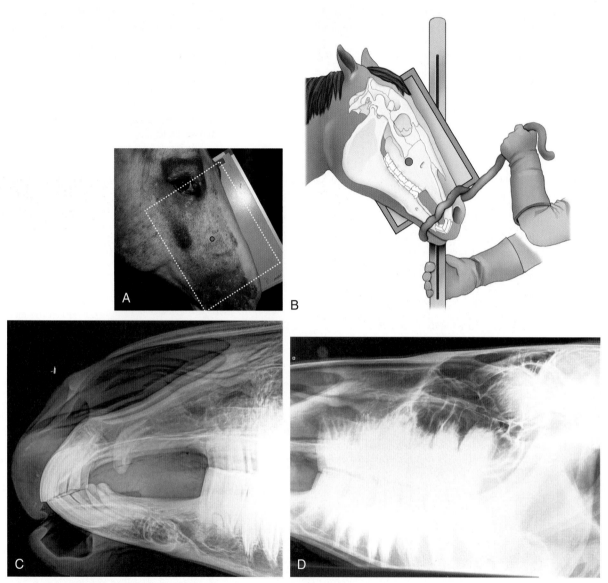

FIG. 24.52 A, Positioning for the lateral view of the skull. **B,** Anatomy of the view of the lateral skull. Radiographs of the lateral skull, cranial aspect **(C)** and caudal aspect **(D)**. (**A** courtesy Shannon Brownrigg; **C** and **D** courtesy Carolyn Bennet, Ontario Veterinary College, Veterinary Teaching Hospital, Diagnostic Imaging at University of Guelph, Ontario.)

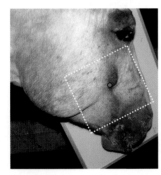

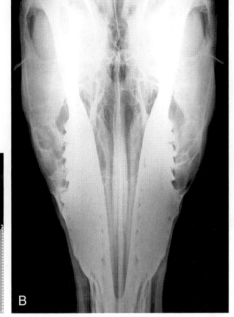

FIG. 24.53 A, Positioning for the dorsoventral view of the skull. **B,** Radiograph of the dorsoventral view of the skull. (**A** courtesy Shannon Brownrigg; **B** courtesy Carolyn Bennet, Ontario Veterinary College, Veterinary Teaching Hospital, Diagnostic Imaging at University of Guelph, Ontario.)

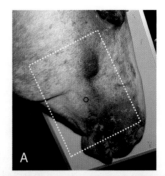

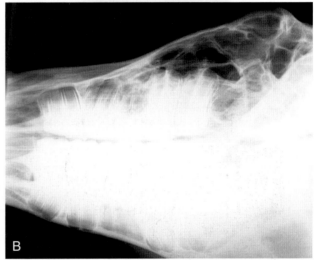

FIG. 24.55 A, Positioning for the oblique view of the teeth. Also referred to as a lateral 30-degree dorsolateroventral oblique. **B,** Radiograph of the oblique projection of the skull. (**A** courtesy Shannon Brownrigg; **B** courtesy Carolyn Bennet, Ontario Veterinary College, Veterinary Teaching Hospital, Diagnostic Imaging at University of Guelph, Ontario.)

FIG. 24.54 Positioning for the oblique view of the skull. (Courtesy Shannon Brownrigg.)

Continued

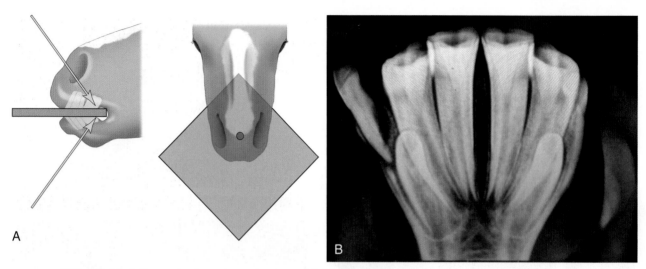

FIG. 24.56 A, The position for an intraoral, rostrocaudal oblique radiograph to evaluate the rostral aspect of the incisive bone and the incisors. The downward arrow is the direction of the central ray for radiography of the maxilla, and the upward arrow indicates the direction of the central ray for the mandibular structures. **B,** Radiograph of the intraoral rostrocaudal mandibular incisors. Note the fractured incisor.

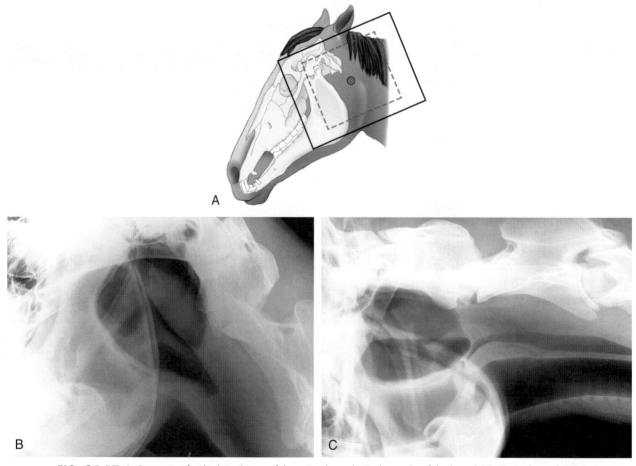

FIG. 24.57 A, Positioning for the lateral view of the guttural pouch. Radiographs of the lateral **(B).** Guttural pouch **(C).** Larynx/pharynx. (**B** and **C** courtesy Carolyn Bennet, Ontario Veterinary College, Veterinary Teaching Hospital, Diagnostic Imaging at University of Guelph, Ontario.)

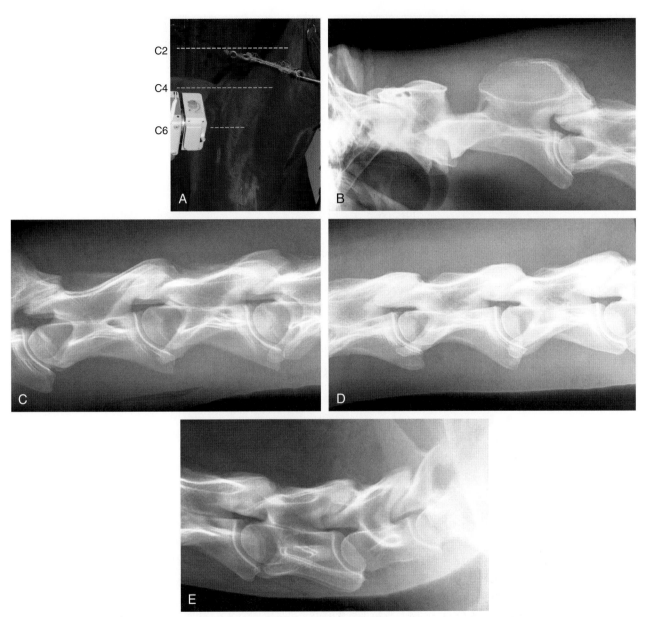

FIG. 24.58 A, Positioning of the cervical vertebrae. Note the three areas of centering, C2, C4, and C6. Radiographs of the lateral cervical spine series: **B,** C1 and C2; **C,** C3 and C4; **D,** C4 and C5; **E,** C6 and C7. (**A** courtesy Dr. Usha Knabe, Knabe Equine Veterinary Services, Orangeville, Ontario; **B** to **E** courtesy Carolyn Bennet, Ontario Veterinary College, Veterinary Teaching Hospital, Diagnostic Imaging at University of Guelph, Ontario.)

Continued

Head, Neck, Thorax, and Abdomen—cont'd

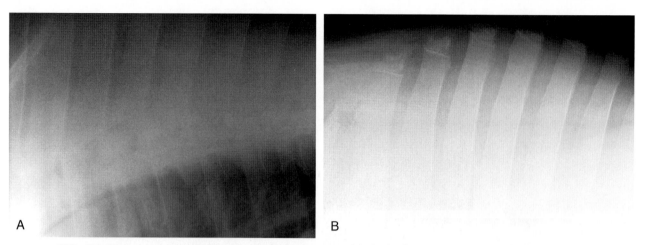

A   B

FIG. 24.59 Radiographs of the thoracic spine. Note the images of the body of the withers **(A)** and **(B)** the tips. (Courtesy Carolyn Bennet, Ontario Veterinary College, Veterinary Teaching Hospital, Diagnostic Imaging at University of Guelph, Ontario.)

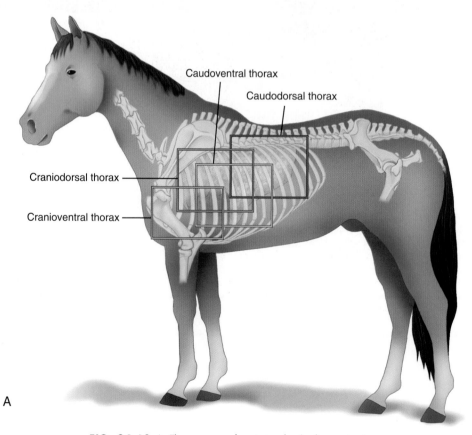

Caudoventral thorax

Caudodorsal thorax

Craniodorsal thorax

Cranioventral thorax

A

FIG. 24.60 A, Thorax areas of centering for the four main views.

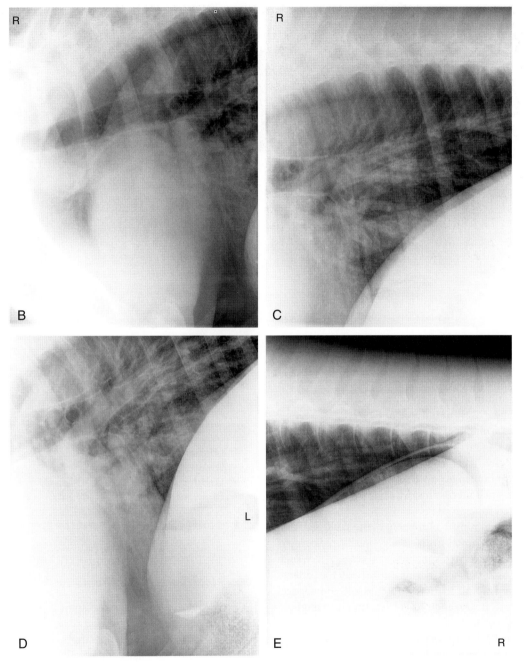

FIG. 24.60, cont'd Lateral radiographs of the cranioventral thorax (B), craniodorsal thorax (C), caudoventral thorax (D), and caudodorsal thorax (E). (B to E courtesy Carolyn Bennet, Ontario Veterinary College, Veterinary Teaching Hospital, Diagnostic Imaging at University of Guelph, Ontario.)

Continued

Head, Neck, Thorax, and Abdomen—cont'd

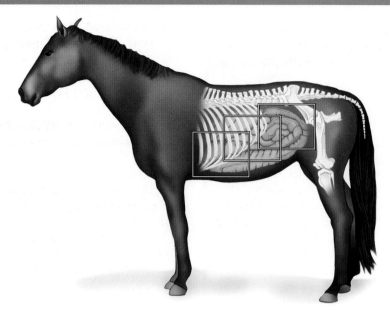

FIG. 24.61 Radiographic quadrants of the equine abdomen.

Skull Comments

- The area of interest must be isolated because of the density of the skull and multiple areas of interest.
- Keep the plate closest to the area of interest.
- For best results, multiple views are recommended, including oblique views.
- Removal of the halter is required to avoid artifacts. A commercial or homemade rope halter may be used. Inspect the rope for small metal clips, which are often present in manufactured rope products.
- It is difficult to minimize movement of the skull. Sedation is crucial for most horses to obtain high-quality radiographs with minimal retakes. Resting the head on a surface such as hay bales or a stand and placing a cover over the patient's eyes may be helpful. Maintaining constant contact will keep the horse at ease and prevent reaction to changes in positioning.
- The head is held without rotation. A lead rope placed under the chin and pulled upward may help stabilize the head.
- Lowering the level of the head by extension or mild pressure allows for easier positioning of the unit and the image receptor.
- Because of the weight of the x-ray unit, it may be difficult and awkward to hold it motionless at the level of the skull. The use of a stand or ceiling-mounted unit may prove more successful.
- Flushing of the oral cavity is required to remove any foodstuffs to prevent artifacts.
- If the patient is sedated, an oral gag may be used to improve the isolation of the selected arcade for oblique views.

- An incisor block can be used for oblique views.
- Barium or malleable metal may be used to mark draining facial tracts.

✎ **TECHNICIAN NOTES**

The dental formula (see Chapter 22 for further explanation) of the horse is:
- Deciduous: 2(di3/3, dc 0/0, dp 3/3) = 24
- Permanent: 2(I3/3, *C1/1, *P3-4/3, M3/3) = 36 to 42

---

*Mares often do not have canine teeth; the first premolars, called *wolf teeth*, may not be present in either gender.

Cervical Spine Comments

- Remember that the cervical spine is located in the ventral portion of the neck.
- If the patient is in lateral recumbency, positioning devices are required to position the spine parallel to the table.
- An increase in exposure factors is needed.
- Flexed lateral, ventrodorsal, and oblique views are optional.
- Consider placing radiopaque markers dorsal to the vertebrae for identification and repeat radiographs.
- Collimate to the bones.

Thoracic Spine Comments

- A lower-powered unit can be used to visualize the dorsal spinous processes (withers) of the thoracic spine (Fig. 24.59).
- For the ventral portion of the thoracic vertebrae, a high-powered x-ray apparatus and a grid are needed.

Head, Neck, Thorax, and Abdomen—cont'd

- Patient positioning is similar to that for radiographs of the thorax, except that the central ray is over the thoracic spine.
- Mobile equipment may be used with smaller patients (i.e., foals).

Thorax Comments
- High kVp with a grid is used.
- The SID is usually increased to 200 cm (80 inches).
- The caudodorsal region could be imaged with low-output equipment, short SID, and fast intensifying screens.
- Radiographs are generally taken at full inspiration.
- In a natural standing position, the elbows of a horse are superimposed over the cranial region of the thorax. Extend the forelimbs to prevent superimposition.
- Center for the following regions in an average-size horse. Use a large image receptor and collimate to within the margins[1] (Fig. 24.60):

- Craniodorsal: 10 to 15 cm (4-6 inches) ventral to the most caudal point of the scapula.
- Caudodorsal: 20 cm (8 inches) caudal to and 15 cm (6 inches) ventral to the most caudal part of the scapula.
- Cranioventral: 15 cm (6 inches) caudal to the shoulder joint.
- Caudoventral: 20 cm (8 inches) ventral to and 10 cm (4 inches) caudal to most caudal point of the scapula.

Abdomen Comments
- Equipment and preparation are as for the thorax, with high-powered equipment being needed to penetrate the thick tissue.
- The abdomen of the horse can be radiographed in standing or recumbent position.
- Diagnostic ultrasound is generally used in lieu of abdominal radiographs.

Other Large-Animal Radiography

Bovine

Even if they are frequently handled, bovine patients have little to no experience of manipulation of their lower extremities, which poses a challenge to perform these radiographs. Maintaining image receptor placement close to the limb without proper restraint devices is almost impossible in most conditions. It is because of these challenges, as well as economic concerns, that radiographs are generally completed only in high-quality or high-producing livestock.

The use of stocks, ropes, and pulley, or ideally, a lift table, will aid in the production of quality radiographs of cattle. The use of stocks provides reduced mobility of the patient; however, they do not limit the mobility of the limbs. Securing the affected limb or, if weight-bearing, rigging an alternate limb through ropes, may be required. The use of a lift table enables the limbs to be secured in a motionless fashion and increases positioning options because the patient can be lifted and tilted off the ground. The lifting of the alternate limb may increase the safety of maneuvering around distal extremities. Sedation or rapid general anesthesia may be used with the bovine patient. The combined use of restraint devices and sedation can significantly increase the safety of personnel, equipment, and the patient for bovine radiographs. Care must be taken to consider the stage of gestation, if applicable, and the potential for recovery trauma.

Equipment requirements and positioning techniques for bovine radiography are the same as those for equine radiography. Handling restrictions may hinder the options and available positions. See Table 24.4 for the common views.

Center: On the area of interest.

Include: Up to one-third of the bones proximal and distal for a joint; for a bone, include the joints proximal and distal.
Collimate: Tightly to include the area of interest, ensuring that labels are included and borders are visible.

Pelvis, skull, spine, thorax, and abdomen radiographs are completed much like those in horses. In the case of a small calf, radiographs may be performed in the clinic with use of positioning and techniques similar to those used for a large dog. A mobile x-ray machine can be used to take thoracic or abdominal radiographs in a small calf (Fig. 24.62).

Ovine/Caprine/Porcine

Small ruminant patients (sheep/goats) and swine can be radiographed much like small animals (Fig. 24.63). Because they can be easily transported, small ruminant patients are often radiographed within the clinic setting.

Because of their minimal handling experience, however, care must be taken to prevent injury due to patient response to fear (i.e., thrashing of limbs). If the patient is horned, special precautions to prevent injury to staff must be taken. Sedation is recommended to produce quality radiographs in an efficient manner.

The fleece of the ovine patient is dense and may contain dirt and debris (i.e., twigs, clumps of mud/stones). Before imaging, carefully inspect for and remove debris that may produce artifacts within the image.

> **TECHNICIAN NOTES**
> Think of positioning cattle for x-rays as being similar to horses with exceptions due to limb angles or anatomy; positioning of sheep and swine is similar to the dog. Restraint is different for all species.

TABLE 24.4 Suggested Views for the Bovine Limb Examination

STRUCTURES	COMMON NAME	SPECIFIC TERMINOLOGY[a]	POSITION[b]	CENTRAL RAY IS POSITIONED
Digit/foot: P-III (distal phalanx, coffin bone) P-II (middle phalanx) P-I (proximal phalanx-pastern) Proximal interphalangeal joint (pastern joint) joint	DP (Standard) (Fig. 24.62B,C)	Dorsal 45-degree proximal–palmarodistal (D45Pr-PaDi)	Foot slightly forward on image receptor.	Perpendicular to foot axis at MSP (midsagittal plane) at area of interest with beam angled ~45 degrees to ground
	Lateral (Standard) (Fig. 24.62D)	Lateromedial	On a block to elevate limb for P-III; resting on ground for other views.	90 degrees lateral to MSP, parallel to ground on area of interest: coronary band for PIII
	Lateral-interdigit (Optional)	Lateromedial (mediolateral) with interdigital film	Receptor between digits. Easiest with patient in lateral recumbency but can be completed standing with foot raised.	90 degrees laterally from MSP to radiograph the lateral claw. 90 degrees medially from MSP medially to radiograph the medial claw.
	DLPMO (Optional) (Fig. 24.62E)	Dorsoproximal 45-degree lateral–palmarodistomedial oblique (DPr45L-PaDiMO)/ (DPr45M-PDiLO)	As for the lateral view for P-III.	45 degrees to ground on the area of interest
	DMPLO (Optional)	Dorsoproximal 45-degree medial–palmarodistolateral oblique (DPr45M-PaDiLO) (DMPLO)	As for the DP view for P-II and P-I	45 degrees lateral to MSP directed either laterally (DLPMO) or medially (DMPLO)
Fetlock joint and proximal sesamoid bones	Dorsopalmar: DP (Standard)	Dorsoproximal-palmarodistal (DPr-PaDi)	Foot on ground, full weight-bearing and cassette against palmar aspect.	On MSP parallel to the ground, centered at the fetlock
Metacarpophalangeal/ metatarsophalangeal articulation	Lateral (Standard)	Lateromedial extended (LM)	Foot on ground, full weight-bearing, and cassette against medial aspect.	90 degrees laterally from MSP parallel to the ground directed toward the fetlock joint.
	DLPMO (Optional)	Dorsoproximal 30-degree lateral–palmarodistomedial oblique (DPr30L-PaDiMO) (DLPMO)	Foot on ground, full weight-bearing, and cassette against medial aspect of palmar surface	45 degrees lateral to MSP directed either laterally (DLPMO).
	DMPLO (Optional)	Dorsoproximal 30-degree medial–palmarodistolateral oblique (DPr30M-PaDiLO) (DMPLO)	Foot on ground, full weight-bearing, and cassette against lateral aspect of palmar surface	Or medially (DMPLO) and parallel to ground on the fetlock joint or the proximal sesamoid bones.
Carpus[c]	DP (Standard)	-Dorsoproximal-palmarodistal (DPr-PaDi)	Weight-bearing with limbs evenly on ground and cassette on palmar aspect of limb.	Parallel to the ground, centered on palpable intercarpal joint space; slightly lateral to MSP since legs are slightly rotated externally when standing.
	Lateral (Standard)	Lateromedial extended (LM)	Weight-bearing with limbs evenly on ground and cassette against medial aspect of limb.	90 degrees lateral to MSP; parallel to ground just distal and dorsal to prominence of accessory carpal bone.

TABLE 24.4	Suggested Views for the Bovine Limb Examination—cont'd			
STRUCTURES	**COMMON NAME**	**SPECIFIC TERMINOLOGY**[a]	**POSITION**[b]	**CENTRAL RAY IS POSITIONED**
Elbow joint	CdCr (Standard)	Caudoproximal-craniodistal- standing (CdPr-CrDi)	Weight-bearing with limbs evenly on ground and cassette against cranial aspect of joint at angle to the x-ray beam.	Caudal to joint; parallel to ground so beam perpendicular to radius.
	Lateral (Standard)	Lateromedial standing (LM)	Weight-bearing with limbs evenly on ground; cassette against medial aspect of joint at angle to the x-ray beam.	90 degrees lateral to MSP, parallel to ground on either the elbow joint or olecranon if required.
	CrCd (Optional)	Cranioproximal-caudodistal standing (CrPr-CdDi)	Weight-bearing with limbs evenly on ground and cassette parallel against caudal aspect of olecranon and perpendicular to the lateral chest wall.	Directed upward at 20 degrees-30 degrees craniodistal to caudoproximal.
Shoulder	Tangential oblique (Standard)	Caudomedial-Craniolateral oblique[d]	Weight-bearing with limb in normal position and image receptor placed vertically cranial to shoulder and pushed medially to ensure that the lateral tuberosity of the humerus will be imaged.	Caudally and is lateral and slightly dorsal to middle of thorax, angled downward, centered at the craniolateral aspect of the proximal humerus.
	Lateral (Optional since lateral recumbency required)	Mediolateral recumbent (ML)	In lateral recumbency with affected limb down and pulled cranially with the humeral head superimposed over the soft tissue of the neck.	Above the patient with the beam perpendicular to the ground and centered on the shoulder joint or area of interest.
Tarsus	DP (two views) (Standard)	Horizontal dorsoplantar (1) 10 degrees dorsoproximal-plantarodistal (2)	For both views: full weight-bearing with digit pointing slightly outward so beam is not under the patient. image receptor against plantar aspect of tarsus parallel with calcaneus.	Dorsally and slightly laterally on MSP centered on palpable trochlea. For view 1: beam is parallel to ground (shows tarsometatarsal joint space) For view 2: angle 10 degrees downward in dorsoproximal to plantarodistal angle (for intertarsal joint space).
	Lateral (Standard)	Lateromedial	Weight-bearing with limbs evenly on ground and cassette against medial aspect of limb.	10 cm (4 inches) distal to point of hock.

Continued

TABLE 24.4	Suggested Views for the Bovine Limb Examination—cont'd			
STRUCTURES	**COMMON NAME**	**SPECIFIC TERMINOLOGY**[a]	**POSITION**[b]	**CENTRAL RAY IS POSITIONED**
Stifle	Caudocranial CdCr (Standard)	Caudoproximal-craniodistal standing (CdPr-CrDi)	Weight-bearing with limbs evenly on ground and vertical cassette against cranial aspect of patella at right angle to body wall, placed as far proximal and pushed as far medially as abdomen permits.	Caudal to the joint and directed downward to obtain a "tunnel" view of the distal femur.
	Lateral (Standard)	Lateromedial	Weight-bearing with limbs evenly on ground and cassette against medial aspect of joint.	Laterally, parallel to the ground and centered distal and caudal to the patella.
	Lateral patella (Optional)	Lateromedial (LM) patella	Weight-bearing with limbs evenly on ground and cassette against medial aspect of patella further proximally and cranially than for regular LM view.	Parallel to the ground and centered on the patella.

[a]*Palmar(o)* is used with the understanding that *plantar(o)* can be substituted when referring to the hind limb.
[b]Further specifications with preparation and positioning for the digit: Before a digit radiograph is taken in the bovine patient, the interdigital space and both claws should be cleansed thoroughly and lightly trimmed. If this step is not taken, false images or shadows may mask abnormalities present in the claws. The digits can be viewed radiographically using four angles or projections.[6]
[c]Optional views for the carpus include the lateromedial flexed, dorsolateral-palmaromedial oblique (DLPMO), and dorsomedial-palmarolateral oblique (DMPLO). The oblique views are also possible for the elbow joint.
[d]Usually only the area of the acromion process of the scapula and lateral tubercles of the humerus are visualized on the oblique views and not the character of the shoulder joint. There is extensive scatter radiation due to increased soft tissue. The oblique view is best combined with the lateral view in a recumbent patient.

Further studies of the bovine include pelvis (dorsal recumbency only with hind limbs extended laterally as much as possible); the head (please see the equine for similar positioning); and the spine, thorax, and abdomen (also see as per the equine patient).
Data from Morgan JP: *Techniques of Veterinary Radiography,* Ames, IA, 1993, Iowa State University Press.

FIG. 24.62 A, Preparation for the imaging of a calf with the use of a horizontal beam. **B,** Positioning for the dorsopalmar (plantar) radiography of the distal phalanx (PIII). Positioning is similar to that used in equine limb studies. Technically this view would be called a dorsoproximal-palmarodistal oblique (DPr-PaDiO) view. The accurate description is D45Pr-PaDiO because the beam is 45 degrees to the ground.

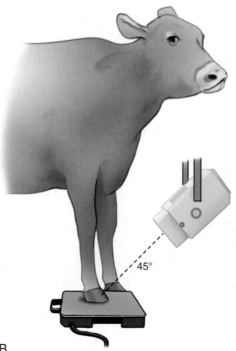

45°

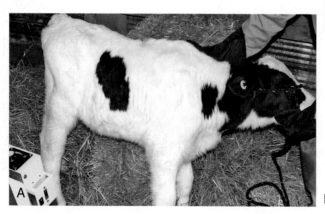

A

B

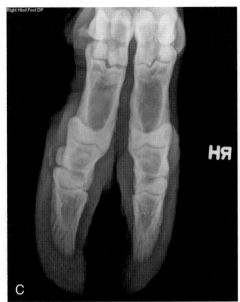

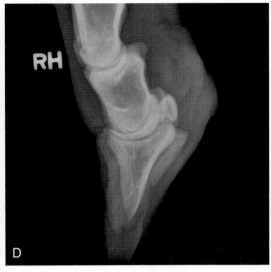

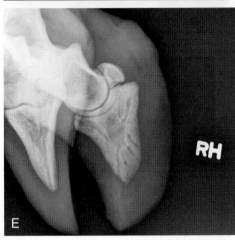

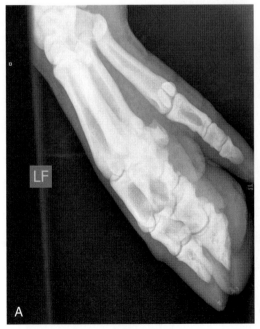

FIG. 24.62, cont'd C, Radiograph of cattle DP view of the foot. **D,** Radiograph of cattle lateral view of phalanx. As per the equine limb, the beam is parallel to the ground and 90 degrees to the MSP (midsagittal plane). **E,** Oblique view of a cattle foot. (**C** to **E** courtesy Carolyn Bennet, OVC. University of Guelph, Ontario.)

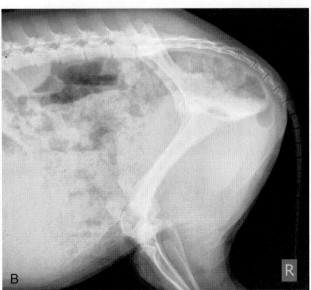

FIG. 24.63 A, Radiograph of lateral view of digits/metacarpus of a swine. **B,** Radiograph of caprine abdomen. (Courtesy Carolyn Bennet, OVC. University of Guelph, Ontario.)

Alternate Modality Images

It is beyond the scope of this text to discuss alternate modalities (Fig. 24.64) in this edition. Additional imaging, such as nuclear scintigraphy, infrared thermal imaging, and MRI, show more features for diagnosis but are considerably more expensive than imaging with the use of x-radiation.

Fig. 24.65 is a mystery radiograph. Review it and answer the question presented with it.

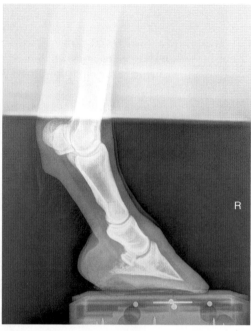

FIG. 24.65 Mystery radiograph. What body part and position is this? Where is the image receptor placed?

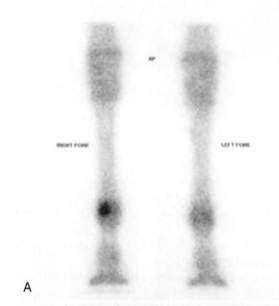

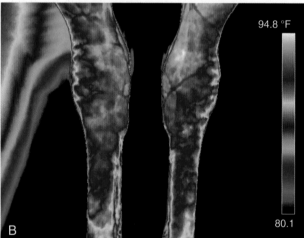

FIG. 24.64 A, Nuclear scintigraphy of the front limbs indicating dark areas known as "hot spots" or inflammation on the carpus. **B,** Infrared thermal image of another horse. The red areas indicate "hot spots" or inflammation. (**A** courtesy Jill McFadden Surette, Toronto Equine Hospital, Mississauga, Ontario; **B** courtesy Vetel Diagnostics San Luis Obispos, California; and Seth Wallack, DVM, DACVR, AAVR, Director and CEO.)

✳ KEY POINTS

1. Patience, planning, proper preparation, and knowledge of anatomy and directional terms are all required for diagnostic large-animal radiographs.
2. Large animals generally stand for radiography, which necessitates the use of a horizontal beam.
3. Radiation, patient, and human safety need to be kept in mind at all times.
4. Because of the unique anatomy of the equine limb, a minimum of four views is required: dorsopalmar/ dorsoplantar, lateromedial, and two oblique views, one on either side of the midsagittal plane taken between the DP and lateromedial positions.
5. If joints are to be examined, further positions may include a flexed lateral, skyline, or flexor view.
6. The same principles of radiography apply to all species. Thus the angle of the beam is always perpendicular to the area of interest. In the equine patient, the angle of the beam to the ground for dorsopalmar/dorsoplantar and oblique radiographs may vary according to the foot trimming and anatomy. For lateromedial views, the beam is always parallel to the ground.
7. Standard radiographs for cloven-footed large animals are generally the dorsopalmar/dorsoplantar and lateromedial views with occasional oblique projections for joints.

REVIEW QUESTIONS

1. Safety is a priority when taking radiographs. To keep personnel away from the central ray when the metacarpus of large animals is being radiographed, you should:
   a. Use a cassette tunnel
   b. Use a foot block with a cassette slot
   c. Use a cassette holder with a clamp and long handle
   d. Hold the cassette

2. When viewing a DMPLO radiograph of the equine fetlock, you should place the image on the viewer so that the proximal cannon bone is positioned:
   a. Down with the dorsal aspect to your left
   b. Up with the dorsal aspect to your left
   c. Up with the dorsal aspect to your right
   d. Down with the dorsal aspect to your right

3. To prevent air artifacts when radiographing the equine foot, it is best to use:
   a. Play-Doh
   b. Sand
   c. Styrofoam
   d. Plaster

4. The dorsal 65-degree proximal–palmarodistal oblique (D65Pr-PaDiO) view of the distal phalanx means that the beam is angled:
   a. To the ground, 65 degrees palmaroproximal
   b. 65 degrees from the MSP and to the ground
   c. 65 degrees to the limb, dorsoproximal
   d. To the ground 65 degrees dorsoproximal

5. The dorsal 65-degree proximal–palmarodistal oblique (D65Pr-PaDiO) view of the digit is also known as a:
   a. True DP view
   b. Lateral oblique view
   c. High coronary view
   d. Upright pedal view

6. A human wrist is equivalent to the equine:
   a. Proximal phalanx
   b. Metacarpal interphalangeal joint
   c. Carpus
   d. Fetlock joint

7. For the upright pedal route of the navicular bone the foot will be:
   a. Pointed on a block with the beam parallel to the ground
   b. Placed flat on the tunnel cassette with the beam angled
   c. Placed flat on a block with the beam angled to the ground
   d. Placed flat on the tunnel cassette with the beam parallel to the ground

8. For a true DP view of the navicular bone, you need to include the:
   a. Navicular only
   b. P3, navicular, and P2
   c. P1, navicular, and P2
   d. Coffin bone, navicular, and long pastern

9. The descriptive terminology for a DLPMO is:
   a. Dorsal 45-degree proximal lateral–palmarodistomedial oblique
   b. Dorsoproximal 45-degree lateral–palmarodistomedial oblique
   c. Dorsoproximal 45-degree medial–palmarodistolateral oblique
   d. Dorso 45-degree proximal medial–palmarodistolateral oblique

10. You are preparing to image the DMPLO of the digit of a Thoroughbred. The image receptor should be placed at the _____ oblique aspect of the limb and the beam directed dorsal 65-degree proximal and _____
    a. lateral; 45-degree at the lateral
    b. lateral; 45-degree at the medial
    c. medial; 45-degree at the medial
    d. medial; 45-degree at the lateral

11. The veterinarian will request that you complete the DMPLO view of the digit to visualize the _____ wing of the coffin bone, which will appear _____ on the image.
    a. lateral; smaller and denser
    b. lateral; larger and less dense
    c. medial; smaller and denser
    d. medial; larger and less dense

12. To image the fetlock, the image receptor should be placed against the:
    a. Medial aspect of the limb, perpendicular to the ground for a flexed lateral view
    b. Medial aspect of the limb, perpendicular to the ground for a DP view
    c. Medial aspect of the limb, parallel with the ground for a flexed lateral view
    d. Lateral side of the limb, perpendicular to the ground for a lateromedial view

13. The splint bones are the:
    a. First and fifth metacarpus/metatarsus
    b. Second and fourth metacarpus/metatarsus
    c. Second and third metacarpus/metatarsus
    d. Third and fourth metacarpus/metatarsus

14. You are required to complete a lateromedial view of the metacarpals of an Arabian. The central ray is:
    a. On the medial aspect and angled 90 degrees from the MSP
    b. Angled to the ground and 90 degrees from the MSP
    c. Parallel to the ground and angled 90 degrees from the MSP
    d. Parallel to the ground and angled 45 degrees from the MSP

15. To position for the craniocaudal view of the elbow, place the image receptor on the:
    a. Palmar aspect of the joint
    b. Plantar aspect of the joint
    c. Cranial aspect of the joint
    d. Caudal aspect of the joint

16. Oblique views are necessary for an equine dental survey to avoid:
    a. Increased amount of soft tissue on the head
    b. Superimposition of the guttural pouch
    c. Superimposition of the frontal sinuses
    d. Superimposition of the opposite arcade

17. Pelvic radiographs may be contraindicated in equine patients with a pelvic injury because:
    a. Anesthesia poses a risk to the equine patient
    b. Patient recovery may cause additional injury
    c. Pelvic radiographs are often unsuccessful
    d. Pelvic radiographs are never contraindicated

18. The SID for large animals is generally:
    a. The same as for small animals
    b. Not of concern
    c. Shorter than for small animals
    d. Longer than for small animals

19. You are required to complete a carpus DP view for a Holstein cow (dairy). You should position the central ray:
    a. Parallel to the ground and slightly lateral to the MSP
    b. Parallel to the ground on the MSP
    c. Parallel to the ground slightly medial to the MSP
    d. At a slight angle to the ground on the MSP

20. The view that is completed for cattle but not performed on an equine P3 is the:
    a. Lateromedial view
    b. Dorsal 45-degree proximal–palmarodistal view
    c. Lateromedial (mediolateral) view with interdigital film
    d. Dorsal 45-degree lateral–palmaromedial oblique

Answers to Review Questions can be found on the Evolve website.

References

1. Weaver M, Barakzai S. *Handbook of Equine Radiography*. London: Saunders Elsevier; 2010.
2. Morgan JP. *Techniques of Veterinary Radiography*. Ames, IA: Iowa State University Press; 1993.
3. Butler JA, Coles CM, Dyson SJ, et al. *Clinical Radiology of the Horse*. Osney Mead, Oxford: Wiley-Blackwell; 2008.
4. Han C, Hurd C. *Practical Diagnostic Imaging for the Veterinary Technician*. St. Louis: Elsevier Mosby; 2005.
5. Thrall DE. *Textbook of Veterinary Diagnostic Radiology*. 6th ed. St. Louis: Elsevier; 2013.
6. The Merck veterinary manual. http://www.merckvetmanual.com/mvm/index.jsp?cfile=htm/bc/90504.htm.

Bibliography

American College of Veterinary Radiology (ACVR). Radiology 2—equine; 2009, ACVR.

Aspinall V, Cappello M. *Introduction to Veterinary Anatomy*. London: Butterman-Heineman; 2009.

Bassert JM, McCurnin DM. *McCurnin's Clinical Textbook for Veterinary Technicians*. 7th ed. St. Louis: Elsevier; 2010.

Colville T, Bassert J. *Clinical Anatomy and Physiology for Veterinary Technicians*. 3rd ed. St. Louis: Mosby; 2016.

Crawford SJ. Equine radiography: Positioning techniques and tips for acquiring good images; April 2016. http://www.slideshare.net/ShalynCrawfordGarman/equine-radiography-positioning-techniques-tips-for-acquiring-good-images.

Done SH, Goody PC, Stickland NC, et al. *Color atlas of Veterinary Anatomy, the Dog and Cat*. London: Mosby; 2009.

Douglas SW. *Principles of Veterinary Radiography*. London: Bailliere Tindall; 1980.

Dyce KM, Sack WO, Wensing CJG. *Textbook of Veterinary Anatomy*. 4th ed. St. Louis: Saunders; 2010.

Garrett KS, Berk JT. How to properly position thoroughbred repository radiographs, http://www.ivis.org/proceedings/aaep/2006/pdf/z9100106000600.pdf?origin=publication_detail. Retrieved March 2016.

O'Brien T. *O'Brien's Radiology for the Ambulatory Equine Practitioner*. Jackson, MS: Tewton NewMedia; 2005.

Radiology of the equine limbs; n.d. http://www.quia.com/files/quia/users/medicinehawk/2407-Vet/Radiology-2.pdf.

Redding WR. Radiographic Examination of the Equine Foot. College of Veterinary Medicine, North Carolina State University, Raleigh, NC. http://www.equipodiatry.com/Radio.htm.

Reid CF, Bathurst NW. Large animal radiography nomenclature. 1995, University of Pennsylvania School of Veterinary Medicine. http://cal.vet.upenn.edu/projects/larad/names/name.htm.

Romich J. *An Illustrated Guide to Veterinary Medical Terminology*. 4th ed. Stamford, CT: Cengage Learning; 2015.

Smallwood JE, Shively MJ, Rendano VT, et al. A standardized nomenclature for radiographic projections used in veterinary medicine. *Vet Radiol*. 1985;24:2-9.

Be as a bird perched on a frail branch that she feels bending beneath her, still she sings away all the same, knowing she has wings.
—Victor Hugo, French writer, 1802–1885

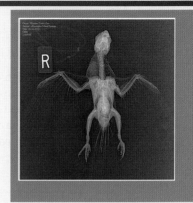

OUTLINE

*Special thanks to Sue Carstairs, DVM, of Seneca College, Toronto Wildlife Centre and Kawartha Turtle Trauma Centre, for her assistance with this chapter in the previous edition.

LEARNING OBJECTIVES

When you have finished this chapter you will be able to:

1. Produce diagnostic high-quality radiographs of birds, exotic companion mammals, and reptiles with special emphasis on patient and machine preparation, centering, and inclusion.
2. Position the body part parallel to the image receptor with the central ray perpendicular to both.
3. Describe the common reasons for imaging, normal views, and protocol for the various species and positions.
4. Describe common anatomical species-specific terms and identify normal avian and exotic species anatomy found on a radiograph.

KEY TERMS

Key terms are defined in the Glossary on the Evolve website.

Amphibian	Coelom	Horizontal beam	Positional terminology
Cloacogram	Gavaging	Orthogonal	Testudine

TECHNICAL NOTE: To preserve space, the radiographs presented in this chapter do not show collimation. For safety, always collimate so that the beam is limited to within the image receptor edges. In film radiography, should see a clear border of collimation (frame) on every radiograph. In some jurisdictions, evidence of collimation is required by law.

Medical imaging is an important diagnostic tool in avian and exotic animal medicine (Table 25.1) because anatomy of the respiratory tract limits auscultation, and palpation of the viscera is difficult.

Radiographs are often required by the veterinarian for avian patients that show obscure clinical signs. Fortunately, the bird's system of air sacs provides enhanced contrast in areas that are not well visualized in mammals.

Very small variations in x-ray output are more noticeable in the avian patient than in cats and dogs because of their smaller size; thus an x-ray unit with uniform output is required. The machine should be capable of producing at least 300 milliamperes (mA), have an exposure time of 1/120 sec or shorter with a kilovolt range from a minimum of 40 kV that should be adjustable in 1-kV increments. Short exposure times are essential to minimize the motion artifacts associated with a rapid respiratory rate and muscle tremors that are common in birds as well as in some exotic companion mammals.

Because of lower bone density than in reptiles or mammals, less exposure is needed for flight birds of the same thickness. Wing radiographs are often overpenetrated, making this area appear excessively dark with low contrast. Unlike with dogs and cats, most exposure charts are based on species and size and not on measurement.

If there is not a specific avian or small mammal chart, the cat abdomen chart for that thickness is useful, especially for the larger small exotics. Decrease the milliampere-seconds (mAs) by at least 50%. Alternatively, the feline extremity chart can be used by halving the exposure. If a measurement is required, do so at the thickest body part of the area to be examined.

The general principles of canine and feline radiography apply to avian and exotic companion mammals imaging. Two orthogonal views should also be taken. A shorter scale of contrast, associated with lower kV in the 40 to 60 kV range, is preferred.

Nonscreen film (larger dental film, size 4) is useful, and high-detail film/screen systems produce images with better detail than digital systems. If available, a mammography cassette with a single screen and with single emulsion film is especially diagnostic. As a guide, about four times the mAs will be required over a regular 400-speed system, 1/120 sec or shorter with a kilovolt range from a minimum of 40 kV.

Digital radiography systems usually use higher kV techniques than the film/screen systems, possibly leading to lower contrast, but incremental changes of 1 kV will help with adjustments to achieve the proper contrast. However, a greater image contrast range, resulting in improved image quality, is more possible in digital radiography than with film imaging. Special algorithms for digital units are required. These are often provided by the manufacturers.[1]

Further detail can also be achieved with smaller focal spots. Grids are not typically used because even for those patients over 10 cm, the air within the air sacs of birds, for example, does not generate noteworthy scatter radiation.

The tube stand should have source-image distance (SID) adjustments that can compensate for changing the mAs to decrease the exposure time. Remember from Chapter 6 that mAs is inversely proportional to the square of the distance from the x-ray source (focal spot). As you decrease the distance from the source, you can also decrease the mAs. As SID decreases, magnification increases. Penumbra is also affected. The minimum SID used should be 76 cm (30 inches) unless a magnification study is required.

Dental units can be used, but to minimize respiratory movement, the patient should be small (typically less than 20 g for birds), the area localized, and the patient anesthetized. Portable units used for large animals typically do not produce

TABLE 25.1	Recommended Views of Exotic Species for Complete Body Study	
SPECIES	**RECOMMENDED VIEW**	**OPTIONAL**
Avian	VD: coelom (whole body) Lateral: coelom (whole body) with wing superimposition	Modified lateral: whole body; wings not superimposed Wing: CdCr and mediolateral Lateral and VD Foot: lateral and CrCd Contrast study for GI tract Urography for urinary tract
Exotic companion mammals	DV: whole body (smaller mammals) Lateral: whole body	VD: whole body or site of interest Extremities: lateral and ventral recumbency Contrast study for GI
Larger exotic companion mammals (rabbits, ferrets, guinea pigs)	VD: site of interest Lateral: site of interest Skull: DV and lateral Extremities: both views	Contrast study for GI Further skull views
Lizards	Whole body: DV with vertical beam Whole body: lateral with horizontal beam	Extremities: vertical beam Contrast study for GI
Chelonian	DV with vertical beam Lateral: horizontal (preferred). Craniocaudal: horizontal beam (preferred)	Contrast study for GI
Snakes	DV: whole body for GI, cranial 2/3 for respiratory Whole body for GI: lateral view, with horizontal beam	Contrast study for GI

Cd, caudal; *Cr,* cranial; *DV,* dorsoventral; *GI,* gastrointestinal; *VD,* ventrodorsal.

sufficient mA values at the required short exposure times without drastically reducing the SID.

Ultrasound, computerized tomography, and magnetic resonance imaging are more diagnostic modalities but are relatively expensive and not always readily available.

Avian Radiography

Patient Preparation

A bird is best fasted so that the crop (for those species that possess one) feels empty on palpation. The time varies greatly with species and can range from 1 hour to multiple hours. The radiographic appearances of the internal organs are affected by digestive tract contents, possibly leading to misdiagnosis.[1] Avoid gavaging before radiography, especially in debilitated birds. Stress associated with the procedure increases the likelihood of regurgitation and airway aspiration. The crop and proventriculus emptying times may be prolonged in dehydrated birds.

Recall that in canine and feline patients, thorax radiographs should be taken at peak inspiration. In the avian patient the effect of the respiratory cycle on the radiographic appearance is less noticeable, as the lungs are nonexpansile, and air is continuously moving into the pulmonary parenchyma and the air sac. Distention of the abdominal air sacs may enhance the contrast of the abdominal viscera, especially those with abundant coelomic fat. Respiratory movements should be minimized, if possible, by trying to coordinate the exposure time during a pause in the respiratory cycle. Positive-pressure ventilation can be applied to an intubated, anesthetized bird for air sac inflation and radiographic exposure timed accordingly to correspond with increased air in the sacs.

Anesthesia and Positioning Devices

Anesthetizing a healthy bird with inhalation gas anesthesia is generally less stressful for the patient than taking radiographs without chemical restraint. Accurate positioning with near-perfect alignment is essential for correct interpretation of avian images. Radiographs are generally of higher quality, and fewer images need to be taken because there is less chance of motion artifacts when the patient is anesthetized. The birds are easily positioned, there is less potential for iatrogenic fractures, and the air sacs can be inflated in the intubated patient.

However, anesthesia and stress may further compromise debilitated patients. Precautions should be taken. Many of these considerations apply not only to birds but also to any species undergoing radiography.

The following suggestions apply particularly to the handling of wild birds that are fully conscious[2]:

- Have everything organized before the procedure to minimize the time required for restraint or anesthesia.
- Wear protective clothing, gloves, and headgear as appropriate with the species. Wear protective eye wear and long protective gloves over the lower arms for raptor

restraint. Never leave talons unrestrained. Once the feet have been radiographed, it is advisable to wrap the talons for added handler safety. A full face shield is suggested for water birds with long beaks. Never leave dangerous beaks such as those of herons unrestrained.

- Work in a dimly lit room, and minimize unnecessary noise and movement.
- Ensure that the area is contained, avoiding escape routes and areas in which the patient can hide or injure itself. Have capture devices, such as nets, on hand in case of escape.
- Cover the bird's head and torso with a towel.
- If taping the bird down, ensure that the tape will not rip out feathers. Using masking tape, transparent medical tape, or a floral Millipore tape causes less damage to the skin and feathers (Fig. 25.1). Always remove tape in the direction the feathers are pointed.

Stress can be fatal, especially for debilitated birds, so reduce stress and minimize handling time. Small birds weighing less than 100 g can be positioned directly on the image receptor.

If anesthetizing, have everything prepared ahead of time, working quickly and accurately to minimize the anesthetic

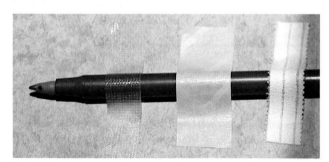

FIG. 25.1 Three types of tape used for avian and exotic restraint. *Left,* Transparent medical tape is best, as it does not pull the feathers off birds. *Center,* Paper masking tape or autoclave tape also minimizes hair and feather loss. *Right,* Adhesive tape could pull off feathers and hair. Floral tape is also effective. (Courtesy Rick Axelson, DVM, Links Road Animal Clinic, North York, Ontario.)

time. An anesthetized or chemically restrained bird should be monitored very closely, regularly, and kept warm.

For small ill birds, such as canaries or budgies, the veterinarian will not likely recommend anesthesia; excessive handling will cause further stress. Consider using a horizontal beam while the bird is either perching or placed in a small box or plasticware (e.g., Tupperware) container, where it can be wedged in the corner with pieces of foam. Make sure the patient's breathing is not compromised in any container in which it is placed. The images are not ideal, but they may be diagnostic enough to indicate the problem. Make sure that the radiographs and the number of views are satisfactory before recovering the patient.

Minimize manual restraint. Bird-positioning devices or restraint boards simplify the positioning and reduce the time required for correct positioning (Fig. 25.2). Use of a Plexiglas or other acrylic restraint device often requires an increase of 2 to 4 kV, especially if the lower range of kV is used. Extensions such as intravenous (IV) tubing, Velcro, rope, or gauze can be used in lieu of tape to attach the limbs to the positioner or to the table. Alternatively, sandbags can be gently placed over the extensions. Radiolucent containers can restrain ill birds that cannot tolerate anesthesia (see Fig. 25.16A). Be mindful of patient stress and possible injury that may result from struggling.

As with mammals, two projections, made at a 90-degree angle (orthogonal projections), are recommended unless the patient is compromised. Standard views include lateral and ventrodorsal (VD) studies of the coelom. If a pectoral extremity is required, the standard is the mediolateral and caudocranial of the wing due to the curvature of the skeletal structures of the wing.

In between imaging and during recovery, ensure that the bird is placed in a normal sternal position to aid breathing efforts. A towel "donut" (twisted towel to support the bird) can aid. Do not place the bird on a perch until the patient is fully recovered. Because recovery can be rapid, keep hands on the patient to prevent a fall.

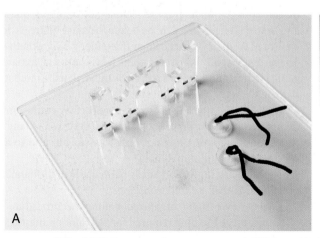
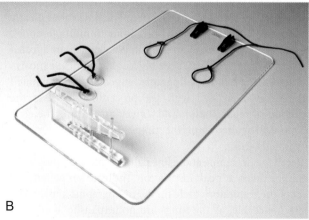

A   B

FIG. 25.2 Two types of avian restrainers. **A,** VSP Avian Neck Restraint and VSP Avian Restraint Board (Veterinary Specialty Products, Shawnee, KS). Different-sized collars or suction cups are available. **B,** VSP Miami Vise Avian Restraint. Another type of positioner is the Auspex Avian Positioner (Jorgensen Laboratories, Inc., Loveland, CO; not shown).

Radiographic Views

Avian Coelom

Lateral View of the Avian Coelom

Positioning for a True Lateral

Place the patient in right lateral recumbency. Use a radiolucent or cardboard sheet on the image receptor to tape the patient to this sheet to facilitate moving the patient if another exposure is required (Fig. 25.3B). Gently extend the bird, and with precut strips of tape, carefully tape the patient on the radiolucent Plexiglas or cardboard sheet in the following order if the patient is not chemically restrained:

Head: Tape is gently placed across the neck at the base of the skull. If the tape is too tight, tracheal collapse may result.

Wings: Extend the wings dorsally in full extension; tape the dependent wing first and then superimpose the upper wing. Avoid excessive pressure to the upper wing to prevent rotation.

Pelvic Limbs: Extend and superimpose the pelvic limbs slightly caudally, secure the tape or gauze to the distal tarsometatarsal bones, and extend the limbs. Tape the dependent limb first.

Tail: Taping of the tail is optional but should be close to the base. Include the correct positional marker, and place it on the cranial aspect of the film.

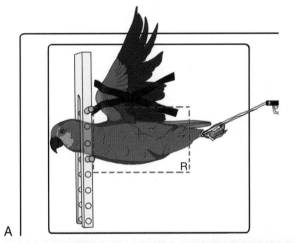

MEASURE: At the thickest part of the chest (over the keel if it is a larger bird) if required. Use the species and size chart otherwise.

CENTRAL RAY: At the level of the xiphoid (caudal tip of keel), between the spine and keel.

BORDERS:

Small Birds: The whole body should be included.

Large and Medium Birds: Include the coelom, proximal extremities, and caudal cervical regions or the area of interest. Multiple exposures are needed for larger birds, especially long-necked patients such as swans.

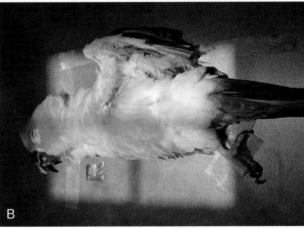

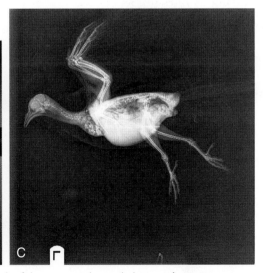

FIG. 25.3 A, Positioning technique for a right lateral radiograph of the avian coelom with the use of a positioning device.[3] **B,** Positioning for a lateral whole-body radiograph of a Sun Conure with the use of tape. If the extremities are superimposed, there will be less rotation of the bird's body. **C,** Radiograph of the lateral view of an adult bird with the wings superimposed. Superimposition of the pelvic limbs would minimize rotation. (**A** courtesy Devon Greves; **B** courtesy Rick Axelson, DVM, Links Road Animal Clinic, North York, Ontario; **C** courtesy Sue Carstairs, DVM, Seneca College, Toronto Wildlife Centre and Kawartha Turtle Trauma Centre.)

Continued

Lateral View of the Avian Coelom—cont'd

If the bird positioner (commercial or homemade guillotine device [bird board]) is being used:

- Place the neck in the cervical restraint portion; then gently move the body caudally to reduce the curvature of the neck (Fig. 25.3A).
- Immobilize the rest of the body as needed to obtain positioning as described previously, using tape, gauze, or tubing to secure the limbs to the cleats.

Comments and Tips

- If the patient is anesthetized, the order of taping or positioning is not important.
- Be gentle; luxation of the shoulder can result if the position is forced. Increasing the plane of anesthesia may be required, but there may be an anatomical inability to position the limb properly.

- Superimposition of the extremities helps minimize rotation (Fig. 25.5). If pelvic limb or wing images are required, the limbs are not superimposed. Instead they are positioned as described later for the modified whole-body/pectoral limb lateral view (Fig. 25.6).
- The pelvic limbs need to be securely pulled and fastened to straighten the femur.
- The sternum and vertebral column can be palpated and should be on the same plane.
- The tail can be taped, and more tape can be placed on either the humeral portions of the wings or on the body if needed.
- Be careful to avoid pressure over the chest area.
- If the lungs are to be examined, it may be beneficial to deliberately underexpose a lateral view. Make sure that the wings are drawn away from the torso.

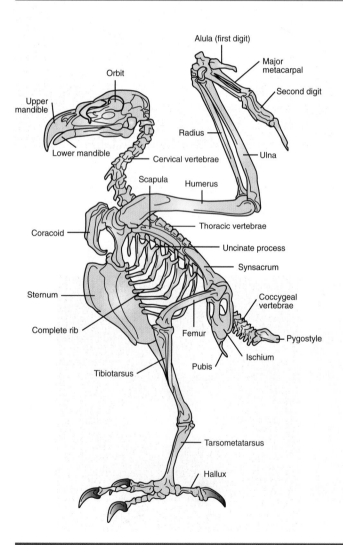

✎ TECHNICIAN NOTES

When working with raptors, make sure to tape the talons or use vet wrap to keep them restrained once the feet have been imaged.

✎ TECHNICIAN NOTES

To ensure that a lateral coelom or whole-body view is symmetrical:
- The head is slightly extended.
- The acetabula, ribs, coracoids, femoral heads, and kidneys are superimposed.
- The sternum and vertebral column are on the same plane.

FIG. 25.4 Skeleton of a hawk. (From Colville T, Bassert JM. *Clinical Anatomy and Physiology for Veterinary Technicians.* 3rd ed. St. Louis: Elsevier; 2016.)

Lateral View of the Avian Coelom—cont'd

Modified Whole-Body/Pectoral Limb Lateral View
Comments and Tips

- If the pectoral or pelvic limbs of small birds need to be radiographed, the limbs and wings can be separated in the lateral view to minimize the number of images needed (see Fig. 25.6).
- Position in lateral recumbency as described previously, with the following exceptions:
  - Do not superimpose the limbs; instead separate both the wings and the legs.

- The extremities on the dependent side should be pulled and taped cranially, with padding placed between the perspective limbs to avoid rotation of the body.
- Secure the contralateral limbs caudally (leg) and dorsally (the wing) to minimize superimposition.
- In this view, the contralateral wing is in a mediolateral view, but there will be increased object-film distance (OFD).
- Thus the patient is best placed in a VD position for the mediolateral pectoral limb.
- There is more rotation of the body when the limbs are not superimposed.

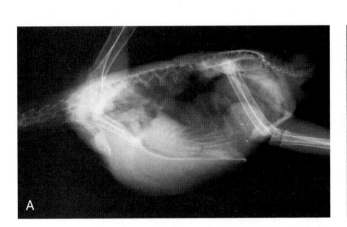

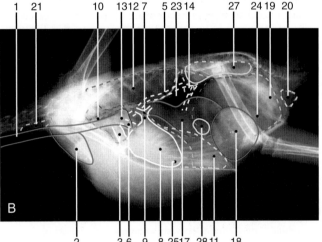

FIG. 25.5 Radiographic anatomy of the lateral view of the adult Lovebird. Projection: Laterolateral (right lateral recumbency). 1, Trachea; 2, crop; 3, brachiocephalic artery and aorta; 4, brachiocephalic artery; 5, aorta; 6, pulmonary artery; 7, pulmonary vein; 8, heart; 9, left atrium; 10 esophagus; 11, liver; 12, lung; 13, syrinx; 14, gonad; 15, ovary; 16, testes; 17, proventriculus; 18, ventriculus; 19, intestines; 20, cloaca; 21, cervical air sac; 22, clavicular air sac; 23, thoracic air sac; 24, abdominal air sac; 25, apex of heart; 26, interface between caudal thoracic and abdominal air sacs; 2,7 kidneys; 28, spleen.

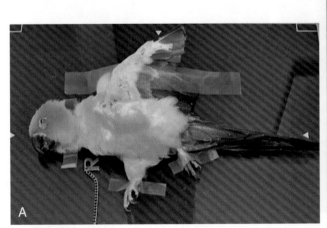

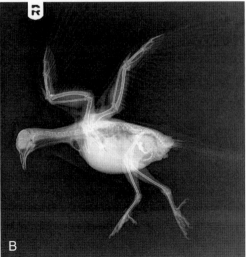

FIG. 25.6 A, Modified positioning technique for a right lateral radiograph of the avian, if separation of the extremities is required. **B,** Radiograph of the modified lateral view of an adult bird with the wings separated. (**A** courtesy Rick Axelson, DVM, Links Road Animal Clinic, North York, Ontario; **B** courtesy Sue Carstairs, DVM, Seneca College, Toronto Wildlife Centre and Kawartha Turtle Trauma Centre.)

Ventrodorsal View of the Avian Coelom

Positioning

Place the patient in dorsal recumbency. Have precut paper tape ready. If the positioning board is used, the Velcro or IV tubing found on the board can be attached to the cleats or suction cups in lieu of tape (Fig. 25.7).

Gently extend and carefully secure the patient in the order described below if the bird is not chemically restrained:

Head: If using a bird-positioning board, gently place the head in the cervical restrainer portion in a true rostrocaudal position. If not using a bird-positioning board, place tape at the mandibular articulation at the base of the skull.

Wings: Open the wings at a 90-degree angle to the body with two pieces of tape crossed at the carpal region of each wing. *Never* tape over the chest. Because of the delicate air sacs, respiration is affected.

Pelvic limbs: Apply tape or tubing separately around each tarsometatarsus and pull caudally and symmetrically.
Tail: Tape close to the base of the tail if needed.

Comments and Tips

- Place an indicator marker on the appropriate side.
- If the patient is anesthetized, the order of taping or positioning is not important.
- To position the leg caudally without moving the bird's body:
  - Gently place a finger at the tip of the sternum for release, making sure not to press dorsally on the sternum while doing so; otherwise the bird could suffocate.

MEASURE: If required, at the thickest part of chest (over the keel if it is a larger bird). Use the species and size chart otherwise.

CENTRAL RAY: Over the midline at the caudal tip of the sternum.

BORDERS:

Small Bird: Include the whole body.

Large or Medium-Sized Bird: Include the coelom, proximal extremities, and caudal cervical regions or the area of interest.

Multiple exposures are needed for larger birds, especially long-necked patients such as swans.

✏ TECHNICIAN NOTES

To ensure that a VD coelom or whole-body view will appear symmetrical:
- The keel (sternum) is directly over the spine.
- The scapula, acetabulum, and femur are parallel, equidistant, and symmetrical.
- The wings are open at 90 degrees to the body.

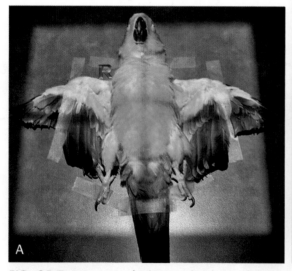

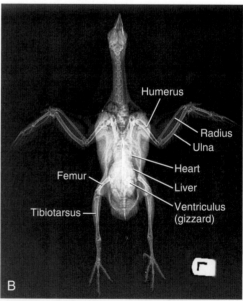

FIG. 25.7 **A,** Positioning for the ventrodorsal view of a Sun Conure with the use of tape. **B,** Radiographic anatomy of the ventrodorsal view of an adult Lovebird. (A courtesy Rick Axelson DVM, Links Road Animal Clinic, North York, Ontario; B courtesy Sue Carstairs, DVM, Seneca College, Toronto Wildlife Centre and Kawartha Turtle Trauma Centre.)

Wing

Mediolateral View of a Wing in Isolation

Positioning

Dorsal recumbency: True mediolateral view of the wing with decreased OFD.

- Position the body as in the VD view of the coelom.
- Place the body to the side of the image receptor to allow the affected wing and area of interest to be centered (Fig. 25.8).
- Tape at the mandibular articulation at the base of the skull.
- Open the wings at a 90-degree angle to the body, with two pieces of tape crossed at the carpal region of each wing.

- Separate and tape the pelvic limbs at the tarsometatarsal bones.
- Tape the tail close to the base.
- Additional tape can be applied to the proximal and distal portions of the affected wing if needed.

Comments and Tips

- Positioning of affected wing is more crucial, but keep the patient's injuries in mind.
- Decrease 2 to 4 kV from the coelomic view to prevent overexposure.

CENTRAL RAY: Midwing or the area of interest.

BORDERS: Include the entire wing, including the scapulohumeral joint.

Large Birds: Position wings diagonally across the image receptor to maximize the x-ray field.

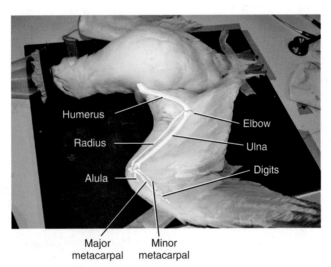

FIG. 25.8 Positioning for a mediolateral view of avian wing in isolation. (Courtesy Sue Carstairs, DVM, Seneca College, Toronto Wildlife Centre and Kawartha Turtle Trauma Centre.)

Caudocranial View of the Avian Wing

This view allows a true orthogonal view, as the lateral and VD coelom positions show the wings in a lateral projection. This CrCd view is also referred to as a *"leading edge or hanging drop view,"*[2] as the cranial edge of the wing is placed just above the image receptor. The patient should be sedated or anesthetized. Unfortunately, to obtain a true caudocranial view, the patient needs to be held (Fig. 25.9).

Positioning
- Carefully position the patient upside down with the head directed to the floor.
- Have the long axis of the body parallel to the vertically directed x-ray beam.

- Extend the wing fully with its cranial edge in contact with the image receptor.[4]

Comments and Tips
- Keep the wing close and parallel to the image receptor to minimize OFD.
- Distortion may occur toward the edges of the radiograph of birds with large wings because of beam divergence.
- For direct digital units, the CdCr view may be difficult because the x-ray sensor may not move to the edge of the table.
- The craniocaudal view is not as practical due to increased OFD because of the length of the flight feathers.

CENTRAL RAY: On the area of interest.

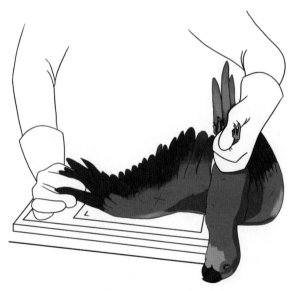

FIG. 25.9 Positioning for a caudocranial view of the avian wing. The patient does need to be sedated and is held to ensure the proper orientation. (Courtesy Devon Greves.)

Avian Head

Lateral View of the Avian Head

Positioning

- Place the patient in right lateral recumbency with the head either positioned through the cervical restrainer of the acrylic positioning board or taped to a sheet or image receptor (Fig. 25.10).
- Collimate and keep the head on the plate, carefully supporting the rest of the body with a towel or other positioner, depending on patient size.

- Secure the head by separately applying tape to the mandible and maxilla.
- A species and size exposure chart will likely be used; otherwise, measure at the thickest part.

CENTRAL RAY: Ventral to the eye.

BORDERS: Include the entire head extending to the cervical region.

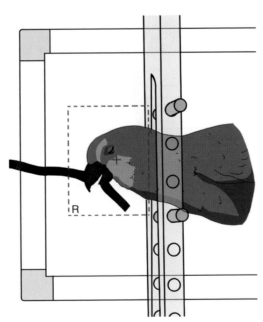

FIG. 25.10 Positioning for a lateral view of the avian head. (Courtesy Devon Greves.)

Ventrodorsal View of the Avian Head

Positioning

- Place the patient in dorsal recumbency as for the VD view of the coelom. Ensure the head is in a true rostrocaudal position.

- Apply radiolucent tape to the ventral aspect of the rhinotheca to bring the maxilla closer to the image receptor (Fig. 25.11).

CENTRAL RAY: Midline between the eyes.

BORDERS: Include the entire head.

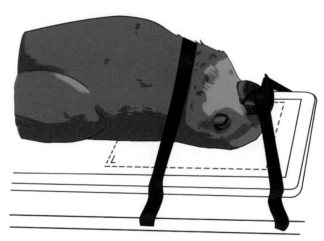

FIG. 25.11 Ventrodorsal positioning for a radiograph of the avian head. (Courtesy Devon Greves.)

Avian Limb

Mediolateral View of the Avian Foot

- Can be combined with the modified whole-body/limb view.
- Larger patients may require a separate film, or a coelom view may not be required.

Positioning

- Place the patient in lateral recumbency on an acrylic positioning board or taped to a sheet or image receptor directly with the affected limb down.
- If the positioning board is utilized, use Velcro or tape, not the cleats, to secure the feet directly to the board.

- Apply radiolucent tape on each toe to separate the digits of the affected limb to minimize superimposition. The tape allows for more precise positioning than gauze.
- Tie and secure the unaffected limb caudally (Fig. 25.12).
- Extend the dependent limb cranially to prevent superimposition.

Comments and Tips

- A decrease of 2 to 4 kV from the coelomic view prevents overexposure.

CENTRAL RAY: On the condyles of the tarsometatarsal bone.

BORDERS: Include all of the phalanges.

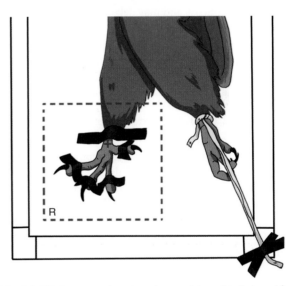

FIG. 25.12 Positioning for a lateral view of the pelvic limb and foot. (Courtesy Devon Greves.)

Craniocaudal View of the Avian Pelvic Limb

Positioning

- Place the patient in dorsal recumbency.
- Position as for the VD view of the coelom, securing the head and pectoral limbs.
- Separate and use tape, gauze, or tubing at the tarsometatarsal bones of the pelvic limbs; caudally extend the pelvic limbs.
- Separate the toes with tape or cotton to prevent superimposition, being careful of any injury.

Comments and Tips

- Place an R or L marker on the appropriate limb.
- Center accordingly.
- If needed, tape the tail close to the base.
- Additional tape can be applied to the proximal portions of the affected limb.

CENTRAL RAY: On the affected limb(s).

BORDERS: Include just beyond the affected area.

Contrast Study of the Gastrointestinal Tract

Due to anatomy and variable rapid digestive tract transit time, a single protocol for a contrast study is limited. Oral contrast media highlights the digestive tract from the esophagus to the large intestine and occasionally the cloaca. For true cloacal studies, contrast medium should be administered retrograde directly into the cloaca.

Preparation

If the bird can tolerate fasting, the crop and the proventriculus should be empty. The fasting period depends on the size, metabolic requirements, and health of the bird. Food in the ingluvies (crop) decreases the volume of contrast media that can be safely administered. Food in the gastrointestinal (GI) tract prevents full contact of the contrast medium with the digestive tract mucosa and may delay passage of the contrast medium.

Birds weighing more than 300 g should not be fed pelleted foods within 4 hours of the contrast study. When food is mixed with the contrast medium, the patterns shown on images are unpredictable.

Anesthesia and Contrast Media

If the health of the bird permits, anesthesia is suggested. Tracheal intubation is ideal to prevent aspiration. Anesthetic masks are used for many small birds.

Anesthetized birds do tend to regurgitate less than nonanesthetized birds, though some birds may vomit upon recovery from anesthesia because of hypersensitivity to the gas anesthetic.[1] If regurgitation does occur, remove the medium immediately from the oropharynx with cotton-tipped applicators to prevent the contrast medium from passing through the choanal slit into the nasal cavity. Monitor the oral cavity carefully for any regurgitated contrast medium. In all situations, the cranial portion of the body should be raised.

Barium sulfate 30% weight to volume (w/v) is recommended at a general calculation of 0.025 to 0.05 mL/g body weight, depending on the species and presence or absence of a crop. The lower dose range is used in larger birds. It is better to estimate the volume of food that can be safely administered via crop gavage and to give the contrast medium at only 50% to 75% of this amount.[1]

Warm the medium to room temperature by immersing the syringe in warm water. Mix the warmed liquid well and test the temperature before administration to prevent crop burn, which can precipitate severe metabolic and fluid imbalances as well as decrease the mucosal detail.

Slowly administer the contrast media via a rigid or soft gavage tube passed into the crop. Verify that the tube is correctly palpated and placed. Keeping a finger over the distal portion of the cervical esophagus may help prevent aspirating barium sulfate during administration. Do not place excessive pressure on the full crop, and slowly remove the tube.

Increase 2 to 4 kV due to the greater opacity of the contrast medium (Fig. 25.13).

Technique for Antegrade GI

Produce survey ventrodorsal and right lateral radiographs just before the contrast study to indicate the current status of the digestive tract. If the esophagus, crop, and proventriculus are of interest, lateral and ventrodorsal radiographs should be taken immediately. There are significant species variations in

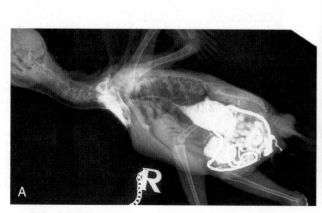
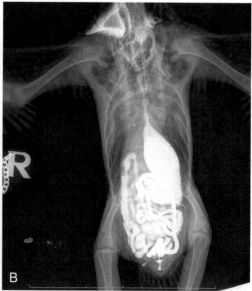

FIG. 25.13 Gastrointestinal barium study with contrast medium administered about 3 hours previously. **A**, Right lateral; **B**, ventrodorsal. Barium is in the crop, proventriculus, ventriculus, intestines, and cloaca. (Courtesy Rick Axelson, DVM, Links Road Animal Clinic, North York, Ontario.)

transit time, so depending on the type of bird, further lateral and ventrodorsal radiographs can be taken at 15 minutes and 30 minutes. Further 30-minute radiographs can be taken as needed and if continued anesthesia allows.

The procedure is technically finished when the contrast medium has entered the colon. Digestive transit time is generally more rapid than in mammals.

Positioning

BORDERS: Include the caudal cervical area and the entire coelom.

Position as for the lateral and ventrodorsal coelom. To prevent retrograde flow of contrast medium, either raise the cranial portion of the body or apply a bandage to the cervical esophagus. Raise the cranial body with a translucent positioning device. A bandage can partially occlude the cervical esophagus to minimize retrograde flow of contrast medium. Ensure bandage material does not occlude the trachea. Diligently monitor the anesthesia level, hypothermia, and any regurgitation.

Double-Contrast Study

A double-contrast study gives superior mucosal detail and usually has a shorter transit time. Anesthesia is frequently required, as gas infused into the crop is immediately expelled in most awake birds.

Less contrast medium is used than in positive-contrast studies, lessening the potential for aspiration into the respiratory tract. If air is regurgitated, further air can be administered to distend the crop.[1]

Cloacagram

Hollow organs are best viewed if properly distended; thus retrograde administration of barium into the vent is best implemented to fully visualize the cloaca.

Procedure

Before administering the barium, gently flush the cloaca with isotonic saline. Positive- and double-contrast cloacagrams can be performed. The common dosage of barium sulfate is 0.025 to 0.05 mL per gram body weight. If a double-contrast study is to be completed, perform the positive-contrast study first and then remove all of the barium pooled in the cloaca before introducing the negative-contrast medium (room air or carbon dioxide). The cloacal mucosal surface is better visualized in this way. Research indicates that carbon dioxide creates less potential for intravascular air emboli to occur. Fecal matter can be refluxed into the ureters when retrograde vent procedures are performed.[1]

CENTRAL RAY: Cranial to the cloaca (vent).
BORDERS: Include the cranial third of the coelom.

Positioning

As described for VD and lateral views of the coelom.

Urography

Urography can also be completed through the use of an intravenous contrast medium to evaluate the urinary tract, especially if an abnormal mass is palpated, the droppings volume and consistency have changed, or there is paresis. Do not complete if anesthesia or sedation cannot be used or if the bird will be stressed out.

Water-soluble iodinated solution (nonionic preferred) is injected, and VD radiographs are rapidly imaged at 10, 60, and 120 seconds after administration. A further VD radiograph can be taken at 5 to 7 minutes to show the contrast agent at the cloaca or rectum.

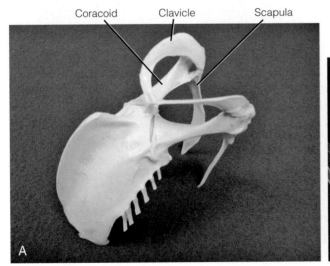

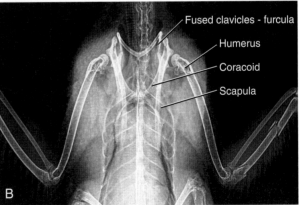

FIG. 25.14 **A,** Anatomy of the pectoral girdle of a rough-legged hawk. **B,** Radiograph showing the pectoral girdle of a red-tailed hawk. (**B** courtesy Sue Carstairs, DVM, Seneca College, Toronto Wildlife Centre and Kawartha Turtle Trauma Centre.)

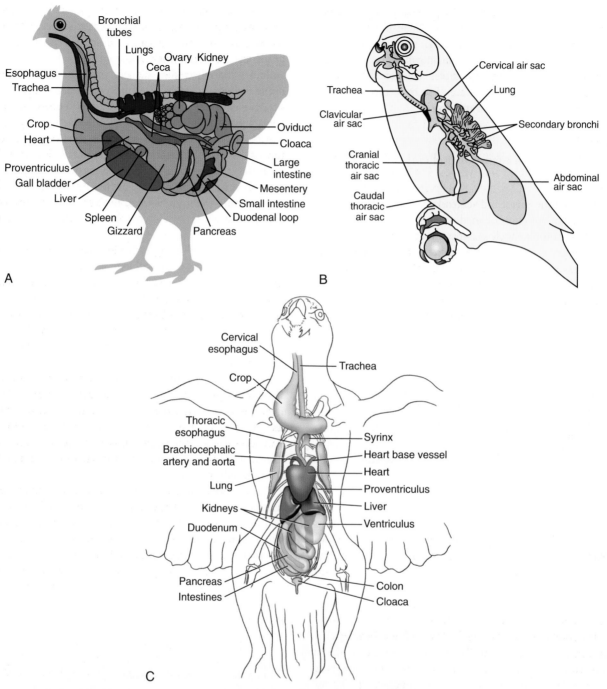

FIG. 25.15 **A,** Anatomical drawing of the viscera of an adult chicken in lateral view. **B,** Diagram of the lateral view of the avian respiratory system. **C,** Anatomical drawing (ventrodorsal view) of the viscera of an adult bird. (**B** from Colville T, Bassert JM. *Clinical Anatomy and Physiology for Veterinary Technicians.* 3rd ed. St. Louis: Elsevier; 2016; **C** from Silverman S. *Radiology of Birds: An Atlas of Normal Anatomy and Positioning.* Philadelphia: Saunders; 2010.)

Radiographic Anatomy

Radiographic anatomy of the avian skeleton (see Fig. 25.4) is very straightforward, but radiographic anatomy and interpretation of the internal structures are more complicated. Radiographically, the viscera are tightly packed together, making it difficult to identify anatomy. There is a minimal amount of perivascular fat and similar soft tissue density, making differentiation difficult.

Due to the lack of a diaphragm, there is no true division of thoracic and abdominal structures. The advantage for birds and reptiles in not having a diaphragm is the ability to expand abdominal contents into the respiratory system without any major compromise.

Anatomically the coelom is not divided in birds, but for discussion purposes, it is often separated into the thoracic and abdominal regions. There are many differences but also some similarities between birds and mammals.

Please see Appendix E on the Evolve website and Figs. 25.14 and 25.15 for avian anatomy and further radiographic concerns.

> ✎ **TECHNICIAN NOTES**
>
> Because of the superimposition of the organs, two perpendicular views, and perhaps an oblique view, may be needed to visualize the larger organs, such as the heart and liver, and the natural contrast of the gizzard and bowel (see Fig. 25.15).

Exotic Companion Mammals

The two orthogonal views generally are the dorsoventral (DV) and lateral in smaller exotic companion mammals such as rats, mice, hamsters, gerbils, or small rabbits and guinea pigs.

In the DV view, the animal is not as stressed, and the patient's small size causes minimum distortion or magnification. Interpretation is easier on the DV view for these species.

A horizontal beam, if available, can be used to obtain a lateral with the patient in the DV position. When using the horizontal beam, the patient and the image receptor may both have to be raised by being placed on a wooden block. The image receptor is placed vertically behind the animal, and the beam is perpendicular to both.

VD recumbency is generally used for larger exotic companion mammals such as rabbits and ferrets.

Anesthesia and Positioning Concerns

Many of the exotic companion mammals can be brought into the x-ray room for the anesthesia induction and recovery. Fasting does not generally occur. Exotic companion mammals are often placed in a properly ventilated "cat anesthesia box" and then connected to an anesthesia mask, or they are directly masked.

These patients can be taped to either the image receptor or a plastic positioner, radiographed, and then allowed to recover. The full process can be completed in 10 minutes. Other chemical restraint can also be used.

Make sure to keep the patients warm and monitor regularly, because they can quickly become hypothermic due to their small size. Plastic containers, cardboard shoeboxes, paper tape, gauze, and IV tubing are all simple positioning devices that are extremely useful in conjunction with anesthesia for radiography of exotic companion mammals (Fig. 25.16). As with the avian patient, it is important to be as quick and efficient as possible to minimize stress to the animal. Masking tape or transparent medical tape is less likely to remove the animal's fur and is less likely to be radiodense at lower kV settings. Velcro is also useful.

If a small guinea pig or rodent cannot be sedated or anesthetized, it can be radiographed while naturally crouched in the DV position in a radiolucent container. Keep in mind that true symmetry will not likely be achieved. If a properly sized container cannot be found to contain the animal, foam blocks can be used to make a corral. The lateral image can also be obtained with this position by using the horizontal x-ray beam.

A clean, loose-fitting stockinet, pinched at both ends to prevent escape, is also effective to restrain the limbs and torso. If needed, a wooden spatula or a tongue depressor can be used to keep the patient in place without the need to hold. Any lumps or subcutaneous masses should be identified by lead or barium marker on the overlying skin, especially in the reptilian species.

Keep species variation in mind when determining the best methods to restrain. For example, the dorsal half of a hedgehog's body is covered by a thick coat of long protective spines. When threatened, hedgehogs roll into a tight ball. If not anesthetized, they are often positioned in a small container with a horizontal beam used for the lateral view, again keeping in mind that true symmetry is not likely to be obtained.

> **TECHNICIAN NOTES**
>
> In smaller exotic companion mammals the views are generally lateral and DV, whereas the radiographic views of larger exotic companion mammals are the VD and lateral.

Ultrasonography Restraint

Ultrasonography is a useful diagnostic tool for exotic companion mammals. Guinea pigs, rabbits, and small rodents are difficult to examine with ultrasound because of their small size and reluctance to keep still. They are often best restrained in an upright position in the lap of or against the body of a restraining assistant. The restrainer will support the upper limbs and head with one hand and the rear limbs with the other. If further support for a larger patient is needed for ultrasonography, the lower limbs can be grasped by another person.

Small Exotic Companion Mammals

The main reason for admitting rats and other pet rodents for treatment is trauma, often due to being stepped on, crushed, or attacked by other pets—mostly cats. Trauma to the chest or diaphragm is often involved. Abdominal distention and tumors are also reasons for medical imaging. Malignant tumors in the form of cranial mediastinal masses are not uncommon, with some tumors being the size of the heart.

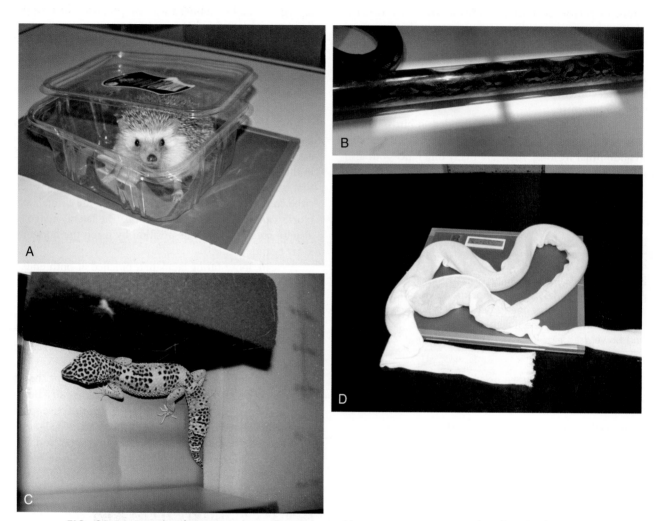

FIG. 25.16 Examples of positioning devices that can be used for exotic companion mammals and reptiles, keeping in mind that true symmetry may not be achieved depending on the device used. **A,** Hedgehog in a deli container for a DV or horizontal beam lateral. **B,** A snake tube, which allows for proper symmetry. **C,** Positioning of a gecko using foam devices to keep it in place. **D,** A stockinette can be tightened and pulled to minimize coiling. (**B** courtesy Ryan Cheeck, RVTg, VTS, [ECC], Veterinary Technology, Gwinnet Technical College.)

Radiographic Views

Dorsoventral View of the Small Exotic Companion Mammal

Positioning

- Place in ventral recumbency (Fig. 25.17).
- Secure the head and neck with precut tape.
- Gently move the limbs away from the body to prevent their superimposition over the abdomen and thorax.
- Tape over the shoulders behind the level of the elbow to stretch the forelimbs.
- Tape over the pelvis.

Comments and Tips

- To ensure that the DV or whole-body view will be symmetrical on the image:
    - The vertebrae are directly over the sternebrae in a vertical plane.
    - The acetabula are symmetrical.
    - The animal is as straight as possible from head to tail.

- For the natural DV position:
    - If too ill to be anesthetized, allow the patient to be in its natural ambulatory position and place in an appropriately sized radiolucent container.
    - Gently corral to a section of the container to limit its movement by using cotton or foam wedges.
    - Place the container with the corralled patient on the image receptor.
    - Use a vertical beam.
    - Depending on the type of container, 2 to 4 kV may need to be added to the original setting.
    - The image will not be as diagnostic as the regular DV due to limb superimposition.

MEASURE AND CENTRAL RAY: Over the thoracolumbar (TL) junction.

BORDERS: Include the whole body or the area of interest.

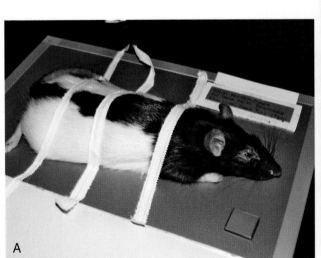
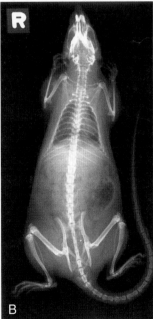

FIG. 25.17 **A,** Positioning for the dorsoventral view of a rat. The patient was anesthetized via a gas anesthetic chamber and quickly positioned and radiographed. Ideally the forelimbs should be extended more. **B,** Dorsoventral radiograph of the rat in A. The artifacts are the adhesive tape, which is more evident at lower exposure factors.

Lateral View of the Small Exotic Companion Mammal

Positioning

- Place in lateral recumbency with the affected side down (Fig. 25.18).
- Secure the head and neck with precut tape.
- Pull the pectoral limbs cranially and the pelvic limbs caudally, superimposing each set.
- Tape or use IV tubing, Velcro, or gauze to secure the patient to the image receptor or sheet.
- Tape over the tail if there is any chance of tail movement.
- Have the sternebrae and vertebrae on the same plane by placing a small sponge under the sternum and some cotton between the limbs, if required.

> ✎ **TECHNICIAN NOTES**
>
> Remember to place an appropriate left or right marker for each radiograph.

CENTRAL RAY: TL junction.

BORDERS: Include the whole body or the area of interest.

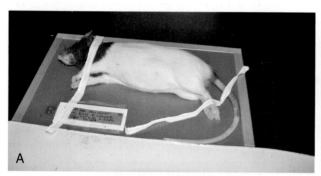 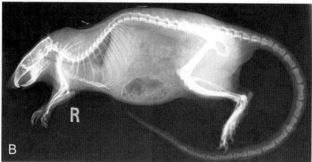

FIG. 25.18 A, Positioning for the lateral view of the full body of a rat. **B,** A lateral radiograph of a rat.

Lateral View of the Small Exotic Companion Mammal—cont'd

Comments and Tips

- Superimposition of the limbs leads to less rotation of the torso. The hind limbs are less in the field of view than if the dependent limb is pulled cranial.
- If radiographs of the limbs are required and extra radiographs are not practical, the limbs can be separated. The dependent limb should be pulled slightly cranially in each case.

- To ensure that the lateral view will be symmetrical on the image:
  - The head is slightly extended.
  - The respective acetabula and ribs are superimposed.
  - The sternum and vertebral column are on the same horizontal plane.

For the lateral view with a horizontal beam (Fig. 25.19):

- If the patient is too ill to be anesthetized, it can be placed in an appropriately sized radiolucent container in its natural ambulatory DV position.

- Gently corral to a section of the container to limit its movement by using cotton or foam wedges.
- Depending on how low the tube head will move, the container may need to be placed on a block or positioning device.
- Move the tube head to the horizontal position.
- Place the image receptor vertically against the side of the container away from the beam.
  - Keep the image receptor as close and parallel to the container as possible to minimize OFD and distortion.
  - The cassette may need to be taped or held in position by a device.
- The horizontally placed beam will be perpendicular to both the image receptor and the patient.
- Due to superimposition of the limbs over the cranioventral viscera and caudal abdomen, this view will not be as diagnostic as the regular lateral.

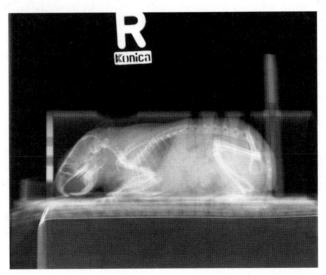

FIG. 25.19 Use of a horizontal beam for the lateral view of a hamster in ventral recumbency. The patient is in a disposable container that was placed on a plastic-covered foam pad.

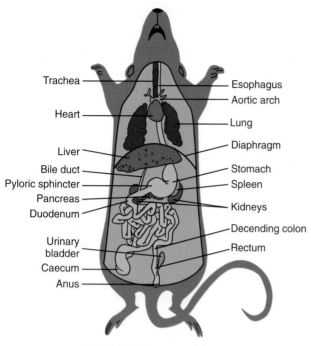

FIG. 25.20 Anatomy of the rat.

Labels (left, top to bottom): Trachea, Heart, Liver, Bile duct, Pyloric sphincter, Pancreas, Duodenum, Urinary bladder, Caecum, Anus

Labels (right, top to bottom): Esophagus, Aortic arch, Lung, Diaphragm, Stomach, Spleen, Kidneys, Decending colon, Rectum

Normal Rat and Other Small Exotic Companion Mammals: Radiographic Anatomy and Concerns

See Appendix E on the Evolve website and Figs. 25.20 and 25.24 for normal rat and other small exotic companion mammal radiographic concerns and anatomy.

> **✐ TECHNICIAN NOTES**
>
> Tape, especially porous or paper masking tape, is very useful in positioning exotic companion mammals, giving the patient the illusion that it is being controlled.

Larger Exotic Companion Mammals: Rabbits, Ferrets, and Guinea Pigs

Rabbit

Common reasons for radiographing rabbits are generally fractures or dislocations of the extremities; pelvic fractures; chest trauma; and bruises, scrapes, and minor lacerations of the face. Dental disease is of concern, and radiographs are often required. Though there are exceptions, most middle ear infections in rabbits appear radiographically normal.

Gastric dilation, often the result of transient atony, is not uncommon on a radiograph, and it is not necessarily a

mechanical obstruction. Massive fluid distension of the stomach can make peritoneal fluid diagnosis difficult.

To minimize radiation exposure for the radiographer, a healthy patient is best anesthetized and positioned according to principles similar to those used for rodents and cats. Rabbits are generally not routinely fasted before anesthesia because they do not regurgitate or vomit. In addition, fasting in the rabbit is not likely to reduce GI volume significantly and can contribute to ileus. Rabbits are generally docile and can be easily handled.

Ferret

Ferrets are often brought in with complaints of trauma, GI obstruction, cancer, or heart disease.[2] As with other small mammals, they often get underfoot and experience limb fractures. Thoracic crush injuries, in which widespread lung bruising is capable of causing severe dyspnea, are often more serious. Ferrets do suffer from various congenital and acquired heart diseases, with cardiomyopathy being the most common. Because of their curiosity and ability to hide in narrow places, ferrets often swallow small objects, many of which can cause obstruction.

Dental radiographs may be needed in ferrets. Occlusal dental film is preferred, but oblique extraoral projections can be made. Follow the same procedure as suggested for the dental radiography of cats (see Chapter 22). At least four views should be taken.

Ferrets are relatively easy to handle because they are friendly and inquisitive, but, as with rabbits, healthy ferrets are best anesthetized or sedated. They can be squirmy and will not remain still in a container similar to that used for smaller exotic companion mammals.

If anesthetized, a ferret should be fasted for 3 to 4 hours beforehand. Check for hidden food in the cage of a ferret that is to be fasted.

Guinea Pig

Guinea pigs often are admitted for injuries, usually caused by a dog or cat or by accidental injuries such as being stepped on, being caught in a door, or being crushed. Suspected bloat and urinary tract calculi are other common reasons for diagnostic imaging.

Guinea pigs are not aggressive but do stress easily and try to escape when scared. They are best sedated or anesthetized for radiography. Generally they are not fasted when anesthetized.

Normal Guinea Pig, Chinchilla, Rabbit, and Ferret Anatomy

See Appendix E on the Evolve website and Figs. 25.24 through 25.29 for some common radiographic anatomy of these species.

Radiographic Positioning

Positioning for radiography is fairly consistent for the slightly larger exotic companion mammals. Depending on the site of interest, variations occur where the patient is measured, centered, and with the peripheral borders. Table 25.2 indicates the differences. See the particular views for how to position.

TABLE 25.2	Where to Measure, Center, and What to Include When Radiographing Slightly Larger Exotic Companion Mammals			
SPECIES	VIEW	WHERE TO MEASURE	WHERE TO CENTER	WHAT TO INCLUDE
Guinea pig, chinchilla, and small rabbits	Ventrodorsal (VD) of full body	At the last rib (thickest part of the body)	Thoracolumbar (TL) junction	Minimum of shoulder joint to caudal to ilium, including the limbs
	Lateral of full body	Last rib (thickest part of the body)	TL junction for a full-body view	Depends on size (similar to small cat)
Ferrets and larger rabbits	VD of abdomen	Last rib (thickest part of the body)	Caudal to last rib	Cranial from xiphoid process to caudal to pubis
	Lateral of abdomen	Last rib (thickest part of the body)	Caudal to last rib	Cranial from xiphoid process to caudal to pubis
	VD of thorax	Last rib (thickest part of the body)	At xiphoid of sternum	Shoulder joint to slightly caudal to last rib
	Lateral of thorax	Last rib (thickest part of the body)	Caudal sternum	Shoulder joint to slightly caudal to last rib

Whole-Body View of Larger Exotic Companion Mammals

Ventrodorsal View of Whole Body/Abdomen/Thorax of a Larger Exotic Companion Mammal

Positioning

- Place the patient in dorsal recumbency, preferably with the patient being chemically restrained.
- Gently extend the pectoral limbs cranially.
- Slightly rotate the pelvic limbs medially and caudally, keeping the limbs equidistant.
- Tape the legs and keep them symmetrical.
- Alternatively, place gauze or tubing around the hocks and elbows extending to either a cleat at each end of the table or a positioning device.
- A sandbag can be placed over the gauze stretching the limbs or on the hind limbs for the larger patients.
- Keep the head straight and secure with tape if needed (Figs. 25.21 and 25.22).

> **✎ TECHNICIAN NOTES**
>
> To ensure that the ventrodorsal/dorsoventral view is symmetrical on the image:
> - The vertebrae are over the sternebrae on the same vertical plane.
> - The spinous processes are aligned in the center of the vertebral bodies.
> - The acetabula are symmetrical and the femurs parallel, if possible.
> - The animal is as straight as possible from the head to its tail, avoiding any rotation.

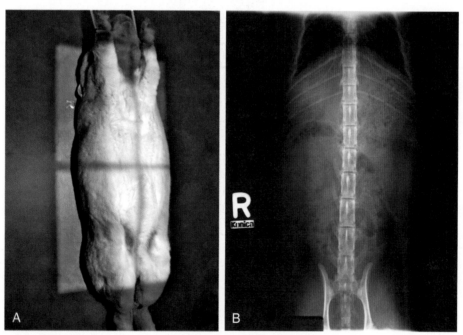

FIG. 25.21 **A,** Positioning for a full-body ventrodorsal (VD) view of a rabbit. The same positioning applies for abdomen, thorax, VD skull, pelvis, and proximal limbs. **B,** Radiograph of the VD view of the abdomen of a rabbit. (**A** courtesy Rick Axelson, DVM, Links Road Animal Clinic, North York, Ontario.)

Ventrodorsal View of Whole Body/Abdomen/Thorax of a Larger Exotic Companion Mammal—cont'd

Comments and Tips

- An acrylic or foam positioning device similar to that used for cats can also be utilized.
- The exposure factors may have to be increased by 2 to 4 kV if a positioning device is used.
- The extended VD can be painful if there is any injury. This pain can be slightly alleviated by not fully extending the legs and by placing the patient on a medium-density foam pad.

- Keep the patient warm, and monitor if anesthetized.
- The same positioning applies for the DV, except that the patient is in sternal recumbency.
- If limb studies are required, either the VD or DV position can be used.
- In the VD position, slightly rotate the patient to the opposite side to minimize soft tissue superimposition. Extend the limbs and secure with tape or tubing so that the affected forelimb is extended cranially and the hind limb caudally.

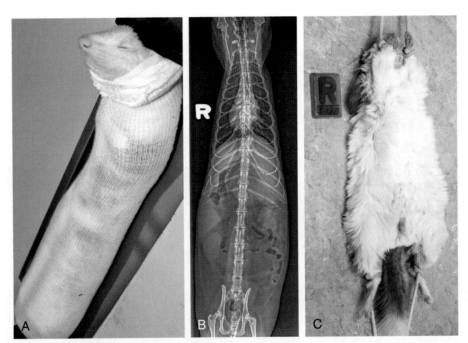

FIG. 25.22 A, Utilizing a stockinet for a ventrodorsal (VD) view of an unanesthetized ferret. Sandbags can be placed at either end and the patient placed on a V-trough. **B,** VD radiograph of the ferret. **C,** Positioning for a VD view of a chinchilla. Place the central ray over the area of interest and collimate appropriately. (B and C courtesy Rick Axelson, DVM, Links Road Animal Clinic, North York, Ontario.)

Lateral View of the Whole Body/Abdomen/Thorax of a Larger Exotic Companion Mammal

Positioning

- Place the patient in lateral recumbency (Fig. 25.23).
- A right lateral view is often preferred, but be consistent.
- Position the head cranially and secure with tape if needed.
- Place a small foam wedge under the sternum to keep the sternum and vertebrae on the same horizontal plane.
- Fully extend and tape the dependent limbs—the pelvic limbs caudally and pectoral limbs cranially.
- Superimpose the contralateral pelvic and pectoral limbs and tape separately.
- Use padding between the legs if needed.
- Use a vertical beam.

Comments and Tips

- If limb radiographs are required and two extra views are not practical, separate the limbs. The dependent limb will be pulled slightly cranial in each case.
- Applying and securing tape around the contralateral limb and rotating the body slightly minimizes superimposition.
- A lateral view can also be obtained with a horizontal beam, if available, as described in small exotic companion mammals.

- Keep the corralled patient in the natural DV position in the container. Place the image receptor vertically against the opposite side close and parallel to the container to minimize OFD and distortion. The horizontal central ray is perpendicular to the image receptor and patient. There will be superimposition of the limbs on the area of interest.

> ### ⬤ TECHNICIAN NOTES
>
> To ensure that the lateral view appears symmetrical on the image:
> - Sternebrae and vertebrae are on the same plane.
> - The ribs are superimposed and straight.
> - Intervertebral foramina are the same size.
> - The acetabula are superimposed.
> - Ventral processes are superimposed.

> ### ⬤ TECHNICIAN NOTES
>
> Be sure to fully extend the front limbs cranially on the lateral projection, especially for a rabbit, so that you have optimum radiographic detail of the cranial thorax. Hind limbs not properly extended interfere with the caudal abdomen viscera.

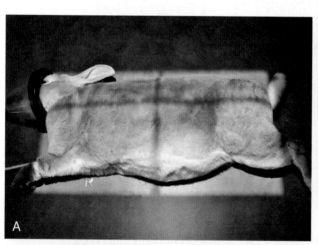

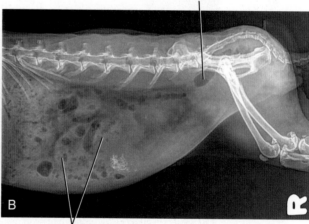

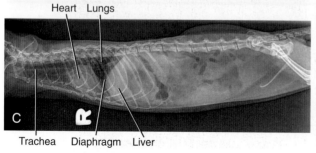

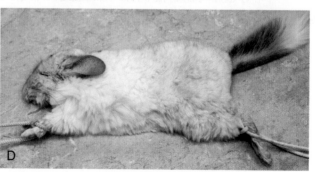

FIG. 25.23 **A,** Positioning for the lateral full-body view of the rabbit. The same positioning applies for abdomen, thorax, skull, pelvis, and limbs (if separated). **B,** Radiograph of the lateral abdomen of a rabbit. **C,** Right lateral view of the thorax and abdomen of a male ferret. **D,** Positioning for a lateral view of a chinchilla. Place the central ray over the area of interest and collimate appropriately. (Courtesy Rick Axelson, DVM, Links Road Animal Clinic, North York, Ontario.)

Skull of a Larger Exotic Companion Mammal

Lateral View of the Skull of a Larger Exotic Companion Mammal

Positioning

- Place the patient in lateral recumbency with affected side down.
- Position the head so that the mandible is parallel to the long edge of the image receptor.
- Use a foam pad or cotton under the nose and neck to superimpose the rami and to prevent rotation of the skull. Tape in place to align the skull parallel to the table.
- Keep the ears dorsal and caudal so they are out of the field of view.
- Place the label dorsal to the nose.

Comments and Tips

- How to ensure a symmetrical image:
  - Draw an imaginary line between the medial canthi, and make sure this line is perpendicular to the table.
  - The left and right halves of a normal skull should be superimposed.
- Malocclusion is common in rabbits. Dental abscesses and resultant osteomyelitis are also of concern.

MEASURE: The thickest part of the skull.

CENTRAL RAY: Midskull just rostral and ventral to the eye.

BORDERS: Include from the tip of the nose to C2 (the base of the skull) (Fig. 25.24).

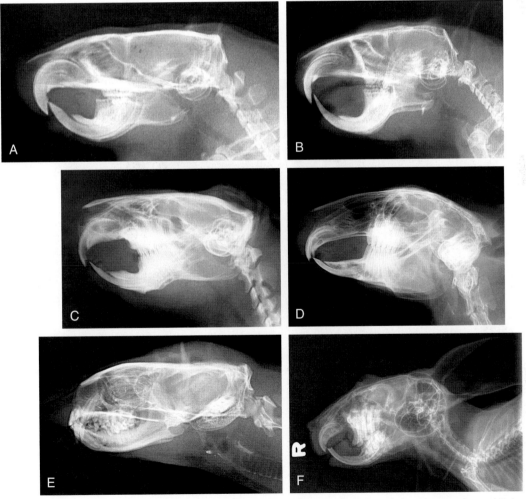

FIG. 25.24 Comparisons of some of the skulls of exotic companion mammals. Right lateral views of a rat **(A)**, hamster **(B)**, guinea pig **(C)**, rabbit **(D)**, ferret **(E)**, and chinchilla **(F)**. (**A** to **E** from Silverman S. *Radiology of Birds: An Atlas of Normal Anatomy and Positioning.* Philadelphia: Saunders; 2010; **F** courtesy Rick Axelson, DVM, Links Road Animal Clinic, North York, Ontario.)

Dorsoventral or Ventrodorsal View of the Skull of a Larger Exotic Companion Animal

Positioning

- Place the patient directly on the table in ventral recumbency for a DV view and in dorsal recumbency for a VD view.
- Sandbags or foam pads can be placed on either side to prevent rotation. Keep radiopaque devices out of the field of view.

For the DV view:
- Position the head flat on the image receptor.
- Place tape across the nasal septum and the cranium to keep the sagittal plane of the head perpendicular to the image receptor.

For the VD view:
- Position a foam pad or cotton under the neck, keeping the hard palate parallel with the image receptor.

- Put tape over the head caudal to the ears.
- Place tape across the mandible to keep the head aligned with the table.

Comments and Tips

- Place the label lateral to the nose.
- Make sure the ears are positioned laterally, equidistant from the head.
- To ensure that the image will be symmetrical:
  - An imaginary line drawn between the medial canthi must be parallel to the table.
  - The left and right halves of a normal skull should be a mirror image of each other when looking at the image (Fig. 25.25).

MEASURE: The thickest part of the skull.

CENTRAL RAY: Midline between the eyes.

BORDERS: Include the tip of the nose to C2 (base of the skull).

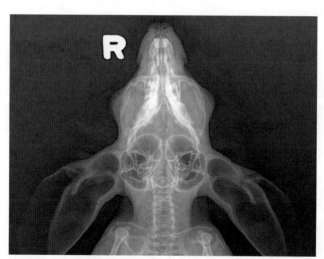

FIG. 25.25 Ventrodorsal view of the skull of a chinchilla. (Courtesy Rick Axelson, DVM, Links Road Animal Clinic, North York, Ontario.)

Lateral Oblique (Oblique Dorsoventral) Views of the Skull for Tympanic Bullae, Dental Arcade, and Temporomandibular Joint of a Larger Exotic Companion Mammal

Positioning

- Place the patient in left or right lateral recumbency.
- Place sponges under the skull, creating a 30-degree angle[5] to the table or receptor, with the nose pointing down and touching the surface.
- This position also produces a radiograph of the lower dental arcade.
- Keep the ears out of the field of view.
- Place a label dorsal to the nose.
- With the patient lying on its right side, the position is technically termed the *LeD30-RtVO* or *right oblique DV view*. (See Chapter 21 for a review of oblique terminology.)

Comments and Tips

- If the upper dental arcade is of interest, place foam pads under the nose, creating a 30- to 45-degree angle to the table, with the back of the skull touching the image receptor and the nose pointing upwards. Secure with tape if needed (Fig. 25.26). If the patient is lying on its right side, this position is technically named the *LeV30-RtDO* or *right oblique VD view*.
- A complete radiographic study of the skull should include extraoral lateral, oblique, dorsoventral (or ventrodorsal), and rostrocaudal head views as well as intraoral views (Table 25.3).[3]
- See Chapters 21 and 22 for further information on radiographing the canine or feline skull and teeth, which can be applied to smaller mammals as well.
- Magnification of rodent and rabbit skulls may be required. This can be obtained by using a small focal spot and increased OFD/decreased SID. The patient can be positioned on a radiolucent foam sponge on top of the image receptor. If the OFD is 12 inches and the SID is 20 inches, the magnification is about 2.0.[5]

MEASURE: The thickest part of the skull.

CENTRAL RAY: Midskull just rostral and ventral to the eye.

BORDERS: Include the tip of the nose to C2 (the base of the skull).

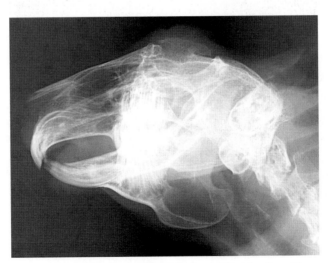

FIG. 25.26 Oblique (30-degree) ventrodorsal view of the skull of an adult rabbit. (From Silverman S. *Radiology of Birds: An Atlas of Normal Anatomy and Positioning.* Philadelphia: Saunders; 2010.)

TABLE 25.3	Dentition of Some Common Rodents and the Rabbit*				
	PERMANENT	**PERMANENT INCISORS**	**PERMANENT CANINES**	**PERMANENT PREMOLARS**	**PERMANENT MOLARS**
Hamsters, gerbils, rodents	16	2/2	0/0	0/0	6/6
Guinea pigs	20	2/2	0/0	2/2	6/6
Rabbits	28	4/2	0/0	6/4	6/6

*Number before slash indicates maxillary teeth; number after indicates mandibular teeth.

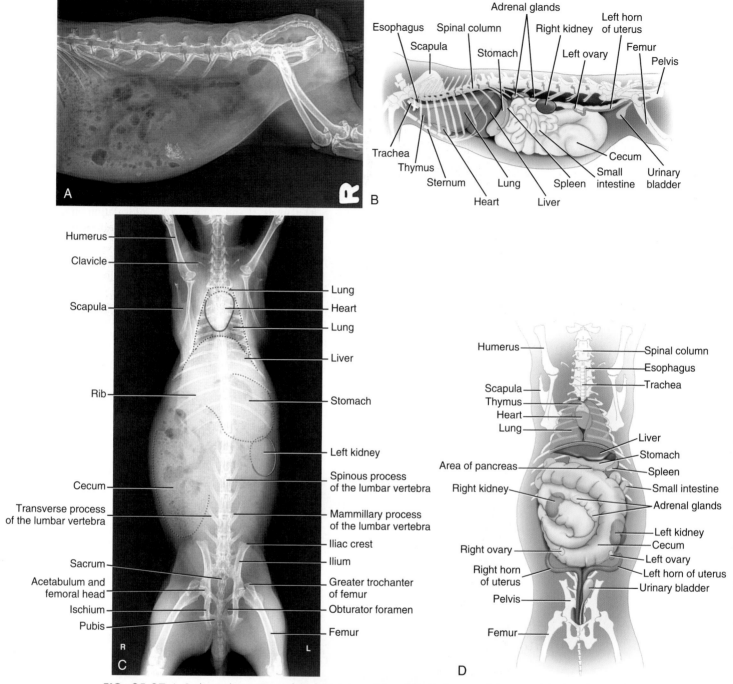

FIG. 25.27 A, Radiographic anatomy of the lateral view of the rabbit. B, Anatomical drawing of the lateral view of the rabbit. C, Radiographic anatomy of the ventrodorsal (VD) view of the rabbit. D, Anatomical drawing of the viscera of the thorax and abdomen of an adult female rabbit in VD view. (A courtesy Rick Axelson, DVM, Links Road Animal Clinic, North York, Ontario; C from Silverman S and Tell L: *Radiology of Rodents, Rabbits, and Ferrets: An Atlas of Normal Anatomy and Positioning.* St Louis: Saunders; 2005.)

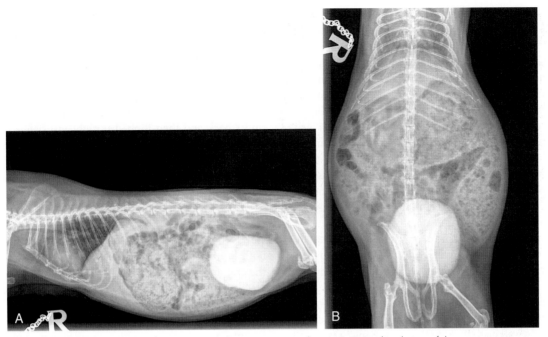

FIG. 25.28 A, Lateral view of a guinea pig showing urinary sediment. **B,** Ventrodorsal view of the same guinea pig. (Courtesy Rick Axelson, DVM, Links Road Animal Clinic, North York, Ontario.)

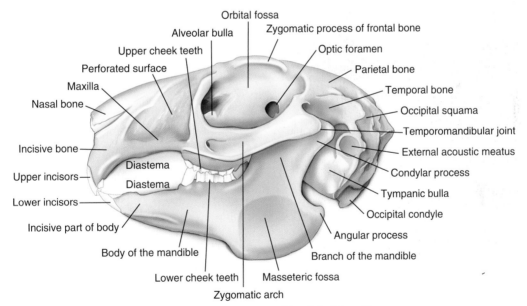

Orbital fossa
Zygomatic process of frontal bone
Alveolar bulla
Optic foramen
Upper cheek teeth
Perforated surface
Parietal bone
Maxilla
Temporal bone
Nasal bone
Occipital squama
Incisive bone
Temporomandibular joint
External acoustic meatus
Diastema
Condylar process
Upper incisors
Diastema
Tympanic bulla
Lower incisors
Occipital condyle
Incisive part of body
Angular process
Body of the mandible
Branch of the mandible
Lower cheek teeth
Masseteric fossa
Zygomatic arch

FIG. 25.29 The anatomy of the skull of the rabbit.

Reptiles

Radiographic imaging is frequently required in pursuing reptile diagnostics. Knowledge of reptiles' unique anatomical characteristics is essential for providing a technically proficient image. Traumatic injuries, gravidity evaluation, impactions, lung evaluation for pneumonia, and urinary calculi are common reasons that a radiograph may need to be acquired in a reptile.

The fused ribs and sternum form the carapace and plastron in chelonians (tortoise and turtles), making coelomic detail difficult to view. Because of constant movement, it may be difficult to obtain a symmetrical lateral view in snakes.

Ultrasound and endoscopy are diagnostic tools in reptilian medicine. Endoscopy is particularly useful. Coelioscopy, or internal examination of the coelomic cavity, provides a direct view of the liver, lungs, kidneys, heart, spleen, bladder, GI tract, pancreas, and gonads, although it requires an incision. In lizards, the incision for coelioscopy is generally made in the lateral body wall just caudal to the last rib. In chelonians, the incision is at the center of the prefemoral fossa, and in snakes, at the junction of the ventral and lateral scales at the expected site of interest. Endoscopy can also be used in reptiles to visualize the trachea and bronchi for evaluation of respiratory disease, to retrieve foreign bodies from the GI tract, and to obtain tissue specimens of diseased organs.[6]

Chelonians/Testudines: Turtle, Tortoise, and Terrapin

Positioning Concerns of Chelonians (Testudines)

The terms *chelonian* and *testudine* are generally interchangeable and refer to shelled reptiles. They are generally easy to restrain for radiography due to the lethargy of many species. Keeping the limbs in extension can be a challenge. Consider using a round device under the plastron so the limbs are not touching the plate (see Fig. 25.30B). Alternatively, tape over the shell caudally to keep the patient from wandering and to encourage chelonians to pull against the force of the tape and extend their limbs (see Fig. 25.30A). The chelonian can be turned on its back and then flipped upright just before taking the image. This may disorient the patient so as to cause momentary extension of the appendages and head.

A short-acting anesthetic agent such as alfaxalone can also facilitate proper positioning.

With turtles, it is important to obtain a craniocaudal (rostrocaudal) view in addition to dorsoventral and lateral views. The craniocaudal view enables unobstructed vision of both lungs. The horizontal beam should be considered for the craniocaudal as well as lateral views if the machine and plate positioning allow. A grid is not likely needed except for the larger species over 10 cm.

Nonscreen dental film or a digital dental unit can be used for smaller patients, and a high-detail system should be used for the larger patients.

A positive-contrast study can be completed if the GI tract is of concern. If GI contrast studies are completed, the time scale for passage of the medium is longer than in mammals.

Radiographic Views

Dorsoventral View of Chelonians/Testudines

Positioning

- Position the patient on its plastron and use tape at the caudal aspect if required (Fig. 25.30).

Comments and Tips

- As long as the central ray is in the center of the shell, most chelonian images show symmetry.

MEASURE: The thickest part of the body.

CENTRAL RAY: The center of the shell.

BORDERS: Include the whole body.

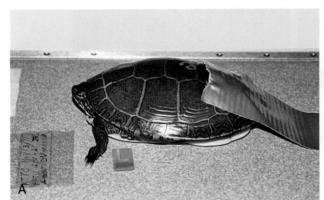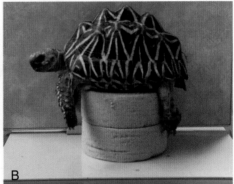

FIG. 25.30 A, Strategic use of tape keeps this turtle in position and may encourage it to extract its limbs as it tries to walk away. **B,** The use of a round positioning device under this Indian Star tortoise (Geochelone elegans) is ideal.

Continued

Dorsoventral View of Chelonians/Testudines—cont'd

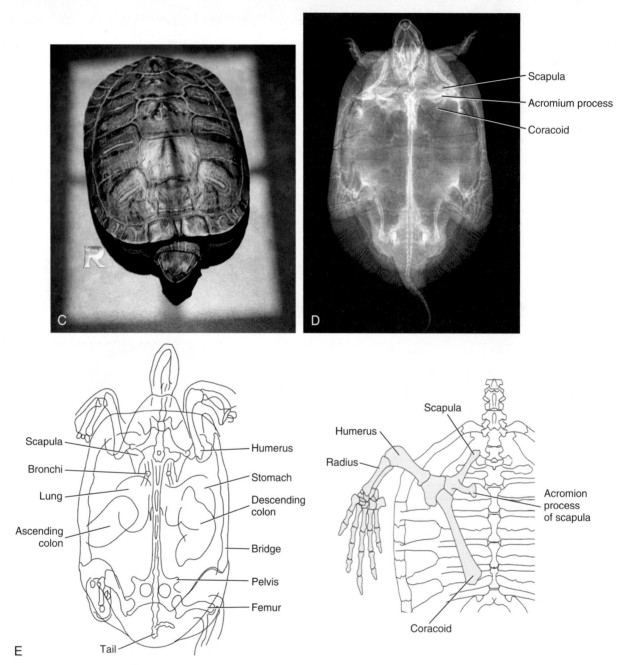

FIG. 25.30, cont'd C, Dorsoventral view of a painted turtle. D, Dorsoventral radiograph of a painted turtle. E, Radiographic anatomy of the snapping turtle. (A and D courtesy Sue Carstairs, DVM, Seneca College, Toronto Wildlife Centre and Kawartha Turtle Trauma Centre; B courtesy Ryan Cheek, RVTg, VTS, (ECC), Veterinary Technology, Gwinnet Technical College; C courtesy Rick Axelson, DVM, Links Road Animal Clinic, North York, Ontario.)

Lateral View of Chelonians/Testudines

Positioning for a Lateral View With a Horizontal Beam of Chelonians/Testudines

- Use of the lateral decubitus view (dorsoventral position with a horizontal beam) is preferred for the lateral view of a chelonian.
- Place the chelonian in ventral recumbency on top of a foam pad or acrylic positioning device or on a small radiolucent object so the legs are exposed (Fig. 25.31).
- Tape over the shell caudally to prevent the patient from wandering or place over a round device.
- Place the image receptor perpendicular to the table directly behind the turtle's lateral side opposite to the beam.
- Position the beam parallel to the table so that the central ray is midway between the plastron and carapace, in full view of the image receptor.
- The beam should bisect the plastron and carapace for the image to be symmetrical.

Positioning for a Lateral View With a Vertical Beam of Chelonians/Testudines

- Place the chelonian in ventral recumbency on its plastron, and securely tape the patient to a foam pad or acrylic positioning device or secure between two devices.
- Turn the pad so that the lateral side of the chelonian is positioned on the image receptor.
  - The chelonian is lying laterally on its "side."
  - The beam passes vertically between the carapace and plastron.
  - The beam should bisect the plastron and carapace for the image to be symmetrical.

> ### ✐ TECHNICIAN NOTES
>
> As with other positions, the lateral decubitus view is labeled according to the side against the image receptor. In a right lateral, the right side is against the plate. Technically this is called a *left to right lateral decubitus view (dorsoventral position) with a horizontal beam.*

MEASURE: The thickest part of the shell.

CENTRAL RAY: The center of the body between the carapace and plastron.

BORDERS: Include the whole body.

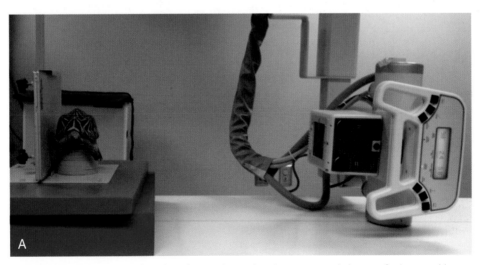

FIG. 25.31 A, Positioning for a lateral view of an Indian Star tortoise with the use of a horizontal beam.

Continued

Lateral View of Chelonians/Testudines—cont'd

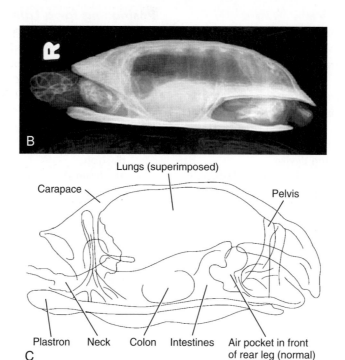

Lungs (superimposed)

Carapace

Pelvis

Plastron Neck Colon Intestines Air pocket in front
of rear leg (normal)

C

FIG. 25.31, cont'd B, Radiograph of a lateral view with the use of the horizontal beam of a painted turtle. C, Lateral radiographic anatomy of a painted turtle. (A courtesy Ryan Cheeck, RVTg, VTS, (ECC), Veterinary Technology, Gwinnet Technical College; B courtesy Sue Carstairs, DVM, Seneca College, Toronto Wildlife Centre and Kawartha Turtle Trauma Centre.)

Craniocaudal View of Chelonians/Testudines

Positioning for a Craniocaudal View With a Horizontal Beam

- Place the chelonian in ventral recumbency on a foam block.
- Have the image receptor caudal to and as close to the patient as possible.
- Direct the beam horizontally from a cranial direction through to the tail (Fig. 25.32).

> ### 🖉 TECHNICIAN NOTES
>
> In female turtles, the caudal vertebrae are short and decrease in size distally, whereas in males, the lateral and dorsal processes are stout. As a general rule, the vent of a female is found at or within the carapace perimeter. The male generally has a long tail, and the vent (cloacal opening) is generally more caudal than in the female or nearer the tip of the tail. Males may have strong curved claws on the second digit, and during mating season the midventral plastron becomes soft. Male painted turtles have very long front toenails.

MEASURE: The thickest area of the body.

CENTRAL RAY: Through the middle of the head.

BORDERS: Include the whole body.

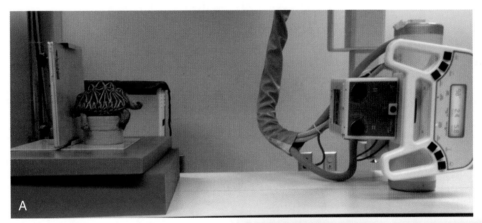

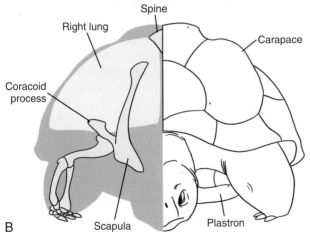

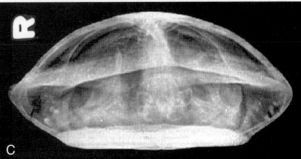

FIG. 25.32 A, A craniocaudal view of an Indian Star tortoise with the use of a horizontal beam. **B,** Radiographic anatomy and overlay of the craniocaudal view of a painted turtle. **C,** Craniocaudal radiograph of a painted turtle. (**A** courtesy Ryan Cheeck, RVTg, VTS, (ECC), Veterinary Technology, Gwinnet Technical College; **C** courtesy Sue Carstairs, DVM, Seneca College, Toronto Wildlife Centre and Kawartha Turtle Trauma Centre.)

Craniocaudal View of Chelonians/Testudines—cont'd

Positioning for Craniocaudal View With a Vertical Beam of Chelonians/Testudines

- Place the chelonian in ventral recumbency, and tape the patient to a foam pad or block.
- Place and position the chelonian and block so that the caudal portion of the body is resting on the cassette and table and the head is pointing up to the beam.
- Direct the beam vertically from the head through the tail.

See Appendix E on the Evolve website and Figs. 25.30 through 25.33 for normal anatomy and radiographic concerns of chelonians.

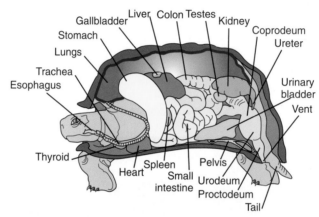

FIG. 25.33 Cross-section of the internal anatomy of a chelonian. (From Colville T, Bassert JM. *Clinical Anatomy and Physiology for Veterinary Technicians.* 3rd ed. St. Louis: Elsevier; 2016.)

Lizards

Radiography Concerns of the Lizard

Positioning of lizards (order Squamata) for radiography employs the conventional DV and lateral views. They are the most straightforward of the reptiles to image, and many of the concepts employed for small mammal radiography can be utilized. Many species can be radiographed awake, although anesthesia aids in obtaining diagnostic radiographs. Strategically placed tape can be employed to stabilize the patient on the plate.

Placing a blindfold of some sort over the eyes of the lizard may minimize movement. This can be achieved by placing eye lubricant in the eyes and wrapping the head with vet wrap.[7] Applying pressure over both eye orbits through closed lids can also be effective. The response to this pressure is the vasovagal reflex, which can induce a drop in heart rate and blood pressure and a catatonic state. Be careful not to pull the patient by the tail, as tail autonomy can occur. Take appropriate precautions with venomous lizards.

Ultrasound Concerns of the Lizard

Ultrasound[6] is more diagnostic and can be used to evaluate various systems, such as the reproductive, as well as the heart and other viscera. The heart, as in most reptiles, is three-chambered. In most lizards it is situated in the pectoral girdle. Place the transducer in the axillary region and rotate it to evaluate all three chambers.

The viscera in the caudal coelom can be examined, and ultrasound can be used to help collect fine-needle biopsy specimens or aspirates. Ovulation can be determined by placing the transducer over the ovary on the lateral body wall just caudal to the last rib and noting the follicle measurement. Both ovaries should be examined. Depending on the species, this comparison may help determine when the male and female should be placed together for breeding.

Normal Anatomy of the Lizard

See Appendix E on the Evolve website for normal anatomy and radiographic concerns of the lizard and snake.

Radiographic Views

Dorsoventral View of the Lizard

Positioning

- Place the lizard in sternal recumbency with limbs lateral to the body (Fig. 25.34).
- Put masking tape over the neck, caudal to the pectoral limbs and over the pelvis, if needed. Use a vertical beam.

> ### ✎ TECHNICIAN NOTES
> How to tell whether the image will appear symmetrical:
> - The spine is superimposed over the sternum.
> - The patient is straight from head to tail.

Comments and Tips

- The limbs are naturally positioned lateral to the body, so superimposition with viscera does not usually occur.
- Be aware of the level of stress of the patient.
- If only the extremities are of interest, tape as described and extend the limb of interest with masking tape, gauze, or Velcro.

MEASURE: The thickest point of the body.

CENTRAL RAY: Over the midline of the body about the level of the TL junction, unless the tail is of interest.

BORDERS: Include the whole body.

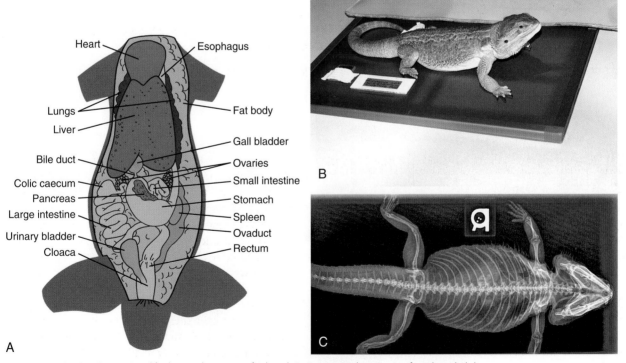

FIG. 25.34 A, Simplified internal anatomy of a lizard. **B,** Dorsoventral positioning for a bearded dragon prior to imaging. To minimize magnification, use tape or Velcro to keep the head and neck more parallel to the cassette. **C,** Dorsoventral radiograph of the bearded dragon. (**A** from Colville T, Bassert JM. *Clinical Anatomy and Physiology for Veterinary Technicians.* 3rd ed. St. Louis: Elsevier; 2016.)

Lateral View of the Lizard

If a lateral view is required, the lateral decubitus (dorsoventral position with horizontal beam) is less stressful for the patient.

Positioning with the Use of a Horizontal Beam

- Place the patient in ventral recumbency on a raised sponge block or plastic sheet.
- Tape the neck, shoulders, and pelvis if needed.
- Position the beam so it is horizontal with the table and perpendicular to the image receptor, which is placed as close as possible to the side of the lizard that is being radiographed (Fig. 25.35).
- Mark the side closer to the cassette.

Comments and Tips

- Keep the body of the patient close to the cassette and the spine straight and parallel to minimize OFD and distortion.
- The tails of larger lizards can be taped.

- To ensure that the image will be symmetrical:
  - The patient should have equal weight on its feet, with the spine parallel to the receptor.
  - The central ray is perpendicular to both.

MEASURE: The thickest part of the body if not using a species chart.

CENTRAL RAY: Over the midline of the body.

BORDERS: Include the whole body.

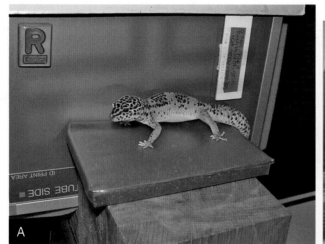

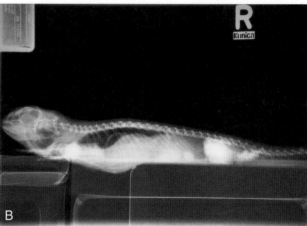

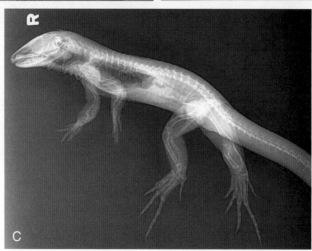

FIG. 25.35 **A,** Horizontal beam for the right lateral view of a gecko. **B,** Lateral view of a bearded dragon on positioning devices with use of a horizontal beam and the patient in ventral recumbency. **C,** Radiograph of a lizard in regular lateral position with the use of a vertical beam.

Snakes[2,8,9]

Radiography Concerns of the Snake

Snake species (order Squamata) are extremely variable in size, and thus restraint devices in many sizes are required. The snake is best placed in a tube (Fig. 25.37A) or stretched and taped to a long plastic sheet or supported in a tubed stockinet. If the stockinet or a tube is used, the position will be fairly well maintained, provided that the patient is not able to rotate its head inside the tube. Keeping the body elongated and not coiled is especially important for the lateral view. It is important to have the body in a straight line, and thus multiple exposures may be required to allow the entire body to be imaged.

Placing metallic pellets may assist with "dividing" the body for easier identification.

Small snakes can be coiled on the image receptor or in a radiolucent container. However, true symmetry will not be obtained with the oblique view.

Manual restraint may be needed for some of the larger species in order to position the body correctly. Consider the use of the bird positioner, especially if the snake is venomous or aggressive.

Knowledge of organ location is essential for proper positioning. The dorsoventral view is more useful for imaging the spine and ribs, and lateral recumbency is more useful for proper visualization of the organs. Reptiles do not tolerate being placed in lateral position, so if this view is required, a horizontal beam for the lateral radiograph with the patient in a tube is recommended.

Normal Snake Anatomy

See Appendix E on the Evolve website and Figs. 25.34A and 25.37C for normal anatomy and radiographic concerns of the lizard and snake.

Radiographic Views

Dorsoventral View of the Snake

Positioning

- Keep the patient in true sternal recumbency, ideally in a plastic tube. Use a vertical beam (Fig. 25.37A).
- For true symmetry, there should be no overlapping of the vertebrae, and the ribs should appear equidistant on each side of the vertebrae.

Comments and Tips

- Multiple handlers may be required for safe radiography of a large snake.

CENTRAL RAY: Over the area of interest.

BORDERS: Include the area of interest (cranial, middle, caudal).

Lateral View of the Snake

Lateral decubitus (dorsoventral position with horizontal beam) (preferred)
* Place the patient in a DV position as described earlier. Use a horizontal beam, placing the image receptor vertically on the side of interest.

Lateral view with a vertical beam
* If the horizontal beam is not available, the snake will need to be placed in lateral position with the aid of a tube or

multiple handlers, depending on the snake size. A vertical beam is used.

* How to tell whether the body is symmetrical:
  * The snake is stretched out, with no coiling of the body.
  * The vertebrae appear on the dorsal aspect.

CENTRAL RAY: Over the area of interest.

BORDERS: Include the area of interest (anterior, middle, caudal end).

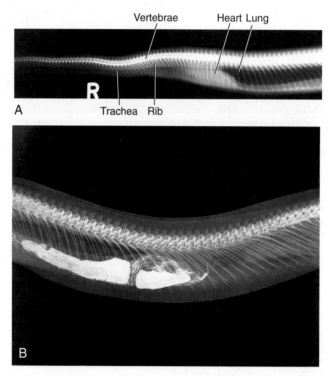

FIG. 25.36 A, Radiographic anatomy of the lateral view of a snake. B, Lateral view taken during a contrast study of a snake. (A courtesy Sue Carstairs, DVM, Seneca College, Toronto Wildlife Centre and Kawartha Turtle Trauma Centre; B courtesy Rick Axelson, DVM, Links Road Animal Clinic, North York, Ontario.)

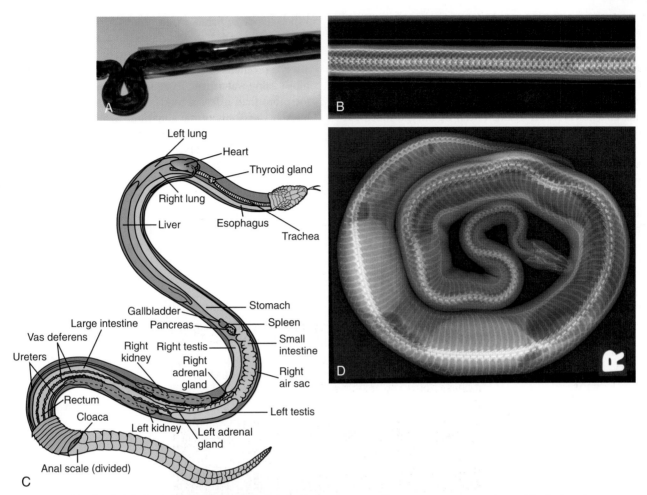

FIG. 25.37 **A,** Positioning for a dorsoventral view of a boa constrictor. The same positioning can be used for the lateral with the use of a horizontal beam. **B,** Radiograph of a dorsoventral view of a boa constrictor. **C,** Ventral view of a male snake showing internal anatomy. **D,** When the patient is allowed to coil naturally, an oblique view, rather than a true DV will be obtained as in this image. (**A** and **B** courtesy Ryan Cheeck, RVTg, VTS, (ECC), Veterinary Technology, Gwinnet Technical College; **C** from Colville T, Bassert JM. *Clinical Anatomy and Physiology for Veterinary Technicians*. 3rd ed. St. Louis: Elsevier; 2016.)

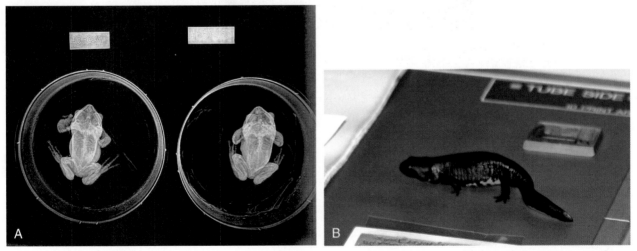

FIG. 25.38 **A,** Dorsoventral views of South American Tree Frogs being restrained in Petri dishes. **B,** Dorsoventral view of a red spotted newt (Caudata species of amphibian).

Amphibians

Radiography Comments and Tips for Amphibians

Amphibians such as toads and frogs (order Anura), salamanders, and newts (order Caudata) can be imaged much like other species. Depending on the size of the species, Petri dishes or containers can be used. When handling amphibians, make sure to use wet, powder-free gloves. Gloves protect the wet mucosal surface on the skin of aquatic amphibians, which is quite sensitive to the chemicals on hands. Gloves also prevent allergic reactions for humans and protects the handler from transmission of bacterial diseases. Anurians are able to prolapse the stomach after eating undesirable food, after some methods of anesthesia, and when they are dying.

The most commonly used view is the DV. If required and if available, lateral views are completed with the patient in a DV position with the use of a horizontal beam (Fig. 25.38).

Fish

Radiography and Positioning Concerns of Fish

Fish medicine is a fast-growing area in veterinary medicine, with ever-increasing knowledge in the area of diagnostics. As such, radiography is more commonly performed.

Common reasons for radiography include trauma, swim bladder issues, and neoplasia.

When handling fish, keep in mind that the skin and scales provide a protective barrier and are quite sensitive to handling. Scales grow continuously throughout the life of the fish and are not regenerated if lost. They must continuously be kept moist using water from its aquarium and not exposed to air for more than a few seconds. If a temporary aquarium or bucket with some of the aquarium water is used, it will be difficult to keep the fish stationary and there will likely be movement artifacts. As with amphibians, make sure to use powder-free gloves.

Generally fish require anesthesia with an agent such as tricaine methanesulfonate (MS-222) in the water to enable proper positioning. Using a moist Baggie with the MS-222 for the procedure will keep the patient comfortable and minimize movement. It is vital that the patient be handled as minimally as possible and returned to its environment as quickly as possible.

Normal Radiographic Anatomy of Amphibians and Fish[9-11]

See Appendix E on the Evolve website and Figs. 25.39 and 25.40 for normal anatomy and radiographic concerns of the amphibian and fish.

Fig. 25.41 is a mystery radiograph. Review it and answer the question presented with it.

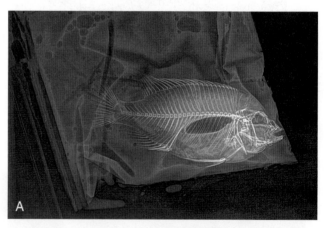
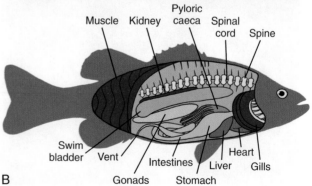

FIG. 25.40 A, Lateral view of a fish radiographed in a bag of water. B, Anatomy of the lateral view of a fish. (B from Colville T, Bassert JM. *Clinical Anatomy and Physiology for Veterinary Technicians.* 3rd ed. St. Louis: Elsevier; 2016.)

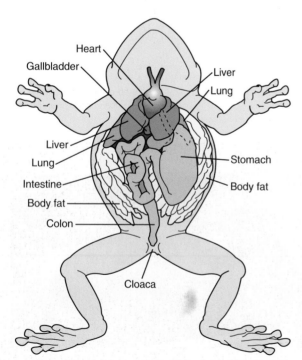

FIG. 25.39 Ventral view of the frog showing internal anatomy. (From Colville T, Bassert JM. *Clinical Anatomy and Physiology for Veterinary Technicians.* 3rd ed. St. Louis: Elsevier; 2016.)

Radiographic Views

Dorsoventral and Lateral Views of Fish

Positioning
- Place the fish in a bag with water from its aquarium (Fig. 25.40A).

- Complete the procedure quickly. For both views, use a vertical beam.
- The lateral view is more practical, but if the DV is required, support the bag so the fish is upright.

CENTRAL RAY: The middle of the body.

BORDERS: Include the whole body.

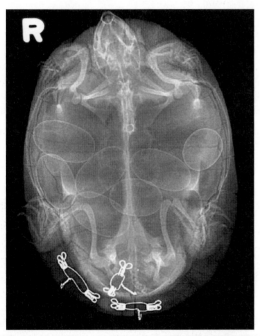

FIG. 25.41 Mystery radiograph: How many eggs does this turtle have? What are the artifacts? (Courtesy Sue Carstairs, DVM, Seneca College, Toronto Wildlife Centre and Kawartha Turtle Trauma Centre.)

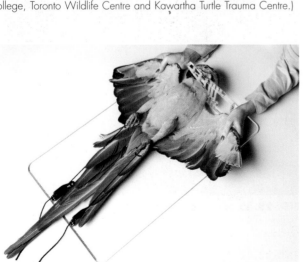

FIG. 25.43 Beginning avian positioning when using a VSP Miami Vise Avian Restraint.

Image Gallery

Figs. 25.42 to 25.55 are additional images to supplement avian and exotic radiographic positioning.

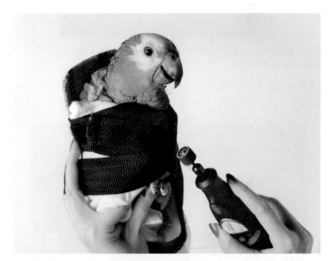

FIG. 25.42 A restraint device such as the avian restraint jacket would not be effective for radiography because of the artifacts and constraints, which would cause superimposition.

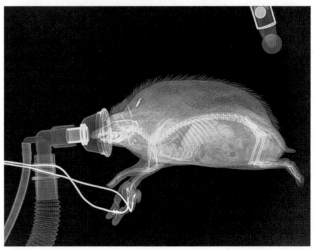

FIG. 25.44 Radiograph of the lateral view of a hedgehog in lateral recumbency with use of a vertical beam.

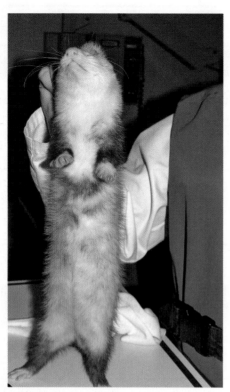

FIG. 25.45 Supporting a ferret by the neck assists in calming it before positioning or sedation.

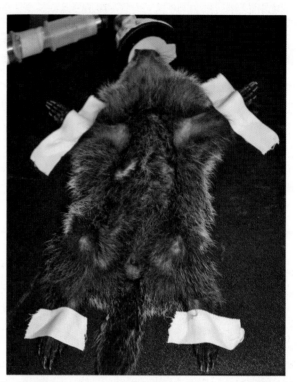

FIG. 25.46 Dorsoventral (DV) view of a woodchuck. The same principles can be applied to any exotic species.

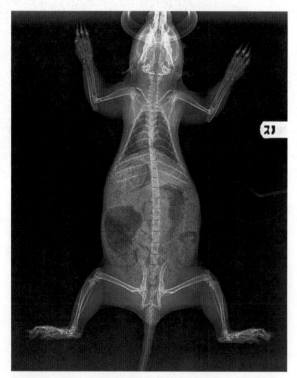

FIG. 25.47 Radiograph of the DV view of the groundhog.

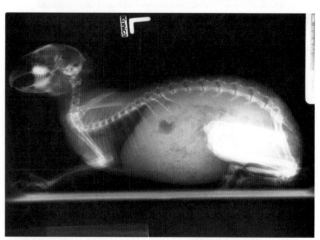

FIG. 25.48 Left lateral view of a rabbit with use of a horizontal beam and the rabbit in a natural position. The hind limbs superimpose over the caudal soft tissue.

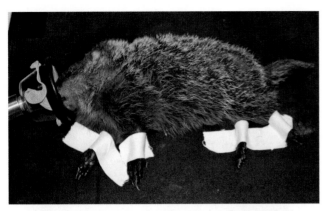

FIG. 25.49 Positioning for a lateral view of a woodchuck.

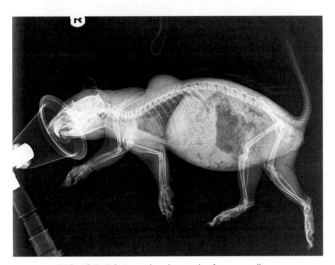

FIG. 25.50 Lateral radiograph of a groundhog.

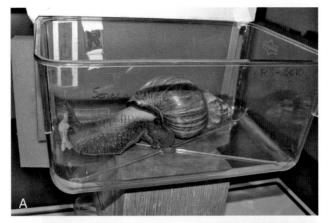

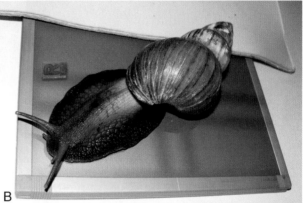

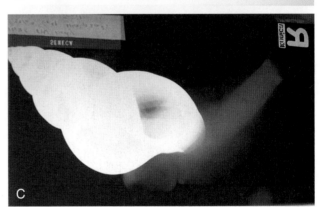

FIG. 25.52 Any species can be restrained with use of common restraint techniques and knowledge of species behavior. Lateral (**A**) and dorsoventral (**B**) views of a giant African land snail. **C,** Dorsoventral radiograph of the giant African land snail.

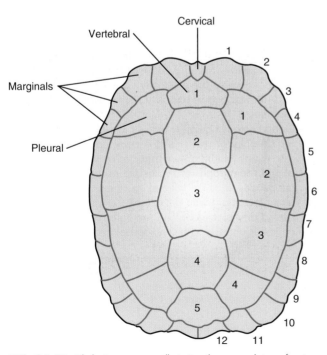

FIG. 25.51 Chelonian carapace illustrating the nomenclature of scutes.

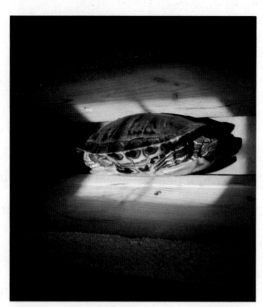

FIG. 25.53 Positioning for a lateral view of a painted turtle with the use of a horizontal beam. (Courtesy Sue Carstairs, DVM, Seneca College, Toronto Wildlife Centre and Kawartha Turtle Trauma Centre, Ontario.)

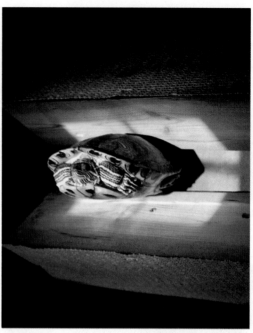

FIG. 25.54 A craniocaudal view of a painted turtle. The beam is coming from the front of patient, which is positioned between two blocks. (Courtesy Sue Carstairs, DVM, Seneca College, Toronto Wildlife Centre and Kawartha Turtle Trauma Centre, Ontario.)

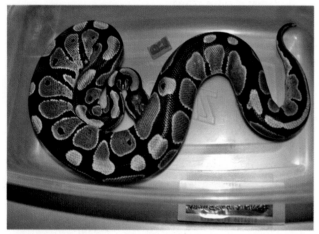

FIG. 25.55 Positioning for a dorsoventral view of a boa constrictor that is often used in practice. This positioning will not result in a true DP image as shown by Fig. 25.37A in the text. If this positioning is used for the lateral view with the use of a horizontal beam, there will be some overlap of the cranial portion in this particular image.

✳ KEY POINTS

1. Generally, avian radiography requires chemical restraint for diagnostic results. Fasting time before anesthesia is variable and species specific.
2. Ensure handler safety when radiographing patients by always restraining their particular weapons, which vary by species.
3. For proper diagnosis, the positions must be exactly perpendicular, especially with the avian ventrodorsal view, to avoid misinterpretation of the radiograph.
4. Exotic companion mammals also generally require chemical restraint for adequate radiographs, but they are not usually fasted before sedation or anesthesia.
5. Dental concerns are extremely common in rodents and rabbits, and so excellent skull radiographs are essential.
6. Good coelomic detail is difficult to visualize during radiography of chelonians. A craniocaudal view is essential to obtain an unobstructed view of the lungs.
7. Lateral radiographs of snakes are necessary to adequately visualize internal structures. Consider use of a horizontal beam if available.
8. Almost any species can be radiographed if the behavior and important radiographic principles are kept in mind.

REVIEW QUESTIONS

1. You are required to obtain an image of a budgerigar. 2.5 mAs is best obtained with:
   a. 300 mA and 1/120 of a sec
   b. 200 mA and 1/80 sec
   c. 100 mA and 1/40 sec
   d. Whatever you can set on your machine

2. A budgerigar is being positioned for a VD whole-body view. To ensure there will be symmetry on the image, the:
   a. Acetabula, ribs, coracoids, and kidneys are superimposed
   b. Keel is directly over the spine and the scapulae, acetabula, and femurs are parallel
   c. Sternum and vertebral column are on the same plane
   d. Patient is in true ventral recumbency

3. You should center for this VD whole-body view of the budgerigar:
   a. Over the midline at the caudal tip of the sternum
   b. Slightly to the left side of the keel
   c. Slightly to the right side of the keel
   d. Over the midline at the cranial part of the sternum

4. An ill cockatoo needs to be gavaged and radiographed. You should obtain a radiograph for this patient:
   a. After the gavaging
   b. Before the gavaging
   c. At any time, as gavaging is not an issue
   d. While gavaging

5. For the VD survey of the cockatoo coelom you should take the image:
   a. At maximum inspiration
   b. At maximum expiration
   c. Whenever there is movement to assist in showing contrast
   d. At any point, as distension of the abdominal air sacs may enhance abdominal viscera

6. A full contrast study is required for the cockatoo patient noted earlier. The images will likely be taken:
   a. Immediately, 15 minutes, 30 minutes, and then half-hourly as needed
   b. Immediately and then half-hourly as needed
   c. Immediately and then hourly as needed
   d. At 15 minutes and then every 15 minutes as needed

7. A blue heron suspected of lead poisoning is to be imaged. When restraining this species, it is particularly important to:
   a. Tape the talons
   b. Wear a full face shield
   c. Keep the room bright
   d. Measure at the thickest part

8. The minimum source-image distance (SID) that should be used when radiographing birds is:
   a. 30 inches
   b. 40 inches
   c. 50 inches
   d. 60 inches

9. To obtain a mediolateral view of the right wing of a swan, the patient should be positioned in:
   a. Dorsal recumbency
   b. Ventral recumbency
   c. Right lateral recumbency
   d. Left lateral recumbency

10. The dorsoventral as opposed to the ventrodorsal position is best utilized for:
    a. All exotic companion mammals and reptiles
    b. Smaller exotic companion mammals such as rats and for reptiles
    c. Small animals such as dogs and cats
    d. Larger exotic companion mammals such as rabbits and ferrets

11. You are looking at the orthogonal image of the rat and know that the image is symmetrical because the:
    a. Acetabula are square and the femurs are bent 90 degrees
    b. Sternebrae and vertebrae are on the same horizontal plane
    c. Spinous processes are to the left of the vertebral bodies
    d. Vertebrae are superimposed over the sternebrae on the same vertical plane

12. A lateral view is needed of a male ferret abdomen. You should center:
    a. Cranial to the xiphoid
    b. Cranial to the pubis
    c. Caudal to the last rib
    d. At the TL junction

13. For this lateral view of the male ferret abdomen, you should include cranial from the:
    a. Shoulder joint and slightly caudal to the last rib
    b. Shoulder joint and caudal to the pubis
    c. Xiphoid process and caudal to the last rib
    d. Xiphoid process and caudal to the pubis

14. When positioning the limbs for this lateral abdomen of the ferret, it is best to:
    a. Superimpose the limbs and pull toward the center as much as possible
    b. Superimpose the limbs, pulling the pectoral limbs cranially and the pelvic limbs caudally
    c. Separate the limbs with the dependent limb positioned more caudally
    d. Separate the limbs with the dependent limb positioned more cranially

15. You are required to obtain a dorsoventral (DV) view for an iguana. It is best to position the patient in:
    a. Lateral recumbency and use a vertical beam
    b. Lateral position and use a horizontal beam
    c. Ventral recumbency and use a vertical beam
    d. Ventral recumbency and use a horizontal beam

16. A lateral radiograph is also required for the iguana. The patient is best placed in:
    a. Lateral recumbency and use a vertical beam
    b. Lateral recumbency and use a horizontal beam
    c. Ventral recumbency and use a vertical beam
    d. Ventral recumbency and use a horizontal beam

17. The view that best illustrates both lung fields when radiographing chelonians is the:
    a. Craniocaudal
    b. Dorsoventral
    c. Lateral
    d. Ventrodorsal
18. The veterinarian wants you to obtain a craniocaudal radiograph of a turtle, but the machine does not allow a horizontal view. After taping the turtle in ventral recumbency to a foam pad or block, you should position both so that the:
    a. Caudal portion is pointing to the beam
    b. Head is pointing to the beam
    c. Lateral surface is pointing to the beam
    d. Beam is horizontal from a cranial direction to the tail.
19. A lateral view is required of a ball python. It is best to:
    a. Use a bird positioner to place it in lateral position and use a vertical beam
    b. Place it in lateral position in a tube and use a vertical beam
    c. Place it in a tube and use a horizontal beam
    d. Allow it to coil in a natural position and use a horizontal beam
20. Fish are best radiographed in position by:
    a. Being taped to a plastic sheet
    b. Placement in a container with tap water
    c. Placement in a moistened small bag
    d. Placement in a small dry container

Answers to Review Questions can be found on the Evolve website.

References

1. Silverman ST. *Radiology of Birds, an Atlas of Normal Anatomy and Positioning.* St. Louis: Elsevier; 2010.
2. Farrow C. *Diagnostic Imaging: Birds, Exotic Pets and Wildlife.* St. Louis: Elsevier; 2009.
3. Gracis MD. Clinical technique: normal dental radiography of rabbits, guinea pigs, and chinchillas. *J Exotic Pet Med.* 2008;17:78-86.
4. Morgan JP. *Techniques of Veterinary Radiography.* Ames, IA: Iowa State University Press; 1993.
5. Silverman S, Tell L. *Radiology of Rodents, Rabbits and Ferrets: An Atlas of Normal Anatomy and Positioning.* St. Louis: Saunders; 2005.
6. Innis CD: Reptile medicine. Cummings School of Veterinary Medicine at Tufts University, 2008. http://ocw.tufts.edu/Content/60/lecturenotes/828884.
7. Mitchell M. Diagnostic imaging of lizards. In: *NAVC Conference: Small Animal and Exotics.* Orlando, FL: North American Veterinary Conference; 2007:1590-1591.
8. Mitchell MA, Tully TN. *Manual of Exotic Pet Practice.* St. Louis: Saunders; 2009.
9. Peterson K. *Biology 453, Comparative Vertebrate Anatomy Course Notes.* Seattle: University of Washington; 2012. http://courses.washington.edu/chordate/453lectures/453lecture_notes.htm. Retrieved 3 March 2016.
10. Colville T, Bassert J. *Clinical Anatomy and Physiology for Veterinary Technicians.* 3rd ed. St. Louis: Elsevier; 2016.
11. Mayer J: Clinical anatomy and physiology of fish. CVC in Kansas City proceedings. Aug 1, 2012. http://veterinarycalendar.dvm360.com/avhc/Veterinary+Exotics/Clinical-anatomy-and-physiology-of-fish-Proceeding/ArticleStandard/Article/detail/738519.

Bibliography

Aspinall V, Cappello M. *Introduction to Veterinary Anatomy.* London: Butterworth Heinemann; 2009.
Avian respiration. (n.d.). Retrieved 3 March 2016. http://people.eku.edu/ritchisong/birdrespiration.html.
Ballard B, Cheek R. *Exotic Animal Medicine for the Veterinary Technician.* Ames, IA: Wiley-Blackwell; 2010.
Dyce KM, Sack WO, Wensing CJG. *Textbook of Veterinary Anatomy.* 4th ed. St. Louis: Saunders; 2010.
Hernandez-Divers S. Reptile radiology: techniques, tips and pathology. In: *NAVC Conference: Small Animal and Exotics.* Orlando, FL: North American Veterinary Conference; 2006:1626-1630.
Hernandez-Divers S. Snake radiology: the essentials. In: *NAVC Conference: Small Animal and Exotics.* Orlando, FL: North American Veterinary Conference; 2008:1772-1774.
Kaufman GD: Avian radiology, Published 2008. http://ocw.tufts.edu/Content/60/lecturenotes/832723. Retrieved 3 January 2016.
McMillan M Imaging techniques, Ch. 12. http://avianmedicine.net/content/uploads/2013/03/12.pdf. Retrieved 3 March 2016.
Quesenberry K, Carpenter J. *Ferrets, Rabbits and Rodents.* 3rd ed. Philadelphia: Saunders; 2012.
Setter M. Ultrasound in reptiles and amphibians. In: *NAVC Conference: Small Animal and Exotics.* Orlando, FL: North American Veterinary Conference; 2003:1232-1233.
Sirois M, Anthony E, Mauragis D. *Handbook of Radiographic Positioning for Veterinary Technicians.* Clifton Park, NY: Delmar Cengage Learning; 2010.
Tighe M, Brown M. *Mosby's Comprehensive Review for Veterinary Technicians.* 4th ed. St. Louis: Elsevier; 2015.

Index

b indicates boxes, *f* indicates illustrations, and
t indicates tables.

Basic Concepts

The important thing in science is not so much to obtain new facts as to discover new ways of thinking about them.

—William Lawrence Bragg, Nobel Prize in Physics, 1915

Fractions

- Numerator—The top of the fraction: 3/8, 2/4
- Denominator—The bottom of the fraction: 3/8, 13/14

APPLICATION: *Setting the technical factors*

Addition and Subtraction

- The denominator = The number of divisions of the whole:

$$1/4 = \text{“1” pie is divided into “4” sections}$$

- To add two fractions with "like" denominators, add or subtract the numerators and maintain the same denominator:

$$1/10 + 2/10 = 3/10$$

Divide the pie into 10 pieces. Subtract 1 piece, then subtract 2 pieces:

$$10 - 1 - 2 = 7 \text{ pieces, or } 7/10 \text{ of the pie remains}$$

- To add two fractions with unlike denominators, find a number that is divisible by both denominators, and then convert both fractions to the same denominator:

$$1/5 + 1/4 = 5/20 + 4/20 = 9/20$$

or

$$1/2 + 1/3 = 3/6 + 2/6 = 5/6$$

APPLICATION: *Using an x-ray generator with fractions on the time setting. Deciding how to increase/decrease the time*

Whole Numbers

Fractions on the timer are replaced by whole numbers representing the mAs.

APPLICATION: *Setting the technical factors on the x-ray generator*

EXAMPLE: *100 mA × 1/4 sec = 25 mAs*

Proportionality (Variation) of Numbers

- Proportionality is defined as the relationship between two numbers.
- There are two types of proportionality: direct and indirect.

APPLICATION: *Choosing the settings on the x-ray machine, calculating distance, measuring chemistry, calculating radiation doses*

Direct Proportionality

- The first quantity is a multiple of the second quantity. For example, I have a basket of 25 apples to use in a pie. If I add an apple each time my friend removes an apple, then the number of apples added is equal to or is "directly proportional to" the number of apples removed.
- Any factor can be applied to a direct proportion, such as 1 apple to 1 apple or 2 apples to 4 apples.

Indirect Proportionality

- As one quantity gets larger, the other quantity gets smaller.
- Thus their product remains the same, but each value is different.

Units of Measurement

The primary fundamental units of measurement are mass, length, and time.

Mass

Standard unit is the pound (lb) [kilogram (kg)].
APPLICATION: *Setting techniques, measuring patients*

Length

Standard unit is the meter (m).
APPLICATION: *Measurement of the thickness of the patient, the distance from the x-ray tube to the patient, and the distance from the x-ray tube to each wall when determining the protection required for the walls of the x-ray room*

Time

Standard unit is the second (s).
APPLICATION: *Time of exposure, time of injection of contrast media, time for processing the image*

Prefixes

The metric system uses various prefixes to denote an increase and decrease of the original value. Common prefixes used in radiography are shown in the table below. The SI units of measurement specific to the field of radiation and radiation dose are described in depth in Chapter 3.

Factors	Prefix (Symbol)	Application
10^6	Mega- (M)	Megavolt
10^3	Kilo- (k)	Kilometer, kilovolt
10^{-1}	Deci- (d)	Decimal
10^{-2}	Centi- [c]	Centimeter
10^{-3}	Milli- [m]	Millimeter